RADIOGRAPHY PREP

EDITION 7

D.A. Saia, MA, RT(R) (M)
Director, Radiography Program
Stamford Hospital
Stamford, Connecticut

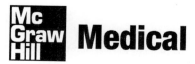

New York   Chicago   San Francisco   Lisbon   London   Madrid   Mexico City
Milan   New Delhi   San Juan   Seoul   Singapore   Sydney   Toronto

The McGraw-Hill Companies

Radiography PREP, Program Review and Examination Preparation, Seventh Edition

Copyright © 2012 by The McGraw-Hill Companies, Inc. All rights reserved. Printed in the United States of America. Except as permitted under the United States Copyright Act of 1976, no part of this publication may be reproduced or distributed in any form or by any means, or stored in a data base or retrieval system, without the prior written permission of the publisher.

Previous editions copyright © 2011, 2009, 2006, 2003 by The McGraw-Hill Companies, Inc.; copyright, 1999, 1996 by Appleton & Lange.

PERMISSION CREDITS: The following figures were originally published in Saia DA, *Lange Q&A Radiography Examination,* 9th ed. New York: McGraw-Hill, 2011 and are reproduced with permission from McGraw-Hill: Figures 8-2, 8-8, 8-10, 11-4, 11-7, 11-11A and B, 11-12, 11-36, 11-38, 11-62, 12-3, 14-10, 14-11, 14-13, 14-15, 14-17, 14-18, and 16-17.

The ARRT does not review, evaluate, or endorse publications. Permission to reproduce ARRT copyrighted materials within this publication should not be construed as an endorsement of the publication by ARRT.

2 3 4 5 6 7 8 9 10   QDB/QDB   14 13 12

ISBN 978-0-07-178704-8
MHID 0-07-178704-6

Notice

Medicine is an ever-changing science. As new research and clinical experience broaden our knowledge, changes in treatment and drug therapy are required. The author and the publisher of this work have checked with sources believed to be reliable in their efforts to provide information that is complete and generally in accord with the standards accepted at the time of publication. However, in view of the possibility of human error or changes in medical sciences, neither the author nor the publisher nor any other party who has been involved in the preparation or publication of this work warrants that the information contained herein is in every respect accurate or complete, and they disclaim all responsibility for any errors or omissions or for the results obtained from use of the information contained in this work. Readers are encouraged to confirm the information contained herein with other sources. For example and in particular, readers are advised to check the product information sheet included in the package of each drug they plan to administer to be certain that the information contained in this work is accurate and that changes have not been made in the recommended dose or in the contraindications for administration. This recommendation is of particular importance in connection with new or infrequently used drugs.

This book was set in Berkeley Book by Aptara®, Inc.
The editors were Catherine A. Johnson and Christie Naglieri.
The production supervisor was Sherri Souffrance.
Project management was provided by Indu Jawwad, Aptara, Inc.
The designer was Mary McKeon.
The cover designer was Eric Myer.
Quad/Graphics was the printer and binder.

This book is printed on acid-free paper.

Library of Congress Cataloging-in-Publication Data

Saia, D. A. (Dorothy A.)
    Radiography PREP : program review and exam prep / D.A. Saia.–7th ed.
        p. ; cm.
    Radiography program review and examination preparation
    Includes bibliographical references and index.
    ISBN 978-0-07-178704-8 (pbk. : alk. paper) — ISBN 0-07-178704-6 (pbk. : alk. paper)
    I. Title.   II. Title: Radiography program review and examination preparation.
    [DNLM: 1. Radiography–Examination Questions.   2. Technology, Radiologic–Examination
Questions. WN 18.2]
    616.07′572076—dc23   2012018428

McGraw-Hill books are available at special quantity discounts to use as premiums and sales promotions, or for use in corporate training programs. To contact a representative, please e-mail us at bulksales@mcgraw-hill.com.
Please tell the author and publisher what you think of this book by sending your comments to radtech@mcgraw-hill.com. Please put the author and title of this book in the subject line.

Dedicated
Spiritus Sancti gratia, illuminet sensus et corda nostra.

Reviewers

Laura Aaron, PhD, RT(R)(M)(QM)
Program Director, Graduate Coordinator and Associate Professor of Radiologic Sciences
Northwestern State University
Shreveport, Louisiana

Christie W. Bolton, MA Ed, RT(R)
Radiologic Technology Program Coordinator
Jefferson State Community College
Birmingham, Alabama

Suzanne E. Crandall, EdD, MHA, RT(R), (ARRT)
Professor/Program Chair
Radiologic Technology Program
Mercy College of Health Sciences
Des Moines, Iowa

Nancy Daugherty, MEd, RT(R)
Pima Medical Institute—Mesa
Mesa, Arizona

Shelley Giordano, DHSc, RT(R)(MR)
Academic Coordinator and Director of Clinical Education
Radiologist Assistant Program
Assistant Professor
Diagnostic Imaging Program
Quinnipiac University
Hamden, Connecticut

Brenda Grant, RN, MPH, CIC, CHES
Infection Preventionist
Stamford Hospital
Stamford, Connecticut

Elaine Halesey, EdD, RT (R)(QM)(ARRT)
Professor and Chairperson
Department of Medical Imaging
Misericordia University
Dallas, Pennsylvania

William F. Hennessy, MHS, RT(R)(M)(QM)
Department Chair and Director
Diagnostic Imaging Program
Quinnipiac University
Hamden, Connecticut

Rebecca Keith, MS, RT(R)(CT)
Assistant Professor,
School of Diagnostic Imaging
Northern Virginia Community College
Medical Education Campus
Springfield, Virginia

Candice Lewis, MSRS, RT(R)(CT)
Radiography Program
Greenville Technical College
Greenville, South Carolina

Bernadette Mele, MHS, RT(R)(ARRT), ROT
Clinical Instructor
Diagnostic Imaging Program
Quinnipiac University
Hamden, Connecticut

David L. North, ScM, DABR
Associate Physicist
Rhode Island Hospital
Providence, Rhode Island

MaryJane S. Reynolds, MAIS, RT(R)(T)
Radiography Program Director
PIMA Medical Institute
Houston, Texas

Theresa D. Roberts, MHS, RT(R)(MR)
Radiographic Technology Program Director
Keiser University - Melbourne
Melbourne, Florida

Bette Schans, PhD, RTR
Professor and Program Director
Radiologic Technology
Mesa State College
Grand Junction, Colorado

Robert Wells MEd, RT(R)(CT)
Program Director, Radiologic Technology
Lanier Technical College
Oakwood, Georgia

Contents

Preface

Radiography PREP (Program Review and Examination Preparation), seventh edition, is useful throughout all phases of radiography education. This text is designed to be useful for regular coursework, helping the student to extract fundamental key concepts from reading assignments and class notes, and for making study and test preparation easier and more productive.

PREP is also useful for students preparing for their American Registry of Radiologic Technologists (ARRT) certification examination. It helps students direct their study efforts toward examination-related material and includes registry-type multiple choice questions designed to help students practice test taking and critical thinking skills they will need for the ARRT radiography examination.

The ARRT's Content Specifications for the Examination in Radiography lists the examination's five content categories and provides a detailed list of the topics addressed in each category. *Radiography PREP* is divided into five parts reflecting each of the five content categories. Part content reflects changes to the ARRT Content Specifications published August 2010 and implemented January 2012. Also included is some basic introductory CT material - an area becoming increasingly important for the entry level radiographer. As this field continues to grow, there is increasing emphasis on its inclusion in the radiography curriculum. Particularly important is updated and expanded information on Digital/Electronic Imaging. Thus, study becomes even more directed and focused on examination-related material. Used with its companion book, *Lange Q&A for the Radiography Examination*, PREP provides a thorough preparation for the certification examination administered by the ARRT.

KEY FEATURES AND USE

- More than 400 ***illustrations and images*** appeal to the visual learner as well as the verbal learner. The essence of radiography is visual and *PREP's* graphics and radiographic images visually express the written words.

- The numerous ***summary boxes*** serve to call the student's attention to the most important facts in a particular section. Students can use summary boxes as an overview of key information.

- ***Inside covers*** list a number of formulae, radiation protection facts, conversion factors, body surface landmarks, digital imaging facts, acronyms, and abbreviations, radiation quality factors, and minimum filtration requirements. A "last-minute cheat sheet" is provided for some things that students often forget because they may not use them on a regular basis.

- The ***final review sections*** allow students to assess chapter material in two ways. The first review section, ***Comprehension Check,*** requires short essay answers; exact page references follow each question, providing answers in chapter material. The second section, ***Chapter Review Questions***, consists of registry-type multiple choice questions followed by detailed explanations.

- Chapter 14 (Equipment) includes a new section on Computed Tomography. As this field continues to grow, there is increasing emphasis on its inclusion in the radiography curriculum.
- Chapter 16 is a practice test; a simulation of the actual certification examination with questions designed to test your problem-solving skills and your ability to integrate facts that fit the situation. The questions are designed to provide focus and direction for your review, thus helping you do your very best on your certification examination.

Following completion of the chapter review questions and the practice test, the student is ready for final self-evaluation by answering more "registry-type" questions in the companion text, *Lange Q&A for the Radiography Examination,* eighth edition, and supplemental study at its website *RADREVIEWEasy.com.*

Acknowledgments

One of my most satisfying tasks is having the opportunity to thank those who have most generously contributed their insights, talents, and concerns to this project. Foremost among those are my teachers and colleagues who have contributed to my knowledge over the years and my students on whom I have the privilege of sharpening my knowledge and skills. I greatly appreciate the friendship, encouragement, and support generously offered by my colleagues Olive Peart, MS, RT(R)(M) and Teresa Whiteside, AS, RT(R)(BD), (CDBT). I am grateful to the professional staff of McGraw-Hill, with special notes of appreciation to Catherine A. Johnson, Christie Naglieri, Midge Haramis, Sherri Soufrance, and Aptara project manager Indu Jawwad for their patience, support, and assistance. Jennifer Pollock deserves a note of appreciation for her development and maintenance of the books' companion Web site, www.RadReviewEasy.com. Her foresight and expertise have brought a successful added dimension to both texts – PREP and the Q&A. Everyone at McGraw-Hill has been helpful in the development of this project; it is always a pleasure to work with their creative and skilled staff.

An outstanding group of reviewers was recruited for these last two editions. Laura Aaron, PhD, RT(R)(M)(QM); Christie W. Bolton, MA Ed, RT(R); Suzanne E. Crandall, EdD, MHA, RT(R), ARRT; Nancy Daugherty, MEd, RT(R); Shelley Giordano, DHSc, RT(R)(MR); Brenda Grant, RN, MPH, CIC, CHES; Elaine Halesey, EdD, RT(R)(QM)(ARRT); William F. Hennessy, MHS, RT(R)(M)(QM); Rebecca Keith, MS, RT(R)(CT); Candice Lewis, MSRS, RT(R)(CT); Bernadette Mele, MHS, RT(R)(ARRT), ROT; David L. North, ScM, DABR; MaryJane S. Reynolds, MAIS, RT(R)(T); Theresa D. Roberts, MHS, RT(R)(MR); Bette Schans, PhD, RTR, and Robert Wells MEd, RT(R)(CT) are all invaluable resources to health care and the radiologic technology community. They reviewed the manuscript and offered suggestions to improve style and remove ambiguities and inaccuracies. Their participation on this project is deeply appreciated. A special note of thanks to Brenda Grant, MPH, BSN, RN, CIC, CHES, Infection Preventionist at Stamford Hospital/Bennett Medical Center for reviewing Infectious Disease material and patiently answering all my questions.

Grateful appreciation goes out to Doug Lofting and his most helpful staff, Tami and Carol, at Shielding International for permission to use images of their protective devices and providing PDF files of the images.

The assistance offered by Rob Fabrizio of Fuji Medical Systems USA is deeply appreciated. He patiently responded to a multitude of questions and provided permission for use of Fuji illustrations. Thank you, Rob!

The support and assistance offered in all previous editions by the late George Spahn of Fuji Medical Systems, USA will always be greatly appreciated. George was instrumental in the introduction and expansion of electronic imaging content in this book. George Spahn is a great loss to Fuji Medical Systems, USA and the radiology community, and is missed by so many.

Another note of thanks goes to Roger Flees, RT (retired), Inside Sales Manager of Philips Healthcare, Dunlee Division. Thank you, Roger, for generously sharing your time and expertise. Our discussions of tube rating and heat storage, and follow-up emails were most helpful. Your help in obtaining permission for use of tube rating charts is appreciated.

I would like to thank the American College of Radiology for the use of radiographs from their teaching file and Stamford Hospital's Department of Radiology for permission to use many of their x-ray images. I would also like to include my appreciation to Conrad P. Ehrlich, MD, for granting permission to use several radiologic images new to this edition; Dr. Ehrlich and his staff at Housatonic Valley Radiological Associates, particularly Joe DeFeo and Angie Dohan, have been most helpful.

The CT section in Chapter 14 could not have been accomplished without the help of several individuals. For answering questions, providing images, and reviewing material, I am extremely grateful to Sarah Bull, MS, DABR, Angie Dohan, RT(R), Conrad Ehrlich, MD, Paula Hill, RT(R)(CT)(CV)(M), Doug Schueler, RT(R)(CT), and Teresa Whiteside AS, RT(R)(BD), (CDBT).

Several people were helpful in securing permission and providing photographs for illustration. Special thanks go to Landauer Inc, especially Judith Mangan, for providing and granting permission to use their dosimeter graphics; Mr. Dick Burkhart at Burkhart Roentgen and Mr. Artie Swayhoover at Nuclear Associates were all very helpful and supportive.

The preparation of this text would have been a far more difficult task without the help and encouragement of my husband, Tony. His patient understanding, support, assistance, and advice are lovingly appreciated.

Master Bibliography

On the last line of each answer/explanation, there appears the last name of the author or editor of one of the publications listed here, along with a number or numbers indicating the correct page or range of pages where information relating to the correct answer may be found. For example, (*Bushong, p 45*) refers to page 45 of Bushong's *Radiologic Science for Technologists*.

Adler AM, Carlton RR. *Introduction to Radiologic Sciences and Patient Care*, 4th ed. St. Louis, MO: Saunders Elsevier, 2007.

ASRT Code of Ethics. http://www.asrt.org/content/RTs/CodeofEthics/Code_Of_Ethics. aspx. Accessed March 21, 2010.

Ballinger PW, Frank ED. *Merrill's Atlas of Radiographic Positions and Radiologic Procedures*, Vols 1, 2, and 3, 10th ed. St. Louis, MO: Mosby, 2004.

BEIR Report VII. www.nap.edu/openbook.php?isbn=030909156x.

Bontrager KL. *Textbook of Radiographic Positioning and Related Anatomy*, 6th ed. St. Louis, MO: Mosby, 2005.

Bontrager KL, Lampignano JP. *Textbook of Radiographic Positioning and Related Anatomy*, 7th ed. St. Louis, MO: Mosby, 2010.

Bushong SC. *Radiologic Science for Technologists*, 8th ed. St. Louis, MO: Mosby, 2004.

Bushong SC. *Radiologic Science for Technologists*, 9th ed. St. Louis, MO: Mosby, 2008.

Bushong SC. *Radiologic Science for Technologists*, 10th ed. St. Louis, MO: Mosby, 2012.

Bushberg JT, Seibert JA, Leidholdt EM, Boone JM. *The Essential Physics of Medical Imaging*, 2nd ed. Baltimore, MD: Lippincott Williams & Wilkins, 2002.

Carlton RR, Adler AM. *Principles of Radiographic Imaging*, 4th ed. Albany, NY: Delmar, 2006.

Carter C, Vealé B. *Digital Radiography and PACS*, 1st ed revised. St. Louis, MO: Mosby/Elsevier, 2010.

Chen MYM, Pope TL, Ott DJ. *Basic Radiology*, 1st ed. New York: McGraw-Hill, 2004.

Dowd SB, Tilson ER. *Practical Radiation Protection and Applied Radiobiology*, 2nd ed. Philadelphia, PA: WB Saunders, 1999.

Ehrlich RA, Daly JA. *Patient Care in Radiography*, 7th ed. St. Louis, MO: Mosby, 2009.

Ehrlich RA, McCloskey ED. *Patient Care in Radiography*, 6th ed. St. Louis, MO: Mosby, 2004.

Fauber TL. *Radiographic Imaging and Exposure*, 2nd ed. St. Louis, MO: Mosby, 2004.

Fauber TL. *Radiographic Imaging and Exposure*, 3rd ed. St. Louis, MO: Mosby; 2009.

Fosbinder RA, Kelsey CA. *Essentials of Radiologic Science*, 1st ed. McGraw-Hill, 2002.

Fosbinder R, Orth D. *Essentials of Radiologic Science*. Baltimore, MD: Lippincott Williams & Wilkins, 2012.

Frank ED, Long BW, Smith BJ. *Merrill's Atlas of Radiographic Positioning and Procedures*, Vols 1, 2, and 3, 11th ed. St. Louis, MO: Mosby, 2007.

Fuji Medical Systems. *CR Users Guide*, Stamford, CT: Fuji Medical Systems, 1999.

Gurley LT, Callaway WJ. *Introduction to Radiologic Technology*, 6th ed. St. Louis, MO: Mosby, 2006.

Haus AG, Jaskulski SM. *Basics of Film Processing in Medical Imaging*, 1st ed. Madison, WI: Medical Physics Publishing, 1997.

Hendee WR, Ritenour ER. *Medical Imaging Physics*, 4th ed. New York: Wiley-Liss, Inc, 2002.

Lazo DL. *Fundamentals of Sectional Anatomy: An Imaging Approach*, 1st ed. Clifton Park, NJ: Thomson Delmar Learning, 2005.

Laudicina P. *Applied Pathology for Radiographers*. Philadelphia, PA: WB Saunders, 1989.

Martini FH, Bartholomew EF. *Essentials of Anatomy & Physiology*, 4th ed. San Francisco, CA: Pearson Education, Inc, 2007.

Mills WR. The relation of bodily habitus to visceral form, tonus, and motility. *Am J Roentgenol* 1917; 4:155-169.

McKinney WEJ. *Radiographic Processing and Quality Control*. Philadelphia, PA: Lippincott Williams & Wilkins, 1988.

NCRP Report No 99. *Quality Assurance for Diagnostic Imaging*. NCRP, 1990.

NCRP Report No 116. *Recommendations on Limits for Exposure to Ionizing Radiation*. NCRP, 1987.

ARRT. New Test Item Format for Radiography Examination. http://www.arrt.org/index.html?content=eduguide/news.htm. Accessed August 2, 2007.

Peart O. *A&L Mammography Review*, 1st ed. McGraw-Hill, 2002.

Peart O. *Mammography and Breast Imaging: Just the Facts*. New York: McGraw-Hill, 2005.

Publication Dissemination, Education and Information Division, National Institute for Occupational Safety and Health, 4676 Columbia Parkway, Cincinnati, OH 45226; 1998.

Purtilo R. *Ethical Dimensions in the Health Professions*, 4th ed. Philadelphia, PA: WB Saunders, 2005.

Romans, LE. *Computed Tomography for Technologists, A Comprehensive Text*. Philadelphia, PA:Wolters Kluwer Health/Lippincott Williams & Wilkins, 2011.

Seeram E. *Radiation Protection*. Philadelphia: Lippincott, 1997.

Seeram E. *Rad Techs Guide to Equipment Operation and Maintenance*. Malden, MA: Blackwell Science, Inc, 2001.

Seeram E. *Digital Radiography: An Introduction for Technologists*. Clifton Park, NJ: Delmar Cengage Learning, 2010.

Selman J. *The Fundamentals of Imaging Physics and Radiobiology*, 9th ed. Springfield, IL: Charles C Thomas, 2000.

Shephard CT. *Radiographic Image Production and Manipulation*, 1st ed. McGraw-Hill, 2003.

Statkiewicz-Sherer MA, Visconti PJ. *Radiation Protection in Medical Radiography*, 5th ed. St. Louis, MO: Mosby, 2006.

Statkiewicz-Sherer MA, Visconti PJ, Ritenour ER. *Radiation Protection in Medical Radiography*, 6th ed. St. Louis, MO: Mosby, 2011.

Thomas CL, ed. *Taber's Cyclopedic Medical Dictionary*, 20th ed. Philadelphia, PA: F. A. Davis, 2005.

Thompson MA, Hattaway MP, Hall JD, et al. *Principles of Imaging Science and Protection*, 1st ed. Philadelphia, PA: WB Saunders, 1994.

Torres LS, Linn-Watson Norcutt TA, Dutton AG. *Basic Medical Techniques and Patient Care in Imaging Technology*, 6th ed. Philadelphia, PA: Lippincott Williams & Wilkins, 2003.

Tortora GJ, Derrickson B. *Principles of Anatomy and Physiology*, 12th ed. Hoboken, NJ: John Wiley & Sons, Inc, 2010.

Tortora GJ, Derrickson B. *Introduction to the Human Body: The Essentials of Anatomy and Physiology*, 8th ed. Hoboken, NJ: John Wiley & Sons, Inc, 2010.

Towsley-Cook DM, Young TA. *Ethical and Legal Issues for Imaging Professionals*, 2nd ed. St. Louis, MO: Mosby, 2007.

Travis EL. *Primer of Medical Radiobiology*, 3rd ed. Chicago, IL: Year Book, 1997.

Wilson BG. *Ethics and Basic Law for Medical Imaging Professionals*. Philadelphia, PA: F. A. Davis, 1997.

Wolbarst AB. *Physics of Radiology*, 2nd ed. Madison, WI: Medical Physics Publishing, 2005.

PATIENT'S RIGHTS

Patient Privacy

Most institutions now have computerized, paperless systems to accomplish information transmittal; these systems must ensure *confidentiality* in compliance with Health Insurance Portability and Accountability Act (HIPAA) of 1996 regulations. The health care professional generally has access to the computerized system only via personal password, thus helping ensure confidentiality of patient information. All medical records and other individually identifiable health information—whether electronic, on paper, or oral—are covered by HIPAA legislation and by subsequent Department of Health and Human Services (HHS) rules that took effect in April of 2001.

All health care practitioners must recognize that their patients comprise a community of people of all religions, races, and economic backgrounds, and that each patient must be afforded their best efforts. Every patient should be treated with consideration of his or her worth and dignity. Patients must be provided *confidentiality* and *privacy*. They have the right to be informed, to make *informed consent*, and to refuse treatment.

Patient Consent

Patient *consent* can be verbal, written, or implied. For example, if a patient arrives for emergency treatment alone and unconscious, implied consent is assumed. A patient's previously granted or presumed consent can be withdrawn at any time. Written patient consent is required before any examination that involves greater than usual risk, for example, invasive vascular examinations requiring the use of injected iodinated contrast agents. For lower risk procedures, the consent given on admission to the hospital is generally sufficient.

It is imperative that the radiographer takes adequate time to thoroughly explain the procedure or examination to the patient. An informed patient is a more cooperative patient, and a better examination is more likely to result. Patients should be clear about what will be expected of

Conditions for Valid Patient Consent

- The patient must be of legal age.
- The patient must be of sound mind.
- The patient must give consent freely.
- The patient must be adequately informed of the procedure about to take place.

3

them and what to expect from the radiographer. This must be considered the *standard of care* for each patient, to fulfill not only legal mandates, but also professional and humanistic obligations.

Bill of Rights/Patient Care Partnership

The American Hospital Association's (AHA) Management Advisory presented a *Patient's Bill of Rights* that was first adopted by the AHA in 1973, then revised and approved by the AHA Board of Trustees in October of 1992. The 1992 Patient's Bill of Rights detailed 12 specific areas of patients' rights and the health care professional's ethical (and often, legal) responsibility to adhere to these rights. The Patient's Bill of Rights was summarized as *the right to*

1. considerate and respectful care;
2. be informed completely and understandably;
3. refuse treatment;
4. have an advance directive (e.g., a living will, health care proxy) describing the extent of care desired;
5. privacy;
6. confidentiality;
7. review his or her records (access to his/her health care information);
8. request appropriate and medically indicated care and services;
9. know about institutional business relationships that could influence treatment and care;
10. be informed of, consent to, or decline participation in proposed research studies;
11. continuity of care;
12. be informed of hospital policies and procedures relating to patient care, treatment, and responsibilities.

The AHA recently replaced the Patient's Bill of Rights with *The Patient Care Partnership—Understanding Expectations, Rights, and Responsibilities.* Their plain-language brochure includes the essentials of the Bill of Rights and reviews what patients can/should expect during a hospital stay.

The Patient Care Partnership statement addresses *high-quality hospital care*—combining skill, compassion, and respect and the right to know the identity of caregivers, whether they are students, residents, or other trainees. It includes *a clean and safe environment*, free from neglect and abuse, and information about anything unexpected that occurred during the hospital stay. The Patient Care Partnership identifies *involvement in your care;* it elaborates on patient discussion/ understanding of their condition and treatment choices with their physician, the patient's responsibility to provide complete and correct information to the caregiver, and understanding who should make decisions for the patient if the patient cannot make those decisions (including "living will" or "advance directive").

The Patient Care Partnership statement also identifies *protection of your privacy*—describing the ways in which patient information is safeguarded. It also describes *help when leaving the hospital*—availability of and/or instruction regarding follow-up care. Lastly, The Patient Care

The Patient Care Partnership

What to expect during your hospital stay:
- High-quality hospital care
- A clean and safe environment
- Involvement in your care
- Protection of your privacy
- Help when leaving the hospital
- Help with your billing claims

Source: The American Hospital Association

Partnership statement addresses *help with your billing claims*—including filing claims with insurance companies, providing patient physicians with required documentation, answering patient questions, and assisting those without health coverage.

The above-mentioned patient rights can be exercised on the patient's behalf by a *designated surrogate or proxy* decision maker if the patient lacks decision-making capacity, is legally incompetent, or is a minor. Many people believe that potential legal and ethical issues can be avoided by creating an *Advance Health Care Directive* or *Living Will*. Since all persons have the right to make decisions regarding their own health care, this legal document preserves that right in the event an individual is unable to make those decisions. An Advance Health Care Directive, or Living Will, names the individual authorized to make all health care decisions and can include specifics regarding *DNR* (do not resuscitate), *DNI* (do not intubate), and/or other end-of-life decisions.

> **Advance Health Care Directive/Living Will:**
>
> - Preserves a person's right to make decisions regarding their own health care.
> - Names the individual authorized to make all health care decisions for them.
> - Can include specifics regarding DNR, DNI, and other end-of-life decisions.

LEGAL ISSUES

It is essential that radiographers, like other health care professionals, be familiar with their *Practice Standards* published by the American Society of Radiologic Technologists (ASRT). The Standards provide a *legal role definition* and identify Clinical, Quality, and Professional Standards of practice—each Standard has its own rationale and identifies general and specific criteria related to that Standard. The student radiographer can access the individual Standards, their rationale, and criteria on the ASRT Web site.

X-Ray Examination Requests

X-ray examinations may be requested by a physician or physician assistant. Request forms for radiologic examinations must be carefully reviewed by the radiographer prior to commencement of the examination. Many hospitals and radiology departments have specific rules about exactly what kind(s) of information must appear on the requisition.

It is important that the radiographer obtain a short but adequate, pertinent patient history of why the examination has been requested. Because patients are rarely examined or interviewed by the radiologist, observations and information obtained by the radiographer can be a significant help in making an accurate diagnosis. The radiographer must be certain to obtain all clinical information in a manner that ensures patient privacy.

The requisition is usually stamped with the patient's personal information (name, address, age, admitting physician's name, and the patient's hospital identification number). The requisition should also include the patient's mode of travel to the radiology department or other imaging facility (e.g., wheelchair vs. stretcher), the type of examination to be performed, pertinent diagnostic information, and any *infection control* or *isolation* information. The radiographer, having access to confidential patient information, must be mindful of compliance with HIPAA regulations.

The radiographer must be certain to understand and, if necessary, clarify the information provided, for example, any abbreviations used and any vague terms such as "leg" or "arm" (femur vs. tibia, humerus vs. forearm). The radiographer must also be alert to note and clarify conflicting information, for example, a request for a left ankle examination when the patient complains of, or has obvious injury to, the right ankle. Computerized systems or department policy may require that there be appropriate and accurate diagnosis information accompanying every request for diagnostic procedure.

Law/Medicolegal Issues

The four primary *sources of law* are the Constitution of the United States, statutory law, regulations and judgments of administrative bureaus, and court decisions.

The *Constitution* expresses the categorical laws of the country. Its impact with respect to health care and health care professionals lies, in part, in its assurance of the *right to privacy*. The right to privacy indicates that the patient's modesty and dignity will be respected. It also refers to the health care professional's obligation to respect the confidentiality of privileged information. Inappropriate communication of privileged information to anyone but the appropriate health care professionals is inexcusable.

Statutory law refers to laws enacted by congressional, state, or local legislative bodies. The enforcement of statutory laws is frequently delegated to administrative bureaus such as the Board of Health, the Food and Drug Administration, or the Internal Revenue Service. It is the responsibility of these agencies to enact *rules and regulations* that will serve to implement the statutory law.

Court decisions involve the interpretation of *statutes* and various regulations in decisions involving individuals. For example, the decision of an administrative bureau can be appealed and the court would decide if the agency acted appropriately and correctly. Court decisions are referred to as common law.

There are two basic kinds of law: *public law* and *private (civil) law*. Public laws are any that regulate the relationship between individuals and government. *Private*, or civil, law includes laws that regulate the relationships among people. *Litigation* involving a radiographer's professional practice is most likely to involve the latter.

A private (civil) injustice, injury, or misconduct is a *tort*, and the injured party may seek reparation for damage incurred. Torts are described as either *intentional* or *negligent/unintentional*.

Examples of *intentional* (misconduct) torts include false imprisonment, *assault* and *battery*, defamation, and invasion of privacy. *False imprisonment* is the illegal restriction of an individual's freedom. Holding a person against his or her will or using unauthorized restraints can constitute false imprisonment.

Assault is to threaten harm; *battery* is the carrying out of the threat. A patient might feel sufficiently intimidated to claim assault by a radiographer who threatens to repeat a difficult examination if the patient does not try to cooperate better. A radiographer who performs an examination on a patient without his or her consent, or after the patient has refused the examination, can be guilty of *battery*. A charge of battery may also be made against a radiographer who treats a patient roughly or who performs an examination on the *wrong* patient.

> **Tort:**
>
> - A private/civil injustice
> - Reparation can be sought
> - Is either intentional or unintentional

A radiographer who discloses confidential information to unauthorized individuals can be found guilty of *invasion of privacy*. A radiographer whose disclosure of confidential information is in some way detrimental to the patient (e.g., causing ridicule or loss of job) can be accused of *defamation*. *Spoken* defamation is *slander*; *written* defamation is *libel*.

The assessment of *duty* (what *should* have been done) is determined by the professional *standard of care* (that level of expertise generally possessed by reputable members of the profession). The determination of whether or not the standard of care was met is usually made by determining what another reputable practitioner would have done in the same situation.

Examples of *negligent/unintentional* torts can include imaging the wrong patient, or patient injury as a result of a fall while unattended on an x-ray table, in a radiographic room, or on a stretcher without side rails or safety belt. Radiographing the wrong patient or opposite limb are other examples of *negligence*.

The term *malpractice* is usually used with reference to *negligence*. Three areas of frequent litigation in radiology involve patient falls and positioning injuries, pregnancy, and errors or delays in *diagnosis*.

Patient falls and positioning injuries. Examples: A sedated patient left unattended in the radiographic room falls from the x-ray table; a patient with a spinal injury is moved from the stretcher to the x-ray table, resulting in irreversible damage to the spinal cord.

Pregnancy. Example: The radiographer fails to inquire about a possible pregnancy before performing a radiologic examination. Some time later, the patient contacts the health care facility, expressing concern about the fetus.

Errors or delays in diagnosis. Example: The patient undergoes an x-ray examination in the emergency department and is sent home. The radiologist interprets the images and fails to notify the emergency department physician of the findings. The physician gets a written report 2 days later. Meanwhile, the patient suffers permanent damage from an untreated condition.

If patient injury results from misperformance of a duty in the routine scope of practice of the radiographer, most courts will apply *res ipsa loquitur*, that is, "the thing speaks for itself." If the patient is obviously injured as a result of the radiographer's/caregiver's actions, it becomes the radiographer's/caregiver's burden to *disprove* negligence. Examples of this include imaging the wrong patient/incorrect limb, surgical removal of a healthy organ or limb, leaving a sponge or clamp in a patient's body after surgery. In many instances, the hospital and/or radiologist will also be held responsible according to *respondeat superior*, or, "let the master answer." The "master," or employer, can be held liable for wrongful acts of the "servant," or employee, in causing injury during employed activities.

ARRT STANDARDS OF ETHICS

The mission of the American Registry of Radiologic Technologists (ARRT) is to promote high standards of patient care by recognizing qualified individuals in medical imaging, interventional procedures,

---

For Negligent Tort Liability, Four Elements Must Be Present

- Duty (what should have been done)
- Breach (deviation from duty)
- Injury sustained
- Cause (as a result of breach)

Legal Doctrines

- *Res ipsa loquitur* "the thing speaks for itself"
- *Respondeat superior* "let the master answer"

and radiation therapy. As every radiography student knows, the ARRT develops and administers examinations that assess the knowledge and skills underlying the intelligent performance of the tasks typically required by professional practice in the modality. In addition, the ARRT adopts and upholds

• standards for educational preparation for entry into the profession
• standards of professional behavior consistent with the level of responsibility required by professional practice

Practitioners of the profession of radiologic technology, like other health care professionals, have an ethical responsibility to adhere to principles of professional conduct and to provide the best services possible to the patients entrusted to their care. These principles are detailed in the ARRT two-part *Standards of Ethics* (Fig. 1–1), which includes the Preamble, the Code of Ethics (Part A) the Rules of Ethics (Part B), and Administrative Procedures. The 10-part *Code* of Ethics is aspirational; the 22 *Rules* of Ethics are enforceable and any violation can result in sanction/injunction. Figure 1–1 includes the Preamble, and Parts A and B.

ARRT® Standards of Ethics

The student should be completely familiar with the ARRT Standards of Ethics. Situations can occur that make us wonder what is the "right" thing to do—circumstances that require us to make ethical decisions. The Standards of Ethics provides guidelines for making these very important decisions; the decision we make could impact our entire professional career.

The ARRT Ethics Committee provides peer review of cases to ensure adherence to standards of professional behavior. Radiographers, like all health care providers, must have the moral character required to practice in the health care professions. If their actions demonstrate that moral character is lacking, that individual can be sanctioned. The sanction can be in the form of a reprimand, a suspension of registration, revocation of registration, ineligibility for certification, or other sanctions deemed appropriate by the Ethics Committee. The student should carefully study the ARRT Rules of Ethics.

For example, if you become aware that one of your coworkers is in violation of one of the Rules of Ethics, what must you do? Your professional obligation is to report your knowledge to your supervisor, then to the ARRT (according to Rule #21, *you* are in violation if you fail to report to the ARRT), *and* you must report to the State if your State has licensing.

The radiographer must remember that failure to disclose a conviction is a violation of Ethical Rules #1 and #19 and involves falsification of ARRT information. ARRT can become aware of an unreported conviction as part of an employment background check. This could actually result in a more serious sanction than the original offense!

The radiographer needs to be familiar with the ARRT Standards of Ethics, as they provide very important information and answers to tough questions that can be encountered during the course of the radiographer's professional practice.

ARRT Standards of Ethics Composed of

• Preamble
• Code of Ethics (aspirational)
• Rules of Ethics (enforceable)
• Administrative Procedures

ARRT® Standards of Ethics

Last Revised: September 1, 2011
Published: September 1, 2011

PREAMBLE

The *Standards of Ethics* of the American Registry of Radiologic Technologists shall apply solely to persons holding certificates from ARRT that are either currently registered by ARRT or that were formerly registered by ARRT (collectively, Certificate Holders), and to persons applying for examination and certification by ARRT in order to become Certificate Holders ("Candidates"). Radiologic Technology is an umbrella term that is inclusive of the disciplines of radiography, nuclear medicine technology, radiation therapy, cardiovascular-interventional radiography, mammography, computed tomography, magnetic resonance imaging, quality management, sonography, bone densitometry, vascular sonography, cardiac-interventional radiography, vascular-interventional radiography, breast sonography, and radiologist assistant. The *Standards of Ethics* are intended to be consistent with the Mission Statement of ARRT, and to promote the goals set forth in the Mission Statement.

STATEMENT OF PURPOSE

The purpose of the ethics requirements is to identify individuals who have internalized a set of professional values that cause one to act in the best interests of patients. This internalization of professional values and the resulting behavior is one element of ARRT's definition of what it means to be qualified. Exhibiting certain behaviors as documented in the *Standards of Ethics* is evidence of the possible lack of appropriate professional values.

The *Standards of Ethics* provides proactive guidance on what it means to be qualified and to motivate and promote a culture of ethical behavior within the profession. The ethics requirements support the ARRT's mission of promoting high standards of patient care by removing or restricting the use of the credential by those who exhibit behavior inconsistent with the requirements.

A. CODE OF ETHICS

The Code of Ethics forms the first part of the *Standards of Ethics*. The Code of Ethics shall serve as a guide by which Certificate Holders and Candidates may evaluate their professional conduct as it relates to patients, healthcare consumers, employers, colleagues, and other members of the healthcare team. The Code of Ethics is intended to assist Certificate Holders and Candidates in maintaining a high level of ethical conduct and in providing for the protection, safety, and comfort of patients. The Code of Ethics is aspirational.

1. The radiologic technologist acts in a professional manner, responds to patient needs, and supports colleagues and associates in providing quality patient care.

2. The radiologic technologist acts to advance the principal objective of the profession to provide services to humanity with full respect for the dignity of mankind.

3. The radiologic technologist delivers patient care and service unrestricted by the concerns of personal attributes or the nature of the disease or illness, and without discrimination on the basis of sex, race, creed, religion, or socio-economic status.

4. The radiologic technologist practices technology founded upon theoretical knowledge and concepts, uses equipment and accessories consistent with the purposes for which they were designed, and employs procedures and techniques appropriately.

5. The radiologic technologist assesses situations; exercises care, discretion, and judgment; assumes responsibility for professional decisions; and acts in the best interest of the patient.

6. The radiologic technologist acts as an agent through observation and communication to obtain pertinent information for the physician to aid in the diagnosis and treatment of the patient and recognizes that interpretation and diagnosis are outside the scope of practice for the profession.

7. The radiologic technologist uses equipment and accessories, employs techniques and procedures, performs services in accordance with an accepted standard of practice, and demonstrates expertise in minimizing radiation exposure to the patient, self, and other members of the healthcare team.

8. The radiologic technologist practices ethical conduct appropriate to the profession and protects the patient's right to quality radiologic technology care.

9. The radiologic technologist respects confidences entrusted in the course of professional practice, respects the patient's right to privacy, and reveals confidential information only as required by law or to protect the welfare of the individual or the community.

10. The radiologic technologist continually strives to improve knowledge and skills by participating in continuing education and professional activities, sharing knowledge with colleagues, and investigating new aspects of professional practice.

B. RULES OF ETHICS

The Rules of Ethics form the second part of the *Standards of Ethics*. They are mandatory standards of minimally acceptable professional conduct for all Certificate Holders and Candidates. Certification and Registration are methods of assuring the medical community and the public that an

Copyright ©2011 by The American Registry of Radiologic Technologists®. All rights reserved.

Figure 1–1. The American Registry of Radiologic Technologists Standards of Ethics. (Reprinted, with permission, from the ARRT. Copyright © 2011 The American Registry of Radiologic Technologists®. All rights reserved. The ARRT does not review, evaluate, or endorse publications. Permission to reproduce ARRT copyrighted materials within this publication should not be construed as an endorsement of the publication by the ARRT.) *(continued)*

individual is qualified to practice within the profession. Because the public relies on certificates and registrations issued by ARRT, it is essential that Certificate Holders and Candidates act consistently with these Rules of Ethics. These Rules of Ethics are intended to promote the protection, safety, and comfort of patients. The Rules of Ethics are enforceable. Certificate Holders and Candidates engaging in any of the following conduct or activities, or who permit the occurrence of the following conduct or activities with respect to them, have violated the Rules of Ethics and are subject to sanctions as described hereunder:

1. Employing fraud or deceit in procuring or attempting to procure, maintain, renew, or obtain or reinstate certification or registration as issued by ARRT; employment in radiologic technology; or a state permit, license, or registration certificate to practice radiologic technology. This includes altering in any respect any document issued by the ARRT or any state or federal agency, or by indicating in writing certification or registration with the ARRT when that is not the case.

2. Subverting or attempting to subvert ARRT's examination process. Conduct that subverts or attempts to subvert ARRT's examination process includes, but is not limited to:
   (i) disclosing examination information using language that is substantially similar to that used in questions and/or answers from ARRT examinations when such information is gained as a direct result of having been an examinee; this includes, but is not limited to, disclosures to students in educational programs, graduates of educational programs, educators, or anyone else involved in the preparation of Candidates to sit for the examinations; and/or
   (ii) receiving examination information that uses language that is substantially similar to that used in questions and/or answers on ARRT examinations from an examinee, whether requested or not; and/or
   (iii) copying, publishing, reconstructing (whether by memory or otherwise), reproducing or transmitting any portion of examination materials by any means, verbal or written, electronic or mechanical, without the prior express written permission of ARRT or using professional, paid or repeat examination takers or any other individual for the purpose of reconstructing any portion of examination materials; and/or
   (iv) using or purporting to use any portion of examination materials that were obtained improperly or without authorization for the purpose of instructing or preparing any Candidate for examination or certification; and/or
   (v) selling or offering to sell, buying or offering to buy, or distributing or offering to distribute any portion of examination materials without authorization; and/or
   (vi) removing or attempting to remove examination materials from an examination room, or having unauthorized possession of any portion of or information concerning a future, current, or previously administered examination of ARRT; and/or
   (vii) disclosing what purports to be, or under all circumstances is likely to be understood by the recipient as, any portion of or "inside" information concerning any portion of a future, current, or

previously administered examination of ARRT; and/or
   (viii) communicating with another individual during administration of the examination for the purpose of giving or receiving help in answering examination questions, copying another Candidate's answers, permitting another Candidate to copy one's answers, or possessing unauthorized materials including, but not limited to, notes; and/or
   (ix) impersonating a Candidate or permitting an impersonator to take or attempt to take the examination on one's own behalf; and/or
   (x) the use of any other means that potentially alters the results of the examination such that the results may not accurately represent the professional knowledge base of a Candidate.

3. Convictions, criminal proceedings, or military court-martials as described below:
   (i) conviction of a crime, including a felony, a gross misdemeanor, or a misdemeanor, with the sole exception of speeding and parking violations. All alcohol and/or drug related violations must be reported. Offenses that occurred while a juvenile and that are processed through the juvenile court system are not required to be reported to ARRT.
   (ii) criminal proceeding where a finding or verdict of guilt is made or returned but the adjudication of guilt is either withheld, deferred, or not entered or the sentence is suspended or stayed; or a criminal proceeding where the individual enters a plea of guilty or nolo contendere (no contest); or where the individual enters into a pre-trial diversion activity.
   (iii) military court-martials related to any offense identified in these Rules of Ethics.

4. Violating a rule adopted by a state or federal regulatory authority or certification board resulting in the individual's license, permit, registration or certification being denied, revoked, suspended, placed on probation, or subjected to any conditions, or failing to report to ARRT any of the violations or actions identified in this Rule.

5. Performing procedures which the individual is not competent to perform through appropriate training and/or education or experience unless assisted or personally supervised by someone who is competent (through training and/or education or experience).

6. Engaging in unprofessional conduct, including, but not limited to:
   (i) a departure from or failure to conform to applicable federal, state, or local governmental rules regarding radiologic technology practice or scope of practice; or, if no such rule exists, to the minimal standards of acceptable and prevailing radiologic technology practice;
   (ii) any radiologic technology practice that may create unnecessary danger to a patient's life, health, or safety.
   Actual injury to a patient or the public need not be established under this clause.

7. Delegating or accepting the delegation of a radiologic technology function or any other prescribed healthcare function when the delegation or acceptance could reasonably be expected to create an unnecessary

Figure 1–1. (*Continued*)

danger to a patient's life, health, or safety. Actual injury to a patient need not be established under this clause.

8. Actual or potential inability to practice radiologic technology with reasonable skill and safety to patients by reason of illness; use of alcohol, drugs, chemicals, or any other material; or as a result of any mental or physical condition.

9. Adjudication as mentally incompetent, mentally ill, a chemically dependent person, or a person dangerous to the public, by a court of competent jurisdiction.

10. Engaging in any unethical conduct, including, but not limited to, conduct likely to deceive, defraud, or harm the public; or demonstrating a willful or careless disregard for the health, welfare, or safety of a patient. Actual injury need not be established under this clause.

11. Engaging in conduct with a patient that is sexual or may reasonably be interpreted by the patient as sexual, or in any verbal behavior that is seductive or sexually demeaning to a patient; or engaging in sexual exploitation of a patient or former patient. This also applies to any unwanted sexual behavior, verbal or otherwise, that results in the termination of employment.

12. Revealing a privileged communication from or relating to a former or current patient, except when otherwise required or permitted by law, or using or releasing confidential patient information in violation of HIPAA.

13. Knowingly engaging or assisting any person to engage in, or otherwise participating in, abusive or fraudulent billing practices, including violations of federal Medicare and Medicaid laws or state medical assistance laws.

14. Improper management of patient records, including failure to maintain adequate patient records or to furnish a patient record or report required by law; or making, causing, or permitting anyone to make false, deceptive, or misleading entry in any patient record.

15. Knowingly assisting, advising, or allowing a person without a current and appropriate state permit, license, or registration certificate or a current certificate of registration with ARRT to engage in the practice of radiologic technology, in a jurisdiction which requires a person to have such a current and appropriate state permit, license, or registration certificate or a current and appropriate registration of certification with ARRT in order to practice radiologic technology in such jurisdiction.

16. Violating a state or federal narcotics or controlled-substance law.

17. Knowingly providing false or misleading information that is directly related to the care of a former or current patient.

18. Subverting, attempting to subvert, or aiding others to subvert or attempt to subvert ARRT's Continuing Education (CE) Requirements for Renewal of Registration. Conduct that subverts or attempts to subvert ARRT's Continuing Education Requirements includes, but is not limited to:
    (i) providing false, inaccurate, altered, or deceptive information related to CE activities to ARRT or an ARRT recognized CE recordkeeper;
    (ii) assisting others to provide false, inaccurate, altered, or deceptive information related to CE activities to ARRT or an ARRT recognized CE recordkeeper;
    (iii) conduct that results or could result in a false or deceptive report of CE completion; or
    (iv) conduct that in any way compromises the integrity of the CE Requirements such as sharing answers to the post-tests or CE self-learning activities, providing or using false certificates of participation, or verifying CE credits that were not earned.

19. Subverting or attempting to subvert the ARRT certification or registration process by:
    (i) making a false statement or knowingly providing false information to ARRT; or
    (ii) failing to cooperate with any investigation by the ARRT.

20. Engaging in false, fraudulent, deceptive, or misleading communications to any person regarding the individual's education, training, credentials, experience, or qualifications, or the status of the individual's state permit, license, or registration certificate in radiologic technology or certificate of registration with ARRT.

21. Knowing of a violation or a probable violation of any Rule of Ethics by any Certificate Holder or Candidate and failing to promptly report in writing the same to the ARRT.

22. Failing to immediately report to his or her supervisor information concerning an error made in connection with imaging, treating, or caring for a patient. For purposes of this rule, errors include any departure from the standard of care that reasonably may be considered to be potentially harmful, unethical, or improper (commission). Errors also include behavior that is negligent or should have occurred in connection with a patient's care, but did not (omission). The duty to report under this rule exists whether or not the patient suffered any injury.

American Registry of Radiologic Technologists ®
1255 Northland Drive
St. Paul, MN 55120

(651) 687-0048, ext. 8580
www.arrt.org

Figure 1–1. (*Continued*)

Honor Code

The word *honor* implies an effective regard for the standards of one's profession, a refusal to lie or deceive, an uprightness of character or action, a trustworthiness and incorruptibility, that is, being incapable of falling short in a trust or responsibility. Other words used to describe these qualities are *honesty*, *integrity*, and *probity*.

Certainly these are qualities required of students and health care professionals. This honor/integrity can only be achieved in an environment where intellectual honesty and personal integrity are highly valued—and where the responsibility for communicating and maintaining these standards is widely shared. The ARRT publishes an important document regarding Honor Code violations (Fig. 1–2).

A student radiographer having any question regarding a violation reportable on their ARRT examination application should contact the ARRT Ethics Requirements Department.

A radiographer (or student radiographer) convicted of a misdemeanor or felony must report that to the ARRT. The Ethics Committee will conduct a peer review of the case and make a determination regarding possible sanction. *One* important consideration will be if

Honor Code Violations

Have you ever been suspended, dismissed, or expelled from an educational program that you have attended in order to meet ARRT certification requirements?

This is a question every primary-pathway candidate for certification must answer on the application, in addition to reading and signing the "Written Consent under FERPA," which allows ARRT to obtain specific parts of their educational records concerning violations to an honor code. If a student has ever been suspended, dismissed, or expelled from an educational program attended in order to meet ARRT certification requirements, he or she should answer "YES" to the question above and include an explanation and documentation of the situation with the completed application for certification.

A list of some of the violations ARRT is concerned about is provided below, but when in doubt contact the ARRT Ethics Requirements Department at (651) 687-0048, ext. 8580.

Reportable Honor Code Violations
Note: This list does not include all reportable infractions. If you are unsure of whether something should be reported, contact a member of the Ethics staff at (651) 687-0048, ext. 8580.

- Cheating and/or plagiarism;
- Falsification of eligibility requirements (e.g., clinical competency information);
- Forgery or alteration of any document related to qualifications or patient care;
- Abuse, neglect, or abandonment of patients;
- Sexual contact without consent or harassment to any member of the community, including patients;
- Conduct that is seriously obscene or offensive;
- Practicing in an unsafe manner or outside the scope of professional training;
- Violating patient confidentiality (HIPAA);
- Attempted or actual theft of any item not belonging to the student (including patients' property); and/or
- Attending class or clinical setting while under the influence of alcohol, drugs, or other substances.

Copyright 1999 - 2011 The American Registry of Radiologic Technologists®

Figure 1–2. ARRT Honor Code Violations. (Reprinted, with permission, from www.arrt.org. Copyright © 2011 The American Registry of Radiologic Technologists®. All rights reserved. The ARRT does not review, evaluate, or endorse publications. Permission to reproduce ARRT copyrighted materials within this publication should not be construed as an endorsement of the publication by the ARRT.)

the actions were job related and could present a risk to the welfare of the patient.

Summary

- Patient consent can be verbal, written, or implied; a valid patient consent includes four conditions.
- Hospital Information Systems must ensure confidentiality in compliance with Health Insurance Portability and Accountability Act (HIPAA) of 1996 regulations.
- The AHA Patient's Bill of Rights details 12 specific areas of patient rights that the health care professional is obligated to respect.
- The AHA has replaced the Patient's Bill of Rights with the six-part Patient Care Partnership.
- An Advance Health Care Directive, or Living Will, names the individual authorized to make all health care decisions and can include specifics regarding DNR, DNI, and/or other end-of-life decisions.
- The ASRT Practice Standards identifies the level of knowledge and skill required of a professional radiographer.
- Radiologic examinations may be requested by a physician or physician assistant.
- The radiographer should examine the requisition carefully prior to bringing the patient to the radiographic room.
- Most health care facilities require that examination requests include pertinent diagnostic information and any infection control or isolation information.
- A civil injustice is a *tort*; a tort can be intentional or negligent.
- Negligence litigation in radiology most frequently involves injuries from falls, positioning injuries, pregnancy, and errors or delays in diagnosis.
- The ARRT Standards of Ethics consists of a Preamble, the Code of Ethics, the Rules of Ethics, and Administrative Procedures.
- The Code of Ethics details guidelines for the radiographer's professional conduct and is *aspirational*. The Rules of Ethics are mandatory and enforceable.
- The ARRT publishes an important document regarding Honor Code violations.

COMPREHENSION CHECK

Congratulations! You have completed this chapter. If you are able to answer the following group of comprehensive questions, you can feel confident that you have mastered this section. You are then ready to go on to the "Registry-type" questions that follow. For greatest success, do not go to the multiple-choice questions without first completing the short-answer questions below.

1. What are the two parts of the ARRT Standards of Ethics? Which part is mandatory and enforceable (p. 8-10)?

2. How can Honor Code violations impact a candidate for an ARRT examination (p. 12)?

3. Discuss the AHA Patient's Bill of Rights with respect to legal considerations pertinent to radiography and relate it to the new AHA Patient Care Partnership (p. 4-6).

4. Describe an Advance Health Care Directive and possible elements that it might address. What is its purpose (p. 5)?

5. Discuss the purpose of the ASRT Practice Standards for the radiographer (p. 5).

6. List the conditions necessary for valid consent (p. 3).

7. Discuss public versus private (civil) law (p. 6).

8. Differentiate between assault and battery, slander and libel (p. 6).

9. Give examples of intentional and unintentional torts (p. 6, 7).

10. List the four elements of a negligent tort (p. 7).

11. Identify the areas of litigation that most frequently involve radiology (p. 7).

12. List the patient information usually found on examination request forms (p. 5, 6).

13. Describe the impact of the 1996 HIPAA regulations on radiologic patient care considerations (p. 3, 5).

14. Identify the kinds of clarification that may be required prior to starting the examination (p. 5, 6).

15. Review the ARRT Rules of Ethics and give an example of how one or more could impact a radiography student (p. 9,10).

CHAPTER REVIEW QUESTIONS

1. The ASRT document that defines the radiographer's role is the:
   (A) Standards of Ethics
   (B) Practice Standards
   (C) Standard of Care
   (D) Legal Standards

2. Honor Code violations that can keep a radiography student from meeting ARRT certification requirements include:
   1. being suspended from a radiography program
   2. being dismissed/expelled from a radiography program
   3. failing one or more courses in their radiography program
   (A) 1 only
   (B) 2 only
   (C) 1 and 2 only
   (D) 1, 2, and 3

3. Violations of the ARRT Rules of Ethics include:
   1. accepting responsibility to perform a function outside the scope of practice
   2. failure to obtain pertinent information for the radiologist
   3. failure to share newly acquired knowledge with peers
   (A) 1 only
   (B) 1 and 2 only
   (C) 1 and 3 only
   (D) 1, 2, and 3

4. Which organization has the authority to impose professional sanction on a radiographer?
   (A) ARRT
   (B) ASRT
   (C) JRCERT
   (D) TJC

5. A radiographer who discloses confidential information to unauthorized individuals may be found liable for:
   (A) assault
   (B) battery
   (C) intimidation
   (D) defamation

6. Patients' rights include the following:
   1. the right to refuse treatment
   2. the right to confidentiality
   3. the right to possess one's medical records
   (A) 1 only
   (B) 1 and 2 only
   (C) 1 and 3 only
   (D) 1, 2, and 3

7. A radiographer who performs an examination on a patient without the patient's consent or after the patient has refused the examination may be liable for:
   (A) assault
   (B) battery
   (C) slander
   (D) libel

8. An individual's legal document that names the person authorized to make all health care decisions, should they be unable to, is called a:
   1. Living Will
   2. Advance Health Care Directive
   3. Last Will and Testament
   (A) 1 only
   (B) 1 and 2 only
   (C) 2 and 3 only
   (D) 1, 2, and 3

9. The legislation that guarantees confidentiality of all patient information is:
   (A) HSS
   (B) HIPAA
   (C) HIPPA
   (D) MQSA

10. If the patient lacks decision-making capacity, their rights can be exercised on their behalf by:
    1. designated surrogate
    2. designated proxy
    3. no one
    (A) 1 only
    (B) 2 only
    (C) 1 and 2 only
    (D) 3 only

Answers and Explanations

1. (B) Radiographers should be familiar with their *Practice Standards* published by the American Society of Radiologic Technologists (ASRT). The Standards provide a legal role definition and identify Clinical, Quality, and Professional Standards of practice—each Standard has its own rationale and identifies general and specific criteria related to that Standard. The student radiographer can access the individual standards, their rationale, and criteria on the ASRT Web site.

The American Registry of Radiologic Technologists (ARRT) establishes principles of *professional conduct* to ensure the best services possible to patients entrusted to our care. These principles are detailed in the ARRT two-part *Standards of Ethics*, which includes the Code of Ethics and the Rules of Ethics. The 10-part *Code* of Ethics is aspirational; the 23 *Rules* of Ethics are enforceable and violation can result in professional sanction.

2. (C) The word *honor* implies regard for the standards of one's profession, a refusal to lie/deceive, an uprightness of character or action, a trustworthiness and incorruptibility. Other words used to describe these qualities are *honesty*, *integrity*, and *probity*.

These are qualities required of students and health care professionals. This honor/integrity can only be achieved in an environment where intellectual honesty and personal integrity are highly valued—and where the responsibility for communicating and maintaining these standards is widely shared. The ARRT publishes an important document regarding Honor Code Violations (Fig. 1–2). In order to meet ARRT certification requirements, candidates for the ARRT examination must answer the question "Have you ever been suspended, dismissed, or expelled from an educational program that you have attended?" . . . in addition to reading and signing the "Written Consent under FERPA", allowing the ARRT to obtain specific parts of their educational records concerning violations to an honor code if the student has ever been suspended, dismissed, or expelled from an educational program attended. If the applicant answers "yes" to that question he/she must include an explanation and documentation of the situation with the completed application for certification. If the applicant has any doubts, he/she should contact the ARRT Ethics Requirements Department at (651) 687-0048, ext. 8580.

3. (A) Accepting responsibility to perform a function outside the scope of practice is a violation of Ethical *Rule #7*, which states that it is a violation to "delegate or accept delegation of a radiologic technology function or any other prescribed health care function when the delegation or acceptance could reasonably be expected to create an unnecessary danger to a patient's life, health, or safety. Actual injury to a patient need not be established under this clause." So, accepting a responsibility outside the scope of practice is a violation of an ARRT *rule*. However, choices 2 and 3 are in violation of the *aspirational Code* of Ethics.

4. (A) The ARRT establishes principles of professional conduct to ensure the best services possible to patients entrusted to our care. These principles are detailed in the ARRT two-part *Standards of Ethics*, which includes the Code of Ethics and the Rules of Ethics. The 10-part *Code* of Ethics is aspirational; the 23 *Rules* of Ethics are enforceable and violation can result in professional sanction. The ARRT Ethics Committee provides peer review of cases (misdemeanor, felony, etc.) to ensure adherence to standards of professional behavior and possession of the moral character required to practice in the health care professions. If the violator's actions demonstrate that moral character is lacking, that individual can be sanctioned—that is, reprimanded, suspended, revoked, ineligible for certification, etc., or other sanctions deemed appropriate by the Ethics Committee.

5. (D) A radiographer who discloses confidential information to unauthorized individuals may be found guilty of *invasion of privacy or defamation*. A radiographer whose disclosure of confidential information is in some way detrimental to the patient may be accused of defamation. Spoken defamation is *slander;* written defamation is *libel. Assault* is to threaten harm; *battery* is to carry out the threat.

6. (B) The AHA identifies 12 important areas in its *Patient's Bill of Rights*. These include the right to refuse treatment (to the extent allowed by law), the right to confidentiality of records and communication, and the right to continuing care. Other patient rights identified are the right to informed consent, privacy, respectful care, *access* to personal medical records, refusal to participate in research projects, and an explanation of one's hospital bill.

7. **(B)** *Assault* is to threaten harm; *battery* is to carry out the threat. A patient may feel sufficiently intimidated to claim assault by a radiographer who threatens to repeat a difficult examination if the patient does not try to cooperate better. A radiographer who performs an examination on a patient without the patient's consent or after the patient has refused the examination may be liable for battery. A charge of battery may also be made against a radiographer who treats a patient roughly or who performs an examination on the wrong patient. A radiographer who discloses confidential information to unauthorized individuals may be found liable for *invasion of privacy* or *defamation*. A radiographer whose disclosure of confidential information is in some way detrimental to the patient may be accused of defamation. Spoken defamation is *slander;* written defamation is *libel*.

8. **(B)** Patient's rights can be exercised on the patient's behalf by a designated surrogate or proxy decision maker if the patient lacks decision-making capacity, is legally incompetent, or is a minor. Many people believe that potential legal and ethical issues can be avoided by creating an *Advance Health Care Directive* or *Living Will*. Since all persons have the right to make decisions regarding their own health care, this legal document preserves that right in the event an individual is unable to make those decisions. An Advance Health Care Directive, or Living Will, names the individual authorized to make all health care decisions and can include specifics regarding *DNR*

(do not resuscitate), *DNI* (do not intubate), and/or other end-of-life decisions.

9. **(B)** Most institutions now have computerized, paperless systems for patient information transmittal; these systems must ensure confidentiality in compliance with Health Insurance Portability and Accountability Act (HIPAA) of 1996 regulations. The health care professional generally has access to the computerized system only via personal password, thus helping ensure confidentiality of patient information. All medical records and other individually identifiable health information, whether electronic, on paper, or oral, are covered by HIPAA legislation and by subsequent Department of Health and Human Services (HHS) rules that took effect in April of 2001.

10. **(C)** Patient's rights can be exercised on the patient's behalf by a *designated surrogate or proxy* decision maker if the patient lacks decision-making capacity, is legally incompetent, or is a minor. Many people believe that potential legal and ethical issues can be avoided by creating an Advance Health Care Directive or Living Will. Since all persons have the right to make decisions regarding their own health care, this legal document preserves that right in the event an individual is unable to make those decisions. An Advance Health Care Directive, or Living Will, names the individual authorized to make all health care decisions and can include specifics regarding *DNR* (do not resuscitate), *DNI* (do not intubate), and/or other end-of-life decisions.

Patient Communication and Safety | 2

COMMUNICATION WITH PATIENTS

The importance of effective patient and professional *communication* skills cannot be overstressed; the interaction between a patient and a radiographer generally leaves the patient with a lasting impression of his or her health care experience. Of course, communication refers not only to the spoken word but also to unspoken/nonverbal communication. *Facial expression* can convey caring and reassurance or impatience and disapproval. Similarly, a radiographer's *touch* can convey his or her commitment to considerate care, or it can convey a rough, uncaring, hurried attitude. Making *eye contact* while speaking is generally considered polite and respectful in the United States, whereas it can be considered just the opposite in other cultures (e.g., Asian, East Indian, Native American). Our *appearance* gives an impression about how we feel about our work and our patients; it is very much a part of communication and we should strive for a professional appearance/image.

Effective communication begins with establishing trust and rapport. The technologist/student introduces himself/herself to the patient and then follows with verification of patient identity. Care must be taken when making the initial patient identification. If the radiographer calls out a name into a rather full waiting room, or asks a patient if he is Mr. so-and-so, an anxious patient might readily respond in the affirmative without actually having heard his or her name called. The radiographer must check the patient's wristband *and* ask the patient for a second verification, such as his or her birth date.

Effective communication with patients should also begin with a review of relevant patient history, often including ascertainment of the patient's current medication(s). The acquisition of pertinent clinical history from the patient is one of the most valuable contributions to the diagnostic process. Because the diagnostic radiologist rarely has the opportunity to speak with the patient, this is a crucial responsibility of the radiographer. For instance, to report that your patient indicates most pain at his or her medial malleolus is far more valuable than simply saying that his or her leg hurts. Review of patient information *before* bringing the patient into the radiographic department also enables the radiographer to have the x-ray room prepared, with all equipment and accessories readily available. *However*, it is exceedingly important to respect patient privacy and HIPAA (Health Insurance Portability and Accountability Act) regulations. Be certain to interview the patient in a manner/place that your conversation cannot be overheard by individuals not involved with that patient's examination.

Verbal/Written and Nonverbal Communication

Scenario #1: Consider the *nonverbal* messages communicated to a patient brought into a disorderly radiographic department, or by a radiographer's sloppy, poorly groomed appearance. What about the grim-faced professional who hurries the patient along to the radiographic department, gives rapid-fire instructions on what to do while searching for missing markers and cassettes, tosses the patient about on the x-ray table, and finally dismisses the patient with a curt "you can go now"?

Scenario #2: Consider another patient, greeted by a smiling professional who introduces himself or herself and brings the patient to a neat and orderly radiographic department, where everything is in readiness for the procedure. The radiographer explains the procedure and answers the patient's questions. At the end of the examination, the patient is escorted back to the waiting area and clear instructions are given for appropriate postprocedural care.

Which scenario provides the patient with a more comfortable, anxiety-free examination? Which patient leaves the hospital or clinic environment with a more favorable impression of his or her health care experience? Which experience would *you* prefer for yourself or a loved one?

The volume of the radiographer's *voice* and rate of speech are also important factors to consider in effective communication. The radiographer should face the patient and make *eye contact* during communication. Loud, rapid speech is particularly uncomfortable for the sick patient. A conscious effort should be made to use a well-modulated tone.

X-ray examinations may be requested by a physician or physician assistant. Written and/or verbal instructions and requests received by the radiographer must be clearly understandable. Request forms for radiologic examinations should be carefully reviewed by the radiographer prior to commencement of the examination. If the radiographer has any question about the examination to be performed, or receives conflicting/questionable information from the patient, it is his or her duty to *clarify all information*. It is the responsibility of the radiographer to *clarify all information and documentation before proceeding*. Many hospitals and radiology departments have specific rules about exactly what kind(s) of information is required on the requisition forms.

Explanation of Procedure

It is imperative that the radiographer takes adequate time to thoroughly explain the procedure or examination to the patient. The radiographer requires the cooperation of the patient throughout the course of the examination; therefore, providing a thorough explanation will alleviate the patient's anxieties and permit fuller cooperation. Effective communications skills require the use of layman's terms and an explanation should be given for any technical terms employed. Patients should be clear about what will be expected of them and what they may expect from the radiographer.

Patients often have questions about other scheduled diagnostic imaging procedures, such as mammography, computed tomography (CT), magnetic resonance imaging, sonography, or nuclear medicine studies. They often inquire about the length of an examination as well as ask other questions relating to safety or contraindications for an examination. The diagnostic radiographer must be well informed and able to effectively respond to questions relating to all types of examinations. If they are unsure about how to answer a patient's concerns, they must know where to get the proper information. Patient concerns relate to diet restrictions or other preparation that may be required for CT or sonography; concerns or contraindications for some examinations such as magnetic resonance imaging; and positioning techniques such as compression used in mammography. The radiographer should also be able to help the patient obtain information about these and other services he or she might require, for example, social services, rehabilitation, and spiritual counseling.

Explanation of Aftercare

Radiographers must be certain to provide patients with appropriate aftercare instructions (e.g., plenty of fluids following barium examinations).

To alleviate the anxiety associated with diagnostic imaging examinations and procedures, patients sometimes need to repeat explanations or instructions (to the radiographer) to be certain they understand; some have an additional question or two they must ask to clarify their thoughts. The radiographer's patience and understanding at these times is greatly appreciated by the anxious patient or relative.

COMMUNICATION CHALLENGES

Cultural and Other

Gaining the patient's confidence and trust through effective communication is an essential part of the radiographic examination. Some patients present challenges and will require a greater use of the radiographer's communication skills—patients who are seriously ill or injured; traumatized patients; patients who have impaired vision, hearing, or speech; infants and children; non–English-speaking patients; the elderly and infirm; the physically or mentally impaired; alcohol and drug abusers, the families of patients—*radiographers must adapt their communication skills to meet the needs of all individuals.*

Misunderstandings between cultures can occur as a result of seemingly innocuous circumstances—such as standing too close while speaking to another, looking directly into someone's eyes, or the use of certain gestures. Gestures have different meanings in different countries. In the United States and Europe, the "thumbs up" gesture has a positive implication. However, it is considered rude in Australia and obscene in the Middle East. Other examples of potentially misunderstood gestures include: if you compliment a Mexican child, you must touch that child's head, while in Asia, it is not acceptable to touch the head of a child; in the Philippines, it is rude to beckon with the index finger. Furthermore, in the United States, people are comfortable speaking about 18 inches apart, while in the Middle East, people stand much closer together when they talk; in England, people stand further apart.

Ethnocentrism is the belief that one's own cultural ways are superior to any other way. Ethnocentrism is common to all cultures and is the most significant barrier to good communication. It is essential that we have an awareness of our own ethnocentrism.

Medical Terminology

Although many individuals today are knowledgeable health care consumers, we cannot assume that all patients understand the medical terminology or technical jargon of radiologic procedures. Patient anxiety can be relieved by explaining procedures and answering questions in a simple, clear, and direct manner, avoiding the use of elaborate medical terminology. Using language that is not comprehensible to patients can make them feel intimidated and cause them more anxiety. Let the patient know you are there for them—not simply to perform the x-ray examination, but to help them understand and to be as comfortable as possible.

Techniques to Improve Communication

Many patients are anxious about their illness/condition and are unfamiliar with the procedure they are about to undergo. Communication difficulties can be simply and significantly improved through explanation. Since *anxious* patients require more time to think and to move, a radiographer who takes the time to explain the procedure, explain unfamiliar terminology, and answer patient's questions will be long remembered and appreciated by that patient.

Elderly patients, for example, dislike being pushed or hurried about. They appreciate the radiographer who is compassionate enough to take the extra few minutes necessary for comfort. Some elderly patients are easily confused; it is best to address them by their full name and to keep instructions simple and direct. The elderly deserve the same courteous, dignified care as all other patients.

Another special population that should be considered carefully in the imaging department is infants and children. Communication and care challenges can be quite different with *children*, depending on their age. Children must be provided with a safe environment and never left unattended. *Infant* care includes minimizing separation anxiety by keeping infant and parent(s) together, keeping a familiar object or two (toy, blanket) with the infant, and limiting the number of staff present in the x-ray room. *Toddlers* should be spoken to at eye level; the radiographer should be cheerful and unhurried. Talking to the child cheerfully and having a playful manner can significantly reduce his or her anxiety and help him or her be more cooperative. *Preschoolers* benefit from simple explanations of what you will be doing and how they can help you. Be honest with *school-age children*, explain what you will be doing and let them help whenever possible. *Adolescents* require privacy and modesty. Establish rapport by striking up conversation about hobbies or other interests.

Communication difficulties can arise with non–English-speaking patients. Most hospitals and large clinics have a list of resource people to assist with interpretation when there is a language barrier. A certified interpreter is most helpful because he or she translates exactly what has been said—rather than a family member or friend who might edit, or try to explain what he or she thinks is implied.

Summary

- Most health care facilities require that examination requests include pertinent diagnostic information and any infection control or isolation information.
- Patients must be identified by checking their wristbands and requesting a second verification such as birth date.
- Verbal communication involves the tone and rate of speech as well as what is being said. It involves personalization and respect.
- Nonverbal communication involves facial expression, touch, eye contact, professional appearance, orderliness of the radiographic department, and the preparation and efficiency of the radiographer.
- The radiographer must clarify any unclear or contradictory information or documentation before proceeding with the examination.
- A thorough explanation of procedures reduces the patient's anxiety, increases cooperation, and results in a better examination.
- The radiographer must be able to provide accurate aftercare information and ably address patient's questions about other imaging studies.
- Patients should receive explanations in a simple, clear, and direct manner, without the use of elaborate medical terminology.
- Communication challenges can arise with many patients; for example, the seriously ill, traumatized; impaired senses; children; non–English-speaking; elderly, infirm; mentally impaired; substance abusers, and patients' families.

EVALUATING PATIENT CONDITION

The radiographer must *assess* a patient's condition prior to bringing the patient to the radiographic department and as the examination progresses. A good place to begin is with a review of the patient's chart. Other useful information includes the admitting diagnosis and recent nurses' notes including information regarding the patient's degree of ambulation, any preparation for the x-ray procedure and how it was tolerated, notes regarding laboratory tests, and saving the patient's urine.

As the radiographer obtains a brief pertinent clinical history, he or she also assesses the patient's condition by observing and listening. To provide safe and effective care, the radiographer must be able to assess the severity of a traumatized patient's injury, the patient's degree of motor control, and the need for support equipment or radiographic accessories. Can the patient move or be moved from the stretcher? Can the part be imaged adequately and with less pain on the stretcher or in the wheelchair? Will the use of sponges and/or sandbags result in a more comfortable, safer, and better-imaged examination?

Physical Signs

When the patient is first approached, and as the examination progresses, the radiographer should be alert to the patient's appearance and condition, and any subsequent changes in them. It is important to notice the color, temperature, and moistness of the patient's skin. Paleness frequently indicates weakness; the *diaphoretic* patient has pale, cool skin. *Fever* is frequently accompanied by hot, dry skin. "Sweaty" palms may indicate *anxiety*. A patient who becomes *cyanotic* (bluish lips, mucous membranes, or nail beds) needs oxygen and requires immediate medical attention.

Vital Signs

If a medical emergency arises, the radiographer may be required to assist by obtaining the patient's vital signs. Although checking vital signs is not a routine function, the radiographer should be proficient and confident if and when the need arises. Practicing the skills associated with taking vital signs during "slow" periods will benefit the patients during an emergency situation and those on whom you practice will learn their baseline signs—which provide valuable information for everyone.

Obtaining vital signs involves the measurement of body temperature, pulse rate, respiratory rate, and arterial blood pressure.

Body temperature varies with the time of day and site of measurement. It can be measured via a thermometer in the mouth, rectum, axilla, bladder, heart chamber, or external auditory canal. Increased body temperature, or fever, usually signifies infection. Symptoms of fever include general malaise, increased pulse and respiratory rates, flushed skin that is hot and dry to the touch, and occasional chills. Patients who experience very high, prolonged fevers can suffer irreparable brain damage.

Normal body temperature varies from person to person depending on several factors, including age. A normal *adult* body temperature taken orally is 98.6°F (37°C). Rectal temperature is generally 0.5° to 1.0° higher, whereas axillary temperature is usually 0.5° to 1.0° lower. A variation of 0.5° to 1.0° is generally considered within normal limits. Body temperature is usually lowest in the early morning and highest at night. Infants and children have a wider range of body temperature (rectal: 97.9°–100.4°F) than do adults; the elderly have lower body temperatures than do others. Infants and children up to 4 years have normal (tympanic) body temperatures of between 96.4°–100.4°F. *Children* aged 5 to 13 years have a normal body temperature range of 97.8° to 98.6°F.

Body areas having superficial arteries are best suited for determination of a patient's pulse rate. The *five most readily palpated pulse points* are the radial, carotid, temporal, femoral, and popliteal pulse. Of these, the radial pulse is the most frequently used. The apical pulse, at the apex of the heart, may be readily evaluated with the use of a stethoscope.

Pulse rate depends on the person's age, sex, body exertion and position, and general state of health. The very young and the very old have higher rates. Pulse rate increases in the standing position, after exertion, and with certain conditions, such as fever, organic heart disease, *shock*, and alcohol and drug use. Certain variations in the regularity and strength of the pulse are characteristic of various maladies. Pulse rates

Normal Body Temperatures

Adult	
Oral	98.6°F
Rectal	99.1°–99.6°F
Axillary	97.6°–98.1°F
Infant to age 4 y	97.9°–100.4°F (rectal)
Child aged 5–13 y	97.8°–98.6°F

Common Pulse Points

Artery	Location
Radial	Wrist; at base of thumb
Carotid	Neck; just lateral to midline
Temporal	In front of upper ear
Femoral	Inguinal region; groin
Popliteal	Posterior knee

vary between men and women and among adults, children, and infants; athletes often have lower pulse rates.

The act of *respiration* serves to deliver oxygen to all the body cells and rid the body of carbon dioxide. The radiographer must be able to recognize abnormalities or changes in patient respiration. The general term used to describe difficult breathing is *dyspnea*. More specific terms used to describe abnormal respirations include *uneven, spasmodic, strident* (shrill, grating sound), *stertorous* (labored, e.g., snoring), *tachypnea* (abnormally rapid breathing), *orthopnea* (difficulty breathing while recumbent), and *oligopnea* (abnormally shallow, slow).

A patient's respirations should be counted after counting the pulse rate, while still holding the patient's wrist. Respiratory action may become more deliberate and less natural in the patient who is aware that his or her respirations are being counted. The normal *adult* respiratory rate is 12 to 18 breaths per minute. The respiratory rate of young *children* is somewhat higher, up to 30 breaths per minute. Although the radiographer is counting respirations, he or she should also be assessing the respiratory pattern (even, uneven) and depth (normal, shallow, deep).

Blood encounters a degree of resistance as it travels through the peripheral vascular system; thus, a certain amount of pressure exists within the walls of the vessels. *Blood pressure* among individuals varies with age, sex, fatigue, mental or physical stress, disease, and trauma. The blood pressure within vessels is highest during ventricular *systole* (contraction) and lowest during *diastole* (relaxation). Blood pressure measurements are recorded with the systolic pressure on top and the diastolic pressure on the bottom, as in 100/80 (read "one hundred over eighty"). Normal *adult* systolic pressure ranges between 100 and 140 mm Hg, whereas the normal diastolic range is between 60 and 90 mm Hg. Prehypertension is present when blood pressure measurements are between 120 and 140 mm Hg systolic and/or between 80 and 90 mm Hg diastolic. Blood pressure consistently above 140/90 mm Hg is considered *hypertension*. Left undiagnosed and untreated, hypertension can lead to renal, cardiac, or brain damage. Hypotension is characterized by a systolic pressure of less than 90 mm Hg. Hypotension is seen in individuals with a decreased blood volume as a result of hemorrhage, infection, fever, and anemia. *Orthostatic* hypotension occurs in some individuals when they rise quickly from a recumbent position.

Blood pressure is measured using a *sphygmomanometer* and stethoscope. The patient may be recumbent or seated with the arm supported. The cuff of the sphygmomanometer is wrapped snugly around the arm, with its lower edge just above the *antecubital fossa*. With the stethoscope earpieces in place, the brachial artery pulse is palpated in the antecubital fossa and the bell (diaphragm) of the stethoscope is placed over the brachial artery. The valve on the bulb pump is closed and the cuff inflated *enough to collapse the brachial artery* (approximately 180 mm Hg). The valve is then opened very slowly. The first sound heard is the systolic pressure; as the valve pressure is slowly released, the sound becomes louder and then suddenly gets softer—this is the diastolic pressure. After the blood pressure measurements are recorded, the stethoscope earpieces and bell should be cleaned.

Normal (resting) Pulse Rates (beats/min)

Men	68–75
Women	72–80
Children	70–100
Infants	100–160

Blood Pressure Is Affected by:

- Cardiac output
- Blood volume
- Vascular resistance

Blood Pressure:

- Measured using a sphygmomanometer and stethoscope
- Cuff inflation sufficient to collapse the brachial artery
- First sound heard is systolic pressure

Summary

- Radiologic examinations can be requested by a physician or physician assistant.
- The radiographer should examine the requisition carefully prior to bringing the patient to the radiographic department.
- Patient condition may be assessed through chart information, observation, questioning, and vital signs.
- A patient's vital signs are temperature, pulse and respiration rates, and blood pressure.
- A normal adult oral body temperature is 98.6°F, axillary temperatures are 0.5° to 1° lower, and rectal temperatures are 0.5° to 1° higher.
- The arterial pulse points include radial, carotid, temporal, femoral, and popliteal.
- The normal adult pulse rate is 70 to 80 beats per minute; infant and children pulse rates are higher.
- The normal adult respiratory rate is 12 to 18 breaths per minute, with children's respirations being higher (up to 30/min).
- Dyspnea refers to difficulty breathing; other terms are used to describe specific respiratory abnormalities. Blood pressure is measured using a sphygmomanometer and stethoscope.
- The average normal adult systolic blood pressure is less than 120 mm Hg, whereas average normal adult diastolic blood pressure is less than 80 mm Hg; blood pressure varies with a person's age, sex, fatigue, mental or physical stress level, disease, and with trauma.
- Systolic pressure (contraction) is the top number, whereas diastolic pressure (relaxation) is the bottom number.

PATIENT SAFETY AND COMFORT

Body Mechanics

Radiographers work with many patients whose capacities for *ambulation* vary greatly. Outpatients are usually *ambulatory*, that is, able to walk and not confined to bed. Ambulatory inpatients generally travel by wheelchair, whereas patients confined to bed must travel by stretcher. It is essential for the radiographer to use proper technique and *body mechanics* when transferring patients, for the safety of the patient and the radiographer.

Not all patients need, or want, well-intentioned assistance. Many prefer to manage on their own. The radiographer should recognize this, but be ever alert and watchful should the patient need assistance. Other patients find it reassuring and feel an added sense of security with an attentive radiographer. The professional radiographer develops a sense of awareness of each patient's needs and concerns.

To transfer the patient with maximum safety, the radiographer must correctly use certain concepts of body mechanics. First, *a broad base of*

Other Rules of Good Body Mechanics

1. When carrying a heavy object, hold it close to the body.
2. The back should be kept straight; avoid twisting.
3. When lifting an object, bend the knees and use leg and abdominal muscles to lift (rather than the back muscles).
4. Whenever possible, push or roll heavy objects (rather than lifting or pulling).

support lends greater stability; therefore, the radiographer should stand with his or her feet approximately 12 in. apart and with one foot slightly forward. Second, stability is achieved when the body's *center of gravity* (center of the pelvis) is positioned over its base of support. For example, leaning away from the central axis of the body makes the body more vulnerable to losing balance; if the feet are close together, balance is even more difficult to maintain.

Even the ambulatory outpatient might be somewhat unsteady, so a ready, supporting hand at the elbow can be very helpful. The radiographer should keep a watchful eye on the patient and assist him or her as needed.

Patient Transfer

Before helping a patient into or out of a wheelchair, it must first be positioned parallel to the bed/x-ray table and locked. The footrests must be moved aside to avoid tripping over them or tilting the wheelchair forward. Once the patient is seated, the footrests should be lowered into place for the patient's comfort. When the patient is transferred from the wheelchair *to* the x-ray table, the patient's *stronger* side should approach the x-ray table *first*, while the radiographer assists his or her weaker side.

If the x-ray tables possess controls to adjust the height, this can greatly facilitate patient transfer and make the process safer for the patient as well as for the radiographer.

It is essential that someone should be responsible for keeping any intravenous (IV) tubing, *catheters*, oxygen lines, or other equipment free from entanglement during wheelchair and/or stretcher transfers.

Once the transfer is complete, the patient may be adjusted into the Fowler position (head higher than feet) for comfort or ease of breathing. The radiographer must be certain that safety belts and/or side rails are appropriately used for any patient on a stretcher.

Transfer Conditions Requiring Special Attention

It is the health care practitioner's responsibility to ensure patient safety and comfort while the patient is in his or her care. The radiographer should make a mental note of what the patient has in his or her possession when he or she enters the department, such as glasses or a purse. Patient belongings should be properly secured according to institution or department policy. The radiographer must be certain that the radiographic department is hazard free, that all equipment and accessories are used properly and safely, and that the patient is as comfortable as possible.

When moving to or from the wheelchair or stretcher, patients should always be assisted or, at least, given careful attention. It is exceedingly unwise to finish a radiographic examination and say "OK, you can get off the x-ray table now," or something to that effect. The x-ray tube must be moved away from the x-ray table, the x-ray table lowered if possible, a footstool must be in place to assist the patient from the table, and the radiographer must be there to guide or assist the patient safely to the correct dressing room.

Should an injured patient require assistance with dressing and undressing, it is important to remember that clothing should be *removed* from the *un*injured side first and *placed* on the *injured* side first.

Safety/Comfort Guidelines

- Belongings secure
- Hazard-free environment *to* avoid unnecessary/painful movement
- Equipment used properly
- Remove clothing first from uninjured side
- Place clothing first on the injured side

Special consideration must be given to each patient according to his or her condition. Elderly and very thin patients, and those who will be required to lie on the x-ray table for a lengthy period of time, benefit greatly from a foam pad between themselves and the x-ray table. Lumbar strain is relieved by a pillow or positioning sponge placed under the knees. An extra pillow for the head or cushioning under the heels or ischial tuberosities can make a big difference in patient care. Special care and attention should be given to the skin of the elderly, as it bruises and bleeds easily.

Patients who are sedated, senile, in shock, or under the influence of alcohol or drugs must never be left unattended. Patients who arrive in the radiology department with restraints in place must never be left alone on the x-ray table, since they are usually active, disoriented, and occasionally, combative. Indeed, many radiology departments have rules stating that *no* patient may *ever* be left unattended in the radiographic department.

Patients with IV *infusions* in place require added attention. The IV standard/bag should be 18 to 24 in. above the level of the vein. The infusion site should be checked periodically for any signs of tissue infiltration. Swelling around the needle site generally indicates that the needle or catheter is no longer in the vein and that the medication is infiltrating the surrounding tissues. The radiographer should turn off the IV and notify the physician or nurse.

Difficulty in communication can be encountered with a patient having a *tracheostomy* in place. These individuals are often anxious because they cannot communicate verbally and they are fearful of choking because they cannot remove the secretions that accumulate in their throats. They require careful attention. The nurse should be available to suction secretions if the patient starts to breathe noisily or with difficulty. The radiographer can relieve much patient anxiety by careful explanation of the examination. The patient can be provided with a pencil and pad to communicate any questions or concerns.

Just as health care practitioners provide for patient safety and comfort, they must ensure their own safety by practicing good body mechanics, infection control, and standard precautions.

Should an accident ever occur and a patient or health care practitioner be injured, no matter how small or insignificant the injury seems, it must be reported to the supervisor and an incident report completed. The risk management team, or similar group, requires all such information for legal documentation and as a means of identifying and resolving potential hazards.

Summary

- Modes of patient transportation include ambulation, wheelchair, and stretcher.
- Patient and radiographer safety requires the use of proper and safe body mechanics.
- Wheelchairs and stretchers must be locked and wheelchair footrests positioned out of the way prior to patient transfer.
- One person should be responsible for the safe transport of IV lines, catheters, and other tubes.

- Patient transfer between the radiographic table and the stretcher should involve pulling, not pushing; a smooth plastic board often helps.
- The knees should be bent when lifting heavy objects; leg and abdominal muscles are used instead of back muscles.
- Heavy objects should be carried close to the body; the back should be kept straight and twisting motions should be avoided.
- Heavy objects should be pushed or rolled (instead of pulled or lifted) whenever possible.
- Patient belongings should be properly secured according to policy while the patient is in the radiographer's care.
- The radiographer must be alert for patient safety and comfort at all times; patients should not be left unattended in the radiographic department.
- Should an accident occur involving the patient and/or radiographer, an incident report should be completed regardless of how minor the incident.

COMPREHENSION CHECK

Congratulations! You have completed your review of this chapter. If you are able to answer the following group of comprehensive questions, you can feel confident that you have mastered this section. You are then ready to go on to "Registry-type" questions that follow. For greatest success, do not go to these multiple-choice questions without first completing the short-answer questions below.

1. Explain the importance of reviewing the examination request and other patient information prior to bringing the patient to the radiographic department (p. 20).

2. Discuss the best way(s) to ensure correct identification of a patient (p. 19).

3. Explain the importance of obtaining patient history (p. 19, 20).

4. Discuss the importance of explaining the procedure to the patient (p. 20, 21).

5. Discuss five ways through which the radiographer communicates verbal messages to the patient (p. 19, 20).

6. Discuss five ways through which the radiographer communicates nonverbal messages to the patient (p. 19, 20).

7. Discuss some qualities of verbal communication likely to evoke a *positive* response from the patient; a *negative* response (p. 20).

8. Explain the value of making as many preparations as possible prior to bringing the patient into the radiographic department (p. 20, 21).

9. Discuss five types of patients who might require special communication efforts on the part of the radiographer (p. 21).

10. List five benefits of effective communication skills (p. 19, 20).

11. Discuss potential sources/causes of cultural misunderstanding (p. 21, 22).

12. Discuss the importance of being alert to the initial patient condition and any subsequent changes in condition (p. 23, 24).

13. Identify the following with respect to body temperature (p. 24).
    A. Normal adult, infant, and child temperature
    B. The significance of fever, that is, what it usually indicates
    C. Symptoms usually associated with fever
    D. Difference among oral, rectal, and axillary temperatures

14. Identify the following with respect to pulse rate (p. 24, 25).
    A. The normal, average adult pulse rate for men and women
    B. Normal and abnormal conditions under which pulse rate will vary/change
    C. The usual site of pulse determination; other possible sites/any special equipment needed

15. Identify the following with respect to respiration (p. 25).
    A. Its function
    B. The ideal time to determine patient respiration rate; why?
    C. The normal, average adult respiratory rate

16. Identify the following with respect to blood pressure (p. 25).
    A. Equipments necessary
    B. Position of patient
    C. Position of cuff and bell
    D. First and second sounds heard
    E. Maximum norms for systolic and diastolic pressures
    F. Prehypertensive and hypertensive pressures

17. Discuss three modes of patient transport (p. 26, 27).

18. Discuss some specials needs that a tracheostomy patient might have (p. 28).

19. Identify, with respect to body mechanics and patient transfer (p. 26, 27).

    A. Position of radiographer's feet (as base of support)

    B. The body's center of gravity (vis-à-vis stability) and when moving heavy objects: push versus pull; use of knees, legs, and back; proximity of object to body

    C. Position of footrests and locks during wheelchair transfers

    D. Position of locks, use of drawsheet and plastic mover, push versus pull in stretcher transfer

    E. Care of IV lines, catheters, O_2, safety belts, and side rails

20. Identify the manner in which patients should be directed onto, and removed from, the x-ray table (p. 27).

21. Explain how clothing should be removed from a patient with unilateral injury (p. 27, 28).

22. Identify techniques used to reduce discomfort of elderly and/or thin patients recumbent on the radiographic table (p. 27, 28).

23. Discuss the types of patients likely to be at greater risk left unattended on the radiographic table (p. 28).

CHAPTER REVIEW QUESTIONS

1. Prehypertension is present when:
   1. Systolic pressure is between 120 and 140 mm Hg
   2. Diastolic pressure is between 80 and 90 mm Hg
   3. Diastolic pressure is consistently 90 mm Hg
   (A) 1 only
   (B) 2 only
   (C) 1 and 2 only
   (D) 1 and 3 only

2. When an injured patient requires assistance with dressing or undressing, the radiographer must remember to:
   1. Place clothing on the injured side first
   2. Remove clothing from the injured side first
   3. Always start with the injured side
   (A) 1 only
   (B) 1 and 2 only
   (C) 3 only
   (D) 1, 2, and 3

3. Instruments needed to assess vital signs include:
   1. Tongue blade
   2. Watch with a second hand
   3. Thermometer
   (A) 1 only
   (B) 1 and 2 only
   (C) 2 and 3 only
   (D) 1, 2, and 3

4. The normal adult rectal temperature is:
   (A) Higher than axillary temperature
   (B) Lower than axillary temperature
   (C) The same as axillary temperature
   (D) The same as oral temperature

5. The period of contraction of the heart chambers is termed:
   (A) Systole
   (B) Diastole
   (C) Hypertension
   (D) Dyspnea

6. A patient who is *diaphoretic* has:
   (A) Pale, cool, clammy skin
   (B) Hot, dry skin
   (C) Dilated pupils
   (D) Warm, moist skin

7. A pulse can be detected only by the use of a stethoscope in which of the following locations?
   (A) Wrist
   (B) Neck
   (C) Groin
   (D) Apex of the heart

8. Which of the following communicate(s) messages to the patient?
   1. Rate of speech
   2. Eye contact
   3. Readiness of radiographic department
   (A) 1 only
   (B) 1 and 2 only
   (C) 3 only
   (D) 1, 2, and 3

9. What number of breaths per minute represents the average rate of respiration for a normal adult?
   (A) 8 to 15
   (B) 10 to 20
   (C) 30 to 60
   (D) 60 to 90

10. To reduce the back strain associated with transferring patients from stretcher to x-ray table, you should:
    (A) Pull the patient
    (B) Push the patient
    (C) Hold the patient away from your body and lift
    (D) Bend at the waist and pull

Answers and Explanations

1. (C) Blood pressure among individuals varies with age, sex, fatigue, mental or physical stress, disease, and trauma. The blood pressure within vessels is highest during ventricular contraction/*systole* and lowest during ventricular relaxation/*diastole.* Blood pressure measurements are recorded with the systolic pressure on top and the diastolic pressure on the bottom. Normal *adult* systolic pressure ranges between 100 and 140 mm Hg, whereas the normal diastolic range is between 60 and 90 mm Hg. *Prehypertension* is present when blood pressure measurements are between 120 and 140 mm Hg systolic and/or between 80 and 90 mm Hg diastolic. Blood pressure consistently above 140/90 mm Hg is considered *hypertension.* Left undiagnosed and untreated, hypertension can lead to renal, cardiac, or brain damage. Hypotension is characterized by a systolic pressure of less than 90 mm Hg. Hypotension is seen in individuals with a decreased blood volume as a result of hemorrhage, infection, fever, and anemia.

2. (A) Special consideration must be given to each patient according to his or her condition. Elderly and very thin patients, and those who will be required to lie on the x-ray table for a lengthy period of time, benefit greatly from a foam pad between themselves and the x-ray table. Should an injured patient require assistance with dressing and undressing, it is important to remember that clothing should be *removed from* the *un*injured side first and *placed on* the *injured* side first.

3. (C) Obtaining vital signs involves the measurement of *body temperature, pulse rate, respiratory rate,* and *arterial blood pressure.* A *thermometer* is used to take the patient's temperature. A *watch* with a second hand is required to time the patient's pulse rate and respirations. To measure blood pressure, a *sphygmomanometer* and *stethoscope* are required. A tongue blade is used to depress the tongue for inspection of the throat and is not part of vital sign assessment.

4. (A) Normal body temperature varies from person to person depending on several factors, including age. Normal adult body temperature taken orally is 98.6°F (37°C). Rectal temperature is generally 0.5° to 1.0° higher, whereas axillary temperature is usually 0.5° to 1.0° lower. Variation of 0.5° to 1.0° is generally considered within normal limits. Body temperature is usually lowest in the early morning and highest at night. Infants and children up to 4 years have normal rectal body temperatures of between 97.4° and 100.4°F. Children aged 5 to 13 years have a normal range of 97.8° to 98.6°F.

Obtaining *vital signs* involves the measurement of *body temperature, pulse rate, respiratory rate, and arterial blood pressure.* Increased body temperature, or fever, usually signifies infection. Symptoms of fever include general malaise, increased pulse and respiratory rates, flushed skin that is hot and dry to the touch, and occasional chills. Very high, prolonged fevers can cause irreparable brain damage.

5. (A) Blood pressure within vessels is highest during ventricular *systole* (contraction) and lowest during *diastole* (relaxation). Blood pressure measurements are recorded with the systolic pressure on top and the diastolic pressure on the bottom, as in 100/75 (read "one hundred over seventy-five"). Normal *adult* systolic pressure ranges between 100 and 140 mm Hg, whereas the normal diastolic range is between 60 and 90 mm Hg. *Prehypertension* is present when blood pressure measurements are between 120 and 140 mm Hg systolic and/or between 80 and 90 mm Hg diastolic. Blood pressure consistently above 140/90 mm Hg is considered *hypertension.* Left undiagnosed and untreated, hypertension can lead to renal, cardiac, or brain damage. Hypotension is characterized by a systolic pressure of less than 90 mm Hg. Hypotension is seen in individuals with a decreased blood volume as a result of hemorrhage, infection, fever, and anemia. *Orthostatic* hypotension occurs in some individuals when they rise quickly from a recumbent position. *Dyspnea* is the medical term used to describe difficulty in breathing.

6. (A) The radiographer must be alert to the patient's appearance and condition, and any subsequent changes in them. Notice the color, temperature, and moistness of the patient's skin: paleness frequently indicates weakness; the *diaphoretic* patient has pale, cool skin; *fever* is frequently accompanied by hot, dry skin; "sweaty" palms may indicate *anxiety*, a patient who becomes *cyanotic* (bluish lips, mucous membranes, nail beds) needs oxygen and requires immediate medical attention.

7. **(D)** Body areas having superficial arteries are best suited for determination of a patient's pulse rate. The five most readily palpated pulse points are the radial, carotid, temporal, femoral, and popliteal pulse. Of these, the radial pulse is the most frequently used. The apical pulse, at the apex of the heart, may be readily evaluated with the use of a stethoscope.

8. **(D)** The interaction between a patient and a radiographer generally leaves a lasting impression on the patient's health care experience. Communication may be verbal or nonverbal. *Verbal communication* involves tone and rate of speech as well as what is being said. It involves personalization and respect. *Nonverbal communication* involves facial expression, professional appearance, orderliness of radiographic department, and preparation and efficiency of the radiographer.

9. **(B)** A patient's respirations should be counted after counting the pulse rate, while still holding the patient's wrist. Respiratory action may become more deliberate, or less natural, in the patient who is aware that his or her respirations are being counted. *The normal respiratory rate is 12 to 18 breaths per minute*. The respiratory rate of young *children* is somewhat *higher*, up to 30 breaths per minute. Although the radiographer is counting respirations, he or she should be assessing the respiratory pattern (even, uneven) and depth (normal, shallow, deep) as well.

10. **(A)** When transferring a patient from the stretcher *to the x-ray table, several rules apply that will help reduce back strain. Pull*, do not push the patient; pushing increases friction and makes the transfer more difficult. *Use the biceps* muscles for pulling; do not bend at the waist and pull, as this motion *increases back strain*.

Infection Control | 3

TERMINOLOGY AND BASIC CONCEPTS

Microorganisms

Living organisms too small to be seen with the naked eye are referred to as *microorganisms*. Most microorganisms do not produce infection or disease, many reside harmlessly, and many are actually *beneficial* for our good health, for example, bacteria, protozoa, and fungi found on/in particular body areas. Specific permanent flora are found, for example, in the mouth, upper respiratory tract, and intestines; many of these microorganisms inhibit the growth of pathogens in their *natural* sites, but can cause infection if introduced into a site where they do not normally reside, or when introduced into an immunocompromised host.

Pathogenic microorganisms are capable of causing infection or disease by destroying cells or tissues, or secreting toxins. Pathogenic microorganisms can be transmitted from one host to another. Since hospitals are places that treat and care for infection and disease, it stands to reason that health care practitioners must be particularly vigilant against transmission of pathogenic microorganisms.

Medical and Surgical Asepsis

Antisepsis is a practice that retards the growth of pathogenic microorganisms. *Medical asepsis* refers to the destruction of pathogenic microorganisms (bacteria) through the process of *disinfection*. Examples of disinfectants are hydrogen peroxide, chlorine, iodine, boric acid, and formaldehyde. *Surgical asepsis* (*sterilization*) refers to the removal of all microorganisms *and* their spores (reproductive cells) and is practiced in the surgical suite. Health care practitioners must practice medical asepsis at all times.

Hand Hygiene

As early as 1843, Dr. Oliver Wendell Holmes advocated handwashing to prevent childbed fever. Holmes's ideas were greeted with disdain by many physicians of his time. Today, we know that *the most important precaution in the practice of aseptic technique is proper handwashing.* The radiographer's hands should be thoroughly washed with soap and warm running water for at least 15 seconds before and after each patient examination, or by using an alcohol sanitizer. If the faucet cannot be operated with the knee, it should be opened and closed using paper towels (to avoid contamination of or by the faucet). The radiographer's uniform should not touch the sink. The hands and forearms should always be kept lower than the elbows; care should be taken to wash all surfaces and between fingers. Hand lotions should be used to prevent hands from chapping; broken skin permits the entry of microorganisms. *Disinfectants, antiseptics, and germicides are substances used to kill pathogenic bacteria;* they are frequently used in handwashing substances. Alcohol-based hand sanitizers have been recommended as an alternative to handwashing with soap and water, except when there is visible soiling or after caring for a patient with *Clostridium difficile* infection.

Personal Care

Uniforms are recommended because clothing worn in patient areas should not be worn elsewhere. Because clothing becomes contaminated in the patient area, a clean uniform should be worn daily. Microorganisms can find safe harbor in jewelry, especially in rings with stones and other crevices; many facilities do not permit health care workers to wear artificial nails, for they can harbor fungi and microbes. The only jewelry a health care practitioner should wear is a wristwatch and simple wedding band. *Many microorganisms can remain infectious while awaiting transmission to another host.*

Sterile technique is employed during invasive procedures, such as biopsies, and for the administration of contrast media via the intravenous (IV) (e.g., urography) and *intrathecal* (e.g., myelography) routes. When radiography is required in the surgical suite, every precaution must be made to maintain the surgical asepsis required in surgical procedures. This requires proper dress, cleanliness of equipment, and restricted access to certain areas. One example of a restricted area is the "sterile corridor," the area between the draped patient and the instrument table. This area is occupied only by the surgeon and the instrument nurse.

CYCLE OF INFECTION

Pathogens

Pathogens are causative agents—microorganisms capable of producing disease. Pathogens termed *opportunistic* are usually harmless, but can become harmful if introduced into a part of the body where they do not normally reside, or when introduced into an immunocompromised host. *Bloodborne* pathogens reside in blood and can be transmitted to an individual exposed to that blood or body fluids of the exposed individual. Common bloodborne pathogens include hepatitis C virus, hepatitis B virus (HBV), and human immunodeficiency virus (HIV).

The control and prevention of infection must be a hospital-wide effort; each department is required to have its own infection-control protocol, designed according to the risks unique to the services provided.

Factors in Infection Transmission/ Cycle of Infection

1. An infectious organism/pathogen
2. A reservoir of infection and environment for pathogen to live and multiply
3. A portal of exit from the reservoir
4. A means of transmission
5. A susceptible host
6. A portal of entry into the susceptible new host

Because radiography often involves exposure to sickness and disease, the radiographer must be aware of, and conscientiously practice, infection control and effective preventive measures.

Reservoir of Infection

The reservoir (source) of infection is any environment where these pathogens can survive and reproduce, and ultimately pose a risk of transmission to a susceptible host. This environment must afford an appropriate temperature, moisture, and nutrients—all conditions found in the human body.

Examples of reservoirs of infection include a patient with active tuberculosis, a visitor with an upper respiratory infection, or a health care professional with conjunctivitis.

Some people, called "carriers," can be healthy yet harbor infectious microorganisms. Some people are unwitting carriers of *Staphylococcus aureus*; they experience no sore throat symptoms, yet a susceptible host (patient or coworker) could become infected with the organism. Probably the most famous example of an unwitting carrier was Mary Mallon ("Typhoid Mary"), a healthy Irish immigrant whose employment as a cook was traced back to 1900. It was found that typhoid outbreaks had followed Mallon's employment from job to job. From 1900 to 1907, Mallon worked at seven places of employment in which 22 people had became ill with typhoid fever shortly after Mallon came to work for them. Once traced, Mallon did not understand how a healthy person could possibly spread disease. But Mallon was tried in court, subsequently ran from health officials, was recaptured, and forced to live in relative seclusion on an island off New York. Mary Mallon was the first healthy carrier of typhoid fever in the United States. An example of today's healthy carriers includes asymptomatic carriers of HIV.

Although we might think of the human body as the typical reservoir for infection, any environment that can provide an appropriate temperature (warm), moisture (damp), and lack of cleanliness will provide welcome accommodations for pathogenic microorganisms. Animals, arthropods, plants, and soil are all potential reservoirs of infection.

Portal of Exit

A portal of exit from the reservoir can be any pathway by which pathogens are able to leave the reservoir. Examples of portals of exit include urine, feces, blood, respiratory droplets, and contaminated solutions.

Susceptible Host

The more susceptible hosts include the sick, infirm, immunocompromised, very young, poorly nourished, weak, or fatigued—all who have a diminished natural resistance to infection. *Health care–acquired infections (HAIs)*, formerly referred to as *nosocomial* infections, are infections acquired by *patients* (susceptible hosts) while they are in the hospital, unrelated to the condition for which the patients were hospitalized.

Hospital personnel can also be susceptible hosts. The most important precaution is proper hand hygiene. Hand lotions should also be used; broken skin permits the entry of microorganisms. Disinfectants, antiseptics, and germicides are substances used to kill pathogenic bacteria and are frequently used in hand hygiene substances. Alcohol-based hand sanitizers have been recommended as an alternative to handwashing with soap and water, and may be used as previously described. Uniforms worn in patient areas should not be worn elsewhere; a clean uniform should be worn daily, and minimal jewelry worn. *Microorganisms can remain infectious while awaiting transmission to another host.*

Portal of Entry

The pathway by which infectious organisms gain entry to the body is termed the *portal of entry*. Potential portals of entry include breaks in the skin, the gastrointestinal tract, mucous membranes of eyes, nose or mouth, the respiratory tract, and the urinary tract. Entry can be accomplished by ingestion, injection, inhalation, and across mucous membrane; the placenta serves as portal of entry between mother and fetus.

Modes of Transmission

Infectious microorganisms can be transmitted from patients to other patients or to health care workers, and from health care workers to patients. There are three main modes of transmission: *droplet*, *airborne*, and *contact*.

Pathogenic microorganisms expelled from the respiratory tract through the mouth or nose can be carried as evaporated *droplets* through the air or on *airborne* dust particles and settle on clothing, utensils, or food. Patients with respiratory tract infections/disease who are transported to the radiology department, therefore, should wear a mask to prevent such transmission during a cough or sneeze; it is not necessary for the health care worker to wear a mask (as long as the patient does).

Many microorganisms can remain infectious while awaiting transmission to another host. A contaminated inanimate object such as a food utensil, doorknob, or IV pole is referred to as a *fomite*—that is, transmission via *indirect contact*.

The Centers for Disease Control and Prevention (CDC) identifies *other sources of infection*. A *vector* is an insect or animal carrier of infectious organisms, such as a rabid animal, a mosquito that carries malaria, or a tick that carries Lyme disease. *Vehicle* transmission includes anything that transmits infectious microorganisms; examples of vehicles include contaminated blood, water, food, and drugs.

Direct contact involves touch. The courteous act of handshaking is a simple way of transmitting infection from one individual to another. Diseases transmitted by direct contact include skin infections such as boils, and sexually transmitted diseases such as syphilis and acquired immunodeficiency syndrome (AIDS).

Modes of Transmission

- Droplet
- Airborne
- Contact:
  - Direct
  - Indirect (e.g., fomite)

Other sources of infection:
- Vector
- Vehicle

Summary

- Most microorganisms do not produce infection or disease; many are harmless and many are beneficial.
- Pathogenic microorganisms can cause infection/disease; pathogenic microorganisms can be transmitted from one host to another.

- Antiseptics retard the growth of bacteria.
- Medical asepsis refers to the destruction of bacteria through the use of disinfectants/antiseptics.
- Surgical asepsis refers to the destruction of all microorganisms and their spores through sterilization.
- The practice of medical asepsis is required at all times, whereas surgical asepsis is required for invasive procedures.
- The single most important component of medical asepsis is proper and timely hand hygiene.
- A clean uniform must be worn daily; uniforms become contaminated and should not be worn elsewhere; pathogenic microorganisms thrive in jewelry crevices and chipped nail polish.
- The six factors in the cycle of infection are the infectious organism, the reservoir of infection, the portal of exit, the susceptible host, the means of transmission, and the portal of entry.
- Modes of transmission of infectious microorganisms are droplet, airborne, and contact (direct and indirect).
- Disinfectants (germicides) are used in handwashing liquids to kill microorganisms.

STANDARD PRECAUTIONS

Infection Control Basic Guidelines

The Centers for Disease Control and Prevention (CDC) and the Hospital Infection Control Practices Advisory Committee (HICPAC) have revised and simplified infection-control guidelines for hospitals and other health care facilities. The various types of isolation techniques, disease-specific precautions, and varied terminology have been reviewed, revised, and updated. All these considerations are now incorporated into *standard precautions* and *transmission-based precautions*.

Exposure to infectious microorganisms is a daily concern for health care professionals, especially with the rapid spread of *HIV*, *AIDS*, and *HBV* infections. HIV-infected individuals may be symptomless and go undiagnosed for 10 years or more, yet they are carriers of the infection and have the potential to spread the disease. *Epidemiologic* studies indicate that HIV infection can be transmitted only by intimate contact with blood or body fluids of an infected individual. This can occur through the sharing of contaminated needles, through sexual contact, from mother to baby at childbirth, and from transfusion of contaminated blood. HIV *cannot* be transmitted by inanimate objects such as water fountains, telephone surfaces, or toilet seats. *Hepatitis B* is another bloodborne infection; it affects the liver. It is thought that more than one million people in the United States have chronic hepatitis B and, as such, can transmit the disease to others.

Because no symptoms may be evident in patients infected with particular diseases, such as HIV, AIDS, and hepatitis B, all patients must be treated as potential sources of infection from blood and other body

Guidelines for Standard Precautions

The radiographer is now legally, as well as ethically, responsible for strict adherence to standard precaution principles identified in the following guidelines:

- Avoid cross-contamination of soiled (with bodily fluids) patient care linens/equipment.
- Clean reusable equipment properly before using on another patient; properly discard single-use items.
- Clean and disinfect environmental surfaces on a routine basis.
- Patients who can contaminate the environment should be placed in private rooms.
- Shielding for the face and eyes must be in place whenever the possibility of blood or body fluid splashes may occur near the face.
- Plastic aprons must be worn whenever the possibility of blood or body fluid splashes may occur on the clothing.
- Gloves must be worn whenever there is a possibility of touching blood or body fluids, and whenever there is a possibility of handling equipment or touching surfaces contaminated with blood or body fluids.
- Hands must be washed/sanitized before applying gloves and before patient contact.
- Gloves must be changed and the hands washed after every patient contact.
- Blood and body fluid spills should be carefully cleaned and disinfected using a solution of 1 part bleach to 10 parts water.
- Used needles must not be separated from the syringe or resheathed, and must be placed in designed puncture-proof containers.
- Prescribed procedures must be followed and sufficient care and attention given to risky tasks to avoid needle sticks and other skin penetrations from cutting instruments ("sharps").
- Emergency cardiopulmonary resuscitation (CPR) equipment must include resuscitation bags and mouthpieces.

fluids. The practices associated with this concept are called *standard precautions*. This rationale treats *all* body fluids and substances as infectious and serves to prevent the spread of microorganisms to other patients by the radiographer, as well as to protect the radiographer from contamination. Body fluids and substances that may be considered infectious include blood, breast milk, vaginal secretions, amniotic fluid, semen, peritoneal fluid, synovial fluid, cerebrospinal fluid, feces, urine, secretions from the nasal and oral cavities, and secretions from the lacrimal and sweat glands.

It is essential, then, that the radiographer makes the practice of blood and body fluid precautions *standard*; that is, they must be practiced on all patients without exception. This involves the use of barriers, such as gloves, to provide a separation between a patient's blood and body fluids and the radiographer or other health care worker. *Special precautions must also be taken with the disposal of biomedical waste*, such as laboratory and pathology waste, all sharp objects, and liquid waste from suction, bladder catheters, chest tubes, and IV tubes, as well as drainage containers.

Biomedical waste is generally packaged in easily identifiable impermeable bags and removed from the premises by an approved biomedical waste hauler.

Health Care–Acquired Infections

Health care–acquired infections (HAIs) are infections acquired by patients while they are in the hospital. These infections are unrelated to the condition for which the patients were hospitalized. The CDC estimates that from 5% to 15% of all hospital patients acquire some type of HAI. Hospital personnel can also become infected. It is somewhat surprising, yet understandable, that many infections can be acquired in the hospital; surprising because hospitals are places where people go to regain their health, yet understandable because individuals weakened by illness or disease are more susceptible to infection than are healthy individuals. Infections acquired in hospitals, especially by patients whose resistance to infection has been diminished by their illness, are termed *HAI*. The most common HAI is the *urinary tract infection*, often related to the use of urinary catheters, that can allow passage of pathogens into the patient's body. Other types of HAIs include sepsis, wound infection, and respiratory tract infection.

Health care practitioners must exercise strict infection-control precautions so that their *equipment* and/or technique will not be the source of HAI. *Contaminated* waste products, soiled linen, and improperly sterilized equipment are all means by which microorganisms can travel. Not every patient will come in contact with these items; however, the health care professional is in constant contact with patients and is therefore a constant threat to spread infection. Microorganisms are most commonly spread by way of the hands; spread of infection can be effectively reduced by proper disposal of contaminated objects and proper hand hygiene before and after each patient. *Disinfectants, antiseptics*, and *germicides* are used in many hand-hygiene liquids to kill microorganisms.

TABLE 3–1. Transmission-Based Precautions

Examples	Protection
Airborne	
TB	Patient: wears surgical string mask; private, negative-pressure room
Varicella	Radiographer: wears N95 particulate respirator mask if patient is not able to wear a mask, gloves; gown
Rubeola	for blatant contamination
Droplet	
Rubella	Patient: wears surgical string mask; private room
Mumps	Radiographer: gown and gloves as indicated; surgical string mask if patient is not able to wear a mask,
Influenza	except for H1N1 Influenza when an N95 particulate respirator mask would be worn.
Contact	
Mumps	Patient: private room; wears mask if required by your facility
Influenza	Radiographer: gloves and gown; mask for MRSA, if required by facility

*MRSA: methicillin-resistant *Staphylococcus aureus*.
†*C. difficile*: *Clostridium difficile*.

TRANSMISSION-BASED PRECAUTIONS

Adherence to standard blood and body fluids and substances precautions in the care of all patients will minimize the risk of transmission of HIV and other blood- and body substance–borne pathogens from the patient to the radiographer and from the radiographer to the patient. The use of standard precautions also minimizes the need for category-specific isolation. These have been replaced by *transmission-based precautions: airborne*, *droplet*, and *contact* (Table 3–1). Under these guidelines, some conditions/diseases can fall into more than one category.

Airborne

Medical asepsis and blood and body fluids precautions are used when performing radiographic examinations on *all* patients, but additional precautions may be required when a patient is suspected or known to have a *particular communicable disease*. For example, *airborne precaution* is employed with patients suspected or known to be infected with the *tubercle bacillus (TB), chickenpox (varicella),* and *measles (rubeola)*. Airborne precaution requires the patient to wear a surgical string mask to avoid the spread of acid-fast bacilli (in bronchial secretions) or other pathogens during coughing, particularly if the patient must be transported. The health care staff must wear personal N95 respirators whenever they enter an airborne isolation room. This special mask requires periodic fit testing. The radiographer should wear gloves, but a gown is required only if flagrant contamination is likely. Patients infected with *airborne diseases* require a *private, specially ventilated (negative-pressure) room* (Table 3–1).

Droplet

A private room is indicated for all patients on *droplet precaution*; that is, diseases transmitted via large droplets expelled from the patient while speaking, sneezing, or coughing. The pathogenic droplets can infect

Airborne Precautions

They are used to prevent airborne disease transmission in the health care setting.

- Patients are isolated in private rooms with special air handling and ventilation systems (negative pressure rooms). If a private room is not available, patients are cohorted.

- Health care personnel must wear personal N95 respirators whenever they enter an airborne isolation room.

- Patient transport must be limited as much as possible; when patient transport is essential, the patient must wear a surgical string mask.

- Health care personnel must wear a surgical string mask when working within 3–6 feet of a patient on droplet precautions.

others when they come in contact with mouth or nasal mucosa or conjunctiva. *Rubella* ("German measles"), *mumps*, and *influenza* are among the diseases spread by droplet contact; *a private room is required* for the patient, and health care practitioners must wear a regular (string) *mask* to enter a droplet-precautions isolation room, except for H1N1 Influenza which requires an N95 particulate respirator mask be worn by the health care worker.

Contact

Any disease spread by direct or close (indirect) contact, such as *MRSA* (methicillin-resistant *Staphylococcus aureus*), *Clostridium difficile (C. difficile)*, and *some wounds*, requires *contact precautions. Contact-precaution* procedures require a *private patient room,* and the use of *gloves and gown* for anyone coming in direct contact with the infected individual or the infected person's environment. Some facilities require health care workers to wear a mask when caring for a patient with MRSA.

Patients in *contact isolation* occasionally have to be transported to the radiology department for examination. When this is the case, the department should be notified first in order to prepare properly. The patient should wash his or her hands first if possible. The wheelchair or stretcher should first be covered with a clean sheet, followed by a second sheet or thin blanket. After transferring the patient to the wheelchair or stretcher, the inner sheet is wrapped around the patient, and the outer sheet over it (thus, the inner sheet is the contaminated one). The radiographic room should be available and ready for the patient to be taken in directly. The x-ray table should be covered with a clean sheet before the patient is transferred to it. One radiographer (wearing gloves) must be responsible for patient positioning and the other for equipment controls and operation (to avoid contamination of equipment and possible transmission of disease to others via indirect contact or fomites).

After the examination is completed, the patient is transferred to the wheelchair or stretcher and wrapped in the same way. Any contaminated *linens* should be placed in a plastic bag and contaminated disposables such as tissues are placed in a separate bag; both are disposed of in a linen hamper.

The radiographic table and other equipment should be cleaned with a disinfectant and hands should be washed carefully when the task is completed.

Mobile radiography performed on patients on *contact isolation* generally requires special precautions and the teamwork of *two* radiographers. The first (or "dirty") radiographer dons gown, gloves (gloves must cover gown cuffs), and mask, usually available just outside the patient's room. The necessary cassette(s) must be placed in a plastic bag or pillowcase to protect them from contamination. This radiographer must remember to bring an extra pair of gloves into the patient room. The mobile x-ray unit is brought into the room, and all possible adjustments must be made before the radiographer touches anything else.

The equipment and cassette are positioned, and the patient is adjusted properly. *At this point, the mobile x-ray unit must not be touched*

Contact Precautions

They are used to prevent contact transmission of disease in the health care setting.

- Patients are isolated in private rooms or cohorted.
- Health care personnel must use gloves and gowns as indicated to prevent unprotected exposure.
- Hands must be disinfected before and after gloving.
- Patient transport should be limited as much as possible; when necessary, special precautions are taken.
- All x-ray imaging requires special precautions and two-radiographer teamwork.
- Equipment should be dedicated to a single patient or cohort, or equipment must be cleaned and disinfected between patients.

until the radiographer disposes of the gloves he or she has on and replaces them with the clean extra pair.

The exposure is then made; the covered cassette is removed from behind/under the patient and brought to the door. The "dirty" radiographer slides the pillowcase or plastic cover away from the cassette and the second member of the team (the "clean" radiographer) grasps the uncovered cassette. Just inside the patient room door, the contaminated gloves should be removed properly and the hands washed/sanitized thoroughly. The mask and gown ties are then untied with clean hands; the gown is removed by placing a clean hand under the cuff and pulling the arm down from underneath. The other sleeve is also removed *by touching only the inside of the gown*. The gown is slipped off and folded forward with the contaminated surfaces touching.

The discarded garments must be placed in the container provided. The radiographer should then carefully rewash his or her hands, dry them with paper towels, and take care not to touch the faucets. After leaving the room, *the mobile unit must be thoroughly cleaned* with a disinfectant and the hands carefully washed once again.

It should be noted that these patients may feel ostracized and relegated to a kind of solitary confinement. The radiographer must remember that these patients have the same needs as other patients (indeed, perhaps greater needs) and be certain to treat them with dignity and care.

Patients Whose Immune Systems Are Compromised

The purpose of that which is still often referred to as *protective, or reverse, isolation* is to keep the susceptible patient/patient whose immune system is compromised from becoming infected. Patients suffering from burns, who have lost their means of protection, their skin, have increased susceptibility to bacterial invasion. Patients whose immune systems are compromised (e.g., transplant recipients, leukemia) are unable to combat infection and are more susceptible to infection. These patients are treated with strict isolation technique, taking care to protect the *patient* from contamination.

The teamwork of two radiographers is also required for care of the patient with compromised immune system, although the purpose and procedure is largely opposite that of the other isolation categories. Preparation for cleanliness and hygiene start *before* entering the patient room. The "clean" radiographer touches only the patient and that which comes in contact with the patient.

Contaminated Material Disposal

Special precautions must be taken with the disposal of biomedical waste, such as laboratory and pathology waste, all sharp objects, and liquid waste from suction, bladder catheters, chest tubes, and IV tubes, as well as drainage containers.

Biomedical waste is generally packaged in easily identifiable impermeable bags and removed from the premises by an approved biomedical waste hauler.

Summary

- Because no symptoms may be evident in patients afflicted with certain diseases such as HIV, AIDS, and hepatitis B, all patients must be treated as potential sources of infection from blood and other body fluids; this is the standard precautions concept.
- The practice of standard precautions helps prevent transmission of infection to the health care professional and to other patients.
- Infections acquired in hospitals are called health care–acquired infections (HAIs); the most common HAI is urinary tract infection.
- The health care professional is legally and ethically responsible for adhering to standard precautions principles; they must be practiced on all patients at all times without exception.
- Biomedical waste (body substances and their containers) must be disposed of in carefully controlled circumstances.
- Transmission-based precautions include airborne, droplet, and contact.
- Airborne precaution requires that the patient wear a surgical string mask and be admitted to a private, specially ventilated, negative-pressure room.
- Droplet precaution and a private room are required for measles, mumps, and influenza; the radiographer requires a mask (if the patient is not wearing one) and may also need to wear gown and gloves. An N95 particulate respirator mask is required for contact with a patient who has H1N1 Influenza.
- Contact precaution (*C. difficile*, MRSA, some wounds) requires that the radiographer use mask, gown, and gloves when in direct contact with the patient.
- Radiography of a patient with contact precaution requires the teamwork of two radiographers.
- Protective, or reverse, isolation is used to keep the susceptible patient from being infected.

COMPREHENSION CHECK

Congratulations! You have completed your review of this chapter. If you are able to answer the following group of comprehensive questions, you can feel confident that you have mastered this section. You are then ready to go on to "Registry-type" questions that follow. **For greatest success, do not go to these multiple-choice questions without first completing the short-answer questions below.**

1. List three disinfectant agents (p. 35).

2. Describe the correct method of handwashing, including *when* hands should be washed, opening/closing faucets, position of hands and forearms (p. 35, 36).

3. Define *pathogen*; describe its types (p. 36).

4. Describe the importance of the radiographer's personal care, related to disease control (p. 36).

5. Identify and differentiate between the three basic means of transmitting infectious microorganisms (p. 38).

6. List three means of indirect transmission of pathogenic microorganisms (p. 38).

7. Identify the most common type of hospital-acquired infection (p. 40).

8. List five possible sources of HAI infection in the radiology department (p. 40).

9. Describe the type of protection required for patients with respiratory infections (p. 38).

10. Identify the means by which microorganisms are spread (p. 38).

11. What substances are added to handwashing liquids to kill microorganisms (p. 36)?

12. Discuss the rationale of body fluid and substance (standard) precautions (p. 39, 40).

13. Discuss each of the following with respect to standard precautions (p. 39, 40):
    A. When a face shield should be used
    B. When a plastic apron should be used
    C. When hands should be washed
    D. When gloves should be used
    E. How body fluid and substance spills should be cleaned
    F. Care of used needles
    G. Special devices available for CPR
    H. On whom standard precautions should be practiced

14. Differentiate between medical and surgical asepsis (p. 35).

15. Identify and explain the most important practice in good aseptic technique (p. 36).

16. Discuss the function of uniforms worn by health care practitioners; the hazards of jewelry and nail polish (p. 36).

17. List the three types of transmission-based precautions (p. 41).

18. Explain the precautionary measures taken in airborne precaution regarding apparel (and for whom) and patient room (p. 41).

19. List three communicable diseases spread by droplet contact that require droplet precaution (p. 41, 42).

20. Describe the method of performing mobile chest radiography on patients with contact precaution, to include (p. 42, 43):
    A. Number of persons needed
    B. Radiographer's apparel
    C. How to protect cassettes from contamination
    D. Why an extra pair of gloves is needed in the patient room
    E. Role played by the second individual
    F. How protective clothing should be removed
    G. Care of x-ray machine at completion of examination

21. Describe the proper method of transporting a contact precaution patient to the radiology department (p. 42).

22. Describe the purpose of reverse isolation (p. 43).

23. Discuss any special needs the isolation patient may have (p. 43).

CHAPTER REVIEW QUESTIONS

1. Pathogens are:
   1. Always harmful
   2. Sometimes harmful
   3. Capable of producing disease
   (A) 1 only
   (B) 2 only
   (C) 1 and 3 only
   (D) 2 and 3 only

2. Diseases that can be transmitted by direct contact include:
   1. Skin infections
   2. Syphilis
   3. Malaria
   (A) 1 only
   (B) 1 and 2 only
   (C) 2 and 3 only
   (D) 1, 2, and 3

3. In which of the following conditions is protective or reverse isolation indicated?
   1. Transplant recipient
   2. Burns
   3. Leukemia
   (A) 1 only
   (B) 1 and 2 only
   (C) 2 and 3 only
   (D) 1, 2, and 3

4. Which of the following is/are means of transmission of microorganisms?
   1. Vector
   2. Fomite
   3. Airborne
   (A) 1 only
   (B) 1 and 2 only
   (C) 3 only
   (D) 1, 2, and 3

5. What is the single most effective means of controlling the spread of infectious microorganisms?
   (A) Wearing gloves
   (B) Wearing masks
   (C) Handwashing
   (D) Sterilization

6. What is the name of the practice that serves to retard the growth of pathogenic bacteria?
   (A) Antisepsis
   (B) Bacteriogenesis
   (C) Sterilization
   (D) Disinfection

7. Which of the following diseases require(s) airborne precaution?
   1. TB
   2. Varicella
   3. Rubella
   (A) 1 only
   (B) 1 and 2 only
   (C) 3 only
   (D) 1, 2, and 3

8. The radiographer must perform the following procedure(s) prior to entering an isolation room with a mobile x-ray unit:
   1. Wear gown and mask
   2. Wear gown, mask, and gloves
   3. Clean the mobile x-ray unit
   (A) 1 only
   (B) 2 only
   (C) 1 and 3 only
   (D) 2 and 3 only

9. Lyme disease is a condition caused by bacteria carried by deer ticks. The tick bite may cause fever, fatigue, and other associated symptoms. This is an example of transmission of an infection by:

(A) Droplet contact

(B) The airborne route

(C) A vector

(D) A vehicle

10. Which of the following can be transmitted via infected blood?

1. TB

2. AIDS

3. HBV

(A) 1 only

(B) 1 and 2 only

(C) 2 and 3 only

(D) 1, 2, and 3

Answers and Explanations

1. (D) *Pathogens* are causative agents—microorganisms capable of producing disease. Pathogens termed *opportunistic* are usually harmless, but can become harmful if introduced into a part of the body where they do not normally reside, or when introduced into an immunocompromised host. *Bloodborne* pathogens reside in blood and can be transmitted to an individual exposed to that blood or body fluids of the exposed individual. Common bloodborne pathogens include hepatitis C virus, hepatitis B virus (HBV), and human immunodeficiency virus (HIV). Because radiography often involves exposure to sickness and disease, the radiographer must be aware of, and conscientiously practice, infection control and effective preventive measures.

2. (B) Infectious microorganisms can be transmitted from one patient to other patients or to health care workers, and from health care workers to patients. They are transmitted by means of either direct or indirect contact. *Direct contact* involves touch. Diseases transmitted by direct contact include skin infections such as boils and sexually transmitted diseases such as syphilis.

Indirect contact involves transmission of microorganisms via airborne contamination, fomites, and vectors. Pathogenic microorganisms expelled from the respiratory tract through the mouth or nose can be carried as evaporated droplets through the air or on dust and settle on clothing, utensils, or food. Patients with respiratory tract infections and disease transported to the radiology department, therefore, should wear a mask to prevent such transmission during a cough or sneeze; it is not necessary for the health care professional or transporter to wear a mask (as long as the patient does). Many such microorganisms can remain infectious while awaiting transmission to another host. A contaminated inanimate object such as a food utensil, doorknob, or intravenous (IV) pole is referred to as a fomite. A vector is an insect or animal carrier of infectious organisms, such as a rabid animal (e.g., rabies; although the rabid animal is the vector, rabies is contracted by contact), a mosquito that carries malaria, or a tick that carries Lyme disease.

3. (D) *Protective, or reverse, isolation is used to keep the susceptible patient from becoming infected.* Burn patients who have lost their means of protection (their skin) have increased susceptibility to bacterial invasion.

Patients whose immune systems are compromised (e.g., transplant recipients, leukemia) are unable to combat infection and are more susceptible to infection. These patients are treated with strict isolation technique, taking care to protect the *patient* from contamination.

4. (D) Microorganisms can be transmitted via *droplet, airborne,* and *contact (direct or indirect)*. Other sources of transmission are *vehicle* and *vector*. Pathogenic microorganisms expelled from the respiratory tract through the mouth or nose can be carried as evaporated droplets through the air or on dust and settle on clothing, utensils, or food. A contaminated inanimate object such as a pillowcase, x-ray table, or IV pole is referred to as a *fomite*. A *vector* is an insect or animal carrier of infectious organisms, such as a rabid animal (rabies), a mosquito that carries malaria, or a tick that carries Lyme disease.

5. (C) Health care practitioners must exercise strict infection-control precautions so that they or their equipment will not be the source of health care–acquired infections (HAIs). Contaminated waste products, soiled linen, and improperly sterilized equipment are all means by which microorganisms can travel. Not every patient will come in contact with these items; however, the health care professional is in constant contact with patients and is therefore a constant threat to spread infection. *Microorganisms are most commonly spread by way of the hands; therefore, handwashing before and after each patient is the most effective means of controlling the spread of microorganisms.* Disinfectants, antiseptics, and germicides are used in many handwashing liquids to kill microorganisms.

6. (A) *Antisepsis* retards the growth of pathogenic bacteria. Alcohol is an example of an antiseptic. *Medical asepsis* refers to the destruction of pathogenic microorganisms through the process of *disinfection*. Examples of disinfectants are hydrogen peroxide, chlorine, and boric acid. *Surgical asepsis (sterilization)* refers to the removal of all microorganisms and their spores (reproductive cells) and is practiced in the surgical suite. *Bacteriogenesis* refers to the formation of bacteria.

7. (B) *Airborne precaution* is employed with patients suspected or known to be infected with the tubercle bacillus (TB), chickenpox (varicella), and measles (rubeola). Airborne precaution requires the patient to wear a surgical string mask to avoid the spread of acid-fast bacilli (in bronchial secretions) and other pathogens during coughing. If the patient is unable or unwilling to wear a mask, the radiographer must wear one. An N95 particulate respirator is the mask required for health care workers. The radiographer should wear gloves, but a gown is required only if flagrant contamination is likely. Patients with airborne precautions require a private, specially ventilated (negative-pressure) room (Table 3–1).

A private room is indicated for all patients on *droplet precaution*, that is, diseases transmitted via large droplets expelled from the patient while speaking, sneezing, or coughing. The pathogenic droplets can infect others when they come in contact with mouth or nasal mucosa or conjunctiva. Rubella ("German measles"), mumps, and influenza are among the diseases spread by *droplet* contact; a private room is required for the patient, and health care practitioners must wear a mask. An N95 particulate respirator mask is required for contact with a patient who has H1N1 Influenza.

8. (B) When performing bedside radiography in an isolation room, the radiographer should wear a gown, gloves, and sometimes a mask. The cassettes are prepared for the examination by placing a pillowcase over them to protect them from contamination. Whenever possible, one person should manipulate the mobile unit and remain "clean," while the other handles the patient. The mobile unit should be cleaned with a disinfectant before *exiting* the patient's room.

9. (C) Lyme disease is a condition that results from transmission of an infection by a vector ("deer" tick). *Vectors* are insects and animals carrying disease. *Droplet contact* involves contact with secretions (from the nose, mouth) that travel via a sneeze or cough. *Airborne* route involves evaporated droplets in the air that transfer disease.

10. (C) Epidemiologic studies indicate that HIV and AIDS (acquired immunodeficiency syndrome) can be transmitted only by intimate contact with blood or body fluids of an infected individual. This can occur through the sharing of contaminated needles, through sexual contact, from mother to baby at childbirth, and from transfusion of contaminated blood. HIV and AIDS cannot be transmitted by inanimate objects. HBV is another bloodborne infection and affects the liver. It is thought that more than one million people in the United States have chronic hepatitis B and, as such, can transmit the disease to others. Acid-fast bacillus isolation is employed with patients suspected or known to be infected with the TB. Acid-fast bacillus isolation requires that the patient wear a mask to avoid the spread of acid-fast bacilli (in bronchial secretions) during *coughing*.

Patient Monitoring, Medical Emergencies, and Contrast Media | 4

ROUTINE MONITORING

The radiographer *assesses* a patient's condition before bringing the patient to the radiographic department and must continue to be alert to patient condition, and any possible change in condition, as the examination proceeds. *Assessment* begins with a review of the patient's chart; useful information includes the admitting diagnosis, nurses' notes, the patient's degree of ambulation, preparation for the radiologic procedure and its effectiveness, results of laboratory tests, any requirements for collecting the patient's urine, etc.

The radiographer obtains a brief pertinent *clinical history*, and assesses the patient's condition by *observing* and *listening*. To provide safe and effectual care, the radiographer will *assess* the severity of a traumatic injury, degree of motor control, and any need for support equipment or radiographic accessories. Is the patient able to move? Can the patient be imaged more effectively and/or less painfully on the stretcher or in the wheelchair? Can the use of sponges, sandbags, or other x-ray accessories result in a more comfortable, safe, and diagnostic examination?

Vital Signs

The radiographer can be required to assist in an emergency situation by obtaining patient's vital signs. Although not a routine function of radiographers, they should be proficient and confident if and when the need arises. Regular review and practice is essential.

Obtaining vital signs involves the measurement of body temperature, pulse rate, respiratory rate, and arterial blood pressure.

Routine monitoring of patient's condition, physical signs, and *vital signs* are discussed in Chapter 2. Routine and continuous monitoring of patient's condition is essential, so that any change in condition can be addressed *before* it becomes a medical emergency.

In review, obtaining *vital signs* involves the measurement of *body temperature, pulse rate, respiratory rate*, and *arterial blood pressure*. Elevated body temperature, or *fever*, often signifies infection. Symptoms include

---

Vital Signs

- Temperature
- Pulse
- Respiration
- Blood pressure

Normal Body Temperatures

Adult
Oral	98.6°F
Rectal	99.1°F–99.6°F
Axillary	97.6°F–98.1°F
Infant to age 4 y	97.9°F–100.4°F
Child aged 5–13 y	97.8°F–98.6°F

---

malaise; increased pulse and respiratory rates; flushed, hot, and dry skin; and occasional chills.

Normal body temperature varies from person to person depending on several factors, including age. Normal adult body temperature taken orally is 98.6°F (37°C). *Rectal* temperature is generally 0.5° to 1.0° *higher*, whereas *axillary* temperature is usually 0.5° to 1.0° *lower*. Slight variation of 0.5° to 1.0° is generally considered within normal limits. Body temperature is usually lowest in the early morning and highest at night. Infants and children have a wider range of body temperature than adults; the elderly have lower body temperatures than others.

Superficial arteries are best suited for determination of *pulse rate*. The five most easily palpated pulse points are the radial, carotid, temporal, femoral, and popliteal pulse. The radial pulse is the most frequently used. The apical pulse, at the apex of the heart, can be evaluated with the use of a stethoscope.

Respirations should be counted after counting the pulse rate while still holding the patient's wrist. *The normal respiratory rate is 12–18 breaths/min.* The respiratory rate of young children is higher, up to 30 breaths/min. Although the radiographer is counting respirations, he or she should be assessing the respiratory pattern (even, uneven) and depth (normal, shallow, deep) as well.

Blood pressure within vessels is greatest during ventricular *systole* (contraction) and lowest during *diastole* (relaxation). Blood pressure is recorded with the systolic pressure on top and the diastolic pressure on the bottom, as in 100/70 (read, "one hundred over seventy"). Normal adult systolic pressure ranges between 100 and 140 mm Hg; the normal diastolic range is between 60 and 90 mm Hg. Blood pressure consistently above 140/90 is considered *hypertension.*

Physical Signs/Symptoms

The radiographer should always be alert of a patient's appearance and condition, and any sudden *changes* in them, such as changes in the color, temperature, and moistness of the patient's skin. Paleness can indicate weakness; the *diaphoretic* patient has pale, cool skin; *fever* is frequently accompanied by hot, dry skin; "sweaty" palms might indicate *anxiety*, a patient who is *cyanotic* (bluish lips, mucous membranes, nail beds) needs oxygen and requires immediate attention. Chronic obstructive pulmonary disease (COPD) patients receive low flow rates of oxygen; acute exacerbations are managed with inhaled bronchodilators.

Respiration delivers oxygen to all body cells and rids the body of carbon dioxide. The radiographer should recognize abnormalities or altered respirations of the patient. The term describing difficult breathing is *dyspnea*. More specific terms used to describe abnormal respirations include *uneven, spasmodic, strident* (shrill, grating sound), *stertorous* (labored, e.g., snoring), *tachypnea* (abnormally rapid breathing), *orthopnea* (difficulty breathing while recumbent), and *oligopnea* (abnormally shallow, slow).

Chronic respiratory conditions such as *emphysema* should be noted by the radiographer during patients' assessment. Some patients' conditions require the upper body to be elevated for easier breathing; the term *orthopnea* describes difficulty breathing while recumbent. Any change in breathing should alert the radiographer of possible onset of respiratory distress.

The *pulse* is felt as a result of regular expansion and contraction of an artery as waves of blood travel through arteries; the pulse felt over arteries is in time with the heart beat as the left ventricle contracts. The average normal adult pulse rate is between 60 and 100 BPM. The term *tachycardia* describes an abnormally fast pulse rate; it can be temporary as a result of exertion or excitement or can be caused by heart disease. Resting pulse is faster in febrile, anemic, or hypovolemic patients, as well as patients who experience shock. An abnormally slow pulse rate is termed *bradycardia* and can result in inadequate circulation of blood to the brain, coronary arteries, and other essential organs.

Pulse *rate* depends on the person's age, sex, body exertion and position, and general state of health. Children and the elderly have higher pulse rates. The pulse rate increases in the standing position and after exertion. The pulse rate also increases with certain conditions, such as fever, organic heart disease, *shock*, and alcohol and drug use. Pulse rates vary between men and women and among adults, children, and infants; athletes often have lower pulse rates.

Blood pressure varies with age, sex, fatigue, mental or physical stress, disease, and trauma. Blood pressure is greatest during ventricular *systole* (contraction) and lowest during diastole (relaxation). Blood pressure measurements are recorded with the systolic pressure on top and the diastolic pressure on the bottom, as in 100/80 (read "one hundred over eighty"). Normal *adult* systolic pressure ranges between 100 and 140 mm Hg; the normal diastolic range is between 60 and 90 mm Hg.

Prehypertension is present when systolic measurements are between 120 and 140 mm Hg and/or between 80 and 90 mm Hg diastolic pressure. Blood pressure consistently more than 140/90 is considered hypertension. Left undiagnosed and untreated, hypertension can lead to renal, cardiac, or brain damage. *Hypotension* is characterized by a systolic pressure of less than 90 mm Hg. Hypotension can be seen in individuals with decreased blood volume as a result of hemorrhage, infection, fever, and anemia. *Orthostatic* hypotension occurs in some individuals when they rise quickly from a recumbent position.

Documentation

The *chart* of a hospitalized patient is a collection of information, records, and laboratory and imaging reports. Information includes the patient's condition, progress, medications, treatments, etc.

Documentation required of the radiographer should be entered directly on the patient's examination *requisition*, or in the radiology computer system *notes*. Notes are made regarding pertinent patient history, patient's illness, or injury.

Any incident, accident, or unusual occurrence that causes injury or potential injury/harm to the patient (or visitor, or staff) must be reported to a radiology supervisor. Once the individual has been appropriately cared for, an "incident report" must be completed. This is very important for the hospital's risk management department—for liability considerations and for possible procedural alterations to prevent future similar incidents.

Blood Pressure is Affected by

- Cardiac output
- Blood volume
- Vascular resistance

Blood Pressure

- Measured using sphygmomanometer and stethoscope
- Cuff inflation sufficient to collapse the brachial a.
- First sound heard is systolic pressure

Common Pulse Points

Artery	Location
Radial	Wrist; at base of thumb
Carotid	Neck; just lateral to midline
Temporal	In front of upper ear
Femoral	Inguinal region; groin
Popliteal	Posterior knee

Normal Pulse Rates (BPM)

Men	68–75
Women	72–80
Children	70–100
Infants	100–160

Note should always be made regarding any unusual, though very minor, occurrence that might not require an incident report. A supervisor should always be consulted to make that decision.

PATIENT SUPPORT EQUIPMENT

Oxygen

One of human being's most basic physiologic needs is an adequate supply of oxygen. Diminished oxygen supply (*hypoxia*) can result from an airway obstructed by *aspirated* material, laryngeal edema as a result of *anaphylaxis*, or a pathologic process such as *emphysema*. The radiographer must be knowledgeable enough to recognize symptoms and respond appropriately. The proper response to respiratory distress might be to perform the *Heimlich maneuver*, to summon the code team, or to check the flow of oxygen already in place.

Oxygen is taken into the body and supplied to the blood to be delivered to all body tissues. Any tissue(s) lacking in, or devoid of, an adequate blood supply can suffer permanent damage or can die. Oxygen may be required in cases of severe anemia, pneumonia, pulmonary edema, and shock.

Symptoms of inadequate oxygen supply include *dyspnea, cyanosis, diaphoresis*, and distention of the veins of the neck. A patient who experiences any of these symptoms will be very anxious and must not be left unattended. The radiographer must *call* for help, assist the patient to a sitting or semi-*Fowler position* (the recumbent position makes breathing more difficult), and have oxygen and emergency drugs available.

In areas that patients will occupy for extended periods (e.g., patient department, operating room, emergency department, and radiology department), oxygen is available through wall outlets at a pressure of 60–80 psi (pounds per square inch) equipped with an easily adjustable flowmeter to regulate the administration of oxygen. It is important to administer *humidified* oxygen to avoid drying and irritation of the respiratory mucosa. In other areas, oxygen will be available in tanks having one valve to regulate its flow and another to indicate the amount of oxygen remaining in the tank.

There are various devices available to deliver oxygen to patients. Their use is determined by the amount of oxygen required by the patient. They are frequently classified as *low* or *high flow*.

The *nasal cannula* is the most frequently used device and is used to supplement the oxygen in room air; its short prongs extend approximately 1 cm into the nares. The nasal cannula is a low-flow small percentage oxygen device. It is convenient and fairly comfortable for the patient, although it can be somewhat easily moved out of position, during sleep, for example.

There are various types of oxygen *masks* available for delivery of oxygen. The *simple face mask* (low flow) is best suited for short-term oxygen therapy. With extended use, the plastic becomes warm and sticky. Communication is difficult, the mask is easily displaced, and it must be removed at mealtime. The *partial rebreathing mask* (low flow) and *nonrebreathing mask* (low flow) deliver more precise concentrations of oxygen to the patient.

Mechanical ventilators (high flow) are most frequently encountered in a hospital critical care unit. Patients on ventilators have an artificial airway in place, while the ventilator controls the respiratory rate and volume.

Although oxygen is not a flammable substance, it does support combustion, so care must be taken to avoid spark or flame where oxygen is in use.

Suction

The use of a *suction* device is occasionally required to maintain a patient's airway by *aspirating* secretions, blood, or other fluids when the patient is unconscious or otherwise unable to do so. Suction is available from a wall outlet, similar to oxygen, or as a mobile apparatus. It is unlikely that the radiographer would be required to suction a patient, but he or she might be needed to assist with the procedure. Suction tubing must have a disposable catheter attached to its end for collection of airway secretions. The radiographer should be familiar with the location of suction equipment and replacement of disposable catheters.

Intravenous Equipment and Venipuncture

Intravenous fluids and/or medication are administered to meet specific patient needs. Medications administered intravenously result in rapid patient response; medications are often delivered in this fashion in emergency and critical situations. Patients who are dehydrated and require fluid and electrolyte replacement will have these (normal saline or D5W) administered intravenously. *Intravenous* (IV) *equipment* includes needles, syringes, fluids such as normal saline or D5W (a solution of 5% dextrose in water), IV catheters, heparin locks, IV poles, and infusion sets.

The diameter of a needle is identified as its *gauge*. As the gauge increases, the *bore* becomes smaller. Hence, a 23-gauge needle has a smaller diameter bore than an 18-gauge needle. Hypodermic needles are generally used for phlebotomy, whereas butterflies and IV catheters are used more frequently for injections such as contrast media. If an *infusion* injection is required, an IV catheter is generally preferred. The *hub* of the hypodermic needle is attached to a syringe, whereas the hub of the butterfly tubing or IV catheter may be attached to a syringe or an IV bottle or bag via an IV infusion set.

Medication or contrast material is often mixed with normal saline or D5W. Some IV medications are given at intervals through an established heparin lock. A *heparin lock* consists of a venous catheter established for a certain length of time to make a vein available for medications that have to be administered at frequent intervals. This helps prevent the formation of scarred, sclerotic veins as a result of frequent injections at the same site. When repeated administrations of medication are needed, an *IV catheter* is often used. This is a two-part device consisting of a solid (without a bore) needle and a flexible plastic catheter. After the needle is introduced into the vein, the catheter is advanced over the needle, secured with tape, and the needle removed.

The IV bottle or bag should be hung 18–24 inches *above the level of the vein.* If placed lower than the vein, the solution will stop flowing and blood will return into the tubing. If hung too high, the solution can run too fast. Occasionally, the position of the needle or catheter in the vein

> ## Needles
>
> - **Gauge:** identifies diameter of needle bore/lumen
> - **Larger gauge:** smaller bore diameter
> - **Smaller gauge:** larger bore diameter
> - **Hub:** part of needle attached to syringe or IV tube

will affect the flow rate. If the bevel is adjacent to the vessel wall, flow may decrease or stop altogether. Often, just changing the position of the patient's arm will remedy the situation.

The term *extravasation* refers to medication or contrast medium that has leaked from a vein rupture or has been inadvertently introduced into tissue outside the vein. The term *infiltration* refers to the diffusion of the injected material further into adjacent tissues. The needle should be removed, pressure applied to prevent formation of a *hematoma*, and *a cold pack* applied to relieve pain and limit further infiltration of area tissue.

The *antecubital* vein is the most commonly used *venipuncture* site for contrast medium administration. It is not used for infusions that take longer than 1 hour because of its location at the bend of the elbow. The *basilic* vein, located on the dorsal surface of the hand, is used when the antecubital vein is inaccessible. The *cephalic* vein may also be used. A *warm compress* can be applied to the area of intended injection to *increase area blood circulation* and improve access to the intended vein. The needle is inserted into the vein at a 15-degree angle; blood will flow back into the tubing when the needle is correctly positioned. Strict aseptic technique must be used for all IV injections.

There are battery-powered peripheral "vein-finder" devices available commercially, They use high-intensity LED lights to transilluminate the patient's subcutaneous tissue; in so doing, the device highlights the veins via their absorption (rather than reflection) of the light. These devices can be particularly useful for locating hard-to-find veins, obese adults, infants, and small children.

Tubes

Following thoracotomy or other thoracic surgery, a *chest tube* may be put in place for the purpose of treating pneumothorax or hemothorax (removing air and/or fluid from the pleural space). The *chest drainage system* usually has three compartments: one is the suction control chamber, another is the collection chamber, and the third is the water seal chamber, which prevents atmospheric air from entering the chest cavity. The drainage system must always be kept below the level of the patient's chest.

Radiographers might encounter chest drainage systems when performing mobile radiographic examinations on postsurgical patients. The radiographer must be careful not to disturb chest tubes during patient or equipment manipulation, and to immediately report any sudden change in the patient's condition and/or patient's complaint of chest pain or discomfort.

Gastrointestinal (GI) tubes can be *nasogastric* (NG), *nasointestinal* (NI), or nasoenteric (NE). NG tubes, such as the Dobbhoff tube, are used as feeding tubes for patients whose condition prevents normal swallowing. NI/NE *tubes* can be used following digestive tract surgery to remove gastric fluids and/or air (decompression; e.g., Levin and Salem-Sump tubes). NG and NI/NE tubes may be single or double *lumen* and can sometimes be temporarily disconnected for radiographic examinations. The *single*-lumen NG or NI/NE tube can be clamped, but the *double*-lumen tube must *never* be clamped. If clamped, the walls of the double-lumen tube could adhere permanently. Instead, the tip of a syringe is inserted into the lumen and the syringe and tube then pinned (open side up) to the

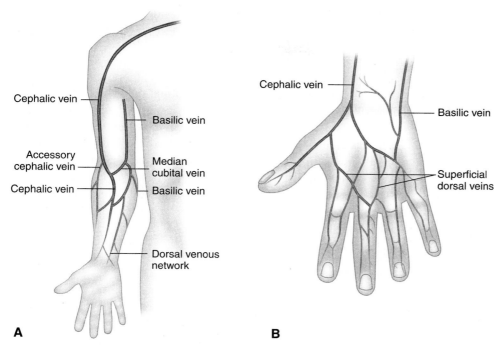

Figure 4–1. Veins commonly used for venipuncture. **(A)** anterior aspect right forearm **(B)** dorsal aspect left hand.

patient's gown. Care must be taken not to disturb the placement of the GI tube. Examples of single-lumen NE tubes are the Cantor and Harris tubes; the Miller–Abbott tube is a double-lumen NE tube.

There are a number of specialized tubes/catheters used to provide regular or *continual access* to the circulatory system long-term care requirements such as dialysis, blood transfusion, drug therapy such as chemotherapy, and parenteral nutrition. They can also be used for laboratory blood draws and for monitoring central venous pressure (CVP). These are referred to as *central venous catheters* (CVC or *central lines*). Examples of these central lines include the Port-A-Cath, the Hickman, the Raaf, and the PICC. For x-ray verification of position placement, they usually have a radiopaque distal tip. The distal tip should be located in the superior or inferior vena cava near the right atrium. During mobile radiography of the chest for tube placement, it is often necessary to *move the radiopaque external wires out of the way* as much as possible to avoid artifacts that can interfere with accurate diagnosis (Fig. 4–1).

Central Lines

Classification	Purpose	Example
Short-term, external/ nontunneled	Admin med, draw blood, monitor RA BP	PICC, CVC
Long-term, external/ nontunneled	Admin med, draw blood	PICC
Long-term, tunneled	Parenteral nutrition, dialysis	Hickman, Raaf,
Long-term implanted venous access	Chemotherapy, blood transfusion	Port-A-Cath

Urinary catheterization may be employed postsurgically to assist in the healing of tissues or to assist an incontinent patient in the elimination of urine. It is essential that equipment used for the catheterization procedure is sterile, and that subsequent care is given to the catheterized patient to prevent infection, as *urinary tract infections* (UTIs) *account for the greatest number of nosocomial infections.* Urinary catheters are made of plastic, rubber, PVC (polyvinylchloride), and silicone. The type selected is dependent on how long it is expected to remain in the bladder. Plastic and rubber are generally employed for short-term use, whereas PVC or silicone catheters can be in place for up to 3 months. The urine collection bag must be *kept below the level of the bladder*; backflow of urine into the bladder can lead to infection. When transporting or transferring the catheterized patient, care must be taken that the catheter does not become entangled or dislodged.

ALLERGIC REACTIONS

Allergy

Medications are administered to meet specific patient needs; medications can have harmless side effects in some individuals. If the *side effect* offsets the benefit, the medication might be discontinued. Medications can also have a *toxic effect.* Toxic effects can occur because of sensitivity, overdose, or poor metabolism. An *antidote* is used to treat a toxic effect.

An *allergy* is an abnormal, acquired immune response to a substance (i.e., *allergen*) that would not usually trigger a reaction. An initial exposure to the allergen (i.e., *sensitization*) is required. Subsequent contact with the allergen then results in an *inflammatory response.* Examples of such responses include hay fever, urticaria, allergic rhinitis, eczema, and bronchial asthma. Allergens can be introduced into the body via contact, ingestion (e.g., food), inhalation (e.g., dust, pollen), or injection (e.g., medication, drugs). Allergic reactions of particular importance to the radiographer involve the use of *latex* products and *contrast media.*

Latex

Latex products are manufactured from a milky fluid derived from the rubber tree and several chemicals are added to the fluid during the manufacture of commercial latex. Some proteins in latex can produce mild to severe allergic reactions. In addition, chemicals added during processing can also cause skin rashes. When *powdered* latex gloves are worn, more latex proteins reach the skin. Also, when gloves are changed, latex protein/powder particles get into the air, where they can be inhaled and come in contact with body membranes. Studies have indicated that when unpowdered gloves are worn, there are extremely low levels of the allergy-producing proteins present.

A wide variety of products contain latex: medical supplies, personal protective equipment, and many household items. The intermittent use of latex products generally causes no health problems. However, workers in the health care industry (physicians, technologists, nurses, dentists, etc.) are at risk for developing *latex allergy* because they use latex gloves frequently. Also at risk are other workers with frequent glove use

Medical Equipment That Could Contain Latex

- Disposable gloves
- Tourniquets
- Blood pressure cuffs
- Stethoscopes
- Intravenous tubing
- Oral and nasal airways
- Enema tips
- Endotracheal tubes
- Syringes
- Electrode pads
- Catheters
- Wound drains
- Injection ports

Types of Reactions to Latex

- Irritant contact dermatitis
- Allergic contact dermatitis (delayed hypersensitivity)
- Latex allergy (immediate hypersensitivity)

(hairdressers, housekeepers, food service workers, etc.) and those involved in the manufacture of latex products.

Irritant Contact Dermatitis. The most common reaction to latex products is *irritant contact dermatitis*. It is characterized by development of irritated dry, itchy areas on the skin, usually the hands. Irritant contact dermatitis is a skin irritation resulting from the use of gloves and/or from exposure to other workplace products and chemicals. Irritant contact dermatitis can also be caused by repeated hand washing, incomplete drying, use of sanitizers, and exposure to glove powder. *Irritant contact dermatitis* is not defined as a true allergy.

Allergic Contact Dermatitis. Allergic contact dermatitis (*delayed hypersensitivity*) results from exposure to the chemicals added to latex during its manufacture. These chemicals can cause skin reactions like those produced by poison ivy, that is, the rash usually begins 24–48 hours following contact and can lead to oozing skin blisters and/or spread to areas away from the area of initial contact. Wearing latex gloves during episodes of hand dermatitis may increase skin exposure and the risk of developing latex allergy.

Latex Allergy. Latex allergy (*immediate hypersensitivity*) can be a much more serious reaction to latex. Certain proteins in latex can cause sensitization and, although the amount of exposure needed to cause this sensitization is unknown, even very low-level exposure can trigger allergic reaction in some sensitized individuals.

Reactions usually begin within minutes of exposure to the latex, but can occur hours later. *Mild* reactions involve skin redness, hives, or itching. *More severe* are respiratory reactions, for example, itchy eyes, runny nose, sneezing, difficulty breathing, and wheezing. A *life-threatening reaction* such as shock is rarely the first sign of latex allergy. Such reactions are similar to those seen in some allergic persons after a bee sting.

Health care professionals should help educate latex-sensitized persons about the latex content of common objects.

Summary

- Obtaining vital signs involves the measurement of body temperature, pulse rate, respiratory rate, and arterial blood pressure.
- The *pulse* represents regular expansion and contraction of an artery as waves of blood travel through it; the average normal adult pulse rate is between 60 and 100 BPM.
- The five most easily palpated pulse points are the radial, carotid, temporal, femoral, and popliteal pulse.
- Normal adult *oral* body temperature is 98.6°F (37°C); *rectal* is generally 0.5° to 1.0° *higher*, *axillary* is usually 0.5° to 1.0° *lower*; infants and children have a wider range of temperature; the elderly have lower body temperatures.
- Normal adult systolic pressure ranges between 100 and 140 mm Hg; the normal diastolic range is between 60 and 90 mm Hg; blood pressure consistently more than 140/90 is considered *hypertension*.

- The normal respiratory rate is 12–18 breaths/min; young children is up to 30 breaths/min higher.
- Symptoms of inadequate oxygen supply include dyspnea, cyanosis, diaphoresis, and neck vein distention; seated and semi-Fowler positions are helpful for dyspneic patients.
- Oxygen is usually available through wall outlets with adjustable flowmeters, or in tanks having a flow-regulation valve and an indicator showing the quantity of oxygen left in the tank.
- Oxygen can be administered via nasal cannula, masks, or mechanical ventilators; oxygen supports combustion so it must be used away from flame.
- Suction devices are used for aspiration of secretions; suction is available from wall outlets or portable suction mechanisms.
- Needle size is indicated by gauge; larger gauge is equal to smaller needle bore.
- Butterfly sets or IV catheters are generally used for IV injection of a contrast medium; the antecubital vein is generally used for injection of contrast material.
- A heparin lock makes a vein accessible for medications administered at frequent intervals.
- IV solutions should be elevated 18–24 inches above the injection site.
- *Extravasation* refers to a leakage of medication or contrast medium from a vein rupture or inadvertent introduction into tissue outside the vein. *Infiltration* refers to diffusion of injected material into adjacent tissues. Treatment includes removing the needle, applying pressure to prevent *hematoma* formation, and *a cold pack* applied to relieve pain and limit further infiltration.
- Chest tubes function to remove fluids or air from the thoracic cavity.
- NG and NI/NE tubes assist in the removal of gastric secretions or air and/or are used for the administration of water-soluble contrast material.
- Urinary collection bags must be kept below the level of the bladder; to prevent UTIs, catheterization procedures must be sterile.
- The radiographer must be alert for any sudden changes in the patient's condition.
- An *allergy* is an abnormal, acquired immune response.
- Allergens can be introduced into the body via contact, ingestion, inhalation, or injection.
- Initial *sensitization* to the allergen is required; subsequent contact results in an *inflammatory response.*
- Proteins in *latex* can produce mild-to-severe allergic reactions.
- Types of reactions to latex include irritant contact and delayed or immediate hypersensitivity.

CONTRAST MEDIA

Terminology and Basic Concepts

Patient History. It is important that the radiographer obtain a short but adequate, pertinent patient history of why the examination has been requested. Because patients are rarely examined or interviewed by the radiologist, observations and information obtained by the radiographer can be a significant help in making an accurate diagnosis.

Routes of Administration. Although radiographic contrast media are usually administered orally or intravenously, there are a number of *routes* and methods of drug administration. Drugs and medications may be administered either *orally* or *parenterally*. *Parenteral* refers to any route other than via the digestive tract and includes *topical, subcutaneous, intradermal, intramuscular, intravenous,* and *intrathecal.*

Purpose. The purpose of a *contrast medium* is to artificially increase subject contrast in body tissues and areas where there is little natural subject contrast. The abdominal viscera, for example, have very little subject contrast; that is, it is very difficult to identify specific organs or distinguish one organ from another. However, if a contrast agent is introduced into a particular organ such as the kidney or stomach, or into a vessel such as the aorta or one of its branches, we may more readily visualize these anatomic structures and/or evaluate physiologic activity.

Types and Properties of Agents. *Contrast media* or *contrast agents* can be described as either positive (radiopaque) or negative (radiolucent). *Positive,* or *radiopaque,* contrast agents have a higher atomic number than the surrounding soft tissue, resulting in a greater attenuation or absorption of x-ray photons. They, therefore, produce higher radiographic contrast. Examples of positive contrast media are *iodinated agents* (both water based and oil based) and *barium sulfate* suspensions. The inert characteristics of barium sulfate render it the least *toxic* contrast medium. On the other hand, iodinated contrast media have characteristics that increase their likelihood of producing *side effects* and reactions.

    Negative, or radiolucent, contrast agents used are *air* and various *gases.* Because the atomic number of air is also quite different from that of soft tissue, high subject contrast is produced. Carbon dioxide is absorbed more rapidly by the body than air.

    Negative contrast is often used *with* positive contrast in examinations termed *double-contrast studies.* The function of the positive agent is usually to *coat* the various parts under study, while the air *fills* the space and permits visualization through the gaseous medium. Examinations that frequently use double-contrast technique are barium enema (BE), upper GI (UGI) series, and arthrography.

Scheduling and Preparation Considerations

Multiple Examinations. When patients are scheduled for multiple x-ray examinations, each requiring the use of a contrast medium, the examinations must be scheduled in the correct sequence. For example, if a particular patient must be scheduled for a UGI series, BE, and intravenous

---

Methods of Administration

Oral
- PO (by mouth), through digestive system

Parenteral
- Topical
- Subcutaneous
- Intradermal
- Intramuscular
- Intravenous
- Intrathecal

Contrast Media

Positive (radiopaque)
- Barium sulfate
- Iodinated

Negative (radiolucent)
- Air
- Other gases

Sequencing and Combining Contrast Examinations

Sequence

IVU

GB

BE

GI

Examinations that can be combined

GB and IVU

IVU and BE

GB and GI

urogram (IVU), what sequence will permit optimal visualization of the required structures? Remember that it is important that residual barium not overlie structures of interest. Radiographic examinations of the gall-bladder (GB) are rarely requested today, but should that examination be requested, the accompanying chart indicates when that examination would be scheduled among the others.

Generally speaking, the examinations with a contrast medium that is excreted quickly and completely should be scheduled first. Therefore, the IVU should be scheduled first, and then the GB, if requested. If the UGI series were scheduled next, residual barium would be in the large bowel the next day, thus preventing adequate investigation. So, the BE should be scheduled third; any residual barium should not interfere with a UGI examination, although a preliminary scout image should first be taken in each case.

If it is desired to expedite the studies, perhaps to reduce the length of hospital stay, some examinations, for example, GB and IVU, can be performed on the same day. If the patient's GB is studied first and a *fatty meal* is used to evaluate its emptying function, there should be little contrast medium left to obscure the right urinary collecting system. Another example of paired examinations is the IVU and BE. IVU contrast medium is excreted rapidly by the kidneys and should not interfere with visualization of the barium- and air-filled large bowel.

Patient Preparation. Patient preparation is somewhat different for each of these examinations. An iodinated contrast agent, usually in the form of several pills, is taken by the patient the evening before a scheduled *GB* examination and only water is allowed the morning of the examination. A patient scheduled for an *UGI* series must receive NPO (nothing by mouth) after midnight. A BE (*lower GI*) requires that the large bowel be very clean prior to the administration of barium; this requires the administration of *cathartics* (laxatives) and cleansing enemas. Preparation for an *IVU* requires that the patient be NPO after midnight; some institutions also require that the large bowel be cleansed of gas and fecal material. Aftercare for BE is very important. Patients are typically instructed to take milk of magnesia, increase their intake of fiber, drink plenty of water, to expect change in stool color until all barium is evacuated, and to call their physician if they do not have a bowel movement within 24 hours. Because water is removed from the barium sulfate suspension in the large bowel, it is essential to make patients understand the importance of these instructions to avoid barium impaction in the large bowel.

Contraindications and Patient Education

Radiopaque contrast media are most frequently employed for radiographic procedures. *Barium sulfate* is one type of radiopaque contrast agent that is used to visualize the GI tract. Mixed with water, it forms a suspension that is usually administered orally for demonstration of the upper GI tract (esophagus, stomach, and progression through the small intestine), and rectally for demonstration of the lower GI tract (large intestine).

Barium sulfate is *contraindicated* if a *perforation* is suspected somewhere along the course of the GI tract (e.g., a perforated diverticulum

---

Patient Preparation

GB

Iodinated contrast evening before examination; water only in AM

UGI

NPO after midnight

BE

Cathartics, cleansing enemas

IVU

NPO after midnight, cleansing enemas, empty bladder before scout film

or gastric ulcer). Barium could escape into the peritoneal cavity and result in peritonitis. A water-soluble (absorbable) iodinated contrast medium is generally used instead of barium in these cases. The water-soluble preparations are available as ready-mixed liquid or as powder requiring appropriate dilution with water. A patient with an NG tube can have the contrast medium administered through it for the purpose of locating and studying any site of obstruction. This procedure is called *enteroclysis*.

Patients can experience constipation following a GI or BE examination unless proper *aftercare instructions* are given to the patient upon completion of the examination. Barium preparations in the large bowel become thickened as a result of absorption of their fluid content, a process called *inspissation*, causing symptoms from mild constipation to bowel obstruction. Constipation can be a serious problem, particularly in the elderly, and fecal impaction or obstruction can result. It is essential that the radiographer provide clear instructions for follow-up care, especially to outpatients. Patients are usually advised to expect light-colored stools for the next few days, to drink plenty of fluids, to increase their intake of fiber, and to take a mild laxative such as milk of magnesia following a barium study.

Iodinated contrast agents are another type of radiopaque contrast medium. They may be *oil based or water based.* Oil-based contrast media are infrequently used today. They are not water soluble, not readily absorbed by the body, and remain in body tissues for lengthy periods of time. Examinations that can employ the use of oil-based contrast agents, though infrequently performed, are lymphangiograms, sialograms, and bronchograms. Water-based contrast media may be *ionic* or *nonionic.* These agents are principally used to delineate the urinary and vascular systems, the GB, and the GI tract when barium sulfate is contraindicated.

Ionic contrast media have a *higher osmolality*, that is, a greater number of particles in a given amount of solution. *Nonionic, or low osmolality*, contrast agents are used especially with children, the elderly, patients with renal disease, patients having a history of *allergic* reaction to contrast media, or patients having multiple allergies. Side effects and allergic reactions are less likely and less severe with these media. Nonionic contrast agents are associated with less injection discomfort, and a lower incidence of *nausea*, vomiting, and cardiovascular complications. Their only disadvantage is their cost, which is far greater than that of ionic contrast agents.

Iodinated contrast agents can become more *viscous* at normal room temperature, making injection more difficult. Warming the contrast to body temperature, in a special warming oven, reduces *viscosity*, permitting an easier and more comfortable injection.

Diabetic patients who are scheduled for a UGI series are generally instructed to withhold their morning insulin until the meal following the examination. Should the patient take insulin before the examination and remain NPO, a reaction might occur, especially if the examinations were delayed for any reason. UGI examinations on diabetic patients should be among the first examinations scheduled each day and priority should be given to these patients.

Qualities of Iodinated Contrast Agents That Contribute to Discomfort, Side Effects, and Reactions

Viscosity. More viscid (thick, sticky) agents are more difficult to inject and produce more heat and vessel irritation; the higher the concentration, the greater the viscosity; viscosity also increases as room temperature decreases.

Toxicity. Potential toxicity is greater with higher concentration agents and ionic agents.

Miscibility. Contrast agents should be readily miscible (able to mix) with blood.

Osmolality. Low-osmolality agents have fewer particles in a given amount of solution and are less likely to provoke an allergic reaction.

Reactions Can Result from

- Ingestion,
- Injection, or
- Absorption ... of the sensitizing agent

Reactions and Emergency Situations

Anaphylaxis is a life-threatening allergic reaction that affects millions of Americans every year and can be caused by a variety of allergens. *Anaphylaxis* can result from the body's sensitivity and allergic reaction to certain foods, insect venom, medications, anesthetics, and latex. The reaction can be the result of *ingestion, injection,* or *absorption* of the sensitizing agent.

Because iodinated contrast media are potentially toxic, the radiographer must be knowledgeable and alert to the possible adverse effects of their use (although the risk of a life-threatening reaction is relatively

TABLE 4–1. Common Medications and Their Application

Type	Effect	Example
Adrenergic	Vasopressor, stimulates sympathetic nervous system: increases BP, relaxes smooth muscle of respiratory system	Epinephrine (Adrenalin)
Analgesic	Relieves pain	Aspirin, acetaminophen (Tylenol), codeine, meperidine (Demerol)
Antiarrhythmic	Relieves cardiac arrhythmia	Quinidine sulfate, lidocaine (Xylocaine)
Antibacterial	Stops growth of bacteria	Penicillin, tetracycline, erythromycin
Anticholinergic	Depresses parasympathetic system	Atropine, scopolamine, belladonna
Anticoagulant	Inhibits blood clotting; keeps IV lines and catheters free of clots	Heparin, warfarin
Anticonvulsant	Prevents/relieves convulsions	Carbamazepine (Tegretol) Phenytoin (Dilantin)
Antidepressant	Prevents/alleviates mental depression	Fluoxetine (Prozac) Paroxetine (Paxil) Sertraline (Zoloft) Nortriptyline (Pamelor, Aventyl)
Antihistamine	Relieves allergic symptoms	Diphenhydramine hydrochloride (Benadryl)
Antipyretic	Reduces fever	Aspirin, acetaminophen
Antitussive	Reduces coughing	Dextromethorphan (Romilar)
Barbiturate	Depresses CNS, decreases BP and respiration, and induces sleep	Phenobarbital sodium (Nembutal), secobarbital sodium (Seconal)
Cardiac stimulant	Increases cardiac output	Digitalis
Cathartic	Laxative, relieves constipation, prepares colon for diagnostic tests	Bisacodyl (Dulcolax), castor oil
Diuretic	Stimulates urine	Furosemide (Lasix)
Emetic	Stimulates vomiting	Activated charcoal; Ipecac
Hypoglycemic	Lowers blood glucose	Insulin, chlorpropamide (Diabinese), metformin (Glucophage)
Narcotic (opioid)	Sedative/analgesic; potentially addictive	Morphine, codeine, meperidine (Demerol)
NSAID	Nonsteroidal pain relief	Aspirin (Bayer, and others) Ibuprofen (Motrin, and others) Naproxen (Aleve, and others)
Stimulant	Stimulates the CNS	Caffeine, amphetamines
Tranquilizer	Reduces anxiety	Diazepam (Valium); alprazolam (Xanex)
Vasodilator	Relaxes and dilates blood vessels, decreases BP	Nitroglycerine, verapamil

rare). Reactions to contrast media generally occur within 2–10 minutes following injection and can affect all body systems.

The body's response to the introduction of contrast material is the production of histamines, which brings about various symptoms. Symptoms of a *mild* reaction include a flushed appearance, nausea, a metallic taste in the mouth, nasal congestion, a few hives (*urticaria*), and, occasionally, vomiting. Treatment of these minor symptoms generally consists of administration of either an *antihistamine* such as diphenhydramine (Benadryl), which blocks the action of the histamine and reduces the body's inflammatory response or an epinephrine to raise the blood pressure and relax the bronchioles (see Table 4–1).

Potentially life-threatening responses include respiratory failure, shock, and death within minutes. A very serious and life-threatening response is an anaphylactic reaction. *Early* symptoms of an anaphylactic reaction include itching of the palms and soles, wheezing, constriction of the throat (possibly caused by laryngeal edema), *dyspnea, dysphagia, hypotension*, and *cardiopulmonary arrest*. The radiographer must maintain the patient's airway, summon the radiologist, and call a "code." The radiographer should then be prepared to stay with the patient and assist until the arrival of the code team.

The diabetic patient requires different and special attention. Metformin (Glucophage) is an antidiabetic agent indicated for the treatment of type 2 diabetes mellitus. Radiologic examinations requiring the use of intravascular-iodinated contrast agents can lead to acute alteration of renal function and have been associated with lactic acidosis in patients taking metformin. The manufacturer recommends that patients taking metformin discontinue it at the time of or prior to the x-ray examination and withhold it for 48 more hours following the examination. The medication should be continued only after *adequate renal function* has been indicated by blood test (blood urea nitrogen, creatinine).

Summary

- Multiple radiologic examinations must be scheduled in a sequence that will allow prompt and adequate visualization of structures of interest.
- Patients must be appropriately prepared for the contrast examination(s) for which they are scheduled.
- Drugs and medications may be administered orally or parenterally.
- *Parenteral* administration includes topical, oral, subcutaneous, intradermal, IM, IV, and intrathecal.
- Artificial contrast media function to increase insufficient subject contrast; artificial contrast media can be positive (radiopaque) or negative (radiolucent).
- Positive contrast media include barium sulfate and iodinated (oil- or water-based) agents.
- Qualities of iodinated contrast media that contribute to their risk include viscosity, toxicity, and miscibility.
- Negative and positive contrast agents are often used together in "double-contrast" studies.

- Water-soluble (absorbable) contrast agents are used in place of barium sulfate when visceral *perforation* is suspected.
- Patients require clear and complete postprocedural instructions, particularly following barium examinations.
- Nonionic iodinated contrast agents produce far fewer side effects than do their ionic counterparts; nonionic contrast agents are more expensive.
- Reactions to ionic agents usually occur within 2–10 minutes following injection.
- Symptoms of a mild reaction include mild urticaria, flushing, nausea, nasal congestion, metallic taste; an antihistamine is usually given to the patient.
- To avoid renal dysfunction, diabetic patients taking metformin must discontinue its use for 48 hours after administration of an intravascular contrast agent.

OTHER MEDICAL EMERGENCIES

The importance of radiographers' careful evaluation of their patients is never more obvious than when an emergency arises. An emergency is defined as *a sudden change in a patient's condition requiring immediate medical intervention*. Most patients arrive in the radiology department in a stable condition; a few arrive for diagnostic evaluation of a medical crisis. The radiographer must note the patient's condition on arrival and be alert to any subsequent sudden change in that condition. The value of continual review of the knowledge and skills required for emergency situations cannot be overemphasized. Many of these emergencies can occur with little or no warning. Many can be life threatening if not dealt with immediately and correctly.

Vomiting

Vomiting patients who are seated or standing should be provided with a basin, tissues, and water for rinsing their mouths. It is essential that recumbent patients have their heads turned to the side to prevent choking from aspiration of vomitus. Patients who report feeling nauseous are often apprehensive and may get some relief by breathing slowly and deeply through their mouths.

Fractures

An *unsplinted* fracture must be moved with great care, with *areas proximal and distal to the fracture site adequately supported*. Any motion is very painful and can result in further injury to tissues surrounding the fracture. Muscle spasm can cause additional pain and can interfere with proper reduction of the fracture. A *splint* should never be removed from an extremity except by or under the direct supervision of the physician. Some splinting devices are not radiolucent and removal may be required before the radiographic examination.

Rib fractures may be associated with lung trauma and sternum fractures with heart lacerations. Rib fractures can be very painful—the patient experiences pain just from breathing. *Pelvic* fractures are often associated with injuries to pelvic and abdominal viscera, and extreme care must be taken to avoid *hemorrhage.*

Spinal Injuries

Patients arriving for radiographic evaluation with possible spinal injuries must not be moved. The position of any sandbags or other supportive mechanisms must not be changed. A *horizontal (cross-table) lateral projection* should be evaluated by the physician first to determine the extent of injury and necessity for further radiographs. If the patient must be placed in a lateral position, the logrolling method is usually advised. *A physician must be present whenever the patient's position is changed.*

Epistaxis

A nosebleed (*epistaxis*) may be a result of any one of many causes, including *hypertension*, dry nasal mucous membranes, sinusitis, or trauma. The patient should be seated or in a Fowler position. The radiographer should place cold cloths over the patient's nose and back of the neck. Compressing the sides of the nose against the nasal septum for 6–8 minutes is also helpful. Continued hemorrhage should be brought to the attention of the physician because cautery or nasal packs might be required.

Postural Hypotension

Orthostatic, or postural, *hypotension* is a decrease in blood pressure that occurs on rising to the erect position. It can be severe enough to cause fainting in individuals who have been confined to bed for several days. The radiographer should assist patients slowly and be watchful for signs of weakness.

Vertigo

Objective vertigo is the sensation of having *objects* (or "the room") spinning about the person; *subjective* vertigo is the sensation of the *person* spinning about. It is usually associated with an inner-ear disturbance. Patients experiencing true vertigo (as opposed to dizziness or lightheadedness) are often very nauseous and must be protected from falls by the use of side rails and/or safety belts.

Syncope

A patient who reports feeling dizzy or faint should be immediately assisted to a chair. Bending forward and placing the head between the knees will often help relieve the lightheadedness as blood flow to the brain increases. In more severe cases, a patient who cannot be assisted to a chair should be *lowered to a recumbent position.* Elevation of the lower legs or use of the Trendelenburg position is helpful. If the patient loses consciousness, the radiographer should make certain that the airway is open and that clothing, especially at the collar, is loose. Once the patient is recumbent, recovery is usually swift; however, a physician should be notified and the cause of *syncope* identified.

Convulsion

Involuntary muscular contractions and relaxations, often associated with epilepsy, characterize a *convulsion*. *Febrile* convulsions are associated with fever, especially in children. During convulsion, no attempt must be made to restrain the patient's movements. The radiographer's responsibility is to keep patients from injuring themselves. Tight clothing can be loosened and objects that could harm the patient should be moved out of the way. A padded tongue blade or other suitable object should be placed between the patient's teeth to prevent biting the tongue.

Unconsciousness

Unconscious patients are unaware of, and unresponsive to, their surroundings. Unconsciousness can be caused by a wide variety of conditions including insulin overdose, uremia, concussion, heat *stroke*, and intoxication.

There are various levels of consciousness and the condition of an acutely ill patient can rapidly deteriorate from being fully aware and responsive to diminished or inappropriate responsiveness, to complete unresponsiveness. The unconscious patient must never be left unattended. The radiographer must be alert to changes in the patient's level of consciousness and notify the physician immediately of any deterioration.

Acute Abdomen

Patients arriving for radiographic evaluation having a diagnosis of "acute abdomen" are usually suffering severe abdominal pain, are nauseous and vomiting, and are frequently close to being in shock. These are indeed very sick patients. The radiographer must perform the examination swiftly and efficiently and remain alert for any sudden changes in patient condition.

Shock

Shock is a general term and is characterized by diminished peripheral blood flow and insufficient oxygen supply to body tissues. Shock can be caused by a number of conditions including allergic reaction, trauma, hemorrhage, myocardial infarction, and infection. The patient is pale and may become cyanotic; the pulse is rapid and weak, breathing is shallow and rapid, and blood pressure drops sharply. The radiographer should keep the patient warm and flat, or in the Trendelenburg position, and be prepared to assist with emergency procedures.

Seizure

The type of *seizure* known as *petit mal* is so subtle as to go unnoticed by the patient and observer. It is characterized by brief loss of consciousness (10–30 seconds) and accompanied by eye or muscle fluttering. A *grand mal* seizure is characterized by loss of consciousness and falling, followed by generalized muscle spasms. The radiographer should remove any objects in the area that could harm the patient and loosen any tight clothing. The patient's head should be turned to the side to allow any secretions to flow from the mouth. A padded tongue blade should be placed between the patient's teeth to help avoid biting the tongue.

Respiratory Failure

The inability of the lungs to perform ventilating functions is respiratory distress and may be described as *acute* or *chronic*. Acute respiratory distress can be caused by impaired gas exchange processes (requiring positive-pressure ventilation) or airway obstruction (requiring the Heimlich maneuver). Chronic respiratory failure is a result of a disease process that impairs breathing, such as emphysema, bronchitis, *asthma*, or cystic fibrosis.

The radiographer should be able to distinguish between respiratory arrest (absence of chest movement and breathing sounds) and cardiopulmonary arrest (absence of pulse and respiration with loss of consciousness) and be able to initiate life-saving actions.

Cardiopulmonary Arrest

The *sudden cessation of productive ventilation and circulation* is called cardiopulmonary arrest. The radiographer should be trained in the ABCs (airway, breathing, and circulation) of cardiopulmonary resuscitation and be able to initiate the appropriate care until the arrival of the emergency team.

Many health care facilities require their employees to be certified in basic life-saving skills. It is wise for radiographers to be familiar with skills such as the Heimlich maneuver (abdominal thrust) and cardiopulmonary resuscitation should the need arise.

Stroke

A *stroke*, or cerebrovascular accident, is an interference with blood supplied to the brain as a result of occlusion or rupture of a cerebral vessel. If the condition results from a partial vessel occlusion, the interference is usually mild and temporary and is referred to as a *transient ischemic attack*. The patient may experience temporary blindness in one eye, *dysphasia* or *aphasia, hemiparesis* or hemiplegia, or anesthesia.

If the cerebral vessel is totally occluded or ruptures into the brain or subarachnoid space, a much more serious event has occurred. The patient frequently experiences sudden loss of consciousness and one-sided paralysis (*hemiparesis*), although the onset can be slower if the *occlusion* is caused by *thrombus* formation. Other symptoms include speech disturbances and cool, sweaty skin. Patients should have their head and shoulders elevated or be in the lateral recumbent position; an open airway must be maintained. Because a stroke can occur without warning at any time, the radiographer should be familiar with the signs of an impending stroke and be able to provide appropriate immediate care.

Summary

- It is essential that the radiographer be alert for *any* sudden changes in patient condition; how well the radiographer recognizes and is prepared to meet the challenges of emergency situations can largely determine the outcome of the emergency.

COMPREHENSION CHECK

Congratulations! You have completed your review of this chapter. If you are able to answer the following group of comprehensive questions, you can feel confident that you have mastered this section. You are then ready to go on to "Registry-type" questions that follow. For greatest success, do not go to these multiple-choice questions without first completing the short-answer questions below.

1. Discuss the importance of careful and accurate patient *assessment*; what are the components of a good assessment (p. 51)?

2. List the four vital signs and identify their adult norms (p. 51, 52).

3. What does the pulse that we feel actually represent? What are some variables that can affect pulse rate? List common pulse points (p. 52, 53)?

4. Define the terms *diaphoretic*, *cyanotic*, *febrile*, *hypertension*, *systole*, *bradycardia*, *and hypoxia* (p. 52-54).

5. Identify illnesses/conditions that might require supplemental oxygen (p. 52, 54).

6. What condition specifically requires a low flow rate of oxygen (p. 54)?

7. List the subjective symptoms of inadequate oxygen; identify the body position frequently helpful for the dyspneic patient (p. 54).

8. Describe four methods of oxygen therapy and identify when each might be indicated (p. 54, 55).

9. Identify any hazards involved in the use of oxygen (p. 55).

10. Describe the circumstance(s) in which suction might be required; identify types of suction devices available (p. 55).

11. Identify how needle bore changes with increasing gauge (p. 55).

12. Describe the function and uses of a heparin lock (p. 55).

13. Identify the height at which IV bottles and bags should be hung (p. 55, 56).

14. Explain how contrast medium extravasation/infiltration should be treated (p. 56).

15. Identify the vein(s) frequently used for introduction of contrast medium (p. 56).

16. Explain the function of chest tubes and precautions that should be taken by the radiographer (p. 56).

17. Describe the function of NG and NI tubes and any precautions that should be taken by the radiographer (p. 56, 57).

18. Identify the classification and purpose of the PICC, Hickman, and Port-A-Cath lines (p. 57).

19. Describe the function of urinary catheters and any precautions that should be taken by the radiographer (p. 58).

20. Identify the level at which urinary collection bags should be kept (p. 58).

21. Define *allergy*; discuss *sensitization* and *inflammatory* response (p. 58).

22. Distinguish between *side effect* and *toxic effect* (p. 58).

23. List the three types of latex reactions; discuss the effect *powder* can have in latex gloves (p. 58).

24. Discuss the difference between *delayed* and *immediate* hypersensitivity (p. 59).

25. Discuss the importance of observing initial patient condition and any subsequent changes (p. 51).

26. Describe the difference between oral and parenteral drug administration; list five types of parenteral administration (p. 61).

27. Explain the purpose of contrast medium (p. 61).

28. Identify the two types of contrast media, describe their characteristics, and give examples of each (p. 61).

29. Explain how best to correctly schedule multiple contrast examinations on the same patient. (p. 61, 62).

30. Explain the appropriate patient preparation for GB, UGI, BE, and IVU/IVP (p. 62).

31. Explain why a diabetic patient who is required to receive nothing by mouth beginning the preceding midnight should be scheduled as the first AM appointment (p. 63).

32. Describe the *risks* associated with iodinated contrast media and identify the type of iodinated media associated with less risk (p. 61, 63).

33. Describe three *qualities* of iodinated contrast media that contribute to the production of side effects (p. 63).

34. Explain how double-contrast examinations can serve to better demonstrate certain anatomic parts (p. 61).

35. Describe *contraindications* to the use of barium sulfate; identify the alternative contrast medium (p. 62, 63).

36. Explain the importance of *aftercare* explanations, especially following barium examinations (p. 62, 63).

37. Distinguish between oil- and water-based iodinated contrast media, their uses, and their characteristics (p. 63).

38. Identify the basic difference between ionic and nonionic contrast media and identify when use of nonionic agents is indicated (p. 63).

39. Describe symptoms a patient having a *mild* reaction to iodinated contrast media might experience and their usual treatment (p. 65).

40. Describe the symptoms of a possible *impending anaphylactic reaction* and the radiographer's responsibilities (p. 65).

41. Describe care provided to the nauseous or vomiting patient; identify the body position required for the recumbent patient (p. 66).

42. Describe precautions the radiographer should take when examining a patient with a fracture (p. 66, 67).

43. Discuss precautions that should be taken with patients having suspected spinal injuries (p. 67).

44. Describe first aid for epistaxis (p. 67).

45. Distinguish between postural hypotension, vertigo, and syncope; discuss precautions taken and care given by the radiographer (p. 67).

46. Describe any precautions that should be taken with the unconscious patient (p. 68).

47. Describe symptoms of *acute abdomen* and *shock*; indicate any precautions that should be taken by the radiographer (p. 68).

48. Distinguish between grand mal and petit mal seizures; discuss the care appropriate for a patient experiencing a grand mal seizure (p. 68, 69).

49. Distinguish between respiratory arrest and cardiopulmonary arrest; discuss the responses appropriate to the radiographer (p. 69).

50. Describe "stroke," to include some symptoms and responses appropriate for the radiographer (p. 69).

51. List/name the three parts of a chest drainage system. (p. 56)

CHAPTER REVIEW QUESTIONS

1. Which of the following is/are symptom(s) of inadequate oxygen supply?
   1. Diaphoresis
   2. Cyanosis
   3. Dyspnea
   (A) 1 only
   (B) 1 and 2 only
   (C) 2 and 3 only
   (D) 1, 2, and 3

2. A patient's feeling of spinning, or the room spinning about him, is called:
   (A) Orthostatic hypotension
   (B) Epistaxis
   (C) Vertigo
   (D) Syncope

3. An example/examples of a negative contrast agent include(s):
   1. Air
   2. Iodine
   3. Barium sulfate
   (A) 1 only
   (B) 1 and 2 only
   (C) 2 and 3 only
   (D) 1, 2, and 3

4. Which of the following gauge needles has the largest bore?
   (A) 12
   (B) 18
   (C) 20
   (D) 23

5. Proper treatment for contrast media extravasation into tissues around a vein includes:
   1. Application of a cold pack to affected area
   2. Application of moist heat to affected area
   3. Application of pressure to injection site
   (A) 1 only
   (B) 2 only
   (C) 1 and 3 only
   (D) 2 and 3 only

6. Parenteral administration of drugs may be performed:
   1. Intrathecally
   2. Intravenously
   3. Orally
   (A) 1 only
   (B) 1 and 2 only
   (C) 3 only
   (D) 1, 2, and 3

7. What is the most frequently used site for intravenous injection of contrast agents?
   (A) Basilic vein
   (B) Cephalic vein
   (C) Antecubital vein
   (D) Femoral vein

8. In what order should the following examinations be performed?
   1. UGI
   2. IVU
   3. Barium enema
   (A) 3, 1, 2
   (B) 1, 3, 2
   (C) 2, 1, 3
   (D) 2, 3, 1

9. A patient's IV bottle or bag should be hung:
   (A) 18–24 inches above the vein
   (B) 18–24 inches below the vein
   (C) 18–24 inches above the heart
   (D) 18–24 inches below the heart

10. The usual patient preparation for an upper GI examination is:
    (A) NPO 8 hours before the examination
    (B) Light breakfast only the morning of the examination
    (C) Clear fluids only the morning of the examination
    (D) Two ounces of castor oil and enemas until clear

Answers and Explanations

1. (D) Symptoms of inadequate oxygen supply include *dyspnea*, *cyanosis, diaphoresis*, and distention of the veins of the neck. The patient who experiences some or all of these symptoms will be very anxious and must not be left unattended. The radiographer must call for help, assist the patient to a sitting or semi-Fowler position (the recumbent position makes breathing more difficult), and have oxygen and emergency drugs available.

2. (C) *Objective vertigo* is the sensation of having *objects* (or "the room") spinning about the person; *subjective vertigo* is the sensation of the *person* spinning about. It is often associated with an inner-ear disturbance. Patients experiencing true vertigo (as opposed to dizziness or lightheadedness) are often very nauseous and must be protected from falls. A patient who reports feeling dizzy or faint (*syncope*) should be immediately assisted to a chair. Bending forward and placing the head between the knees will often help relieve the lightheadedness as blood flow to the brain increases. In more severe cases, *a patient who cannot be assisted to a chair should be lowered to a recumbent position.* Elevation of the lower legs, or use of the Trendelenburg position, is helpful. *Orthostatic, or postural, hypotension* is a decrease in blood pressure that occurs on rising to the erect position. It can be severe enough to cause fainting in individuals who have been confined to bed for several days. A nosebleed (epistaxis) may be a result of any one of many causes, including hypertension, dry nasal mucous membranes, sinusitis, or trauma. The patient should be seated or placed in a Fowler position. The radiographer should place cold cloths over the patient's nose and back of the neck.

3. (A) *Negative, or radiolucent, contrast agents* used are *air* and various *gases*. Because the atomic number of air is also quite different from that of soft tissue, high subject contrast is produced. Carbon dioxide is absorbed more rapidly by the body than air.

Negative contrast is often used *with* positive contrast in examinations termed *double-contrast studies*. The function of the positive agent is usually to *coat* the various parts under study, while the air *fills* the space and permits visualization through the gaseous medium. Examinations that frequently use double-contrast technique are BE, UGI series, and arthrography.

4. (A) The diameter of a needle is identified as its *gauge.* As the diameter of its *bore* decreases, the *gauge* increases. Hence, a 23-gauge needle has a smaller diameter bore than an 18-gauge needle. Hypodermic needles are generally used for phlebotomy (i.e., blood samples), whereas butterflies and IV catheters are used more frequently for injections such as contrast media. If an infusion injection is required, an IV catheter is generally preferred. The hub of the hypodermic needle is attached to a syringe, while the hub of the butterfly tubing or IV catheter may be attached to a syringe or an IV bottle or bag via an IV infusion set.

5. (C) The term *extravasation* refers to medication or contrast medium that has leaked from a vein rupture or has been inadvertently introduced into tissue outside the vein. The term *infiltration* refers to the diffusion of the injected material further into adjacent tissues. The needle should be removed, *pressure* applied to prevent formation of a *hematoma*, and *a cold pack* applied to relieve pain and limit further infiltration of area tissue.

6. (B) Although radiographic contrast media are usually administered orally or intravenously, there are a number of routes or methods of drug administration. Drugs and medications may be administered either *orally* or *parenterally. Parenteral* refers to any route other than the digestive tract (orally) and includes *topical*, *subcutaneous*, *intradermal*, *intramuscular*, *intravenous*, and *intrathecal.*

7. (C) The *antecubital* vein is the most commonly used injection site for contrast medium administration. It is not used for infusions that take longer than 1 hour because of its location at the bend of the elbow. The basilic vein, located on the dorsal surface of the hand, is used when the antecubital vein is inaccessible. The cephalic vein may also be used. Strict aseptic technique must be used for all intravenous injections.

8. (D) When scheduling patient examinations, it is important to avoid the possibility of residual contrast medium overlying areas of interest of later examinations. The IVU should be scheduled first because the contrast medium used is excreted very rapidly. The BE should be scheduled next. The UGI is scheduled last. Any barium remaining from the previous BE is unlikely to interfere with the stomach or duodenum, although a preliminary scout image should be taken in each case.

9. (A) The IV bottle or bag should be hung 18–24 inches *above the level of the vein.* If placed lower than the vein, solution will stop flowing and blood will return into the tubing. If hung too high, solution can run too fast. Occasionally, the position of the needle or catheter in the vein will affect the flow rate. If the bevel is adjacent to the vessel wall, flow may decrease or stop altogether. Often, just changing the position of the patient's arm will remedy the situation.

10. (A) Patient preparation differs for various contrast examinations. To obtain a diagnostic examination of the stomach, it must first be empty. The usual *UGI* preparation is NPO (nothing by mouth) after midnight (approximately 8 hours before the examination). Any material in the stomach can simulate the appearance of disease. An iodinated contrast agent, usually in the form of several pills, is taken by the patient the evening before a scheduled *GB* examination and only water is allowed the morning of the examination. The patient scheduled for a *BE* (lower GI) requires a large bowel that is very clean prior to the administration of barium; this requires the administration of cathartics (laxatives) and cleansing enemas. Preparation for an *IVU* requires that the patient be NPO after midnight; some institutions may require that the large bowel be cleansed of gas and fecal material. *Aftercare* for barium examinations is also very important. Patients are typically instructed to take milk of magnesia and to drink plenty of water. Because water is removed from the barium sulfate suspension in the large bowel, it is essential to make patients understand the importance of these instructions to avoid barium impaction in the large bowel.

PART II

Image Procedures

General Procedural Considerations | 5

The development of positioning skills requires a thorough knowledge of normal *anatomy*, an awareness of *pathologic conditions* and their impact on positioning limitations, and selection of *technical factors*.

A review of basic positioning principles and terminology is essential to an overview of radiographic procedures. Several tables and figures in this chapter summarize body *planes* (Fig. 5–1), body *habitus* (Figs. 5–2 and 5–3), *four quadrants* and *nine regions* of the abdomen (Fig. 5–4), *body surface landmarks* and localization points (Fig. 5–5), and *standard terminology* (Fig. 5–6). The student should be thoroughly acquainted with these before approaching the study of specific positioning skills.

It must be emphasized that patients' condition often impacts their ability to move readily on the x-ray table or maintain positions for lengthy periods of time. Most of the descriptions of *position of part* in Chapter 6 are easily used on patients not severely injured or patients with debilitating pathology; in many instances, suggested modifications for *traumatized* patients are included. One measure of a skillful radiographer is his or her ability to be cautious and resourceful when examining injured or debilitated patients having pathologic or traumatic conditions, such as metastatic bone disease, arthritis, or bone fractures.

The use of *body surface landmarks* and localization points (Fig. 5–5) as external indicators of anatomic structures can increase the ease and accuracy of positioning.

Thoughtful placement of a cushioning sponge, the use of a horizontal beam ("cross-table") for *lateral* projections instead of moving the patient (Fig. 5–7), and performing the examination *erect* if the *recumbent* position is uncomfortable are examples of modifications that a considerate radiographer can make that will result in an appreciative patient, as well as a diagnostic examination. The radiographer must also be alert to changes in technical factors that may be necessitated by various pathologic processes.

BODY PLANES

There are four major *body planes* (Fig. 5–1) that the radiographer regularly uses while performing most radiologic examinations. Positioning

Body Habitus

Hypersthenic and asthenic characterize the *extremes* in body types:

Hypersthenic

- Body large and heavy
- Bony framework thick, short, and wide
- Lungs and heart high
- Stomach transverse (Fig. 5–3A)
- Gallbladder high and lateral
- Colon peripheral

Asthenic

- Body slender and light
- Bony framework delicate
- Thorax long and narrow
- Stomach very low and long ("fish hook") (Fig. 5–3B)
- Gallbladder low and medial
- Colon low, medial, and redundant

Sthenic and hyposthenic types characterize the *more average* body types:

Sthenic

- Build average and athletic
- Similar to hypersthenic, but modified by elongation of abdomen and thorax

Hyposthenic

- Somewhat slighter, less robust
- Similar to asthenic, but stomach, intestines, and gallbladder situated higher in abdomen

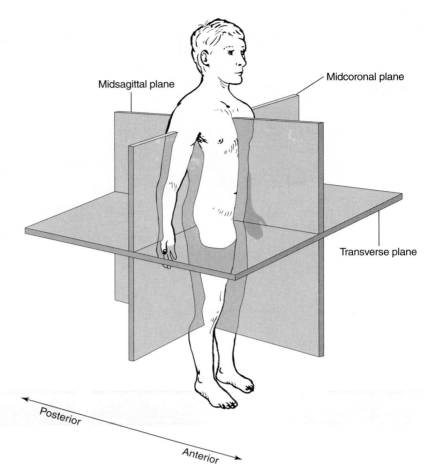

Figure 5–1. Body planes.

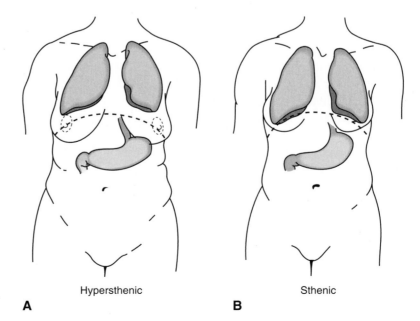

Hypersthenic

A

Sthenic

B

Figure 5–2. The *position*, *shape*, and *motility* of various organs can differ greatly from one *body habitus* to another. Each of the body habitus types is shown and the characteristic variations in shape and position of the diaphragm, lungs, and stomach are illustrated. The radiographer must consider these characteristic differences while performing radiographic examinations on individuals of various body habitus. (*continued*)

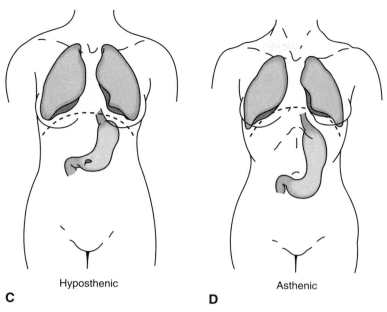

Hyposthenic

C

Asthenic

D

Figure 5–2. (*Continued*)

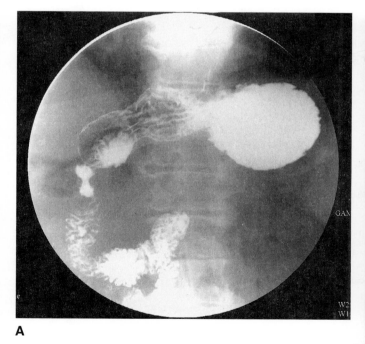

A

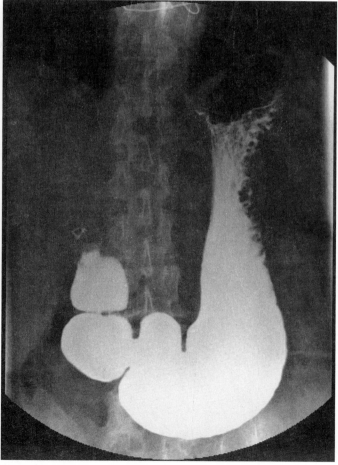

B

Figure 5–3. **A.** Example of hypersthenic stomach.
B. Example of asthenic stomach. (Courtesy of Stamford
Hospital, Department of Radiology.)

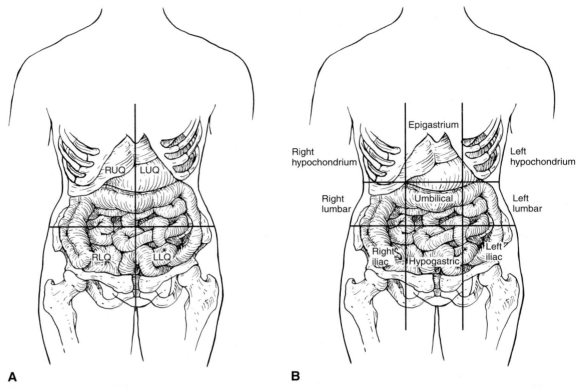

Figure 5–4. A. Four quadrants of the abdomen, illustrating position of major organs. **B.** Nine regions of the abdomen, illustrating position of major organs.

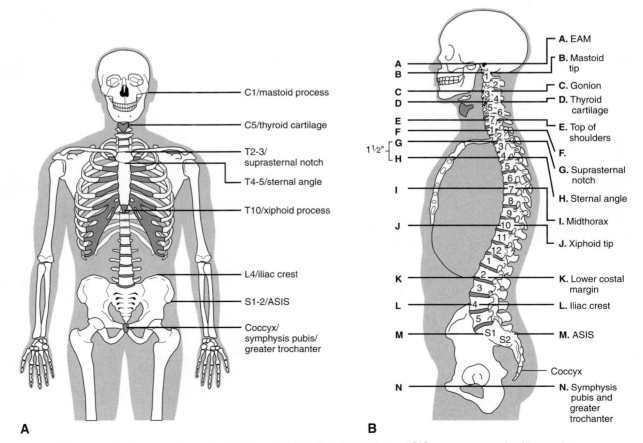

Figure 5–5. Body surface landmarks and localization points. ASIS, anterosuperior iliac spine.

descriptions and methodology always employ these terms. It is essential that the student radiographer knows and understands these body planes and their relationship to each other.

- *Midsagittal or median sagittal plane (MSP):* Divides the body into left and right halves
- *Sagittal plane:* Any plane parallel to the MSP
- *Midcoronal plane (MCP):* Divides the body into anterior and posterior halves
- *Coronal plane:* Any plane parallel to the MCP
- *Transverse/horizontal plane:* Perpendicular to the MSP and MCP, and divides the body axially into superior and inferior portions

BODY HABITUS

Patients come in all shapes and sizes. The term *body habitus* refers to the body's physical appearance (Fig. 5–2). Variations in body habitus have a significant effect on the *shape* and *location* of organs, and can affect their function. It is essential that radiographers are knowledgeable about the characteristics of each body habitus and how to use that knowledge when imaging patients of varying body habitus.

The *hypersthenic* habitus is the largest of the four types. This type is large and heavy; the chest area is short, with a high diaphragm. The viscera (stomach, gallbladder, and colon) are usually high and lateral.

The *sthenic* habitus is defined as an average athletic build. Compared to the hypersthenic, it is characterized by a longer chest and abdomen, with viscera located more medially.

The *hyposthenic* habitus is a slighter version of the sthenic—less athletic/strong.

The *asthenic* habitus is the smallest/slightest of the four types. This habitus can be frail-looking, slender, and slight. The chest is long and the abdominal viscera are located quite low and medial.

Vertebra(e)		Localization Point
Cervical region	C1	Mastoid process
	C5	Thyroid cartilage (Adam's apple)
	C7	Vertebra prominens
Thoracic region	T2–3	Suprasternal (jugular) notch
	T4–5	Sternal angle
	T7–8	Inferior angle of scapula
	T9	Xiphoid (ensiform) process
	T10	Xiphoid tip
Lumbar region	T12–L3	Kidneys
	L1	Transpyloric plane
	L3	Inferior costal margin
	L3–4	Umbilicus
	L4	Iliac crest
Sacral and coccygeal regions	S1–2	Anterosuperior iliac spine (ASIS)
	Coccyx	Symphysis pubis and greater trochanter

Positioning Terminology

Radiographic position
Refers to body's physical position, e.g., recumbent, erect, prone, supine, Trendelenburg, etc.

Radiographic projection
Describes the path of the CR, e.g., PA (CR enters posteriorly, exits anteriorly)

Radiographic view
Describes the body part as seen by the IR, e.g., palmar view of the hand; infrequently used

General Terminology
1. Recumbent/lying down in any position
   - lying on back, face up = *supine*
   - lying on abdomen, face down = *prone*
   - supine, prone, or lateral, using horizontal CR = *decubitus*
2. Erect/upright/standing or sitting up
   - facing the IR = *anterior position*
   - with back toward IR = *posterior position*
3. Oblique position—erect or recumbent
   - *RAO/Right Anterior Oblique:* body rotated, with right anterior aspect nearest the IR
   - *LAO/Left Anterior Oblique:* body rotated, with left anterior aspect nearest the IR
   - *RPO/Right Posterior Oblique:* body rotated, with right posterior aspect nearest the IR
   - *LPO/Left Posterior Oblique:* body rotated, with left posterior aspect nearest the IR

Figure 5–6. Standard terminology provides descriptions and interpretation of accepted radiologic positioning language. (*continued*)

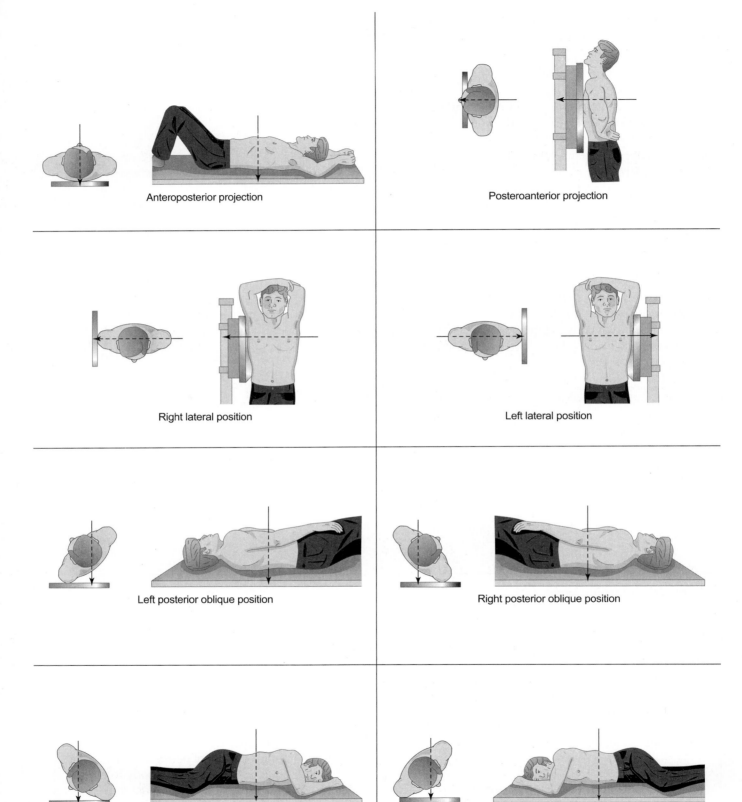

Anteroposterior projection

Posteroanterior projection

Right lateral position

Left lateral position

Left posterior oblique position

Right posterior oblique position

Left anterior oblique position

Right anterior oblique position

Figure 5–6. (*Continued*)

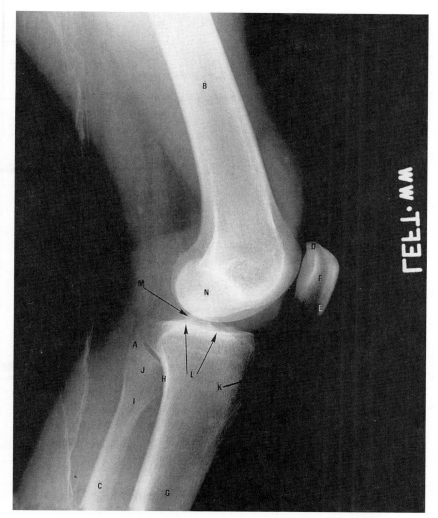

Figure 5–7. *Horizontal beam lateral* projection of the knee performed in supine position on a patient with multiple injuries. A horizontal ("cross-table") x-ray beam was used to reduce discomfort and risk of further injury. Observe the bedsheet artifact from the mattress pad beneath the patient. Use this radiograph to *review the skeletal anatomy* of the knee and correctly identify the lettered parts. A, styloid process of fibula; B, femur; C, fibula; D, patella—base; E, patella—apex; F, patella—body; G, tibia; H, proximal tibiofibular articulation; I, neck of fibula; J, head of fibula; K, tibial tuberosity; L, tibial plateau; M, intercondylar eminence; N, femoral condyle. (Courtesy of Stamford Hospital, Department of Radiology.)

SURFACE LANDMARKS AND LOCALIZATION POINTS

A number of surface anatomic points and particular vertebral levels are effectively used in radiographic positioning (Fig. 5–5A and 5–5B). Knowledge of these relationships can improve patient-positioning accuracy and accuracy of central ray entry/exit points.

SKELETAL MOTION TERMINOLOGY

- *Supination:* Turning of the body or arm so that the palm faces forward, with the thumb away from midline of the body

- *Pronation:* Turning of the body or arm so that the palm faces backward, with the thumb toward midline of the body
- *Abduction:* Movement of a part away from the body's MSP
- *Adduction:* Movement of a part toward the body's MSP
- *Flexion:* Bending motion of an articulation, decreasing the angle between associated bones
- *Extension:* Bending motion of an articulation, increasing the angle between associated bones
- *Eversion:* A turning outward or lateral motion of an articulation, sometimes with external tension or stress applied
- *Inversion:* A turning inward or medial motion of an articulation, sometimes with external tension or stress applied
- *Rotation:* Movement of a part about its central or long axis
- *Circumduction:* Movement of a limb that produces circular motion; circumscribes a small area at its proximal end and a wide area at the distal end

PRELIMINARY STEPS AND PROCEDURAL GUIDELINES

The following are steps and procedures that help ensure high-quality patient care and diagnostic radiographs:

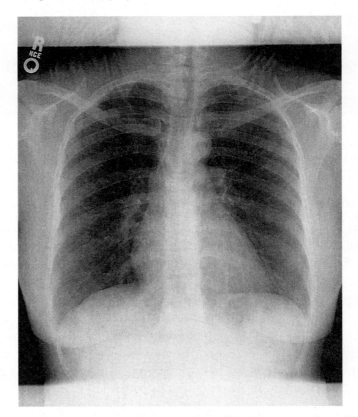

Figure 5–8. The posteroanterior projection of the chest is well positioned and exposed, but observe the braids of hair that extend past the neck and superimpose on the pulmonary apices. Braided hair should be pinned up or otherwise removed from superimposition on thoracic structures. (Courtesy of Stamford Hospital, Department of Radiology.)

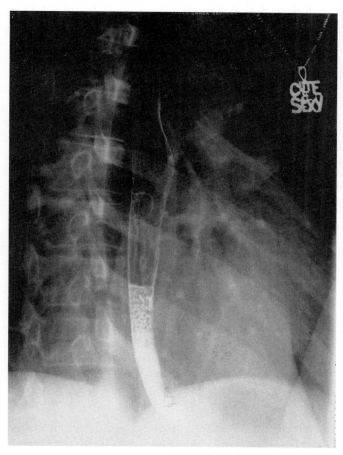

Figure 5–9. Left posterior oblique image of the esophagus with a jewelry artifact near the area of interest. The patient must remove clothing and other objects, such as jewelry, from the area to be examined before donning the dressing gown. (Courtesy of Stamford Hospital, Department of Radiology.)

1. *Read the request carefully*, noting the type of examination, condition of the patient, and mode of travel. (Make mental notes of any modifications or accessory equipment that may be required.)

2. *Prepare the radiographic department*. Be certain that the x-ray room is neat and orderly with a clean x-ray table and a fresh pillowcase. All accessories needed for the examination should be in the department before bringing in the patient.

3. *Identify* the correct patient, quickly evaluating any special needs; *introduce* yourself and establish rapport en route to the radiographic department, *being careful not to discuss confidential issues within earshot of others.*

4. *Instruct* the patient to change into a dressing gown (if necessary), removing appropriate clothing and objects (e.g., jewelry, dentures, and braided hair) that may cast *artifacts* within the area of interest (Figs. 5–8 and 5–9).

5. Speak in a well-modulated voice, give a clear and succinct *explanation* of the procedure, and address any questions or concerns of the patient. Obtain a short pertinent *patient history* of why the examination

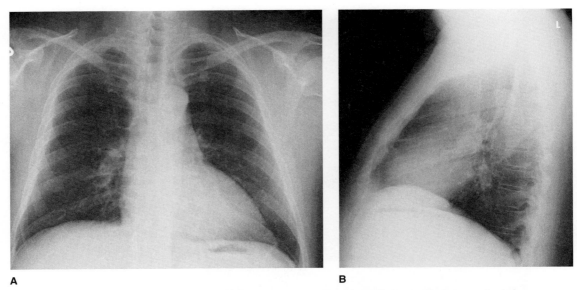

A   **B**

Figure 5–10. A *minimum of two projections*, at right angles to each other, is the usual minimum requirement for radiographic studies. Side-to-side (*left/right*) relationships are demonstrated in the *frontal* projection (**A**), whereas anterior/posterior relationships are seen in the *lateral* projection (**B**). This is especially important in localizing foreign bodies and tumors, and demonstrating fracture displacement or alignment. (Courtesy of Conrad P. Ehrlich, MD.)

has been requested. The radiographer should explain that a number of different positions may be needed to evaluate the area of interest and may require *palpation* of bony landmarks and instructions to turn into various positions.

6. Radiography of most structures *usually requires a minimum of two projections*, usually at right angles to each other. Side-to-side (left/right) relationships are demonstrated in the *frontal* projection (Fig. 5–10A), whereas anterior/posterior relationships are seen in the *lateral* projection (Fig. 5–10B). This is especially important in localizing foreign bodies and tumors, and demonstrating fracture displacement or alignment.

7. It is customary and economical to use the smallest size image receptor that will include all the necessary information. Therefore, the smallest possible anatomic area (consistent with a diagnostic examination) will be irradiated to keep patient dose to a minimum.

8. In radiography of the long bones, every effort should be made to *include both articulations* associated with the injured bone, but it is essential to include at least the articulation nearest the injury.

9. To ensure accurate diagnosis, supplemental radiographs of any anatomic part may be required, for example *oblique*, *axial*, *tangential*, *erect*, or *decubitus*. Exposure factors must be correctly adjusted for each change of position.

10. Each image must be accurately *labeled* with patient information such as *name* or *identification number*, *institution name*, *date of examination*, and *side marker*. Other information may be included according to institution policy.

IMMOBILIZATION AND RESPIRATION

Motion obliterates recorded detail; thus, it is essential that the radiographer be able to reduce patient motion as much as possible. Several means can be employed to reduce motion unsharpness, but good *patient communication* is the most important because it is required before any other means can be effective.

The single most important way to reduce *involuntary* motion is to use the *shortest possible exposure time*. Various types of *immobilization devices* can also be used to effectively reduce motion. Motion from muscular tremors as a result of anxiety or pain is involuntary and can be greatly minimized with good communication, a carefully placed positioning sponge or sandbag, and the use of the shortest exposure time possible.

Suspension of patient respiration for parts other than the extremities is an effective means of reducing *voluntary* motion; patient understanding and cooperation is required, thus making good *communication* the *most effective means of reducing voluntary motion*. The phase of respiration on which the exposure is made can be essential to the diagnostic quality of the radiographic image. Chest radiography, for example normally requires that the exposure be made on inspiration (the second inspiration for better filling of the lungs). Most abdominal examinations are exposed on expiration. The phase of respiration on which the exposure is made can also make a significant difference in the resulting radiographic density (discussed in Part IV).

MODIFIED AND ADDITIONAL PROJECTIONS

Additional projections/positions are often required in order to demonstrate the structure(s) of interest. Since human bodies are not identical and pathologic processes often unpredictable, routine protocols occasionally require supplemental images.

If a patient is unable to assume or maintain the routine position used for a particular examination, the radiographer should be capable of modifying it to provide the required information. This is often a good measure of the radiographer's skill. Skillful maneuvering of the x-ray tube and correct placement of the image receptor can often yield excellent images of an anatomic part difficult or impossible to manipulate.

It is not within the radiographer's scope of practice to supply additional unrequested images, but the radiographer should advise the physician of other positions or modifications that may provide better visualization of the affected area.

COMPREHENSION CHECK

Congratulations! You have completed your review of this chapter. If you are able to answer the following group of comprehensive questions, you can feel confident that you have mastered this section. You are then ready to go on to "Registry-type" questions that follow. For greatest success, do not go to these multiple-choice questions without first completing the short-answer questions below.

1. Discuss how knowledge of anatomy and pathologic conditions relates to positioning skills (p. 77, 81).

2. Identify the sagittal and midsagittal, coronal and midcoronal, and transverse (horizontal) planes; describe their relationship to each other (p. 78, 81).

3. Identify the four types of body habitus and list physical characteristics of each (p. 78).

4. Name, identify, and describe the quadrants and nine regions of the abdomen (p. 80).

5. Identify surface anatomic localization points and their corresponding vertebrae (p. 81).

6. Define and identify various skeletal movement terms (p. 83, 84).

7. Discuss the importance of establishing an orderly sequence of preparation for performing radiologic examinations (p. 85, 86).

8. Explain the importance of obtaining two images at right angles to each other for most radiologic examinations (p. 86).

9. Discuss the inclusion of articulations in radiography of the extremities (p. 86).

10. List the information that must be included on the radiographic image (p. 86).

11. What is the most effective means of reducing *voluntary* and *involuntary* motion? (p. 87).

12. Why/When might the radiographer be required to modify the routine projections? (p. 87)

CHAPTER REVIEW QUESTIONS

1. The plane that passes vertically through the body dividing it into left and right halves is termed the:
   - (A) Midsagittal plane
   - (B) Midcoronal plane
   - (C) Sagittal plane
   - (D) Transverse plane

2. The position of the asthenic gallbladder, as compared to the position of the sthenic gallbladder, is more:
   - (A) Superior and lateral
   - (B) Superior and medial
   - (C) Inferior and lateral
   - (D) Inferior and medial

3. What is the relationship between the midsagittal and midcoronal planes?
   - (A) Parallel
   - (B) Perpendicular
   - (C) 45 degrees
   - (D) 70 degrees

4. With the patient recumbent and head positioned at a level lower than the feet, the patient is said to be in the:
   - (A) Trendelenburg position
   - (B) Fowler position
   - (C) Decubitus position
   - (D) Sims position

5. Prior to x-ray examinations of the skull and cervical spine, the patient should remove:
   1. Dentures
   2. Earrings
   3. Necklaces
   - (A) 1 only
   - (B) 1 and 2 only
   - (C) 2 and 3 only
   - (D) 1, 2, and 3

6. Image identification markers should include:
   1. Patient's name and/or ID number
   2. Date
   3. A right or left marker
   - (A) 1 only
   - (B) 1 and 2 only
   - (C) 1 and 3 only
   - (D) 1, 2, and 3

7. The radiographer should be able to:
   1. Take a short patient history prior to the examination
   2. Modify routine protocol to obtain similar images in patients unable to move
   3. Evaluate patient condition and needs
   - (A) 1 only
   - (B) 1 and 2 only
   - (C) 1 and 3 only
   - (D) 1, 2, and 3

8. The best way to control voluntary motion is:
   - (A) Immobilization
   - (B) Careful explanation
   - (C) Short exposure time
   - (D) Physical restraint

9. Before bringing the patient into the radiographic room the radiographer should:
   1. Be certain that the x-ray room is clean and orderly
   2. Check that all necessary accessories are available in the room
   3. Check that x-ray table is clean and pillowcases are fresh
   - (A) 1 only
   - (B) 1 and 2 only
   - (C) 2 and 3 only
   - (D) 1, 2, and 3

10. The lower portion of the costal margin is approximately at the same level as that of the:
    - (A) Midthorax
    - (B) Umbilicus
    - (C) Xiphoid tip
    - (D) Third lumbar vertebra

Answers and Explanations

1. (A) The *midsagittal* (or median sagittal) plane passes vertically through the midline of the body, dividing it into left and right halves. Any plane parallel to the MSP is termed a *sagittal* plane. *The midcoronal plane is perpendicular to the MSP* and divides the body into anterior and posterior halves. A *transverse* plane passes across the body, also perpendicular to a sagittal plane. These planes, especially the MSP, are very important reference points in radiographic positioning.

2. (D) The position, shape, and motility of various organs can differ greatly from one body habitus to another. The position of the diaphragm, lungs, stomach, gallbladder, and large and small intestines vary greatly with body habitus. The individuals with small extreme habitus (*asthenic*) have structures *lower* and *more medial*, whereas these structures in individuals of the large extreme habitus (*hypersthenic*) have structures *high* and *lateral* (Figs. 5–2 and 5–3).

3. (B) The *midsagittal* plane passes vertically through the midline of the body, dividing it into left and right halves. Any plane parallel to the MSP is termed a *sagittal* plane. The *midcoronal* plane is *perpendicular* to the MSP and divides the body into anterior and posterior halves. The *transverse* plane passes across the body, also *perpendicular* to a sagittal plane. These planes, especially the MSP, are very important reference points in radiographic positioning.

4. (A) When the patient is recumbent with his or her head *lower* than the feet, the patient is said to be in the *Trendelenburg* position. In the *Fowler* position, the patient's head is positioned *higher* than his or her feet. The *decubitus* position is used to describe the patient as recumbent (prone, supine, or lateral) with the central ray directed horizontally. The *Sims* position is the left anterior oblique position assumed for enema tip insertion.

5. (D) The patient must remove any metallic objects if he or she is within the area of interest. Dentures, earrings, necklaces, and braided hair can obscure bony details in the skull or cervical spine. The radiographer must be certain that the patient's belongings are cared for properly and returned following the examination (Figs. 5–8 and 5–9).

6. (D) Correct and complete patient information on every radiograph is of paramount importance. Each radiographic image must be accurately labeled with such patient information as *name* or *identification number*, *institution name*, *date of examination*, and *side marker*. Other information may be included according to institution policy.

7. (D) The acquisition of pertinent *clinical history* is one of the most valuable contributions to the diagnostic process. Because the diagnostic radiologist rarely has the opportunity to speak with the patient, this is a crucial responsibility of the radiographer. As the radiographer obtains a brief pertinent clinical history, the radiographer also *assesses the patient's condition* by observing and listening. To provide safe and effective care, the radiographer must be able to assess the severity of a traumatized patient's injury, his or her degree of motor control, the need for support equipment, or radiographic accessories. In patients too injured or ill to move, the radiographer should be capable of modifying routine positions to obtain images with the required anatomic part/information.

8. (B) Motion obliterates recorded detail; it is therefore essential that the radiographer be able to reduce patient motion as much as possible. Even the slightest movement can cause severe degradation of the radiographic image. Suspension of patient respiration for parts other than the extremities is an effective means of reducing *voluntary* motion; patient understanding and cooperation is required, thus making good *communication* the most effective means of reducing *voluntary* motion. The single most important way to reduce *involuntary* motion is to use the *shortest possible exposure time*.

9. (D) A patient will naturally feel more comfortable and confident if brought into a clean, orderly x-ray room that has been prepared appropriately for the examination to be performed. A disorderly, untidy room and a disorganized radiographer hardly inspire confidence; more likely, they will increase anxiety and apprehension.

10. (D) Surface landmarks, prominences, and depressions are useful to the radiographer in locating anatomic structures not visible externally. The *lower costal margin* is at about the same level as L3. The *umbilicus* is at the same approximate level as the L3 to L4 interspace. The *xiphoid tip* is at about the same level as T10. The fourth lumbar vertebra is at the same approximate level as the *iliac crest*.

Image Procedures: Anatomy, Positioning, and Pathology | 6

THE SKELETAL SYSTEM

Radiographers frequently deal with bone imaging and are required to have a good knowledge of osteology. *Osteology* is the study of bones; there are 206 bones in the human adult skeleton. The skeletal system of bones serves many functions. Bones form the *supporting* framework of the body. Bones serve as a *reservoir for minerals* such as calcium and phosphorus, storing them until the body requires them. The design of the skeletal framework is such that it provides *protection* to underlying critical and delicate structures. Most bones have prominences and/or depressions that have either *articular* or *attachment* functions; that is, they provide a surface for articular (joint) formation or serve as attachment for muscles, providing leverage for movement. Bone marrow, particularly red, is important in the production of blood cells—a process called *hematopoiesis*.

Bone tissue, or *osseous* (*os* = bone) tissue, is a specialized type of dense connective tissue. This tissue consists of bone cells (*osteocytes*) embedded in a nonliving matrix composed of calcium and collagen fibers. There are two types of osseous tissue: *cancellous* (spongy) and *compact* (hard, cortical) (Fig. 6–1A).

The structural unit of *compact* bone tissue is the haversian (osteon) system. One haversian system, or osteon, consists of a central haversian canal surrounded by concentric cylinders of osteocytes within the calcium matrix.

Cancellous, or spongy, bone tissue has a reticular or latticework-type structure. This network of lattice-like bone is referred to as *trabeculae*. These trabeculae form little spaces/septa filled with red bone marrow.

The site of close approximation of two or more bones is an *articulation*, or *joint*. The study of bony articulations is termed *arthrology*. There are three classifications of bony articulations. *Synarthrotic* joints are *immovable*; since fibrous tissue connects the bony contiguous surfaces, they are also described as *fibrous* articulations. The sutures of the cranium are examples of synarthrotic joints. *Amphiarthrotic* joints, also described as *cartilaginous*, are *partially* movable. The intervertebral joints (between

> **Functions of Skeletal System**
>
> - Support
> - Reservoir for minerals
> - Muscle attachment/movement
> - Protection
> - Hematopoiesis

> **Bone Tissue Types**
>
> - Cortical (hard, compact)
> - Cancellous (spongy)

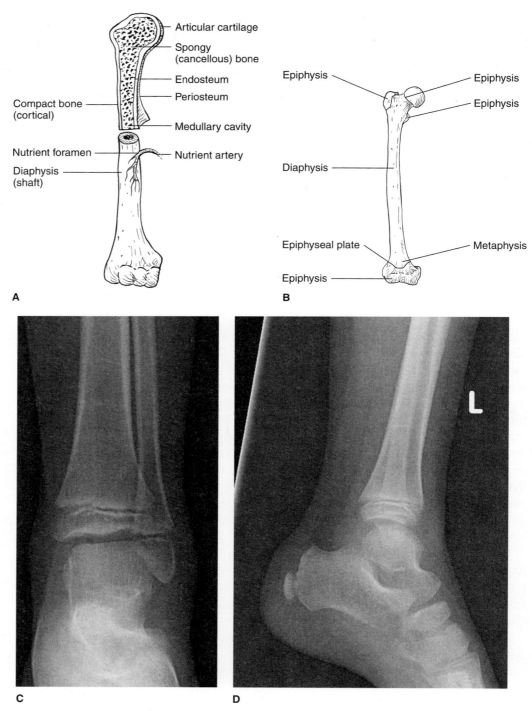

Figure 6–1. (A) and (B). Characteristics and ossification centers of long bones. (C) and (D) demonstrate epiphyseal plates of distal tibia and fibula (C) and calcaneal tuberosity (D). (Courtesy of Stamford Hospital, Department of Radiology.)

vertebral bodies) and the symphysis pubis are examples of amphiarthrotic joints. *Diarthrotic* joints, also described as *synovial*, are *freely movable*. The majority of human articulations are the diarthrotic/synovial type, and there are several *types* of diarthrotic articulations (their names describe their movements). The following list identifies types of diarthrotic joints, describes their movement(s), and gives examples of each:

Gliding (plane)

- The simplest motion, least movement, smooth/sliding motion
- Intercarpal and intertarsal joints, acromioclavicular, and costovertebral joints

Pivot (trochoid)

- Permits rotation around a single axis
- Proximal radioulnar joint and atlantoaxial joint

Hinge (ginglymus)

- Permits flexion and extension
- Elbow, interphalangeal joints, knee, and ankle

Ball and socket (spheroid)

- Permits flexion, extension, adduction, abduction, rotation, and circumduction with more motion distally and less proximally
- Shoulder and hip

Condyloid (ellipsoid)

- Permits flexion, extension, abduction, adduction, and circumduction (no rotation)
- Radiocarpal joint and metacarpophalangeal joints (2–5)

Saddle (sellar)

- Permits flexion, extension, adduction, adduction, and circumduction (no rotation)
- First carpometacarpal joint (thumb)

Arthritis is defined as inflammation of a joint; it is a common affliction often accompanied by pain, swelling, stiffness, and/or deformity. It always involves damage to articular cartilage, but the causes are numerous; that is, there are many types of arthritis. The most common type of arthritis is *osteoarthritis*, or *degenerative arthritis*. The incidence of osteoarthritis increases with age, but is not considered a normal part of aging.

The term *osteoporosis* describes a condition characterized by loss of bone mass, predisposing bones to fracture. Throughout life, healthy bone undergoes growth and resorption—at appropriate times and in appropriate places, as the bones adapt themselves to muscular activity, growth, mechanical pressures, etc. In osteoporosis, this remodeling fails to occur normally and more bone is resorbed than is replaced; thus, the skeleton loses strength as a result of demineralization. *Risk factors* for osteoporosis include being female, postmenopausal, Caucasian or Asian, having a small skeletal frame, a family history of osteoporosis, a sedentary lifestyle, and others.

Articular Classifications

Category	Structure	Function
Synarthrosis	Fibrous	Immovable
Amphiarthrosis	Cartilaginous	Partially moveable
Diarthrosis	Synovial	Freely moveable

THE APPENDICULAR SKELETON

The *appendicular* skeleton (Fig. 6–2; unshaded areas) consists of the *extremities* (appendages or limbs), the arms, legs, and the shoulder and pelvic girdles. Most of these bones serve as *attachment* for muscles, thereby creating leverage for movement.

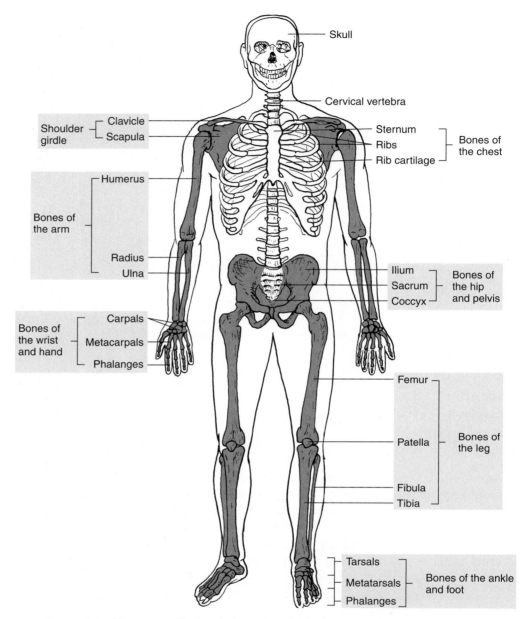

Figure 6–2. The *appendicular* skeleton (unshaded); the *axial* skeleton (shaded).

Bones are classified as *long, short, flat,* and *irregular*. Many of the bones comprising the extremities are long bones. Long bones have a *shaft* (or *body*) and *two extremities* (proximal and distal ends). The shaft (or *diaphysis*) (Fig. 6–1B) of long bones is the *primary ossification center* during bone development. It is composed of compact tissue and covered with a membrane called *periosteum*.

Within the shaft of a long bone is the *medullary cavity*, containing *bone marrow* and lined by a membrane called *endosteum*. In adults, yellow marrow occupies the shaft, and red marrow is found within the *proximal* and *distal* extremities of long bones.

The *secondary ossification center*, the *epiphysis* (Fig. 6–1B, C, and D), is separated from the diaphysis in early life by a layer of cartilage, the *epiphyseal plate*. As bone growth takes place, the epiphysis becomes part of the larger portion of bone. The epiphyseal plate disappears, but

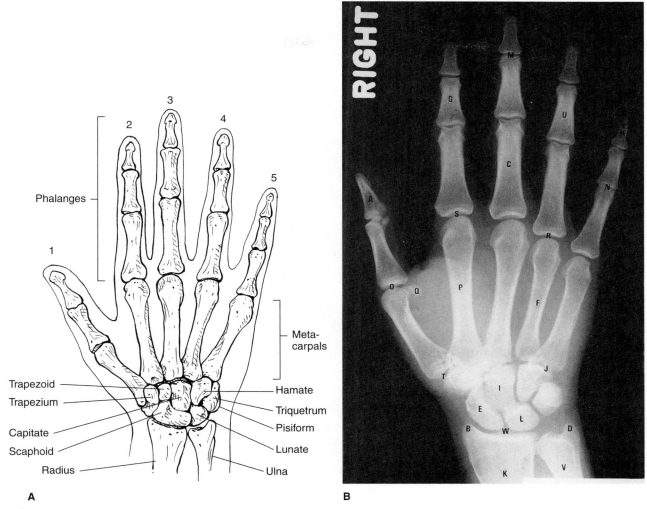

Figure 6–3. **(A)** Posterior aspect of the right hand and wrist. **(B)** PA projection of the hand; note that an oblique projection of the first metacarpal and phalanges is obtained. A, distal phalanx, first digit (thumb/pollex); B, radial styloid process; C, proximal phalanx, third digit; D, ulnar styloid process; E, scaphoid; F, shaft, fourth metacarpal; G, middle phalanx, second digit; H, distal phalanx, fifth digit; I, capitate/os magnum; J, carpometacarpal articulation; K, distal radius; L, lunate/semilunar; M, distal interphalangeal joint, third digit; N, proximal interphalangeal joint, fifth digit; O, metacarpophalangeal joint, first digit (thumb/pollex); P, shaft, first metacarpal; Q, sesamoid bone; R, metacarpophalangeal joint, fourth digit; S, metacarpophalangeal joint, second digit; T, carpometacarpal joint (base of first metacarpal with trapezium/saddle joint); U, middle phalanx, fourth digit; V, distal ulna; W, radiocarpal (wrist) joint. (Courtesy of Bob Wong, RT.)

a characteristic line remains and is thereafter recognizable as the *epiphyseal line*. The articular ends of bones are covered with *articular (hyaline) cartilage*.

Upper Extremity and Shoulder Girdle

Hand, Fingers, and Thumb. The hand (Fig. 6–3A and B) is composed of five *metacarpal* bones, corresponding to the palm of the hand, and 14 *phalanges*, the fingers. The second through fifth fingers have three phalanges each (proximal, middle, and distal rows) and the first finger, or thumb (*pollex*), has two phalanges (proximal and distal). The rows of phalanges articulate with each other forming proximal and distal *interphalangeal joints* (IPJ) (hinge/ginglymus joints), permitting flexion and extension motion.

The *bases* of the proximal row of phalanges articulate with the heads of the metacarpals to form the (condyloid/ellipsoid) *metacarpophalangeal joints* (MCP), which permit flexion and extension, abduction and adduction, and circumduction. The bases of the metacarpals articulate with each other and the distal row of carpals at the *carpometacarpal joints*. The first carpometacarpal joint (thumb) is a saddle/sellar joint, permitting flexion and extension, abduction and adduction, and circumduction.

Wrist. The wrist (Fig. 6–3A and B) is composed of eight carpal bones arranged in two rows (proximal and distal). The proximal row consists of, from lateral to medial, the *scaphoid*, the *lunate/semilunar*, the *triangular/triquetrum*, and the *pisiform*. The distal row, from lateral to medial, consists of the *trapezium/greater multangular*, the *trapezoid/lesser multangular*, the *capitate/os magnum* (the largest carpal), and the *hamate/unciform* (which has a hook-like process, the hamulus).

The joints of the wrist include the articulations between the carpals (*intercarpal joints*), which provide a gliding motion, and the *radio-carpal joint* (between the distal radius and scaphoid), which provides flexion and extension as well as abduction and adduction.

Traumatic *fractures* of the hand and wrist are common. Fractures of the distal (ungual) phalangeal tufts usually occur from crushing injuries, such as being closed in car doors or struck with a hammer. Metacarpal and phalangeal fractures are common fractures and are often accompanied by dislocations of the MCP and IPJ. In fractures of the metacarpal shafts, the bony fragments are usually displaced posteriorly and can be rotated as well.

Scaphoid fractures are common and often result from a fall onto an outstretched hand. Symptoms include tenderness and swelling over the "anatomic snuff box." Delayed or nonunion of these fractures occurs due to damage to the nutrient artery during the initial trauma event. Special projections can be used to detect scaphoid fractures.

Carpal tunnel syndrome is a painful condition of the wrist. If the anteroposterior (AP) diameter of the tunnel is diminished, the *median nerve*, which passes through the tunnel, is impinged upon, thus causing severe pain and disability in the affected hand and wrist. Surgical decompression of the carpal tunnel can provide significant relief.

Forearm. The bones of the forearm, or antebrachium (Fig. 6–4), consist of the *radius* (laterally) and *ulna* (medially), which participate in the formation of the elbow joint proximally and the wrist distally.

The distal ulna presents a *head* and *styloid process* and articulates with the distal radius to form the *distal radioulnar joint*. The ulna is slender distally but enlarges proximally and becomes the larger of the two bones of the forearm. At its proximal end, the ulna presents the *olecranon process* (posteriorly) and *coronoid process* (anteriorly) that are joined by a large articular cavity, the *semilunar*, or *trochlear*, *notch*. The coronoid process fits into the humeral *coronoid fossa* during flexion and the olecranon process fits into the humeral *olecranon fossa* during extension. Just distal and lateral to the semilunar notch is the *radial notch*, which provides articulation for the radial head to form the *proximal radioulnar articulation*. Just as the ulna is the principal bone associated with the elbow joint, the radius is the principal bone associated with the wrist joint. Fracture of the distal radius is one of the most common skeletal fractures.

Carpal Bones

Proximal Row, Lateral to Medial
- Scaphoid
- Lunate/semilunar
- Triangular/triquetrum
- Pisiform

Distal Row, Lateral to Medial
- Trapezium/greater multangular
- Trapezoid/lesser multangular
- Capitate/os magnum
- Hamate/unciform

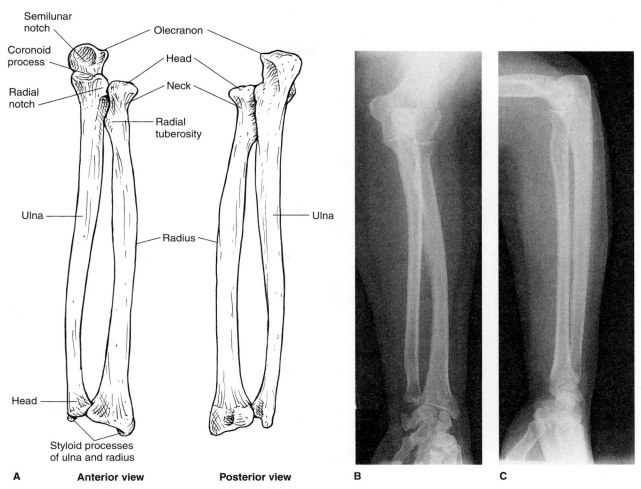

Figure 6–4. **(A)** Bones of the left forearm. **(B)** AP projection right forearm. Arm in extension with *hand supinated* to avoid overlap of radius and ulna. **(C)** Lateral projection right forearm. Elbow flexed 90 degree with hand and wrist in lateral position; humeral epicondyles are superimposed. (Courtesy of Conrad P. Ehrlich, M.D.)

The distal radius presents a *styloid process* laterally; the *ulnar notch* is located medially, helping form the *distal radioulnar articulation*. The distal surface of the radius (carpal articular surface) is smooth for accommodating the scaphoid and lunate in the formation of the *radiocarpal joint*. The proximal radius has a cylindrical *head* with a medial surface that participates in the *proximal radioulnar joint*; its superior surface articulates with the capitulum of the humerus.

Fractures of the radial head and neck frequently result from a fall onto an outstretched hand with the elbow *partially flexed*. Severe fractures are often accompanied by posterior dislocation of the elbow joint. *Colles fractures* of the distal radius usually result from a fall onto an outstretched hand with the arm *extended*. Fractures of the ulnar styloid occur usually due to hyperabduction of the hand.

Elbow. The distal *humerus* articulates with the radius and ulna to form the elbow joint (Figs. 6–5 and 6–6). The lateral aspect of the distal humerus presents a raised, smooth, rounded surface, the *capitulum*, which articulates with the superior surface of the *radial head* (Fig. 6–4).

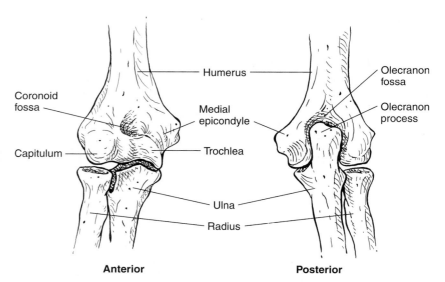

Figure 6–5. Anterior and posterior aspects of the bony articulation of the right elbow joint.

The *trochlea* is on the medial aspect of the distal humerus and articulates with the semilunar notch of the ulna. Just proximal to the capitulum and trochlea are the *lateral* and *medial epicondyles*; the medial is more prominent and palpable. The *olecranon fossa* is found on the posterior distal humerus and functions to accommodate the olecranon process with the elbow in extension (Fig. 6–7).

Lateral epicondylitis ("tennis elbow") is a painful condition caused by prolonged rotary motion of the forearm. *Dislocations* of the elbow can also occur from a fall onto an outstretched hand. One or both bones of the forearm can be involved; a posterior dislocation is the most common and is frequently accompanied by a radial head fracture. Rotation of the radial head can be palpated on the posterior lateral surface of the elbow, with elbow in extension.

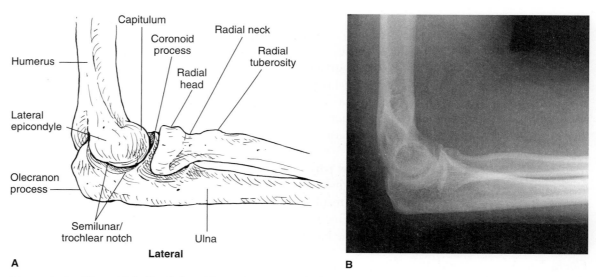

Figure 6–6. **(A)** and **(B)**. Medial and lateral aspects of the bony articulation of the right elbow joint. (Courtesy of Stamford Hospital, Department of Radiology.)

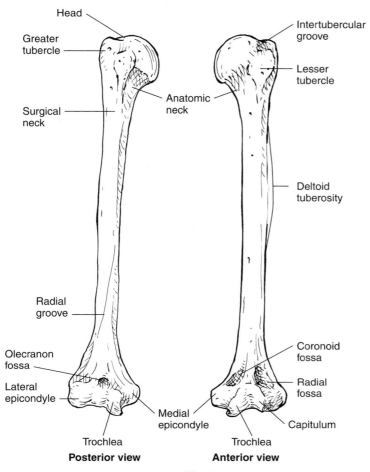

Figure 6–7. The humerus.

There are three important *fat pads* associated with the elbow. The anterior fat pad is comprised of the (superimposed) radial and coronoid fat pads located just anterior to the distal humerus. The supinator fat pad/stripe is located at the proximal radius just anterior to the head, neck, and tuberosity. These fat pads can be demonstrated in the 90 lateral projection of the normal elbow, and become more apparent if injury causes fluid buildup to displace them. The posterior fat pad is located within the olecranon fossa at the distal posterior humerus and is not radiographically visible in the normal elbow; its radiographic visualization is a good indication of injury/pathology.

Humerus. The *deltoid tuberosity* is found on the anterolateral surface of the humeral shaft. The large, round *humeral head* is covered with hyaline cartilage and articulates with the scapula's glenoid fossa. The *anatomical neck* marks the location of the fused epiphyseal plate in the adult and separates the head and metaphysis. The proximal humerus presents two protuberances on its anterior surface; the *greater tubercle* is lateral and the *lesser tubercle* is medial. Between the tubercles is the *bicipital*, or *intertubercular, groove*. The humeral shaft narrows just distal to the tubercles at the point of the *surgical neck*.

Humeral *fractures* usually involve the surgical neck or the distal end of the bone. Fractures of the proximal humerus usually find the shaft

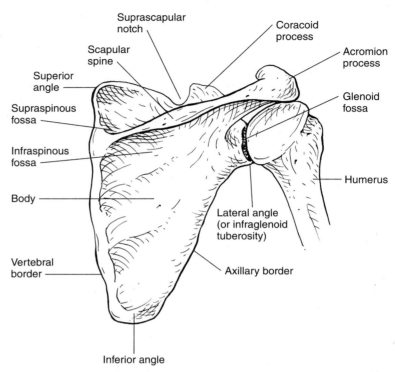

Figure 6–8. Posterior aspect of the right scapula.

Articulation Summary: Upper Extremity and Shoulder Girdle

- Acromioclavicular
- Sternoclavicular
- Shoulder (glenohumeral)
- Elbow—three articulations:
  - b/w humeral trochlea and semilunar/trochlear notch
  - b/w capitulum and radial head
  - proximal radioulnar joint
- Distal radioulnar
- Radiocarpal (distal radius with scaphoid and lunate)
- Intercarpal
- Carpometacarpal
- Metacarpophalangeal
- Interphalangeal

impacted into the head. Fractures of the greater tubercle can result from a direct blow or as a consequence of pull from the associated muscles.

Shoulder. The shoulder (pectoral) girdle consists of the scapulae (Fig. 6–8) and clavicles (Fig. 6–9). The S-shaped *clavicle* ("collar bone") is usually the last bone to completely ossify, at approximately 21 years, and is one of the most commonly fractured bones in young people. Its

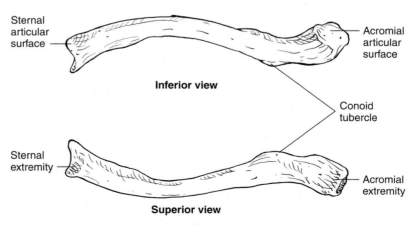

Figure 6–9. The right clavicle.

medial end articulates with the sternum to form the *sternoclavicular joint*; the clavicle articulates laterally with the scapula's acromion process, forming the *acromioclavicular joint*. Superior *dislocation* of the *acromioclavicular joint* is a common athletic injury.

The *scapula* is a flat bone, shaped like a triangle, with a *costal surface* that lies against the upper posterior rib cage. The scapula has a *superior* (or medial) *angle,* a *superior border*, a *medial* (or *vertebral*) *border*, a *lateral* (or *axillary*) *border*, and an *inferior angle*, or *apex*. Its superior border presents a *scapular notch* and, projecting anteriorly just medial to the humeral head is the palpable *coracoid process*. The *scapular spine* divides the posterior surface into a *supraspinatus fossa* and *infraspinatus fossa*; the *acromion process* is the lateral extension of the scapular spine. The *glenoid fossa* is on the lateral aspect of the scapula and, with its articulation with the humeral head, forms the (ball and socket) *shoulder joint*. The shoulder *labrum* is a ring of fibrocartilage that extends from the rim of the glenoid cavity, acting like a suction cup and deepening the joint "socket".

The *rotator cuff* is largely responsible for abduction and internal rotation movements and is composed of the supraspinatus, infraspinatus, teres minor, deltoid, and subscapularis muscles. *Rotator cuff injuries* are a result of acute injury or chronic wear and tear. The articular capsule of the shoulder is loose, permitting a great range of movement but also making it susceptible to dislocation.

Positioning. Positioning of the upper extremity and shoulder girdle requires a thorough knowledge of the anatomy concerned as well as an awareness of possible pathologic conditions and their impact on positioning limitations and technical factors.

Radiopaque objects such as watches, bracelets, and rings should be removed whenever possible because they can obscure important anatomic information. The patient must be instructed regarding the importance of remaining still, and immobilization devices such as sandbags or sponges should be used as required. The shortest possible exposure time should be employed, especially when involuntary motion can be a problem, as with trauma, pediatric, or geriatric patients.

Most upper extremity examinations are more comfortably and accurately positioned with the patient seated at the end of the x-ray table, with the forearm and elbow resting on the x-ray table. Most can be performed tabletop (i.e., without a Bucky grid); the humerus sometimes requires a grid, while the shoulder, clavicle, and scapula usually do. *Suspended respiration* is suggested for radiography of the proximal portion of the upper extremity and shoulder girdle. Patients must be adequately *shielded*.

The use of just a few important bony landmarks and their correct placement with respect to the IR are the basis for accurate positioning. Rotation of the arm and placement of the humeral epicondyles in correct relationship to the IR is the foundation of forearm, elbow, and shoulder positioning. Positioning of the wrist and hand uses the radial and ulnar styloid processes, bending maneuvers (i.e., radial and ulnar flexion), MCP, and IPJ.

Tables 6-1 through 6-11 provide a summary of routine and frequently performed special positions/projections of the upper extremity and shoulder girdle:

List of Abbreviations and Symbols Used in the Tables

AC	Acromioclavicular
∠	Angle
ASIS	Anterior superior iliac spine
AP	Anteroposterior
≈	Approximately (about)
b/w	Between
CMC	Carpometacarpal joint
CR	Central ray
°	Degrees
dist	Distal
EAM	External auditory meatus
fx	Fracture
>	Greater than
"	Inches
IOML	Infraorbitomeatal line
IPJ	Interphalangeal joint
IR	Image receptor
jt	Joint
kV	Kilovoltage
lat	Lateral
LAO	Left anterior oblique
LPO	Left posterior oblique
<	Less than
MCP	Metacarpophalangeal joint
MTP	Metatarsophalangeal joint
MSP	Midsagittal plane
m/w	Midway
OID	Object-to-image receptor distance
Obl	Oblique
OML	Orbitomeatal line
∥	Parallel to
⊥	Perpendicular to
PA	Posteroanterior
proj	Projection
prox	Proximal
RAO	Right anterior oblique
RPO	Right posterior oblique
SID	Source-to-image receptor distance
w/	With
w/o	Without

TABLE 6–1. The Hand

Hand	Position of Part	Central Ray Directed	Structures Included/ Best Seen
PA	Pronated, elbow flexed 90 degree, fingers extended and slightly spread	⊥ 3rd MCP	PA carpals, metacarpals, phalanges, and their articulations (Fig. 6–10A); provides oblique proj of thumb
This projection is often performed to include the wrist for *bone age* studies; 30 degree SID is sometimes recommended, with the CR entering the head of the third metacarpal.			
Oblique	Prone, elbow flexed 90 degree, hand and forearm obliqued 45 degree	⊥ 3rd MCP	Oblique proj carpals, metacarpals, phalanges, and their articulations; use of a "finger sponge" places jts ‖ IR and opens jt spaces (Fig. 6–10B)
Lateral *in extension*	Elbow flexed 90 degree fingers extended, wrist, lateral, ulnar surface down	⊥ MCPs	*Superimposed* carpals, metacarpals, phalanges, and their articulations; decrease 10 kV for foreign body
Lateral *in flexion*	Elbow flexed 90 degree, fingers slightly flexed and superimposed	⊥ MCPs	Superimposed carpals, metacarpals, phalanges, and their articulations; *shows ant/post fx displacement*
A *fan lateral* with the fingers separated is often performed to better visualize each phalange.			

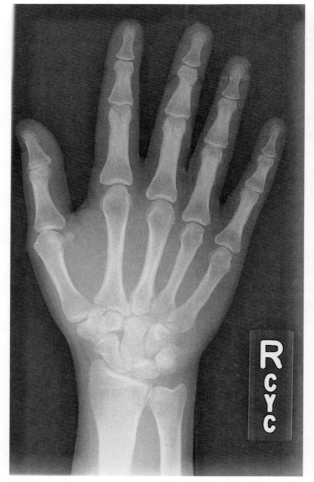 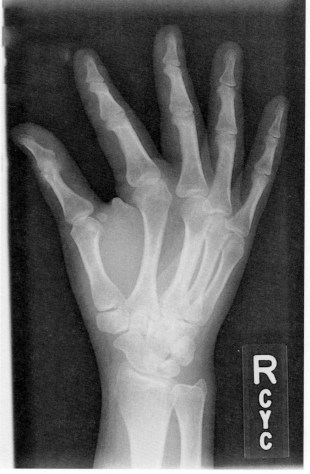

A   B

Figure 6–10. PA and oblique projections of the hand. (Courtesy of Stamford Hospital, Department of Radiology.)

TABLE 6–2. The Thumb

Thumb	Position of Part	Central Ray Directed	Structures Included/Best Seen
AP	Dorsal surface adjacent and ∥ IR	⊥ MCP	
PA	Palmar surface ∥ IR, *OID is increased*	⊥ MCP	
Lateral	Lat surface adjacent to IR, fingers elevated and resting on sponge	⊥ MCP	AP, PA, or lat projection of first digit; *three articulations should be seen:* CMC, MCP, and IPJ

TABLE 6–3. The Fingers

Fingers	Position of Part	Central Ray Directed	Structures Included/Best Seen
PA	Hand pronated and fingers extended, elbow flexed 90 degree	⊥ proximal IPJ	PA proximal, middle, and dist phalanges (usually entire hand examined in this position)
Lateral	Elbow flexed 90 degree, forearm lat, finger(s) extended and ∥ IR	⊥ proximal IPJ	Lat of proximal, middle, and distal phalanges; second and third digits are done *radial side down*; fourth and fifth digits are done *ulnar side down*

TABLE 6–4. The Wrist

Wrist	Position of Part	Central Ray Directed	Structures Included/Best Seen
PA	Hand pronated w/ MCPs slightly flexed and elbow flexed 90 degree	⊥ midcarpal	PA carpals, prox region metacarpals, dist radius, and ulna (Fig. 6–11A); *flexion of MCPs reduces OID*
Lateral	Elbow flexed 90 degree, ulnar surface down, radius and ulna superimposed	⊥ midcarpal region	Lat carpals, superimposed prox metacarpals and dist radius and ulna (Fig. 6–11B)
PA *semi-pronation oblique*	Elbow flexed 90 degree, wrist 45 degree w/ IR, ulnar surface down	⊥ midcarpal region	Useful for scaphoid and for other *lat carpals* (trapezium and trapezoid) *and their interspaces* (Fig. 6–11C)
AP *semiarm supination oblique*	Extended, 45 degree w/ IR, ulnar surface down	⊥ midcarpal	Useful for pisiform, region triquetrum, and hamate *medial carpals and their interspaces*
PA ulnar flexion/deviation	Position as PA wrist, evert hand (laterally) without moving forearm	⊥ scaphoid	Scaphoid and other lat carpal interspaces; *reduces foreshortening of scaphoid*
PA radial flexion/deviation	Position as PA wrist, move elbow toward body w/o moving hand/wrist	⊥ midcarpal region	*Medial* carpal interspaces (Fig. 6–12)
Scaphoid (*Stecher*)	Forearm (a) pronated *or* (b) pronated and elevated 20 degree	(a) 20 degree toward elbow entering scaphoid *or* (b) ⊥ scaphoid	Scaphoid w/o *foreshortening* and self-superimposition
Carpal canal (*Gaynor–Hart*)	Hyperextend wrist w/palm vertical	25–30 degree into long axis of hand	Carpal canal (*tunnel*); trapezium, scaphoid, capitate, triquetrum, and pisiform

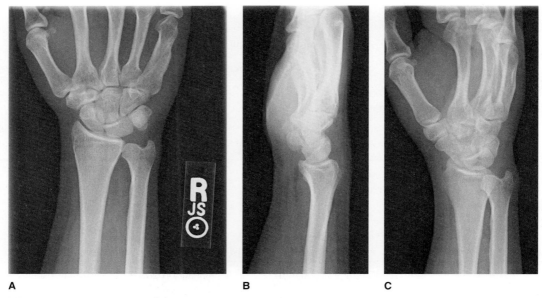

A   **B**   **C**

Figure 6–11. (**A**) PA projection of wrist. Flexion of the metacarpophalangeal joints reduces OID. (**B**) Lateral projection of the wrist. (**C**) Semipronation oblique projection of the wrist. (Courtesy of Conrad P. Ehrlich, MD)

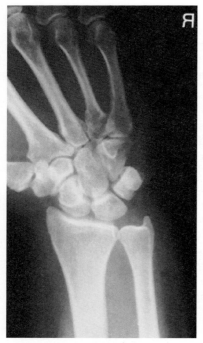

Figure 6–12. Radial flexion/ deviation maneuver of left wrist. Radial flexion/deviation is used to better demonstrate the medial carpals (pisiform, triangular, hamate, and medial aspect of capitate and lunate). (Courtesy of Stamford Hospital, Department of Radiology.)

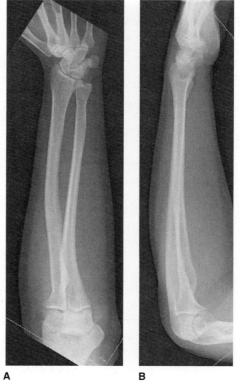

A   **B**

Figure 6–13. (**A**) AP projection of the forearm. The hand must be supinated to avoid overlap of the proximal radius and ulna. (**B**) Lateral projection of the forearm. Humerus should be on same plane as forearm to superimpose humeral epicondyles. (Courtesy of Conrad P. Ehrlich, MD)

TABLE 6–5. The Forearm

Forearm	Position of Part	Central Ray Directed	Structures Included/Best Seen
AP	Supinated and extended, epicondyles ‖ IR; *shoulder and elbow on same plane*	⊥ midforearm	AP radius and ulna, including wrist and elbow jts (Fig. 6–13A); *arm must be supinated to avoid overlap of radius and ulna*
Lateral	Elbow flexed 90 degree, epicondyles superimposed and ⊥ IR, hand lat; *shoulder and elbow on same plane*	⊥ midforearm	Radius and ulna superimposed distally, lat proj of radius and ulna, elbow and wrist jts (Fig. 6–13B)

TABLE 6–6. The Elbow

Elbow	Position of Part	Central Ray Directed	Structures Included/Best Seen
AP	Extended, supinated; epicondyles ‖ IR	⊥ elbow jt m/w b/w epicondyles	AP elbow jt (Fig. 6-14A), proximal radius and ulna, dist humerus; radial head and tuberosity partially superimposed on ulna

Note: An elbow in AP partial flexion, unable to be extended, requires two projections to achieve an AP elbow: (1) humerus is placed ‖ the IR (with elbow still in partial flexion) and the CR is ⊥ elbow jt; (2) forearm is placed ‖ the IR (with elbow still in partial flexion) and the CR is ⊥ elbow jt. Thus, an AP of the dist humerus and proximal forearm are obtained separately. (An AP with the CR directed through the flexed elbow demonstrates a "closed" jt space.)

Elbow	Position of Part	Central Ray Directed	Structures Included/Best Seen
Lateral	Flexed 90 degree, epicondyles ⊥ IR, forearm, and wrist lat	⊥ elbow jt at the epicondyles	Lat elbow jt, prox radius, and ulna and dist humerus; *radial head partially super imposed on ulna*; olecranon process in profile (Fig. 6–14B)
Internal (*medial*) oblique	Arm extended, palm down, epicondyles 45 degree to IR	⊥ elbow jt midway b/w epicondyles	Oblique elbow jt; *coronoid process in profile* (Fig. 6–14C)
External (*lateral*) oblique	Forearm extended and rotated laterally, radial surface down, epicondyles 45 degree to IR	⊥ elbow jt midway b/w epicondyles	Oblique elbow jt; *radial head, neck, and tuberosity free from superimposition* of ulna
Trauma axial lateral (*Coyle*)	(1) Elbow flexed 90 degree, hand pronated	(1) To elbow, at 45 degree *toward* shoulder	These replace lat and med obliques when patient unable to extend arm
	(2) Elbow flexed 80 degree, hand pronated	(2) *From* shoulder *to* elbow, at 45 degree	(1) For *radial head* (2) For *coronoid process*

TABLE 6–7. The Humerus

Humerus	Position of Part	Central Ray Directed	Structures Included/Best Seen
AP	Arm extended and supinated; epicondyles ⊥ IR	⊥ midhumerus	AP humerus, includes shoulder and elbow jts; *greater tubercle in profile*; epicondyles ‖ IR
Lateral	Elbow flexed 90 degree; epicondyles ‖ IR	⊥ midhumerus	Lat humerus including shoulder and elbow jts; *lesser tubercle in profile*; epicondyles superimposed and ⊥ IR

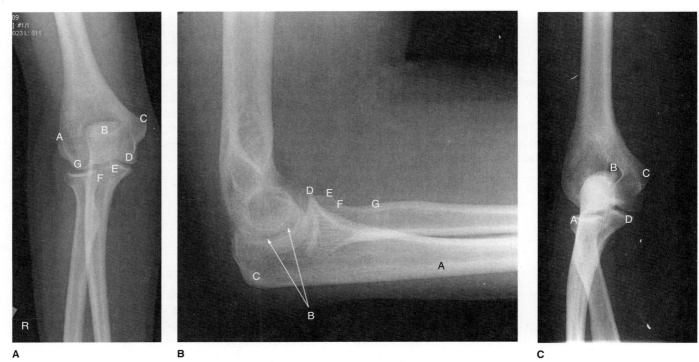

A   **B**   **C**

Figure 6–14. (**A**) AP projection of elbow; radial head and tuberosity has correct partial superimposition on ulna. A, lateral epicondyle; B, olecranon process; C, medial epicondyle; D, trochlea; E, coronoid process; F, proximal radioulnar articulation (or radial notch of ulna); G, capitulum. (Courtesy of Conrad P. Ehrlich, MD.) (**B**) Lateral projection elbow, elbow flexed 90 degree, and humeral epicondyles superimposed. A, shaft of ulna; B, semilunar/trochlear notch; C, olecranon process; D, coronoid process; E, radial head; F, radial neck; G, radial tuberosity. (**C**) Medial (internal) oblique view of elbow; the coronoid process is seen free of superimposition. A, radial head; B, olecranon fossa; C, medial epicondyle; D, coronoid process.(B and C Courtesy of Stamford Hospital, Department of Radiology.)

TABLE 6–8. The Shoulder

Shoulder	Position of Part	Central Ray Directed	Structures Included/Best Seen
AP *rotational projections*	Arm extended and (1) supinated, w/ epicondyles ‖ IR, (2) palm against thigh, epicondyles 45 degree to IR, and (3) elbow slightly flexed, back of hand against thigh	⊥ coracoid process	(1) External rotation: true AP humerus, shows greater tubercle in profile (Fig. 6–15A), (2) neutral position: good for calcific deposits, trauma, and (3) internal rotation: lat of humerus, shows lesser tubercle in profile

Note: In case of trauma, the humerus and shoulder must be examined in a *neutral* position to avoid unnecessary pain and additional injury.

Posterior oblique *Grashey Method*	Patient. RPO or LPO (erect or recumbent), MSP 35–45 degree to affected side; scapula ‖ IR border; suspendrespiration	⊥ 2″ medial and 2″ inferior to superior and lat shoulder	Glenohumeral jt and glenoid cavity (Fig. 6–15B)
Transthoracic lateral	Patient erect lat w/ affected surgical neck centered to IR; unaffected arm over head	Affected surgical neck	Lat shoulder and proximal humerus through thorax
PA oblique *scapular Y*	Affected shoulder centered with MCP 60 degree to IR	⊥ shoulder jt	Oblique shoulder; especially good for *demonstration of dislocations* (Fig. 6–16)
Inferosuperior (*non-trauma*)	Patient supine w/ shoulder elevated from table ≈2″, arm abducted 90 degree, in external rotation	Horizontally to axilla	Lat of prox humerus, glenohumeral jt; coracoid process and lesser tubercle in profile

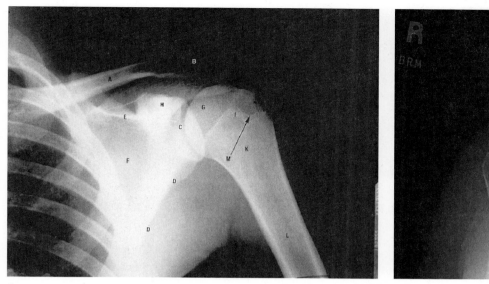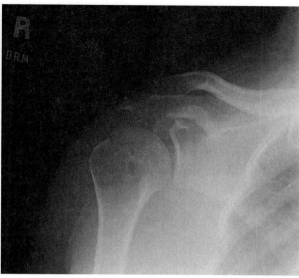

A   B

Figure 6–15. **(A)** Shoulder in external rotation places humerus in a true AP position and places the greater tubercle (J) in profile. A, shaft of clavicle; B, acromioclavicular joint; C, glenoid cavity; D, lateral/axillary border of scapula; E, scapular spine; F, body of scapula; G, head of humerus; H, coracoid process; I, lesser tubercle; J, greater tubercle; K, surgical neck of humerus; L, shaft of humerus; M, anatomical neck of humerus. (Courtesy of Bob Wong, RT.) **(B)** Posterior oblique (Grashey method) for glenoid cavity. (Courtesy of Stamford Hospital, Department of Radiology.)

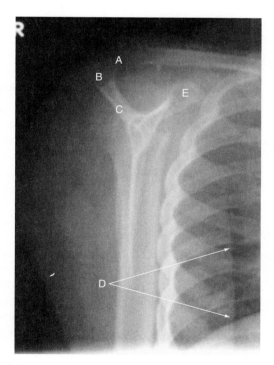

Figure 6–16. PA oblique projection; scapular Y view of the shoulder. Useful for demonstration of dislocations. Humeral head displaced inferior to coracoid process indicates *anterior dislocation*, while humeral head displaced inferior to acromion process indicates *posterior dislocation.* A, acromioclavicular joint; B, acromion process; C, scapular spine; D, medial/vertebral border of scapula; E, coracoid process. (Courtesy of Stamford Hospital, Department of Radiology.)

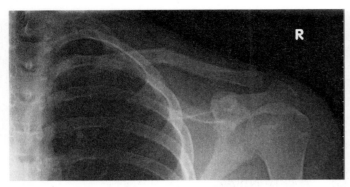
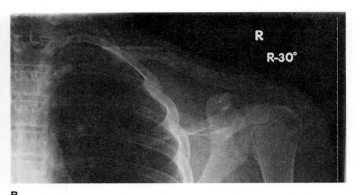

A   **B**

Figure 6–17. (**A**) AP projection of fractured clavicle. (**B**) AP axial projection of fractured clavicle, better illustrating extent of fracture. (Courtesy of Conrad P. Ehrlich, MD)

TABLE 6–9. The Clavicle

Clavicle	Position of Part	Central Ray Directed	Structures Included/Best Seen
PA or AP	Patient recumbent or erect; center affected clavicle to IR; less OID in PA projection	⊥ midshaft	Entire length of clavicle and articulations, best done PA erect or AP recumbent for patient comfort (Fig. 6–17A)
PA or AP axial	Patient PA or AP, affected clavicle centered to IR	To supraclavicular fossa 15–30 degree *caudad for PA*; *cephalad for AP*	Axial projection of clavicle; can demonstrate fxs not seen in direct PA or AP (Fig. 6–17B)

Note: PA best for optimum detail (less OID); erect PA or recumbent AP usually best for comfort (less discomfort to injured part).

TABLE 6–10. The Acromioclavicular Joints

Acromio–clavicular Joints	Position of Part	Central Ray Directed	Structures Included/Best Seen
AP	Patient AP erect, MSP to mid-IR, arms at sides (always bilateral for comparison). Two images are made in the same position: one w/o and one w/ *weights* (images must be properly identified)	⊥ midline at level of AC jts	AP projection of AC jt and soft tissues; demonstrates *dislocation/separation* when performed erect (see Fig. 6–39)

TABLE 6–11. The Scapula

Scapula	Position of Part	Central Ray Directed	Structures Included/Best Seen
AP	AP upright or recumbent; scapula centered w/ arm abducted and elbow flexed	⊥ midscapula, ≈2″ inferior to coracoid process	AP scapula with lat portion away from ribs; exposure may be made during quiet breathing to blur lung markings (see Fig. 6–18A)
Lateral (*anterior oblique*)	Erect PA 45–60 degree (Oblique w/ affected anterior side *toward* IR and (1) arm across chest for acromion and coracoid or (2) palpate scapular borders and rotate body to superimposed	⊥ to midvertebral border	Lat scapula, (1) acromion and coracoid processes, (2) superimposed vertebral and axillary borders (Fig. 6–18B) free of rib cage
Lateral (*posterior oblique*)	Recumbent oblique w/ affected posterior surface *away* from IR; palpate scapular borders and rotate patient till borders are superimposed	⊥ to mid axillary border	Lat scapula, medial and lateral scapular borders superimposed, and humerus away from scapula

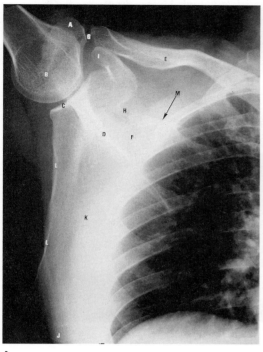
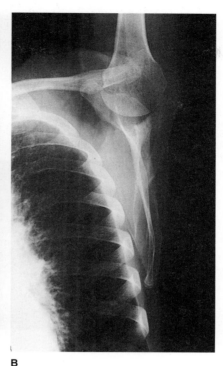

A   **B**

Figure 6–18. (A) AP projection of scapula. Note that arm abduction moves scapula away from rib cage, revealing a greater portion of the scapular body. A, acromion process; B, humeral head; C, glenoid fossa; D, scapular spine; E, clavicle (shaft); F, supraspinatus fossa; G, acromioclavicular articulation; H, scapular notch; I, coracoid process; J, inferior angle/apex of scapula; K, body/costal surface of scapula; L, axillary/lateral border scapula; M, superior border of scapula. (Courtesy of Bob Wong, RT.) (B) Lateral projection of scapula. It is taken with arm elevated and forearm resting on head. It demonstrates scapular body with vertebral and axillary borders exactly superimposed. (Courtesy of Stamford Hospital, Department of Radiology.)

Lower Extremity and Pelvis

Foot and Toes. The bones of the foot (Fig. 6–19A and B) include the 7 *tarsal bones*, 5 *metatarsal bones*, and 14 *phalanges*. The *calcaneus* (os calsis), or heel bone, is the largest tarsal. It serves as attachment for the Achilles tendon posteriorly, articulates anteriorly with the *cuboid bone*, presents three articular surfaces superiorly for its articulation with the *talus*, and has a prominent shelf on its anteromedial edge called the *sustentaculum tali*.

The inferior surface of the talus (*astragalus*) articulates with the superior calcaneus to form the three-faceted *subtalar joint*. The talus also articulates anteriorly with the navicular. Articulating anteriorly with the navicular are the three *cuneiform bones*: medial/first, intermediate/second, and lateral/third. The navicular articulates laterally with the cuboid.

Fractures of the calcaneus can occur, especially as a result of a fall from a height directly onto the heel; these fractures can be comminuted and impacted. The calcaneus can also be associated with painful *spur* formation.

Stress (fatigue, march) fractures can occur in the metatarsal shafts; x-ray examination can "miss" these fractures until callus appears during bony repair process. Phalangeal fractures are common and usually occur as a

Tarsal Bones

- Calcaneus/os calsis
- Talus/astragalus
- Navicular
- Cuboid
- First/medial cuneiform
- Second/intermediate cuneiform
- Third/lateral cuneiform

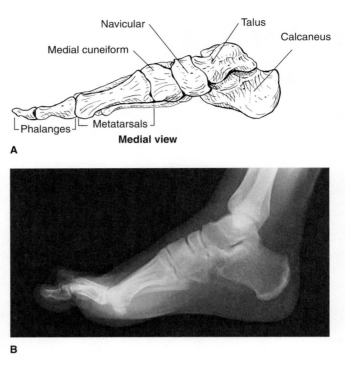

Figure 6–19. (A) Bones of the foot (medial view). **(B)** Mediolateral projection of the foot. (Courtesy of Conrad P. Ehrlich, MD)

result of a stubbing or crushing force. A common deformity of the first metatarsophalangeal joint is *hallux valgus*. The first ("great") toe, referred to as the *hallux*, slowly adducts (medially), resulting in an inflamed first metatarsophalangeal joint (*bunion*). The condition is relieved surgically.

The metatarsals and phalanges of the foot are similar to the metacarpals and phalanges of the hand. The bases of the fourth and fifth metatarsals articulate with the cuboid. The fifth (most lateral) metatarsal projects laterally and presents a large *tuberosity* at its base, making it susceptible to fracture. *Stress fractures* are common to the metatarsals (Fig. 6–19).

The *hallux* has *two* phalanges; the second through fifth toes have *three* phalanges each. The phalanges of the toes are shorter than those of the fingers. Stubbing- and crushing-type injuries are common causes of fractured phalanges. The articulations of the foot are named/numbered similarly to those of the hand.

Ankle. The ankle joint (*mortise*) is formed by the articulation of the talus and distal portions of the tibia and fibula (Fig. 6–20). The medial and lateral malleoli are the most frequently *fractured* components of the ankle joint; severe fractures can disrupt the integrity of the joint and lead to permanent instability and/or arthritis.

Lower Leg. The *tibia* and *fibula* (Fig. 6–21) compose the bones of the lower leg. The tibia is larger and is situated medially. It articulates superiorly with the femur and inferiorly with the talus, forming a portion of the ankle joint. The tibia consists of a shaft and two expanded extremities. Its distal extremity has a prominence, the *medial malleolus*, which also participates in the formation of the ankle *mortise*. The fibular notch provides articulation for the fibula to form the *distal tibiofibular joint*.

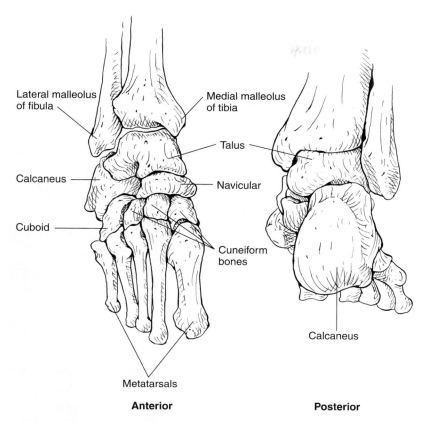

Figure 6–20. Ankle and foot: anterior and posterior views.

The proximal end of the tibia presents a *medial* and a *lateral condyle*, on whose *superior* surfaces there are facets for articulation with the femur. The articular facets form a smooth surface called the *tibial plateau*, which provides attachment for the cartilaginous *menisci* of the knee joint. Between the two articular surfaces is a raised prominence, the *intercondylar eminence* (*tibial spine*).

The proximal *anterior* surface of the tibia presents the *tibial tuberosity*, which provides attachment for the patellar ligament. *Osgood–Schlatter disease* is a chronic *epiphysitis* of the tibial tuberosity that occurs in some active young adults. Its symptoms include pain and tenderness, and it is manifested radiographically by bony separation at the epiphysis.

The fibula is the slender, lateral non–weight-bearing bone forming the lower leg; it also consists of a shaft and two expanded extremities. The bulbous *distal* end is the *lateral malleolus* (projects more distally than the medial), which helps form the ankle joint and has a facet for articulation with the tibia (*distal tibiofibular joint*). The expanded *proximal* portion of the fibula is the *head*, which articulates with the lateral tibial condyle, forming the *proximal tibiofibular joint*. A *styloid* process extends *superiorly* from the head of the fibula. The *neck* is the constricted portion just distal to the fibular head. The fibula is most commonly fractured at the malleolus, just above the ankle joint.

Knee. The knee is formed by the proximal tibia, the patella, and the distal femur, which articulate to form the *femorotibial* (hinge joint) and

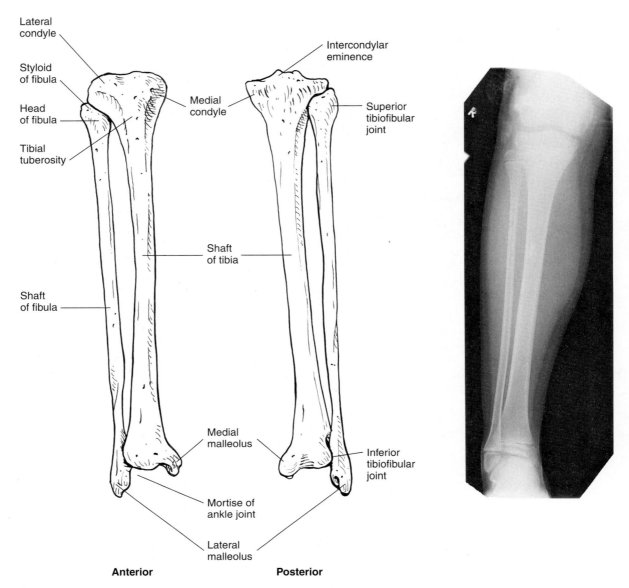

Lateral
condyle

Styloid
of fibula

Head
of fibula

Tibial
tuberosity

Intercondylar
eminence

Medial
condyle

Superior
tibiofibular
joint

Shaft
of fibula

Shaft
of tibia

Medial
malleolus

Inferior
tibiofibular
joint

Mortise of
ankle joint

Lateral
malleolus

Anterior   **Posterior**

Figure 6–21. Right tibia and fibula.

femoropatellar (gliding joint) joints. The distal posterior femur presents two large *medial* and *lateral condyles* separated by the deep *intercondyloid fossa*. Two small prominences, the *medial* and *lateral epicondyles*, are just superior to the condyles. The femoral and tibial condyles articulate to form the *femorotibial joint.*

Semilunar cartilages, the *menisci*, lie medially and laterally between these articulating bones and, together with the *cruciate* and *collateral ligaments*, help form the *articular capsule* of the knee (Fig. 6–22A).

The *patella* is a triangular bone with its *base* superior and *apex* inferior. The *patella* is the largest *sesamoid* bone and is attached to the tibial tuberosity by the patellar ligament and glides over the patellar surface of the distal femur (femoropatellar joint) during flexion and extension of the knee. Simple patellar fractures are usually *transverse* (Fig. 6–22B).

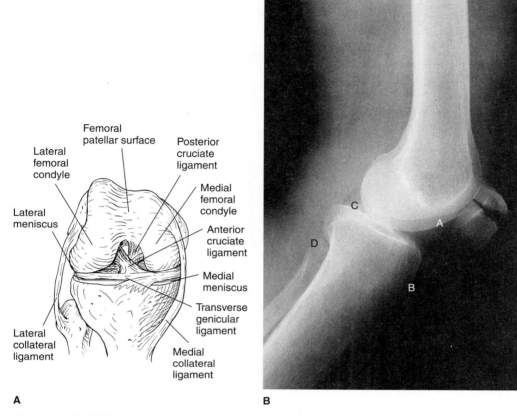

Femoral
patellar surface

Lateral
femoral
condyle

Posterior
cruciate
ligament

Medial
femoral
condyle

Lateral
meniscus

Anterior
cruciate
ligament

Medial
meniscus

Transverse
genicular
ligament

Lateral
collateral
ligament

Medial
collateral
ligament

A

B

Figure 6–22. **(A)** Ligaments of the knee joint. **(B)** The knee should not be flexed more than 10 degree when transverse fracture of patella is known or suspected; flexion can cause pain, fragment separation, and fracture complication. The CR can be angled 5 degree cephalad to superimpose the magnified medial femoral condyle on the lateral condyle and permit better visualization of the joint space; angulation was not employed in this projection and the joint space is obscured by the magnified medial femoral condyle. A, medial femoral condyle; B, tibial tuberosity; C, tibial plateau; D, head of fibula. (Courtesy of Stamford Hospital, Department of Radiology.)

Fractures of the patella can also be *stellate* or comminuted; the more complex fractures can require a patellectomy.

The congenital anomaly, *bipartite patella*, can be misinterpreted as a fracture. Just opposite the *patellar surface*, on the posterior distal femur, is the smooth *popliteal surface*, which accommodates the popliteal artery.

Femur. The *femur* (Fig. 6–23) is the longest and strongest bone in the body. The femoral *shaft* is bowed slightly anteriorly. The proximal end of the femur consists of a *head*, which is received by the *acetabulum* of the pelvis. The femoral head has a small notch, the *fovea capitis femoris*, for ligament attachment. The ligament of the femoral head, or *ligamentum teres*, connects the fovea capitis femoris to the acetabulum. The *femoral neck*, which joins the head and shaft, angles upward approximately 120 degree and forward (in *anteversion*) approximately 15 degree. The *greater* (lateral) and *lesser* (medial) *trochanters* are large processes on the posterior proximal femur. The greater trochanter is a prominent positioning landmark that lies in the same transverse plane as the public

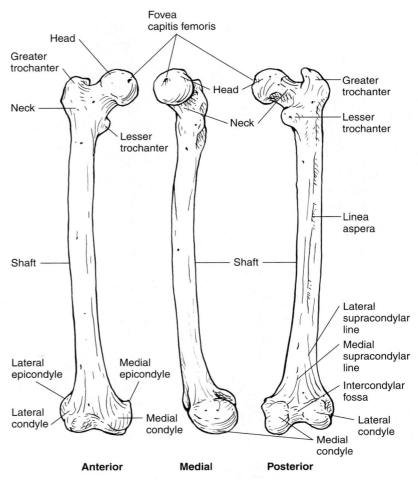

Figure 6–23. The right femur.

symphysis and coccyx. The (posterior) *intertrochanteric crest* runs obliquely between the trochanters; the (anterior) *intertrochanteric line* runs anteriorly parallel to the crest. The femoral shaft presents a long narrow ridge posteriorly called the *linea aspera*.

Its distal anterior portion presents the *patellar surface*—a triangular depression over which the patella glides during flexion.

The distal posterior surface presents the *popliteal surface*—a depression that houses the popliteal artery. The medial and lateral femoral condyles are very prominent posterior structures, and between them is the deep intercondyloid fossa. Just above the condyles are the medial and lateral femoral epicondyles.

The femoral neck is the most commonly *fractured* portion of the femur (Fig. 6–24). Fractures of the femoral shaft are usually the result of a direct blow; fracture *displacement* is dependent on muscular pull and traumatic impact. Dislocations of the hip joint are fairly uncommon because of the very strong pelvic and hip musculature. Disturbance of the fovea capitis femoris or disruption of the nutrient arteries supplying the femoral neck can result in *avascular necrosis* of the femoral head.

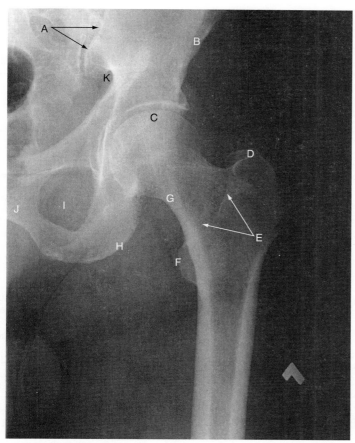

Figure 6–24. AP projection of the left hip. Leg is internally rotated, placing femoral neck parallel to the IR. A, sacroiliac joint; B, anterior inferior iliac spine; C, femoral head; D, greater trochanter; E, intertrochanteric crest; F, lesser trochanter; G, femoral neck; H, ischial tuberosity; I, obturator foramen; J, pubis; K, greater sciatic notch. (Courtesy of Stamford Hospital, Department of Radiology.)

Pelvis. *Pelvis* is the Latin word for a "basin" that is the pelvis was named for its shape. The pelvic girdle consists of two *innominate* (hip, or *coxal*) bones, one on each side of the sacrum. Each innominate bone consists of three fused bones: the *ilium, ischium,* and *pubis* (Fig. 6–25).

Parts of these three bones contribute to the formation of the *acetabulum* (Latin word for "little vinegar cup")—the socket articulation for the femoral head. The *labrum* is a ring of fibrocartilage along the outer rim of the acetabulum, which acts like a suction cup. Any tear or other injury to the labrum causes pain, clicking, or "catching" sensation.

The *ilia* are the large, superior bones whose medial auricular surfaces form the *sacroiliac joints* bilaterally. The broad, flat portion of each ilium is the *ala,* or wing; the upper part of the ala forms a ridge of bone called the *iliac crest,* which terminates in *anterior* and *posterior iliac spines.* The *arcuate line* of the ilium is a smooth rounded border on the internal surface of the ilium. It is immediately inferior to the *iliac fossa.*

The *ischium* forms the posteroinferior portion of the pelvis. The posterior part of the ischium forms the major portion of the *greater* and

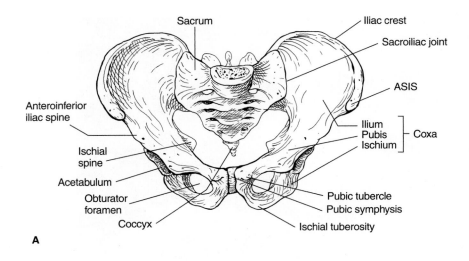

A

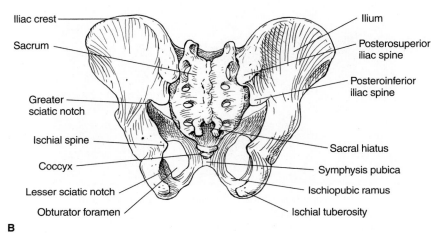

B

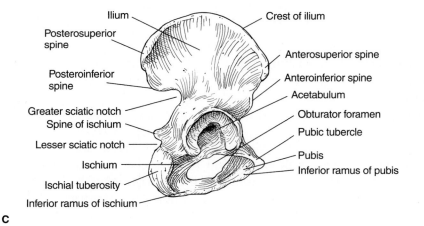

C

Figure 6–25. (**A**) The pelvis (anterior view). (**B**) The pelvic girdle (posterior view). (**C**) The right hip bone (lateral view), showing the acetabulum. (*continued*)

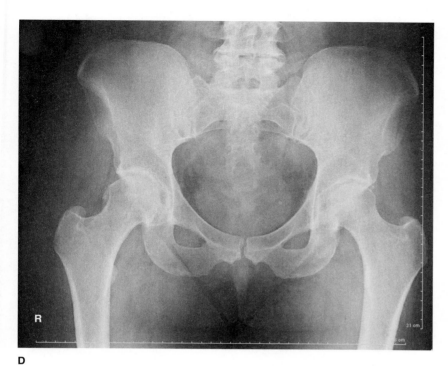

D

Figure 6–25. (*Continued*) **(D)** AP projection of the pelvis. The femoral necks are seen in their entirety: internal rotation of the feet/legs places them parallel to the IR. Note fractures of the public and ischial rami on the left. (Courtesy of Stamford Hospital, Department of Radiology.)

lesser sciatic notches separated by the *ischial spine*. The most inferior portion is the *ischial tuberosity*—a large, rough prominence that provides attachment for posterior thigh muscles. The inferior *ramus* of the ischium extends medially from the tuberosities to unite with the inferior ramus of the pubis.

The pubic bones form the anterior portion of the pelvis. Their bodies unite to form the *pubic symphysis*; just lateral to each superior margin of the symphysis are the prominent *pubic tubercles*. The superior pubic *ramus* fuses with the ilium and inferior pubic *ramus* with the ischium to form the large *obturator foramen*. The *pectineal line* of the pubis is a ridge on the superior rami of the pubic bones. In combination with the *arcuate*, it comprises the *iliopectineal line*.

The superior circumference of the *lesser pelvis* forms the *brim* of the pelvis, or the *pelvic inlet*. The *edge* of the inlet is known as the *pelvic brim*. The terms are often used interchangeably.

Pelvic fractures can cause disturbance of the urinary bladder or urethra; an *intravenous urogram* (IVU) or abdominopelvic CT may be required to diagnose any urinary leakage. The normal *female (gynecoid) pelvis* differs from the normal *male (android) pelvis* in that it is shallower and its bones are generally more delicate. The pelvic outlet is wider and more circular in the female; the ischial tuberosities and acetabula are further apart; and the angle formed by the pubic arch is also greater in the female. All these bony characteristics facilitate the birth process (Fig. 6–26).

Normal Male/Android Pelvis

- Narrower, more vertical
- Deeper from anterior to posterior
- Pubic angle less than 90 degree
- Pelvic inlet narrower and heart-shaped/round

Normal Female/Gynecoid Pelvis

- Wider, more angled toward horizontal
- Shallower from anterior to posterior
- Pubic angle greater than 90 degree
- Pelvic inlet larger and rounder

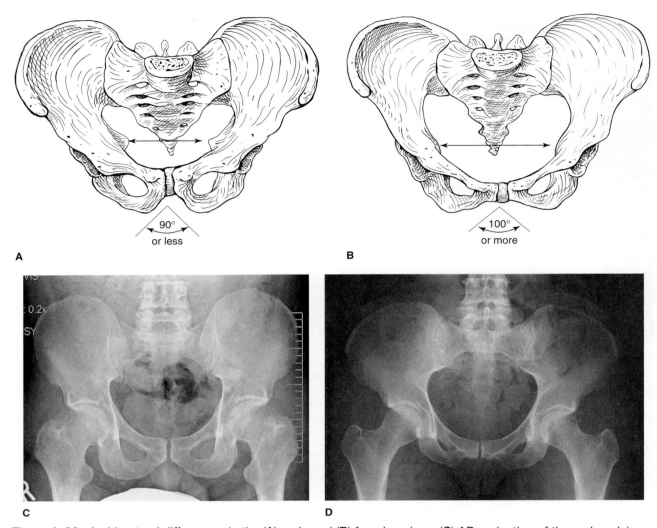

Figure 6–26. Architectural differences in the (**A**) male and (**B**) female pelves. (**C**) AP projection of the male pelvis. (**D**) AP projection of the female pelvis. Femoral necks are parallel to the IR and greater trochanters are seen in profile. (Courtesy of Stamford Hospital, Department of Radiology.)

Positioning. Positioning of the lower extremity and pelvis requires a thorough knowledge of the skeletal anatomy—an awareness of possible pathologic conditions and their impact on positioning and technical factors.

Clothing having radiopaque objects such as buttons, snaps, or zippers should be removed if possible. Bulky or bunched clothing can produce undesirable radiographic artifacts and should therefore be removed whenever possible and replaced with a hospital dressing gown. Elastic-waisted garments can contribute to nonuniform density on abdominal radiographs.

The patient must be instructed about the importance of remaining still, and immobilization devices such as radioparent sponges and sandbags should be used as required. The shortest possible exposure time should be employed, especially when involuntary motion is a potential problem.

Many lower extremity examinations can be performed tabletop (i.e., non-Bucky); the knee frequently requires a grid; and femur, hip, and pelvis almost always do. *Suspended respiration* is suggested for radiography of the proximal portion of the lower extremity and the pelvis. Patients must always be appropriately *shielded.*

Some of the lower leg projections can be performed either AP or PA, depending on the condition and comfort of the patient. Lateral projections can be easily obtained using a horizontal (cross-table lateral) beam when extremity or patient movement is contraindicated.

Tables 6-12 through 6-23 provide a summary of routine and frequently performed special positions/projections of the lower extremity and pelvis.

TABLE 6–12. The Foot

Foot	Position of Part	Central Ray Directed	Structures Included/Best Seen
Dorsoplantar (AP)	Knee flexed ≈45 degree, plantar surface on IR	⊥ or 10 degree toward heel to base of third metatarsal	Tarsals (except calcaneus and part of talus), metatarsals and phalanges with their articulations, in frontal projection
Note: A 10 degree posterior angulation may be used to better demonstrate jt spaces.			
Medial Oblique	Start as dorso-plantar, rotate medially 30 degree; plantar surface and IR form 30 degree angle.	⊥ base of third metatarsal	Most tarsals and metatarsals (except the most medial) and their articulations, sinus tarsi, tuberosity of fifth metatarsal (see Fig. 6–27)
Note: lateral oblique foot demonstrates interspaces b/w the first and second metatarsals and b/w the first and second cuneiforms.			
Lateral (*mediolateral or lateromedial*)	Patient lateral, patella ⊥ tabletop, foot slightly dorsiflexed w/plantar surface ‖ IR	⊥ metatarsal bases	Lateral foot and ankle jt; dist tibia and fibula; superimposed tarsals, tibia, and fibula (see Fig. 6–28)
Note: The lateral projection is more *accurately* obtained in the *lateromedial* (rather than mediolateral) position.			
Note: Lateral weight-bearing feet are occasionally requested to demonstrate the status of the *plantar arches.*			

TABLE 6–13. The Toes

Toes	Position of Part	Central Ray Directed	Structures Included/Best Seen
Dorsoplantar (*AP*)	Knee flexed ≈45 degree, plantar surface on IR	⊥ or 10 degree toward heel, to second MTP	Phalanges, their articulations and dist metatarsals in frontal projection (usually entire foot examined in this position)
Medial Oblique	Start as dorsoplantar, rotate medially 30–45 degree	⊥ 3rd MTP	Oblique projection of phalanges, and their articulations and dist metatarsals
Lateral	Turn to side that brings affected toe(s) closest to IR; unaffected toes may be taped back	⊥ proximal IPJ	Lateral projection of toe(s) and associated articulations
Sesamoids (*tangential*)	Patient prone, *foot* dorsiflexed 15–20 degree, toes dorsiflexed 15–20 degree and resting on cassette	⊥ or ≈10 degree caudad to IR to first MTP	Sesamoids in profile, free of superimposition

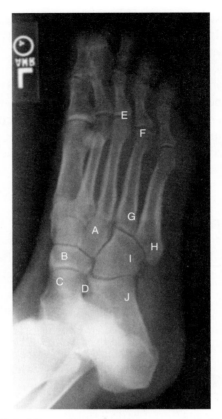

Figure 6–27. Medial oblique view of left foot demonstrates the articulations of the cuboid with the calcaneus, fourth and fifth metatarsals, and lateral cuneiform. The talonavicular articulation and sinus tarsi are also demonstrated. A, lateral/third cuneiform; B, navicular; C, talus/astragalus; D, sinus tarsi; E, 3rd metatarsophalangeal joint; F, head of 4th metatarsal; G, base of 4th metatarsal; H, base/tuberosity of 5th metatarsal; I, cuboid; J, calcaneus/os calsis. (Courtesy of Stamford Hospital, Department of Radiology.)

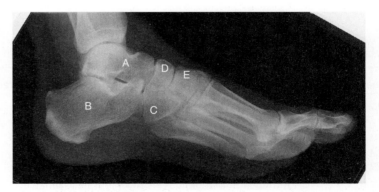

Figure 6–28. Lateral projection of foot demonstrates superimposed tarsals, metatarsals, and phalanges; a little more of the distal tibia and fibula should be visualized. A, talus/astragalus; B, calcaneus/os calsis; C, cuboid; D, navicular; E, medial/first cuneiform. (Courtesy of Stamford Hospital, Department of Radiology.)

TABLE 6–14. The Calcaneus

Calcaneus (Os Calcis)	Position of Part	Central Ray Directed	Structures Included/Best Seen
Plantodorsal Axial	Patient seated on table with leg extended, plantar surface ⊥ tabletop (immobilize w/ strip of tape/gauze held by patient)	40 degree *cephalad* to base of third metatarsal	Axial projection of calcaneus; trochlear process, sustentaculum tali, talocalcaneal jt (see Fig. 6–29)
Dorsoplantar Axial	Patient prone, plantar surface ⊥ tabletop; IR placed against plantar surface	40 degree *caudally* to level of base of second	Axial proj of calcaneus; trochlear process, sustentaculum tali, talocalcaneal jt
Lateral	Patient on affected ⊥ side, patella ⊥ tabletop, foot, and ankle lateral	midcal-caneus	Lateral calcaneus, talus, navicular, ankle jt, and sinus tarsi (see Fig. 6–30)

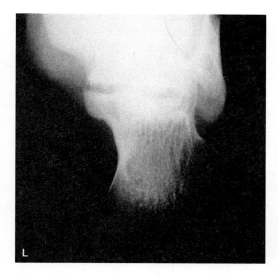

Figure 6–29. Plantodorsal projection of calcaneus; sustentaculum tali, trochlear process, and calcaneal tuberosity are well visualized. (Courtesy of Stamford Hospital, Department of Radiology.)

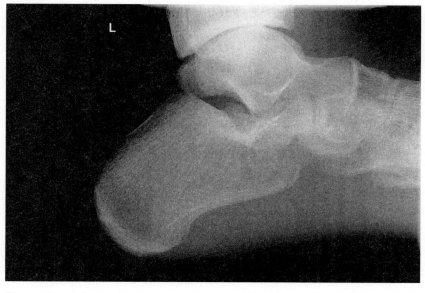

Figure 6–30. Lateral calcaneus; sinus tarsi is well visualized. (Courtesy of Stamford Hospital, Department of Radiology.)

TABLE 6–15. The Ankle

Ankle	Position of Part	Central Ray Directed	Structures Included/Best Seen
AP	Leg extended AP, plantar surface ⊥ IR	⊥ midway b/w malleoli through tibiotalar jt	AP ankle jt, dist tibia/fibula, talus (see Fig. 6–31A)
AP mortise; *medial obl*	Leg extended AP, rotated 15–20 degree medially until intermalleolar plane ⊥ IR	⊥ midway b/w malleoli, ⊥ intermalleolar plane	AP ankle mortise, talotibial and talofibular jts well seen; all three aspects of mortise jt seen in profile (see Fig. 6–31B)

Note: A 45 degree *medial oblique* is often used in ankle surveys. It demonstrates the distal tibia and fibula with perhaps some superimposition on the talus.

Lateral (*medio-lateral or lateromedial*)	Patient turned on to affected side, patella ⊥ tabletop, foot dorsiflexed (≈90 degree)	⊥ ankle jt	Lateral dist tibia/fibula, ankle jt, talus, calcaneus, navicular

Note: The lateral projection is more *accurately* obtained in the *lateromedial* (rather than mediolateral) position.

AP stress views	Leg extended, ankle true AP, foot dorsiflexed, plantar surface ⊥ • One exposure w/ jt in stressed inversion • One exposure w/ jt in stressed eversion	⊥ midway b/w malleoli	AP ankle jt in inversion and eversion—to evaluate jt separation or ligament tear

Note: If someone (e.g., the MD) must hold the ankle in position for the stress views, be certain that appropriate radiation precautions are taken.

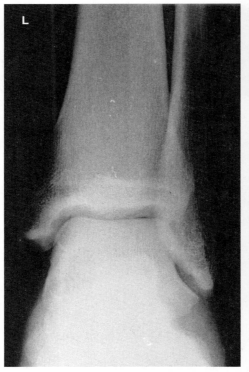
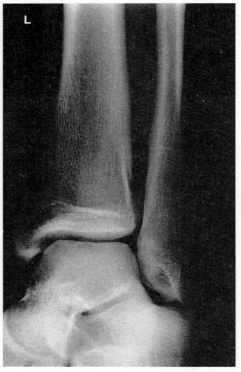

A   B

Figure 6–31. (A) AP projection of the ankle joint. (Courtesy of Stamford Hospital, Department of Radiology.) (B) The 15 degree to 20 degree medial oblique projection of the ankle is used to demonstrate the ankle mortise. An oblique projection of the distal tibia/fibula, proximal talus, and their articular surfaces is also demonstrated. (Courtesy of Stamford Hospital, Department of Radiology.)

TABLE 6–16. The Lower Leg (Tibia/Fibula)

Lower Leg (Tibia/ Fibula)	Position of Part	Central Ray Directed	Structures Included/Best Seen
AP	Leg extended AP, no pelvic rotation, foot dorsiflexed	⊥ midshaft tibia	AP lower leg, both jts should be included (Fig. 6–32A)
Lateral	Patient on affected side, patella ⊥ tabletop, ankle, and foot lat	⊥ midshaft	Lat tibia/fibula, both jts should be included (Fig. 6–32B)
AP Oblique (*medial and lat rotation*)	Leg extended w/ foot dorsiflexed; leg rotated 45 degree medially or laterally	⊥ midshaft tibia	Medial rotation shows proximal and dist tibiofibular articulations

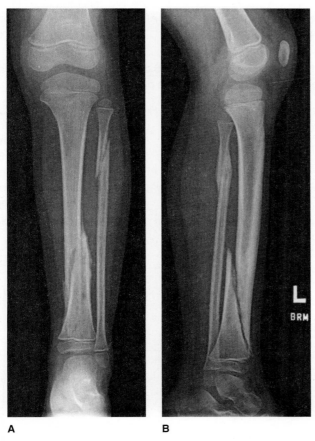

A   B

Figure 6–32. Demonstrates fractures and their degree of displacement **(A)** AP projection tibia and fibula. **(B)** Lateral projection tibia and fibula. Both joints should be included whenever possible. These images demonstrate how AP/PA projections demonstrate medial/lateral relationships and how lateral projections demonstrate anterior/posterior relationships. (Courtesy of Stamford Hospital, Department of Radiology.)

TABLE 6–17. The Knee

Knee	Position of Part	Central Ray Directed	Structures Included/Best Seen
AP	Leg extended AP, no pelvic rotation (leg may be rotated 3–5 degree internally)	To 1/2″ below patellar apex (knee jt); direction of CR depends on distance b/w ASIS and tabletop: up to 19 cm (thin pelvis) 3–5 degree caudad; 19–24 cm 0 degree CR; >24 cm (thick pelvis) 3–5 degree cephalad	AP knee jt, dist femur, and proximal tibia/fibula, patella seen through femur
Lateral	Patient on affected side, patella ⊥ tabletop, knee flexed 20–30 degree	5 degree cephalad to knee jt	Lat proj of knee and femoropatellar jts; superimposed femoral condyles; *knee should not be flexed > 10 degree with known or suspected patellar fx* (see Fig. 6–22B)
AP *weight bearing (bilateral)*	Patient AP erect against upright Bucky, weight evenly shared on legs	⊥ CR midway b/w knees at level of patellar apices	AP weight-bearing knee jts particularly useful for evaluation of *arthritic conditions* (see Fig. 6–41)

Note: If the oblique projections of the knee are requested, they are performed using a 45 degree oblique. The *proximal tibiofibular articulation* is best demonstrated in a 45 degree internal/medial oblique knee position.

Intercondyloid fossa (*Camp Coventry/PA axial*)	Patient PA recumbent, knee flexed so tibia forms 40 degree w/ tabletop and foot rested on support	CR 40 degree caudad (⊥ long axis of tibia) to knee jt	*PA axial* (superoinferior) proj of intercondyloid fossa, tibial plateau, and eminences; "tunnel view" (see Fig. 6–33A and B)
Intercondyloid fossa (Bècleré)	Patient AP w/ knee flexed ≈20–30 degree resting on supported IR	CR cephalad (⊥ long axis of tibia) to knee jt	AP *axial* (inferosuperior) proj of intercondyloid fossa, tibial plateau, and eminences; "tunnel view"

Note: The *Holmblad* PA axial method of intercondyloid fossa is performed w/ the patient in the kneeling position. The affected knee is centered, and CR forms a 20 degree angle w/ femur.

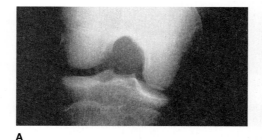
A

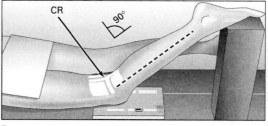
B

Figure 6–33. **(A)** Intercondyloid fossa, using the Camp–Coventry method. The tibial plateau and eminences are well visualized. (Courtesy of Stamford Hospital, Department of Radiology.) **(B)** Patient and CR positioning for Camp–Coventry method.

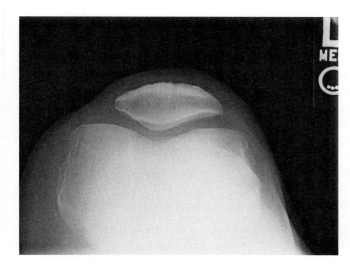

Figure 6–34. Tangential "sunrise" (Settegast) projection of the patella. The femoropatellar joint is well demonstrated. (Courtesy of Stamford Hospital, Department of Radiology.)

TABLE 6–18. The Patella

Patella	Position of Part	Central Ray Directed	Structures Included/Best Seen
PA	Patient prone, leg rotated ≈5–10 degree laterally to place patella ⏊ tabletop	⏊ patella (enters popliteal region)	PA patella, including knee jt; better detail than the AP position (less OID)
Lateral (*mediolateral*)	Patient on affected side, patella ⏊ tabletop, *knee flexed only 5–10 degree*	⏊ IR and mid-femoropatellar jt	Lat proj of patella and femoropatellar jt
Tangential (*Settegast/prone flexion 90 degree*)	Patient prone (or seated) on x-ray table; knee flexed at least 90 degree	Directed to mid-femoropatellar jt	*Tangential* projection of the patella, femoropatellar articulation; useful for demonstrating *vertical* fx; *must not be attempted* in known or suspected transverse fx of patella
Tangential (*Hughston/prone flexion 55 degree*)	Patient prone (or seated) on x-ray table; knee flexed approximately 55 degree	Directed to mid-femoropatellar jt	*Tangential* projection of the patella (Fig. 6–34), femoropatellar articulation; demonstrates *vertical* fx; *must not be attempted* in known or suspected transverse fx of patellas

Note: It has been suggested that the *Settegast and Hughston methods* be modified to *lesser degrees of flexion*, in order that the patella not be pulled into the femoropatellar groove.

Note: The *tangential projection/Merchant method* of demonstrating the patella and femoropatellar jts can require the use of special equipment. However, the essential components of the method include relaxed quadriceps muscles, ≈45 degree knee flexion, ≈30 degree caudal CR angle, at a 6-feet SID to reduce magnification.

TABLE 6–19. The Femur

Femur	Position of Part	Central Ray Directed	Structures Included/Best Seen
AP	Patient supine, affected femur centered to midline of grid w/ leg internally rotated 15 degree	⏊ midfemoral shaft (to include hip and possibly knee jt)	AP proj femur, including hip jt; leg rotation *overcomes anteversion* of femoral neck and places neck IR
Lateral (*mediolateral*)	Patient recumbent lateral w/ affected leg centered to grid; patella ⏊ tabletop	⏊ midshaft	Lateral proj femur, from knee jt up; may be performed w/ horizontal beam if suspected fx or pathologic disease

Note: If an orthopedic appliance is present, the x-ray image should include the entire appliance and the articulation closest to it.

TABLE 6–20. The Hip

Hip	Position of Part	Central Ray Directed	Structures Included/Best Seen
AP	Patient supine, sagittal plane 2″ medial to ASIS centered to midline of grid, no pelvic rotation, leg rotated 15 degree internally	Sagittal plane 2″ medial to ASIS at level of greater trochanter	AP hip jt, femoral neck and proximal femur; a portion of the pelvic bones is included; *the greater trochanter should be seen in profile*

Note: Another method of hip localization is to bisect the ASIS and pubic symphysis: this is the peak of the femoral head. A point ≈2.5″ dist and ⊥ is the midpoint of the femoral neck (see Fig. 6–24).

Note: Leg inversion *must never be forced and is contraindicated in cases of known or suspected fx or destructive disease.*

| AP oblique (*unilateral frog-leg, non-trauma; modified cleaves*) | Patient supine, ASIS of affected side centered to grid, knee and hip acutely flexed, thigh(s) abducted 40 degree | ⊥ the affected hip at a level 1″ above the pubic symphysis | AP oblique proj hip jt; lesser trochanter should be seen on the medial aspect of the femur (see Fig. 6–35). |

Note: *Bilateral* examination can be performed by positioning both hips and directing the CR to the MSP at a point 1″ above the pubic symphysis.

Note: The above position *must not be attempted* when fx is suspected.

| Axiolateral infero-superior (*cross-table lateral; Danelius-Miller*) | Patient supine, unaffected leg elevated; leg rotated internally 15 degree, grid placed against thigh to femoral neck | ⊥ femoral neck and grid | Lateral proj of proximal femur and its articulation with the acetabulum; *the lesser trochanter will be prominently seen on the posterior aspect of the femur* |

Note: Leg inversion must never be forced and is contraindicated in cases of known or suspected fx or destructive disease. This position requires localization of the long axis of the femoral neck. First, *mark* the midpoint b/w the ASIS and pubic symphysis of affected side; next, *mark* a point 19 dist to the prominence of the greater trochanter. A line b/w these 2 points parallels the long axis of the femoral neck.

Trauma axiolateral inferosuperior, trauma (*Clements-Nakayama*)	Patient supine, legs extended; affected side to *edge* of table (Bucky side). Cassette placed on extended Bucky tray, and tilted back ≈15–20 degree, CR ⊥	CR angled 15–20 degree posteriorly, entering proximal medial thigh, ⊥ mid-femoral neck	Lateral oblique of proximal femur, hip jt
Acetabulum posterior obl. (*Judet*)	Patient semisupine recumbent, 45 degree post obl	If affected side *down,* CR ⊥ 2″ medial and dist to (down side) ASIS	*Downside* shows anterior rim of acetabulum
		If affected side *up,* CR ⊥ 2″ dist to (upside) ASIS	*Upside* shows posterior rim and obturator foramen

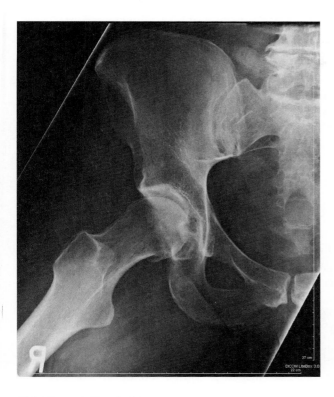

Figure 6–35. AP oblique (modified Cleaves) view of hip. The femoral neck and greater and lesser trochanters are well defined; the lesser trochanter is seen medially.

TABLE 6–21. The Pelvis

Pelvis	Position of Part	Central Ray Directed	Structures Included/Best Seen
AP	Patient supine, MSP ⊥ tabletop, no pelvic rotation, legs rotated internally 15 degree	⊥ midline at a level 2″ above greater trochanter; top of IR 1–2″ above iliac crest	AP proj pelvis and upper femora w/ femoral necks IR and greatertrochanters free of superimposition (Fig. 6–36)
Pelvic bones *outlet/ inlet projections*	Patient supine, no pelvic rotation	*Outlet:* CR to pubic symphysis/ greater trochanter at 20–35 degree cephalad (*males*), 30–45 degree cephalad (*females*)	*Outlet:* shows ischial body and ramus, pubic superior and inferior rami
		Intlet: CR 40 degree caudad, entering m/w b/w ASISs	*Inlet:* shows entire (upper) pelvic unlet

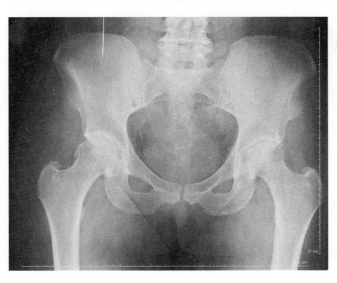

Figure 6–36. AP projection of the pelvis. The femoral necks are seen in their entirety: internal rotation of the feet/legs places them parallel to the IR. Note fractures of the public and ischial rami on the left. (Courtesy of Stamford Hospital, Department of Radiology.)

TABLE 6–22. The Ilium

Ilium	Position of Part	Central Ray Directed	Structures Included/Best Seen
AP	Patient supine, sagittal plane passing through hip jt of affected side centered to grid, patient obliqued 40 degree toward affected side	⊥, enters the sagittal plane 2″ medial to ASIS at level m/w b/w crest and greater trochanter	AP proj of ilium, patient obliquity "opens" the ilium by placing it to the IR

TABLE 6–23. The Sacroiliac Joints

Sacroiliac Jts	Position of Part	Central Ray Directed	Structures Included/Best Seen
AP axial	Patient supine, MSP centered	30–35 degree cephalad, to the midline approxi-mately 2 in. below level of ASIS	Sacrum, SI joints, and L5–S1 articulation
AP oblique (*LPO and RPO*)	Patient supine and obliqued 25–30 degree *affected side up* with sagittal plane passing 1″ medial to ASIS centered to grid	⊥ a point 1″ me-Sacroiliacdial to ASIS	(SI) jt of the elevated side; the opposite obl is similarly obtained; SI jt is placed ⊥ IR (Fig. 6–37A and B)
PA oblique (*LAO and RAO*)	Patient prone and obliqued 25–30 degree *affected side down* with sagittal plane passing 1″ medial to ASIS centered to grid	⊥ a point 1″ Sacroiliac medial to ASIS	(SI) jt of the "down" side; the opposite obl is similarly obtained; SI jt is placed ⊥ IR–35 degree cephalad.

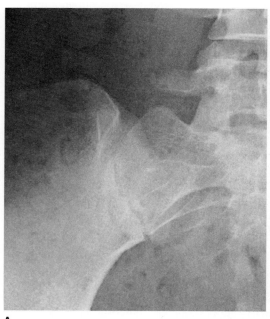
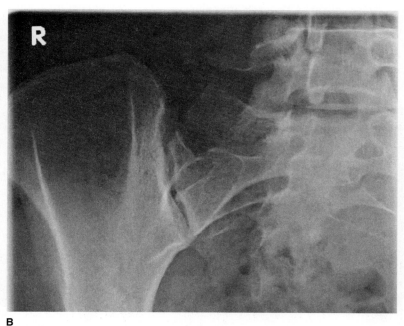

A   B

Figure 6–37. **(A)** AP right SI joint with perpendicular CR. (Courtesy of Conrad P. Ehrlich, MD.) **(B)** LPO right SI joint with perpendicular CR; 25 degree obliquity opens SI joint nicely. (Courtesy of Conrad P. Ehrlich, MD.)

TABLE 6–24. Long-Bone Measurement

Long Bone Measurement	Position of Part	Central Ray Directed	Structures Included/Best Seen
AP (leg)	Patient supine, leg extended and centered to grid w/ metal ruler taped alongside; one exposure each at hip, knee, and ankle jts (on one IR)	⊥ hip, knee, ankle jts	Tightly collimated AP projections of hip, knee, and ankle jts with metallic ruler alongside

Note: For bilateral examination, ruler is placed b/w legs, there must be no rotation, and if one knee is somewhat flexed, the other must be identically flexed for the exposure.

Long Bone Measurement. Accurate measurement of long bones, usually lower extremities, is occasionally required to evaluate abnormal growth patterns in children or lower back disorders in adults (see Table 6–24).

Arthrography. *Arthrography* is a contrast examination performed to evaluate soft-tissue joint structures, such as articular cartilages, menisci, ligaments, and bursae. The examination is most often performed as *double* contrast, with a *positive contrast agent* (water-soluble iodinated) coating the structures and a *negative* contrast agent (air) filling the joint cavity. Fluoroscopic images are made during the examination while applying various *stress maneuvers.* Overhead radiographs could be requested as supplemental images. The knee is the most common joint to be examined in this way, although the hip, wrist, shoulder (Fig. 6–38A), and temporomandibular joint (TMJ) can also be evaluated with contrast arthrography.

Many arthrographic procedures have been supplemented or replaced by magnetic resonance (MR) imaging studies, which have the advantage of being *noninvasive* and provide excellent soft-tissue diagnostic value (Fig. 6–38B). Another option is to perform traditional arthrography using gadodiamide (gadolinium) as the contrast agent. The arthrogram is followed up immediately with an MR examination of the affected joint.

To Locate Joints

Hip: Bisect the ASIS and pubic symphysis; center 1″ distal and lateral to that point

Knee: Center immediately below the patellar apex

Ankle: Center midway between the malleoli

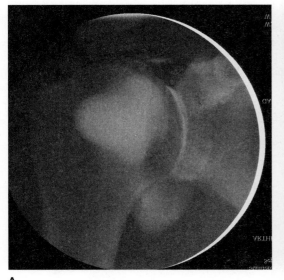

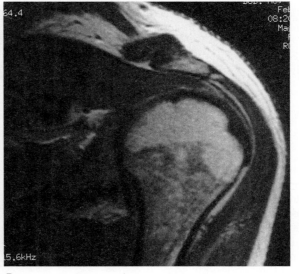

A

B

Figure 6–38. **(A)** A shoulder arthrogram. **(B)** MR imaging of the shoulder is accomplished noninvasively and provides visualization of structures having subtle differences in tissue density. (Courtesy of Stamford Hospital, Department of Radiology.)

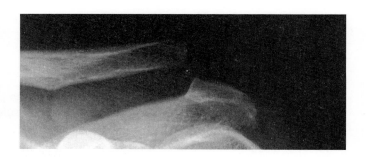

Figure 6–39. Acromioclavicular separation. The examination must be performed erect (in the recumbent position, small separations may not be seen). (Reproduced with permission from Haig SV, Flores CR. *Orthopedic Emergencies: A Radiographic Atlas*. New York: McGraw-Hill, 2005.)

Terminology and Pathology. Some of the radiologically significant skeletal disorders or conditions of upper and lower extremities with which the student radiographer should be familiar are listed as follows:

- Acromegaly
- Battered child syndrome
- Bone metastases
- Bursitis
- Carpal tunnel syndrome
- Epicondylitis
- Fracture (Figs. 6–17, 6–22, 6–32, and 6–42)
- Gout
- Osgood–Schlatter disease
- Osteoarthritis
- Osteochondroma
- Osteomalacia
- Osteomyelitis
- Osteoporosis
- Paget disease (Fig. 6–40)
- Rickets
- Slipped femoral capital epiphysis
- Subluxation
- Talipes
- Tendonitis

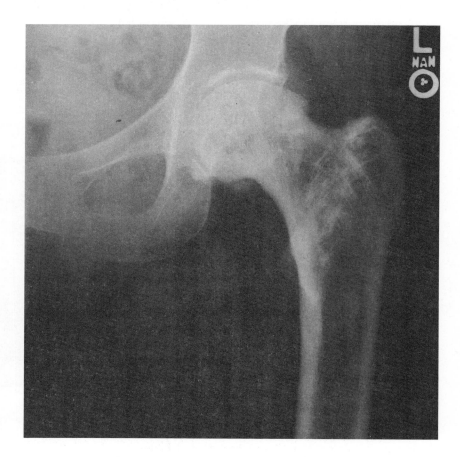

Figure 6–40. AP projection of the hip and proximal femur demonstrates Paget disease. Early lytic changes are seen throughout the bone; observe the beginning of typical "cotton wool" appearance in the region of the head and trochanters. The hip is well positioned, the femoral neck is parallel to the image receptor (not foreshortened), and the greater trochanter is seen in profile. (Courtesy of Stamford Hospital, Department of Radiology.)

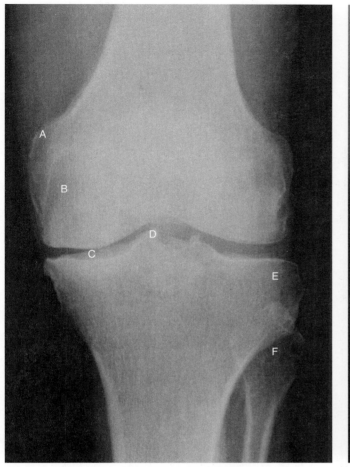

A

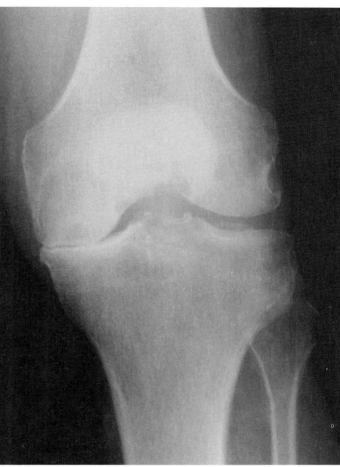

B

Figure 6–41. **(A)** AP knee joint, recumbent. **(B)** The same knee joint taken weight bearing. Note demonstration of significant joint narrowing. A, medial femoral epicondyle; B, medial femoral condyle; C, tibial plateau; D, medial intercondylar tubercle/tibial intercondylar eminence; E, lateral tibial condyle; F, head of fibula. (Reproduced with permission from Miller TT, Schweitzer ME. *Diagnostic Musculoskeletal Imaging.* New York: McGraw-Hill, 2005.)

Types of Fractures

- *Simple:* an undisplaced fracture (fx)
- *Compound:* fractured end of bone has penetrated skin (open fx)
- *Incomplete:* fx does not traverse entire bone; little or no displacement
- *Greenstick:* break of cortex on one side of bone only; found in infants and children
- *Torus/buckle* (see Fig. 6–42): greenstick fx with one cortex buckled/compacted and the other intact
- *Stress/fatigue:* response to repeated strong, powerful force (e.g., jogging, marching)
- *Avulsion:* small bony fragment pulled from bony prominence as a result of forceful pull of the attached ligament or tendon (chip fracture)
- *Hairline:* faint undisplaced fx
- *Comminuted:* one fracture composed of several fragments
- *Butterfly:* comminuted fx with one or more wedge or butterfly wing–shaped pieces

Some Conditions Requiring Adjustment in Exposure

Decrease in Exposure Factors	Increase in Exposure Factors
Arthritis	Acromegaly
Ewing sarcoma	Chronic gout
Osteomalacia	Multiple myeloma
Osteoporosis	Osteochondroma
Rickets	Osteopetrosis
Thalassemia	Paget disease (osteitis deformans)

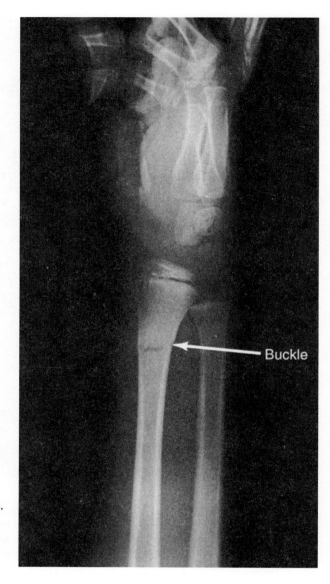

Figure 6–42. Torus/buckle-type greenstick fracture. (Reproduced with permission from Simon RS, Koenigsknecht SJ. *Emergency Orthopedics: The Extremities*, 3rd ed. East Norwalk, CT: Appleton & Lange, 1995, Figure X-ray 32–X5, p. 511.)

- *Spiral:* long fx encircling a shaft; result of torsion (twisting force); especially lower leg (distal tibia and proximal fibula)
- *Oblique:* longitudinal fx forming an angle (approximately 45 degree) with the long axis of the shaft
- *Transverse:* fx occurring at right angles to long axis of bone
- *Boxer:* fx just proximal to head of fifth metacarpal
- *Monteggia:* fx proximal third of ulnar shaft with anterior dislocation of radial head
- *Colles:* transverse fracture of distal third of radius with posterior angulation and associated avulsion fx of ulnar styloid process
- *Trimalleolar:* fx lateral malleolus, fx medial malleolus on medial and posterior surfaces
- *Jones:* fx base of fifth metatarsal
- *Potts:* fx distal tibia and fibula with dislocation of ankle joint
- *Pathologic:* fx of bone weakened by pathologic condition, for example, metastatic bone disease.

COMPREHENSION CHECK

Congratulations! You have completed a large portion of this chapter. If you are able to answer the following group of very comprehensive questions, you should feel confident that you have really mastered this section. You can refer back to the indicated pages to check your answers and/or review the subject matter.

1. Identify the bony structures composing the appendicular skeleton (p. 93, 94).

2. Describe the (a) method of positioning, (b) direction and point of entry of the CR, (c) principal structures visualized, and (d) pertinent traumatic or pathologic conditions and any technical adjustments they may necessitate relative to the appendicular skeleton, to include routine and special views of the

A. Hand and wrist (p. 102-104).
B. Forearm and elbow (p. 105).
C. Humerus and shoulder (p. 105-107).
D. Clavicle and scapula (p. 108).
E. Foot and ankle (p. 119-122).
F. Lower leg and knee (p. 123, 124).
G. Femur and hip (p. 125-127).
H. Pelvis and sacroiliac joints (p. 127-128).
I. Long bone measurement (p. 129).
J. Arthrography (p. 129).

THE AXIAL SKELETON

The axial skeleton (Fig. 6–43A; shaded) consists of the facial and cranial bones of the *skull*, the five sections of the *vertebral column*, and the sternum and ribs of the *thorax*.

Vertebral Column

The vertebral column (Fig. 6–43B) is composed of 33 bones divided into 7 cervical, 12 thoracic, 5 lumbar, 5 (fused) sacral, and 4 (fused) coccygeal regions, with each region having its own characteristic shape. The vertebral bodies gradually increase in size through the lumbar region. The vertebrae are joined by ligaments and cartilage; the first 24 are separate and movable, while the last 9 are fixed. *Intervertebral disks* between the vertebral bodies form *amphiarthrotic* joints.

The cervical and lumbar regions form *lordotic* (convex anteriorly) curves; the thoracic and sacral regions form *kyphotic* (convex posteriorly) curves (Fig. 6–43B, lateral). An exaggerated thoracic curve is called *kyphosis* ("hunchback"); an exaggerated lumbar curve is *lordosis* ("swayback"). Lateral curvature of the vertebral column is called *scoliosis*.

The typical vertebra has a *body* and a *neural/vertebral arch* surrounding the *vertebral foramen*. The neural arch is composed of two *pedicles*, two laminae that support four articular processes, two transverse processes, and one spinous process. The pedicles are short, thick processes extending back from the posterior aspect of the vertebral body, each one sustaining a *lamina*. The laminae extend posteriorly to the midline and join to form the *spinous process* (lack of union, or malunion, results in *spina bifida*). Each pedicle has notches superiorly and inferiorly (*superior* and *inferior vertebral*

Neural/Vertebral Arch

Composed of
• Two pedicles
• Two laminae

Encloses
• Vertebral foramen

Supports Seven Processes
• Two superior articular processes
• Two inferior articular processes
• Two transverse processes
• One spinous process

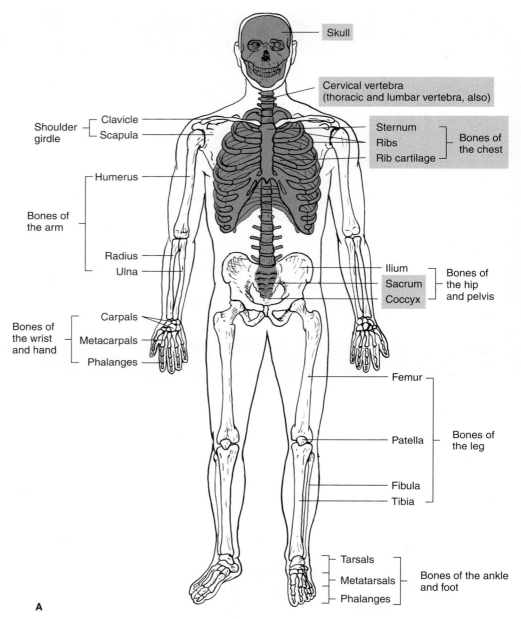

Figure 6–43. (A) The axial skeleton. (Modified with permission from Rice J. *Terminology with Human Anatomy*, 3rd ed. East Norwalk, CT: Appleton & Lange, 1995.) (*continued*)

notches) that—with adjacent vertebrae—form the *intervertebral foramina*, through which the spinal nerves pass. The neural arch also has lateral *transverse processes* for muscle attachment and *superior* and *inferior articular processes* for the formation of *apophyseal joints* (classified as *diarthrotic*). The consecutive vertebral foramina form the *vertebral, or spinal, canal*—through which the spinal cord is enclosed. The vertebral column permits flexion, extension, lateral, and rotary motions through its various articulations.

The bodies of consecutive vertebrae articulate with each other and are separated by *intervertebral disks*. The outer portion of the intervertebral disks is the fibrous *annulus fibrosus*, which encloses a central portion, the *nucleus pulposus*. Rupture of the intervertebral disk, or *herniated nucleus*

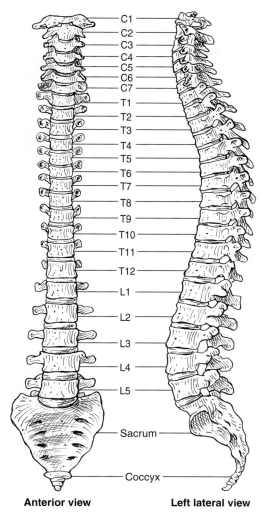

B   Anterior view   **Left lateral view**

Figure 6–43. (*Continued*) (**B**) AP and lateral views of the vertebral column.

pulposus (HNP), can push into the spinal canal or adjacent spinal nerve roots. This condition can cause back pain and even loss of neurological function in the areas that the affected spinal nerves are distributed.

Cervical Spine. There are seven cervical vertebrae (Fig. 6–44). The *atlas* (C1) is a ring-shaped bone having no body and no spinous process; it is composed of an *anterior and posterior arch*, two *lateral masses*, and two *transverse processes*.

The anterior arch has a *tubercle* at its midpoint and has a *facet* on its posterior surface for articulation with the anterior portion of the odontoid process/dens. The posterior arch has a tubercle as well. The lateral masses have *superior articular processes* that articulate with the skull at the *atlanto-occipital joint*, where flexion and extension occurs. Its lateral masses articulate inferiorly with the *axis* (C2).

The axis (C2) has a superior projection, the *dens*, or *odontoid process*. The axis articulates superiorly with the atlas at the *atlantoaxial joint*, a *pivot* joint where rotation of the head takes place, and inferiorly with C3 at the apophyseal articulation. The dens has a *facet* on its anterior

Articulation Summary: *Vertebral*

- Occipitoatlantal
- Atlantoaxial
- Costovertebral
- Costotransverse
- Lumbosacral
- Sacroiliac
- Sacrococcygeal
- Intervertebral
- Apophyseal/interarticular

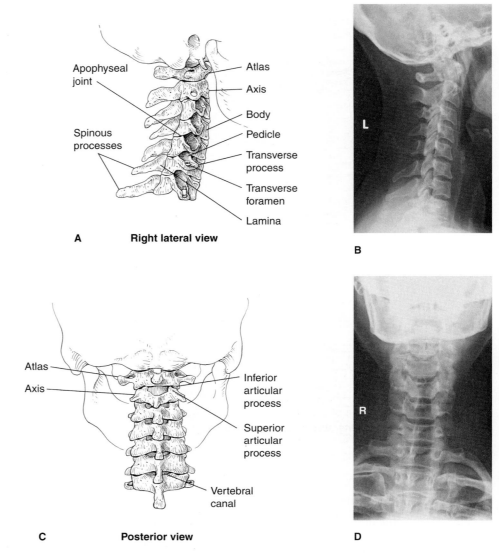

Apophyseal joint

Atlas

Axis

Body

Pedicle

Transverse process

Transverse foramen

Spinous processes

Lamina

A   **Right lateral view**

L

B

Atlas

Axis

Inferior articular process

Superior articular process

Vertebral canal

C   **Posterior view**

R

D

Figure 6–44. (**A**) Right lateral view of the cervical spine. (**B**) Lateral projection, cervical spine. (**C**) Posterior view of the cervical spine. (**D**) AP projection of the cervical spine. (B and D: Courtesy of Conrad P. Ehrlich, MD.)

surface for articulation with the posterior aspect of the anterior arch of C1. The spinous process of C2 is particularly large and strong.

The typical cervical vertebra is small and has a *transverse foramen* in each transverse process for passage of the vertebral artery and vein. The cervical laminae are thin and narrow; they meet at midline to form a short spinous process. Cervical spinous processes are almost horizontal and usually *bifid*. The spinous process of C7 (*vertebra prominens*) is not bifid, is larger and more horizontal, and is a useful positioning landmark.

Fractures and/or dislocations of the cervical spine are usually due to acute *hyperflexion* or *hyperextension* as a result of indirect trauma. *Whiplash* injury is caused by a sudden, forced movement in one direction and then the opposite direction (as in rear-end automobile impacts). Whiplash symptoms frequently include neck pain and stiffness, headache, and pain and numbness of the upper extremities. Whiplash is often evidenced radiographically by straightening or reversal of the normal lordotic curve. Lateral projections of the cervical spine are sometimes performed to evaluate whiplash injury—by demonstrating the degree of anterior and posterior motion.

Osteoarthritis is characterized in the cervical and lumbar spine by chronic, progressive degeneration of cartilage and *hypertrophy* of bone along the articular margins, characterized radiographically by narrowed joint spaces, and *osteophytes*. Osteoarthritis is often observable in the articulations of the fingers, toes, hips, and knees, as well.

Table 6–25 provides a summary of positions/projections of the cervical spine.

TABLE 6–25. Cervical Spine

Cervical Spine	Position of Part	Central Ray Directed	Structures Included/Best Seen
AP	Patient supine, MSP ⊥ table; adjust flexion so mastoid tip and occlusal plane are aligned	15–20 degree cephalad to thyroid cartilage	AP of *lower 5* cervical vertebrae and intervertebral disk spaces
AP *Atlas and Axis* (open mouth)	Patient supine, MSP ⊥ table, w/ patient's mouth open, adjust flexion so mastoid tips and upper occlusal plane are aligned ⊥ IR (‖ CR)	⊥ center of opened mouth	AP proj of C1 and C2 (atlas and axis) (Fig. 6–45A) and their articulations; *too much flexion* superimposes teeth on odontoid; *too much extension* superimposes base of skull on odontoid

Note: If the upper portion of the odontoid process is not seen, the AP (Fuchs) or PA (Judd) projection may be attempted if upper cervical fx or degenerative disease is not suspected. The PA is similar to a Waters position; the AP similar to the reverse Waters. The odontoid is seen projected within the foramen magnum. Since extension of the neck is required, this position must not be attempted if upper cervical fx or degenerative disease is suspected.

Lateral	Patient erect w/ L side adjacent to IR, chin slightly elevated, shoulders depressed, MSP ‖ IR centered, at level of C4	⊥ C4	Lateral proj of all seven vertebrae (Fig. 6–45B). Shows intervertebral jt spaces, apophyseal jts, spinous processes, bodies; due to the unavoidable OID, a 72 degree SID should be used

Note: Lateral flexion and extension projections (Fig. 6–46) may be obtained in this position in cases of whiplash injury.

Note: A recumbent cross-table/horizontal beam lateral must be performed as the first radiograph for trauma or suspected subluxation patients. The patient's neck must not be moved and any cervical collar in place must stay in place until images have been reviewed for fx, subluxation, etc.

Oblique (*LAO and RAO*)	Patient PA erect, MSP 45 degree to IR centered to C5 (1″ inferior to thyroid cartilage), chin slightly raised	15–20 degree caudad to center of IR	Oblique cervical spine; best view of intervertebral foramina *closest* to IR; a similar view can be obtained w/ the patient *LPO* and *RPO*, CR ed cephalad, and showing the foramina *farthest* from the IR (see Fig. 6–45C)

Note: Oblique cervical spine may be performed in the recumbent position on patients whose trauma prohibits moving them. The CR is directed 45 degree medially for one oblique and 45 degree laterally for the other.

Lateral *cervico-thoracic* (*Swimmer's lateral*)	Patient erect (or recumbent) lat *w/ midaxillary line* centered to grid, MSP, arm adjacent to IR over head, depress opposite shoulder farthest from grid	⊥ T2	Lat proj of lower cervical and upper thoracic vertebrae; particularly useful for broad-shouldered individuals

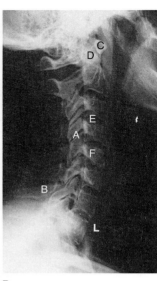

A

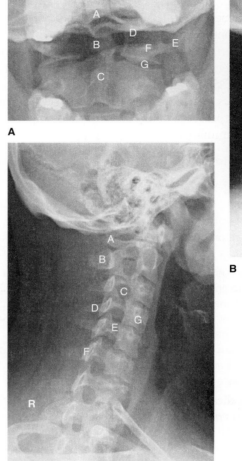

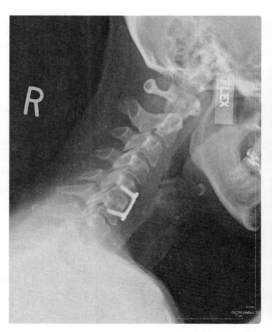

B

Figure 6–45. **(A)** Open-mouth projection of C1–C2. Locate and identify the bony structures shown particularly well in this projection. A, occlusal plane/maxillary incisors; B, odontoid process/dens; C, body, C2/axis; D, base of skull; E, transverse process, C1; F, body, C1; G, atlantoaxial articulation. **(B)** Lateral projection of the cervical spine. A, zygapophyseal articulation; B, spinous process C7/vertebra prominens; C, tubercle of anterior arch, C1; D, odontoid process/dens; E, intervertebral joint/disc space; F, vertebral body, C5. **(C)** An RPO cervical spine. Locate and identify the bony structures shown particularly well in each projection. A, posterior arch, C1; B, spinous process, C2; C, intervertebral foramen, C3; D, spinous process, C4; E, pedicle, C5; F, transverse process, C4; G, body, C4. (Courtesy of Conrad P. Ehrlich, MD)

C

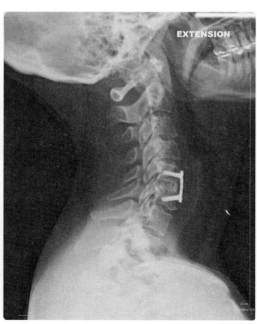

Figure 6–46. Lateral projections of the cervical spine in flexion and extension—used to demonstrate degree of anterior and posterior motion. (Courtesy of Conrad P. Ehrlich, MD)

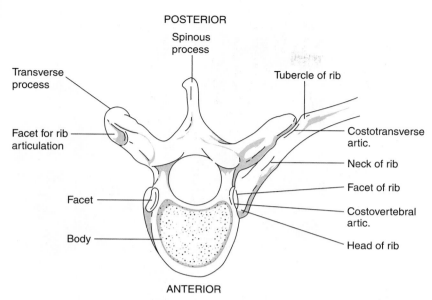

Figure 6–47. Thoracic vertebra and its articulation with rib (superior view).

Thoracic Spine. There are 12 thoracic vertebrae, which are larger in size than cervical vertebrae and which increase in size as they progress inferiorly toward the lumbar region. Thoracic spinous processes are fairly long and sharply angled caudally (T8 usually has the longest vertical spinous process). The bodies and transverse processes have *articular facets* for the *diarthrotic* rib articulations (see Fig. 6–47).

A common metabolic bone disorder frequently noted in radiographic examinations of the thoracic spine is osteoporosis. *Osteoporosis* is characterized by bone demineralization and can result in compression fractures of the vertebrae. The condition is most common in sedentary and postmenopausal women.

Table 6–26 provides a summary of positions/projections of the thoracic spine.

TABLE 6–26. The Thoracic Spine

Thoracic Spine	Position of Part	Central Ray Directed	Structures Included/Best Seen
AP	Patient supine, MSP ⊥ tabletop, top of IR 1″ above shoulders	⊥ T7	AP proj of thoracic vertebrae and intervertebral spaces; it is helpful to use the anode heel effect and/or compensating filtration to provide more uniform density (see Fig. 6–48A)
Note: To demonstrate *apophyseal jts, 70 degree obliques* are performed.			
Lateral	Patient L lat recumbent, midaxillary line cen-tered to table, arms ⊥ long axis of body, top of IR 1″ above shoulders	5–15 degree cephalad (⊥ long axis of spine)	Lat proj of thoracic vertebrae, especially bodies, intervertebral spaces and foramina; a vertical CR may be used if MSP is the tabletop (see Fig. 6–48B)
Note: This exposure can be made at the end of *expiration.* Or, a long exposure time (with low mA) can be used while the patient *breathes* quietly. This has the effect of blurring vascular markings and superimposed ribs.			

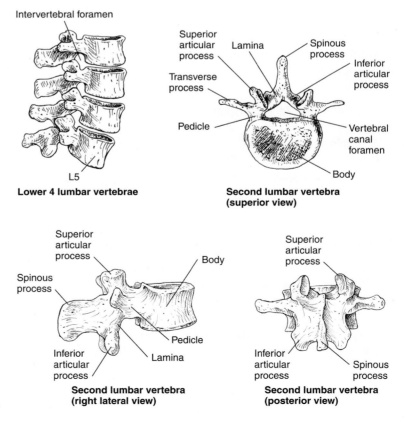

Figure 6–48. **(A)** AP projection of the thoracic spine. Note density difference between upper and lower spine; this can be improved by using the anode heel effect to advantage (placing cathode over lower spine). **(B)** Lateral projection of thoracic spine. "Breathing technique" has helped blur pulmonary vascular markings and provided good visualization of nearly all the thoracic vertebrae. (Courtesy of Stamford Hospital, Department of Radiology.)

A   **B**

Lumbar Spine. The five lumbar vertebrae are the largest of the vertebral column and increase in size toward the sacral region. The spinous processes are short and horizontal and serve as attachment for strong muscles (see Fig. 6–49). The causes of lumbar pain are numerous.

Intervertebral foramen

L5

Lower 4 lumbar vertebrae

Superior
articular
process

Lamina

Spinous
process

Transverse
process

Inferior
articular
process

Pedicle

Vertebral
canal
foramen

Body

**Second lumbar vertebra
(superior view)**

Superior
articular
process

Body

Spinous
process

Pedicle

Inferior
articular
process

Lamina

**Second lumbar vertebra
(right lateral view)**

Superior
articular
process

Inferior
articular
process

Spinous
process

**Second lumbar vertebra
(posterior view)**

Figure 6–49. Lateral view of the lower lumbar vertebrae. Superior, right lateral, and posterior views of L2.

Trauma, fracture, spasm of the paralumbar muscles, herniated intervertebral disk, and osteoarthritis are a few causes of low back pain.

Some of the disorders that can be detected radiographically include *osteoarthritis*, *spondylolysis*, *spondylolisthesis*, and *ankylosing spondylitis*. Myelography and especially MRI are used to evaluate *herniated intervertebral disks*.

Table 6–27 provides a summary of positions/projections of the lumbar spine.

TABLE 6–27. The Lumbar Spine

Lumbar Spine	Position of Part	Central Ray Directed	Structures Included/Best Seen
AP	Patient supine, MSP ⊥ tabletop, knees flexed, feet flat on table	⊥ to L3	AP proj of lumbar vertebrae L1–L4, intervertebral spaces, transverse processes; *flexion of the knees reduces lumbar curve and OID (see Fig. 6–50)*
Note: The AP projection of the lumbar spine is most comfortable for very thin patients and those with low-back pain. The PA projection has the advantages of delivering lower gonadal dose and of placing the intervertebral jts more closely parallel with the divergent x-ray beam.			
AP (L5–S1)	Patient supine, MSP ⊥ tabletop, legs extended	To MSP at 30–35 degree Cephalad to MSP, ≈1¹/₂″ above pubic symph	AP of lumbosacral articulation not seen on AP lumbar
Oblique (*RPO and LPO*)	Patient AP recumbent, obliqued 45 degree w/ spine centered to grid	⊥ L3	Obl proj of lumbar vertebrae, especially for apophyseal articulations (L1–L4) of side *adjacent* to table; opposite obl is done to show opposite articulations (see Fig. 6–51).
Note: This proj demonstrates the characteristic "scotty dogs" (see Fig. 6–51); obl lumbar spine may also be performed in the PA position and demonstrates the apophyseal articulations away from the IR.			
Note: L5–S1 apophyseal articulations shown in 35 degree obl.			
Lateral	Patient L lat recumbent, midaxillary line centered to grid	5–8 degree caudad L3	Lat proj, especially for vertebral bodies, interspaces, intervertebral foramina, spinous processes; *if MSP adjusted tabletop, CR is vertical* (Fig. 6–52A)
Note: Lateral lumbar spine in flexion and extension is often used to demonstrate presence or absence of motion in area(s) of spinal fusion.			
Lateral (L5–S1)	Patient L lat ⊥ recumbent, center plane 1.5″ posterior to midaxillary line to grid, adjust MSP ∥ tabletop	Coronal lat plane at level m/w b/w crest and ASIS	Proj L5–S1; *if MSP not adjusted tabletop, CR is ∠ed 5–8 degree caudad* (Fig. 6–52B)

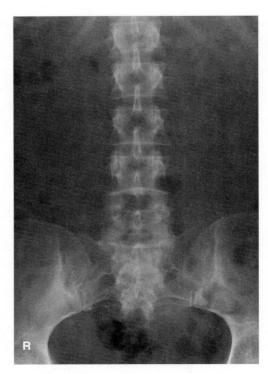

Figure 6–50. AP projection of the lumbar spine. Flexion of the knees reduces lumbar curve and OID and relieves strain on lower back muscles; patients are most comfortable with sponge or pillow support placed under knees. (Courtesy of Stamford Hospital, Department of Radiology.)

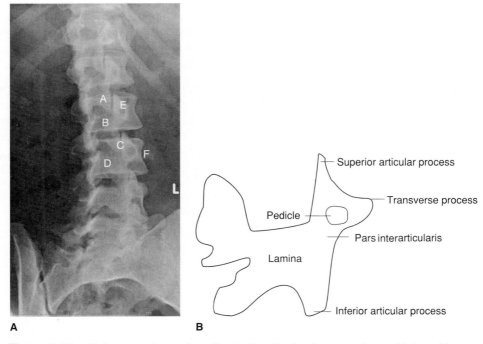

Figure 6–51. Oblique lumbar spine, illustrating the lumbar apophyseal joints. Note "scotty dog" images. The scotty "ear" (C) corresponds to the *superior articular process*, his "nose" to the *transverse process* (F), his "eye" is the *pedicle* (E), his "neck" the *pars interarticularis* (B), his "body" is the *lamina* (D), and his "front foot" is the *inferior articular process* (A). (Courtesy of Stamford Hospital, Department of Radiology.)

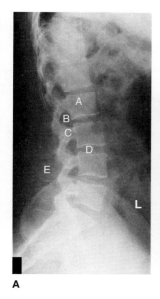

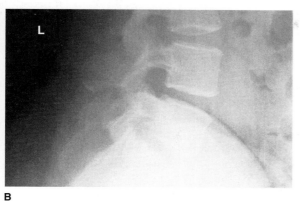

A   **B**

Figure 6–52. (A) Lateral projection of the lumbar spine. If MSP is adjusted parallel to tabletop, CR angulation is unnecessary. A, body, L2; B, intervertebral foramen; C, pedicle; D, intervertebral disc space; E, spinous process, L4. (B) Lateral projection L5–S1. (Courtesy of Stamford Hospital, Department of Radiology.)

Sacrum. There are five fused sacral vertebrae (Fig. 6–53A); the fused *transverse processes* form the *alae*. The anterior and posterior *sacral foramina* transmit spinal nerves. The *sacrum* articulates superiorly with the fifth lumbar vertebra, forming the L5–S1 articulation and inferiorly with the *coccyx* to form the *sacrococcygeal joint*.

Table 6–28 through 6–31 provide a summary of positions/projections of the sacrum, sacroiliac joints, coccyx, and scoliosis series:

TABLE 6–28. The Sacrum

Sacrum	Position of Part	Central Ray Directed	Structures Included/Best Seen
AP	Patient AP supine, MSP ⊥ tabletop	15–25 degree cephalad to midline, to point m/w b/w pubic symphysis and ASIS	AP proj of sacrum; CR < parallels sacral curve and provides less distorted visualization (see Fig. 6–53B)
Note: See sacroiliac jts on page 127.			
Lateral	Patient L lat recumbent, 3″ posterior to MCP centered to grid	⊥ a point 3″ post to ASIS	Lateral proj of sacrum

TABLE 6–29. The Sacroiliac Joints

Sacro Iliac Jts	Position of Part	Central Ray Directed	Structures Included/Best Seen
AP axial	Patient supine, MSP centered	30–35 cephalad, to the midline approxi-mately 2 in. below level of ASIS	Sacrum, SI joints, and L5–S1 articulation
AP Oblique (*LPO and RPO*)	Patient supine and obliqued 25–30 degree *affected side up* with sagittal plane passing 1″ medial to ASIS centered to grid	⊥ a point 1″ me-sacroiliac dial to ASIS	(SI) jt of the elevated side; the opposite oblique is similarly obtained; SI jt is placed ⊥ IR (see Fig. 6–37A and B)
PA Oblique (*LAO and RAO*)	Patient prone and obliqued 25–30 degree *affected side down* with sagittal plane passing 1″ medial to ASIS centered to grid	⊥ a point 1″ sacroiliac medial to ASIS	(SI) jt of the "down" side; the opposite oblique is similarly obtained; SI jt is placed ⊥ IR–35 degree cephalad.

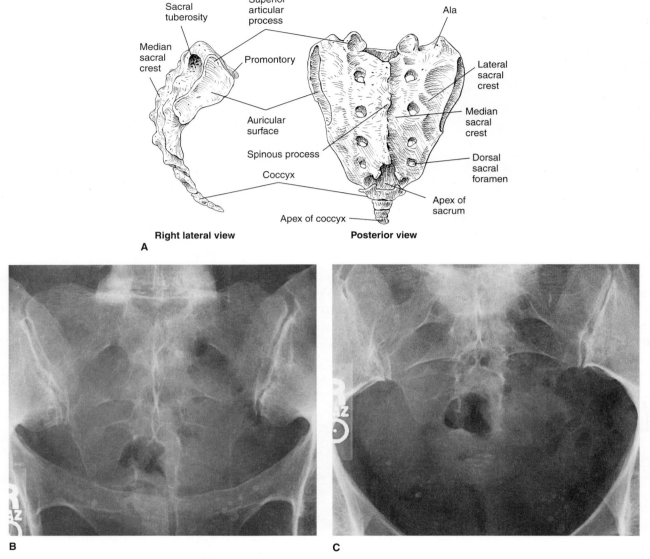

Figure 6–53. **(A)** Sacrum and coccyx. **(B)** AP projection of the sacrum. Cephalad angulation "opens" the sacral foramina. **(C)** AP projection of the coccyx. Caudal angulation "opens" the coccygeal curve. (A: Reproduced with permission from Chusid JG. *Correlative Neuroanatomy & Functional Neurology*, 19th ed. East Norwalk, CT: Appleton & Lange, 1985. B and C: Courtesy of Stamford Hospital, Department of Radiology.)

Coccyx. (See Table 6–30.) There are four or five fused coccygeal vertebrae (see Fig. 6–53A). Fracture of the coccyx usually results from a fall onto it, landing in a seated position. Fracture displacement is fairly common and occasionally requires removal of the fractured fragment to relieve the painful symptoms.

TABLE 6–30. The Coccyx

Coccyx	Position of Part	Central Ray Directed	Structures Included/Best Seen
AP	Patient AP supine, MSP ⊥ tabletop	10–20 degree caudad to midline to point 2″ above pubic symphysis	AP proj of coccyx; CR < parallels coccygeal curve and provides less distorted visualization (see Fig. 6–53C)
Lateral	Patient L lateral recumbent, 5″ post. to MCP centered to grid	⊥ a point 5″ post to MCP at level of mid-coccyx	Lat proj of coccyx and its articulation with the sacrum

Scoliosis Series See Table 6-31 for positioning for a scoliosis series.

TABLE 6–31. Scoliosis Series Positioning

Scoliosis Series	Position of Part	Central Ray Directed	Structures Included/Best Seen
PA bending	14″ × 17″ or 14″ × 36″ IR of vertebrae to include 1″ of iliac crest/L5–S1. Four exposures made: PA recumbent, PA erect, PA/bending L, and R	⊥ center of IR	*Radiation dose is reduced when gonadal, breast, and thyroid shields are used* and *when examination is performed PA rather than AP* (Fig. 6–54)
PA or AP Ferguson method	14″ × 17″ or 14″ × 36″ IR of vertebrae to include 1 of iliac crest/L5–S1; three exposures made with *no rotation*: PA(or AP), PA w/ (3″–4″) block under one foot, PA w/ (3″–4″) block under *opposite* foot	⊥ center of IR	Images used to distinguish primary curve from compensatory curve; protective shielding must be utilized

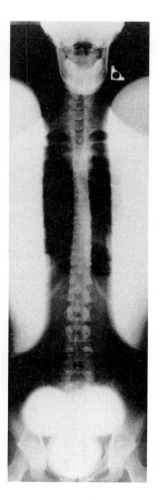

Figure 6–54. AP scoliosis series with protective shielding in place. (Courtesy of Nuclear Associates.)

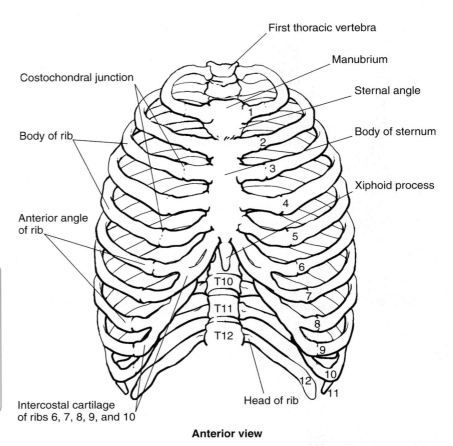

Anterior view

Figure 6–55. The thoracic cage, anterior aspect.

Articulation Summary: *Thorax*

- Sternoclavicular
- Sternochondral
- Costochondral
- Costovertebral
- Costotransverse

Radiographically Significant Skeletal Disorders and Conditions of the Axial Skeleton

Achondroplasia

Ankylosing spondylitis

Cervical rib

Degenerative disk disease

Flail chest

Herniated disk

Hydrocephalus

Kyphosis

Lordosis

Osteophyte

Osteoporosis

Pectus excavatum

Scoliosis

Spina bifida

Spondylolisthesis

Spondylolysis

Transitional vertebra

Whiplash

Thorax

Sternum and Sternoclavicular Joints. (See Tables 6–32 and 6–33.) The bones of the *thorax* (sternum, ribs, thoracic vertebrae; Fig. 6–55) function to protect the vital organs within heart, lungs, and major blood vessels. The *sternum* forms the anterior central portion of the thorax and is composed of three major divisions: the *manubrium, body,* and *xiphoid process.* Sternal fractures are uncommon; when they do occur, fracture displacement is rare, but the possibility of traumatic injury to the heart must still be considered.

Ribs. (See Table 6–34) The *rib* cage (see Fig. 6–55) consists of 12 pairs of ribs. Ribs 1 to 7 articulate with thoracic vertebrae and the sternum and are called *vertebrosternal* or "true" ribs. The first pair of ribs lies under the clavicles and is not palpable; the remaining 11 pairs of ribs are usually palpable. Ribs 8 to 10 articulate with thoracic vertebrae and the super-jacent costal cartilage to form the anterior costal margin and are called *vertebrochondral* or *false ribs.* The last two pairs of false ribs articulate only with thoracic vertebrae and are referred to as *floating ribs.* The spaces between the ribs are called *intercostal spaces* and are occupied by two sets of intercostal muscles.

Rib fractures are a common injury in thoracic trauma because of their relative thinness and exposed position. Their fracture may be complicated by *pneumothorax, hemothorax,* liver laceration (right lower ribs), or spleen laceration (left lower ribs).

TABLE 6–32. The Sternum

Sternum	Position of Part	Central Ray Directed	Structures Included/Best Seen
PA Oblique (RAO)	Patient 15–20 degree RAO; greater obliquity for thin patients, sternum centered to midline of table	⊥ midsternum	obl–frontal proj RAO projects sternum into heart shadow for *uniform density.*
	Note: A long exposure can be used during quiet breathing to blur pulmonary vascular markings, or exposure can be made on expiration (Fig. 6–56).		
Lateral	Patient erect L lateral, shoulders rolled back, MSP vertical, IR top 1.5″ above manubrial notch	⊥ midsternum	Lat proj of sternum free of superimposition of ribs; exposure made on deep inspiration to move sternum away from ribs

TABLE 6–33. The Sternoclavicular Joints

Sternoclavicular Joints	Position of Part	Central Ray Directed	Structures Included/Best Seen
PA	Patient prone, MSP centered to grid, IR centered at T3 (suprasternal notch)	⊥ T3	Bilateral PA proj of sternoclavicular jts visualized through superimposed vertebrae and ribs
PA Oblique (*LAO and RAO*)	Patient prone, MSP centered to grid, rotate body ≈15 degree *affected side down*	⊥ affected jt	Obl proj of sternoclavicular jt *closest to IR*; similar results can be obtained w/a ⊥ MSP and w/ CR 15 degree toward midline from the affected side

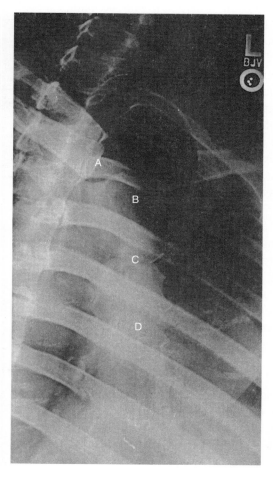

Figure 6–56. RAO sternum. A, medial extremity of clavicle B, manubrium; C, sternal angle; D, body/gladiolus. (Courtesy of Stamford Hospital, Department of Radiology.)

TABLE 6–34. The Ribs

Ribs	Position of Part	Central Ray Directed	Structures Included/Best Seen
AP	Patient supine or AP erect, MSP ⊥ midline of table, top of IR 1″ above shoulder	⊥ center of IR, about level of T7	AP proj, upper posterior ribs best delineated; do PA for better detail of anterior ribs
PA Oblique (*LAO, RAO*)	Patient prone or erect PA, rotate 45 degree, *unaffected side down*	⊥ center of IR, about level of T7 (at T10 to T12 for below diaphragm)	Obl shows *axillary* portions of ribs, RAO shows left ribs, LAO shows right ribs
AP Oblique (*LAO, RAO*)	Patient supine or erect AP, rotate to 45 degree affected side toward the IR	⊥ center of IR, about level of T7 (at T10–T12 for below diaphragm)	LPO shows *left* posterior ribs and their axillary portions, RPO shows *right* ribs and their axillary portions

Note: Above-diaphragm ribs are exposed on deep *inspiration* or during quiet breathing (long exposure). *Below-diaphragm* ribs are exposed on forced *expiration*.

Head and Neck

Skull. The *skull* has two major parts: the *cranium*, which is composed of eight bones and houses the brain, and the 14 irregularly shaped *facial bones* (Figs. 6–57 and 6–58). The eight cranial bones are the paired *parietal* and *temporal* bones and the unpaired *frontal, occipital, ethmoid,* and *sphenoid* bones. The 14 facial bones include the paired *nasal, lacrimal, palatine, inferior nasal conchae, maxillae,* and *zygomatic* bones and the unpaired *vomer* and *mandible*.

The average-shaped skull is termed *mesocephalic* (petrous pyramids and MSP form ≈47 degree), the broad skull is termed *brachycephalic* (petrous pyramids and MSP form ≈54 degree), and the elongated skull is termed *dolichocephalic* (petrous pyramids and MSP form ≈40 degree). These deviations are readily observable in axial CT and MR images. The inner and outer compact tables of the skull are separated by cancellous tissue called *diploë*. The internal table has a number of branching *meningeal grooves* and larger *sulci* that house blood vessels.

The bones of the skull are separated by immovable (*synarthrotic*) joints called *sutures*. The major sutures of the cranium are the *sagittal*, which separates the parietal bones; the *coronal*, which separates the frontal and parietal bones; the *lambdoidal*, which separates the parietal and occipital bones; and the *squammosal*, which separates the temporal and parietal bones (see Figs. 6–57 and 6–58). The articular surfaces of these bones have serrated-like edges with small projecting bones called *wormian* bones that fit together to form the articular sutures.

The sagittal and coronal sutures meet at the *bregma*, which corresponds to the fetal anterior fontanel. The sagittal and lambdoidal sutures meet posteriorly at the *lambda*, which corresponds to the fetal posterior fontanel. The parietal, frontal, and sphenoid bones meet at the *pterion* (see Fig. 6–57), the location of the anterolateral fontanel. The highest point of the skull is called the *vertex*.

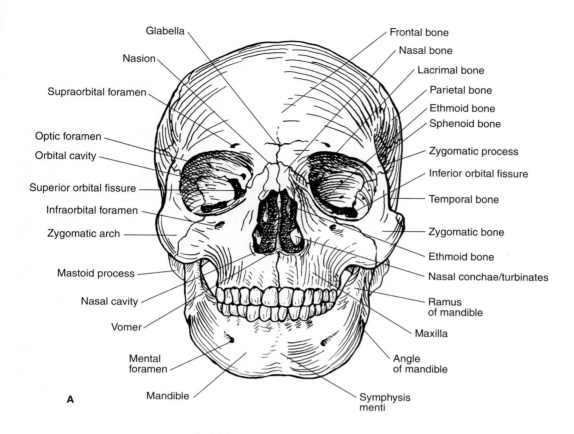

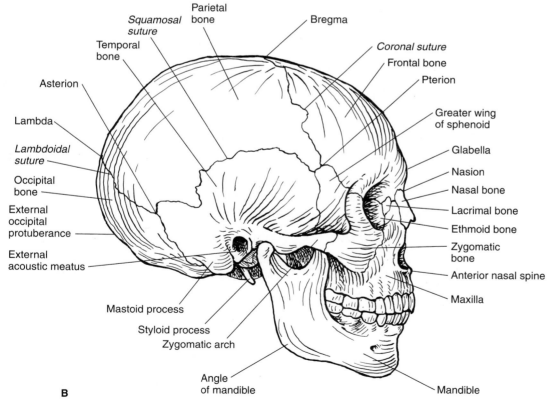

Figure 6–57. (**A**) Anterior view of the skull, labeled. (**B**) Lateral view of the skull, labeled.

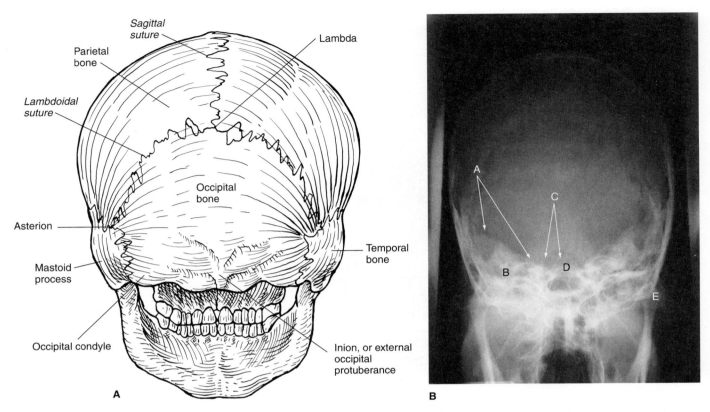

Figure 6–58. **(A)** Posterior view of the skull, labeled. **(B)** AP axial skull (Towne) demonstrates the occipital bone. A, petrous ridge; B, petrous portion of temporal bone; C, foramen magnum; D, dorsum sella and posterior clinoid processes; E, mandibular condyle. (Courtesy of Stamford Hospital, Department of Radiology.)

Cranial Bones (8)
(1) Frontal
(2) Parietal
(2) Temporal
(1) Occipital
(1) Ethmoid
(1) Sphenoid

Cranial Bones

Frontal Bone

- The frontal bone corresponds to the forehead region (Fig. 6–57)
- *Orbital plates* (2): horizontal part of frontal bone; forms much of superior aspect of bony orbit
- *Frontal eminences* (2): on anterior surface of frontal bone, lateral to MSP
- *Glabella:* smooth prominence between eyebrows
- *Frontal sinuses* (2): directly behind glabella, between the tables of the skull
- *Superciliary arches/ridges* (2): ridge of bone under eyebrow region
- *Supraorbital margins* (2): upper border/rim of bony orbit
- *Supraorbital notches/foramina* (2): midportion of supraorbital margin; passage for artery and nerve to forehead
- *Frontonasal suture:* where frontal bone articulates with nasal bones (corresponds exteriorly with *nasion*)

Parietal bones

- Paired; form the vertex and part of lateral portions of cranium
- Meet at midline to form sagittal suture; other borders help form coronal, squammosal, and lambdoidal sutures (Fig. 6–58)

- *Parietal eminences:* rounded prominence on lateral surface of each parietal bone

Ethmoid bone

- Located between orbits; helps form parts of nasal and orbital walls (Figs. 6–57 and 6–60)
- *Cribriform plate:* porous, passage for olfactory nerves; horizontal portion between orbital plates of frontal bone
- *Crista galli:* extends superiorly from midportion of cribriform plate
- *Perpendicular plate:* extends downward from crista galli to form major portion of nasal septum
- *Superior and middle nasal turbinates/conchae:* cartilaginous; within nasal cavity, attached to perpendicular plate
- *Ethmoidal labyrinths/lateral masses:* help form medial wall of orbit; ethmoidal sinuses within

Sphenoid bone

- Wedge- or bat-shaped bone located between frontal and occipital bones (Figs. 6–59, 6–60, and 6–61)
- Anchor for eight cranial bones
- Forms small part of lateral cranial wall and part of skull base
- Consists of body, two lesser wings, two greater wings, two pterygoid plates/processes, and hamuli
- *Body:* central portion; midline of skull base; anterior part joins ethmoid bone; contains the two sphenoid sinuses
- *Lesser (minor) wings:* anterior portion, articulates with orbital plates; contain optic canals for passage of optic nerves and ophthalmic arteries
- *Anterior clinoid processes:* formed by medial aspect of lesser wings
- *Tuberculum sellae:* ridge of bone between anterior clinoid processes; anterior boundary of sella turcica
- *Optic (chiasmic) groove:* horizontal depression crossing body of bone in front of sella turcica, where optic nerves cross
- *Optic foramen and canal:* passage for optic nerve and ophthalmic artery at the orbit's apex
- *Sella turcica:* deep depression in sphenoid bone; houses pituitary gland
- *Dorsum sellae:* posterior boundary/wall of sella turcica
- *Posterior clinoid processes:* extend laterally from dorsum sellae
- *Clivus:* basilar portion; slopes down and posteriorly from dorsum sellae; articulates with basilar portion of occipital bone
- *Superior orbital fissures:* large spaces between greater and lesser wings; for passage of four cranial nerves
- *Greater (major) wings:* larger, posterior portion of sphenoid bone; contains the foramina rotundum, ovale, and spinosum for transmission of cranial nerves
- *Pterygoid processes:* extend inferiorly from junction of body with great wing; each has a medial and lateral *plate* that articulates with posterior part of adjacent maxillae

Types of Fractures

Linear fx

  A skull fx, straight and sharply defined

Depressed fx

  A comminuted skull fx, with one or more portions pushed inward

Hangman fx

  Fx of C2 with anterior subluxation of C2 on C3; result of forceful hyperex-tension

Compression fx

  Especially of spongy (cancellous) bone; diminished thickness or width as a result of compression-type force (e.g., vertebral body)

Blowout fx

  Fx of orbital floor as a result of a direct blow

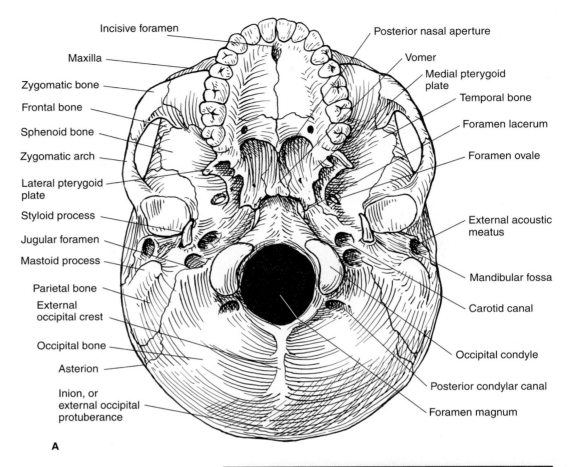

A

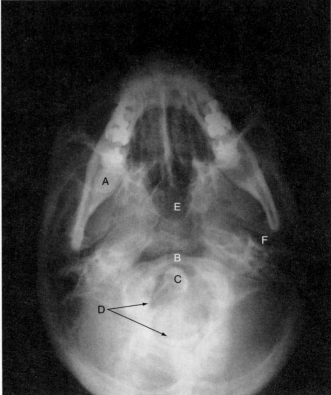

B

Figure 6–59. **(A)** Basal view of the skull (external aspect, inferior view). **(B)** SMV skull demonstrates the base of the skull. A, mandible; B, anterior arch C1; C, odontoid process/dens; D, foramen magnum; E, sphenoid sinuses; F, auditory canal. (Courtesy of Stamford Hospital, Department of Radiology.)

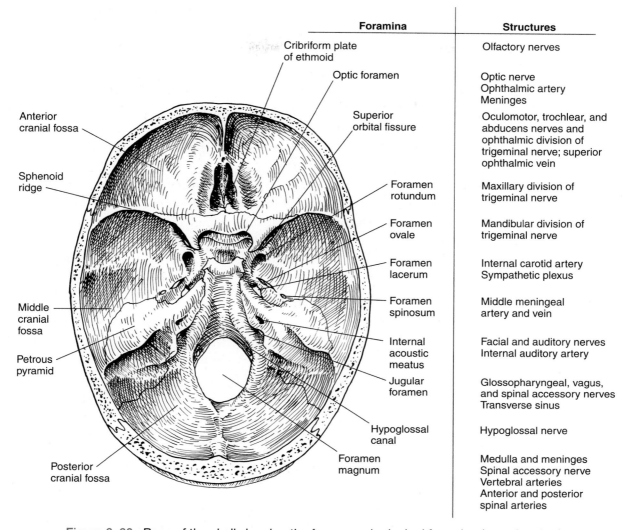

Foramina	Structures
Cribriform plate of ethmoid	Olfactory nerves
Optic foramen	Optic nerve Ophthalmic artery Meninges
Superior orbital fissure	Oculomotor, trochlear, and abducens nerves and ophthalmic division of trigeminal nerve; superior ophthalmic vein
Foramen rotundum	Maxillary division of trigeminal nerve
Foramen ovale	Mandibular division of trigeminal nerve
Foramen lacerum	Internal carotid artery Sympathetic plexus
Foramen spinosum	Middle meningeal artery and vein
Internal acoustic meatus	Facial and auditory nerves Internal auditory artery
Jugular foramen	Glossopharyngeal, vagus, and spinal accessory nerves Transverse sinus
Hypoglossal canal	Hypoglossal nerve
Foramen magnum	Medulla and meninges Spinal accessory nerve Vertebral arteries Anterior and posterior spinal arteries

Other labels on illustration: Anterior cranial fossa, Sphenoid ridge, Middle cranial fossa, Petrous pyramid, Posterior cranial fossa

Figure 6–60. Base of the skull showing the fossae and principal foramina (superior view).

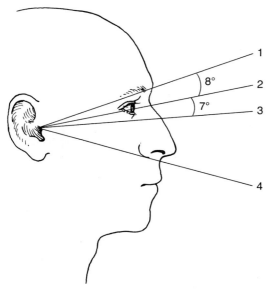

Figure 6–61. Four fundamental baselines are used in skull radiography: (1) the glabellomeatal (GML), (2) the orbitomeatal (OML, also known as canthomeatal or radiographic baseline), (3) the infraorbitomeatal (IOML), and (4) the acanthiomeatal line. There is approximately a 7 degree difference between the OML and IOML and 8 degree between the OML and GML.

- *Inferior orbital fissures:* large openings, lie between the greater wings and the maxilla

Occipital bone

- Forms part of posterior wall and inferior part of cranium (Figs. 6–58A and B and 6–60)
- Upper portion of each side articulates with parietal bones to form lambdoidal suture
- *Basilar portion:* articulates anteriorly with basilar portion (clivus) of sphenoid bone
- *Lateral portions* (2): bilateral to foramen magnum; occipital condyles, hypoglossal canals, and jugular foramina located here
- *Foramen magnum:* large opening; transmits inferior portion of brain (medulla oblongata), which is continuous with spinal cord
- *Squammosal portion:* posterior, superior portion; presents the external occipital protuberance (inion, occiput)

Temporal bones

- Irregularly shaped bones forming lateral aspects of cranium
- Located between greater wings of sphenoid bone and occipital bone (Figs. 6–57 and 6–59A and B)
- Dense, *petrous portions* form ridges and contain the organs of hearing
- Contain internal auditory meati and carotid canals
- *Zygomatic processes:* extend from flat, squammous portion; articulate with zygomatic (facial) bones
- *Mandibular fossae:* articulate with mandibular condyles to form temporomandibular joints (TMJs)
- *Temporal styloid processes:* sharp, slender processes extending anteriorly and inferiorly to mastoid processes
- *External auditory meatus (EAM):* external openings of the ear canal
- *Mastoid processes:* inferior to EAM; contain numerous air cells; communicate with tympanic cavity (middle ear) at mastoid antrum

Facial Bones

Nasal bones

- Small, rectangular (Fig. 6–57)
- Form bridge of nose
- Movable part of nose is composed of cartilage
- Articulate with each other at midline to form nasal suture
- Frontonasal suture: formed by articulation with frontal bone; corresponds to nasion externally

Lacrimal bones

- Smallest of facial bones
- Form part of medial orbital wall (Fig. 6–57)
- Lacrimal groove: accommodates lacrimal (tear) duct

Zygomatic (malar) bones

- Inferior and lateral to outer canthus of eye; cheek bones

Facial Bones (14)

(2) Nasal
(2) Lacrimal (smallest)
(2) Palatine
(2) Inferior nasal conchae
(2) Zygomatic/malar
(2) Maxillae
(1) Vomer
(1) Mandible (largest; only movable)

- Have four processes: frontosphenoidal, orbital, temporal, and maxillary (Fig. 6–57)

Maxillae

- Second largest of facial bones (Fig. 6–57 and 6–59)
- Articulate with each other to form most of upper jaw (hard palate)
- *Palatine processes:* plates of bone that articulate at midline to form two-thirds of the hard palate
- Form most of roof of mouth (hard palate) and floor of nasal cavity
- Contain the maxillary sinuses (maxillary antra; antra of high-more) just superior to bicuspid teeth; the thin floor of the maxillary sinus is formed by the alveolar process
- *Alveolar ridge/process:* contains sockets for teeth; spongy ridge of bone
- *Anterior nasal spine:* corresponds to *acanthion* externally
- *Infraorbital foramen:* located below orbit, lateral to nasal cavity

Palatine bones

- Small bones; form posterior one-third of hard palate (Fig. 6–59)
- L-shaped; have vertical and horizontal processes
- *Horizontal parts:* articulate with palatine processes of maxillae to complete the hard palate
- *Vertical parts:* project superiorly from horizontal part to articulate with the sphenoid bones

Inferior conchae (nasal turbinates)

- Completely osseous (Fig. 6–57)
- Placed inferiorly on each lateral wall of nasal cavity

Vomer

- Inferior to perpendicular plate of ethmoid bone
- Forms posterior bony septum (Fig. 6–57A)
- *Choanae:* posterior opening into nasopharynx; separated by posterior portion of vomer

Mandible

- U-shaped bone; largest facial bone (Fig. 6–57)
- Only movable facial bone
- *Mandibular symphysis:* where two halves fuse after birth
- *Mental tubercles:* prominences at inferolateral margin of symphysis
- *Mental protuberance:* protuberance at lower portion of symphysis
- *Alveolar process/ridge:* spongy ridge of bone with sockets for teeth
- *Body:* horizontal position
- *Ramus:* posterior vertical portion
- *Angle:* junction of vertical and horizontal parts: corresponds to external landmark: *gonion*
- *TMJ:* articulation of head of condyle with mandibular fossa of temporal bone; only movable articulation in skull
- *Coronoid process:* extends anterior and superior from ramus and has no articulation; serves as muscle attachment

- *Mandibular notch:* deep notch between condyloid and coronoid processes
- *Mental foramen:* small opening on outer surface of body, approximately below second premolar; passage for mandibular nerve
- *Mandibular foramen:* opening on inner side of ramus for mandibular nerve

Tables 6–35 through 6–41 provide a summary of positions/projections of the cranium and all facial bones.

Cranium (Table 6–35)

TABLE 6–35. The Cranium

Cranium	Position of Part	Central Ray Directed	Structures Included/Best Seen
PA	Patient prone, MSP ⊥ midtable, OML ⊥ IR (see Fig. 6–62)	⊥ nasion	PA proj of skull, *petrous pyramids should fill the orbits;* demonstrates frontal bone, lateral cranial walls, frontal sinuses, crista galli (see Fig. 6–62)

Note: General survey cranium can be obtained with CR ed 15 degree caudad to nasion (ridges fill lower 1/3 orbits). Similar projections of the same structures may be obtained in the AP position with the OML vertical if the CR is directed in the opposite direction. Anterior structures will be somewhat magnified and eye/lens dose will be greater.

PA axial (*Caldwell*)	Patient PA, MSP centered to grid, OML ⊥ grid, IR centered to nasion	15 degree caudad to nasion	PA axial of cranium, petrous portions in lower third of orbits, frontal and ethmoid sinuses (see Fig. 6–70)
AP axial (*Towne*)	Patient supine, MSP midtable, OML vertical, top of IR 1.5″ below vertex	30 degree caudad to a point ≈1.5″ above glabella (or 37 degree to IOML)	AP axial of skull, especially for *occipital bone,* symmetrical proj of petrous pyramids, projects dorsum sella and posterior clinoid processes within the foramen magnum (Fig. 6–63A)

Note: Excessive tube/or neck flexion will project posterior arch of C1 in foramen magnum. A collimated proj of the sella turcica can be obtained in this proj; an AP axial of the zygomatic arches can be obtained by directing the CR to the glabella and decreasing the technical factors. Similar results can be obtained in the PA position (PA axial; Haas method) with the CR ed 25 degree cephalad to the OML—the CR enters 1½″ below the inion and exits 1½″ above the nasion; it is particularly useful for hypersthenic or kyphotic patients although some magnification of the occipital bone must be expected.

Lateral	Patient PA oblique w/ skull MSP ∥ grid, interpupillary line vertical, IOML ∥ transverse axis of IR	⊥ a point 2″ superior to EAM	Lat proj of skull demonstrating superimposed cranial and facial structures; anterior and posterior clinoid processes and supraorbital margins should be superimposed (see Fig. 6–63B)
Full basal proj submento vertical (SMV)	Patient supine or seated AP, neck hyperextended to place IOML ∥ IR and CR, MSP ⊥ IR ⊥	⊥ IOML and IR, enters MSP at level of sella	Full basal proj of skull, useful for many foramina (spinosum, ovale, carotid canals), sphenoid and maxillary sinuses, dens through foramen magnum, symmetrical proj of petrous pyramids w/ mandibular condyles projected anterior to petrosae and symphysis superimposed on frontal bone (see Figs. 6–59B and 6–64)

Note: A decrease of 10 kV will demonstrate a bilateral axial projection of the zygomatic arches (see Figs. 6–64B and 6–65).

AP (*trauma*)	Patient supine, MSP ⊥ mid-table, OML ⊥ IR	⊥ nasion	AP proj of skull, petrous pyramids should fill the orbits
AP axial (*trauma*)	Patient AP, MSP centered to grid, OML ⊥ grid, IR centered to nasion	15 degree cephalad to nasion	AP axial of cranium, petrous portions in lower third of orbits; facial structures somewhat magnified
Lat (*trauma*)	Patient supine, head supported on sponge, grid IR vertical adjacent to side of interest. MSP ⊥ interpupillary line ⊥ IR.	⊥ IR, 2″ lat superior to EAM.	Lat proj of skull in dorsal decubitus position; can demonstrate sphenoid sinus effusion as the only sign of basal skull fx

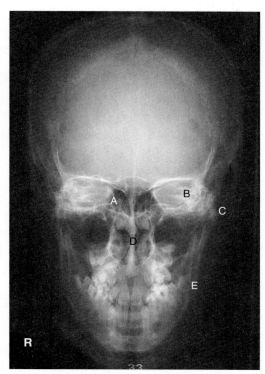

Figure 6–62. PA skull radiograph; the correct amount of flexion places the petrous pyramids within the orbits. A, ethmoid sinuses B, petrous portion of temporal bone; C, mastoid air cells/process; D, vomer; E, mandibular angle. (Courtesy of Stamford Hospital, Department of Radiology.)

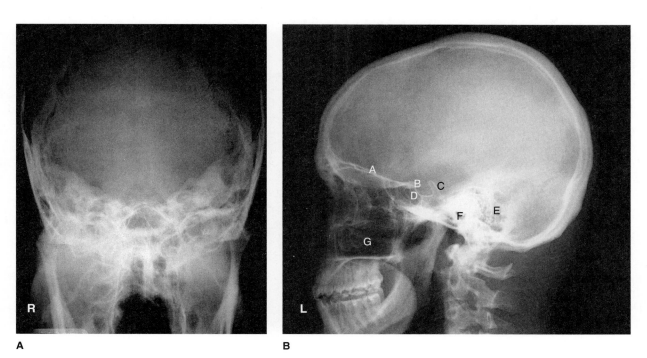

A

B

Figure 6–63. (**A**) AP axial (Towne method) projection of the skull; demonstrates the dorsum sella and posterior clinoid processes within the foramen magnum; useful for demonstration of the occipital bone. (**B**) Lateral projection of the skull. A, supraorbital margins; B, anterior clinoid processes; C, dorsum sella; D, sphenoid sinus; E, mastoid air cells; F, external auditory meatus; G, maxillary sinus. (Courtesy of Stamford Hospital, Department of Radiology.)

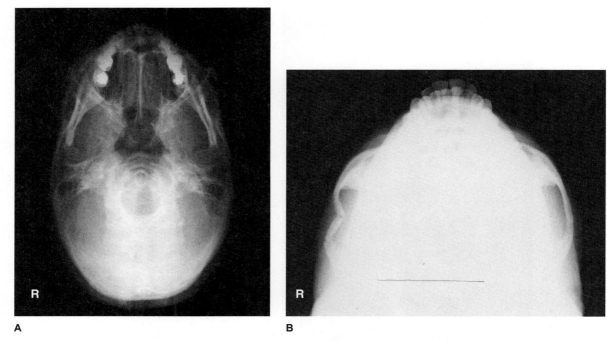

A   B

Figure 6–64. (**A**) Submentovertical (SMV) skull. The success of this projection depends on positioning the CR ⊥ the IOML and IR. (**B**) SMV projection of the skull, collimated and exposure factors adjusted to demonstrate zygomatic arches. Note fracture of right zygomatic arch. (Courtesy of Stamford Hospital, Department of Radiology.)

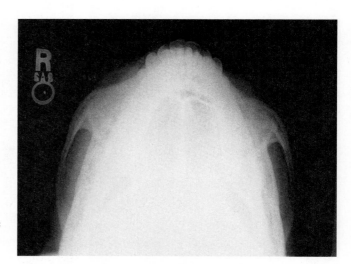

Figure 6–65. SMV projection of bilateral zygomatic arches. (Courtesy of Stamford Hospital, Department of Radiology.)

Orbits. The orbital cavities are formed by seven bones (frontal, sphenoid, ethmoid, maxilla, palatine, zygoma/malar, and lacrimal). The orbital walls are fragile and the orbital floor is subject to traumatic *blowout* fractures—the second most common facial fracture (nasal fx is #1). Orbital fractures can be accompanied by injury to adjacent structures—bone, muscle, other soft tissue. Leakage of air from the adjacent maxillary sinuses can cause orbital edema. Orbital floor fractures can be demonstrated using the *parietoacanthial (Waters)* projection; CT is often indicated for further evaluation (see Table 6–36).

TABLE 6–36. The Orbits

Orbits	Position of Part	Central Ray Directed	Structures Included/Best Seen
Parietoa-canthial (*Waters*)	Patient PA, MSP ⊥ Centered to grid, chin extended so OML is 37 degree to IR	⊥ to parietal region, exiting at acanthion	Axial proj of facial bones, especially orbits, zygomas, and maxillae; best single proj for *facial bones*
Note: X-ray beam may be collimated to orbital region, with CR passing through MSP, and exiting midorbits.			
PA axial (*Caldwell*)	Patient PA, skull MSP centered to grid, OML ⊥ grid, IR centered to nasion	15 degree caudad to nasion	PA axial of orbits, nasal septum, maxillae, and zygomas. Petrous pyramids are seen in the *lower one-third of the orbits*
Note: X-ray beam may be collimated to orbital region, with CR passing through MSP, and exiting midorbits.			
Lateral	Patient PA oblique w/ skull MSP ∥ grid, interpupillary line vertical, IOML ∥ transverse axis of IR	⊥ a point 2″ superior to EAM	Lat proj of skull demonstrating super-imposed cranial and facial structures; anterior and posterior clinoid processes and supraorbital margins should be superimposed
Note: X-ray beam may be collimated to orbital region, with CR passing parallel to interpupillary line.			

Facial Bones, Zygomatic Arches, and Nasal Bones (Tables 6–37 through 6–39)

TABLE 6–37. The Facial Bones

Facial Bones	Position of Part	Central Ray Directed	Structures Included/Best Seen
Parietoa-canthial (*Waters*)	Patient PA, MSP ⊥ centered to grid, chin extended so OML is 37 degree to IR	⊥ to parietal region, exiting at acanthion	Axial proj of facial bones, especially orbits, zygomas, and maxillae; best single proj for *facial bones*
Note: Patient should be upright to demonstrate air/fluid levels.			
Lateral	Patient PA obl, MSP of skull ∥ table, interpupillary line ⊥ IOML ∥ to transverse axis of IR	⊥ zygoma	Lat proj of superimposed facial bones
PA axial (*Caldwell*)	Patient PA, MSP centered to grid, OML ⊥ grid, IR centered to nasion	15 degree caudad to nasion	PA axial of facial bones, petrous portions in lower third of orbits
AP axial *trauma* (*Reverse Waters*)	Patient supine, MSP ⊥ midtable	30 degree ∥ mentomeatal line, entering acanthion	Axial, but *magnified*, proj of facial bones
Lateral *trauma*	Patient supine, performed "crosstable," horizontal beam	CR enters 2″ superior to EAM; grid cassette placed adjacent to lateral aspect of patient skull	

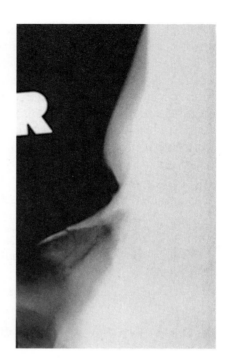

Figure 6–66. Lateral nasal bones demonstrating fracture. (Courtesy of Stamford Hospital, Department of Radiology.)

TABLE 6–38. The Zygomatic Arches

Zygomatic Arches	Position of Part	Central Ray Directed	Structures Included/Best Seen
Full basal position/ submentovertical proj (SMV)	Patient supine or seated AP, neck hyperextended to place IOML ∥ IR and ⊥ CR, MSP ⊥ IR	⊥ IOML and IR, enters MSP at level of sella	SMV proj of skull, useful for many foramina, sphenoid, and maxillary sinuses; a decrease of 10 kV will demonstrate a bilateral axial projection of the zygomatic arches (Figs. 6–64B and 6–65)

Note: In this projection, the skull may be rotated 15 degree *toward the affected side* to better "open up" the zygomatic arches in individuals having flat cheekbones or a depressed fx.

AP axial (*Towne)*	Patient supine, MSP ⊥ midtable, OML vertical	30 degree caudad to glabella (or 37 degree to IOML)	AP axial of zygomatic arches free of superimposition
Parietoacanthial (*Waters*)	Patient PA, MSP ⊥ centered to grid, chin extended so OML is 37 degree to IR	⊥ to parietal region, exiting at acanthion	Axial proj of facial bones, especially orbits, zygomas, and maxillae; best single proj for *facial bones*

Note: Patient could be examined in the upright position to demonstrate air/fluid levels.

TABLE 6–39. The Nasal Bones

Nasal Bones	Position of Part	Central Ray Directed	Structures Included/Best Seen
Lateral	Patient PA obl, MSP of skull ∥ table, interpupillary line ⊥ IOML ∥ to transverse axis of IR	⊥ a point 3/4″ dist to nasion; include nasofrontal suture through anterior nasal spine of maxilla	Lat proj of superimposed nasal bones and their associated soft tissue (see Fig. 6–66)

Note: The *parietoacanthial* (modified Waters) and *PA axial* (Caldwell) from *facial bone* series are most often included in the *nasal bone* series.

Mandible and Temporomandibular Joints (TMJs) (See Tables 6–40 and 6–41).

TABLE 6–40. The Mandible

Mandible	Position of Part	Central Ray Directed	Structures Included/Best Seen
PA	Patient PA, nose and forehead on table, MSP ⊥ IR centered to tip of nose	⊥ the lips	PA proj of mandible, especially body and rami (Fig. 6–67A)
PA axial	Patient PA, nose and forehead on table, MSP ⊥ IR centered to glabella	20–25 degree cephalad to center of IR	PA axial mandible, especially for rami and condyles
Axiolateral oblique	Patient PA, MSP of skull, IR centered 1/2″ anterior and 1″ inferior to the EAM	25 degree cephalad, enters at mandibular angle of unaffected side	Axiolateral mandible, especially for body and ramus; rotate MSP 15 degree forward to better demonstrate body (see Fig. 6–67B)
AP axial (*Towne*)	Patient supine, MSP ⊥ midtable, OML vertical	30 degree caudad through midramus (or 37 degree to IOML)	AP axial of mandibular rami free of superimposition
Basal proj/ submen- tovertical (SMV)	Patient supine or seated AP, neck hyperextended to place IOML ∥ IR and CR, ⊥ MSP ⊥ IR	⊥ IOML and IR, enters MSP at level of sella	Full basal proj of skull; useful for odontoid process through foramen magnum, symmetrical proj of petrous pyramids w/ mandibular condyles projected anterior to petrosae and symphysis superimposed on frontal bone (see Fig. 6–64)

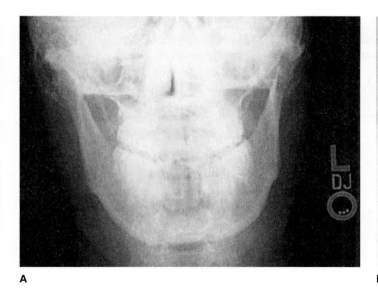
A

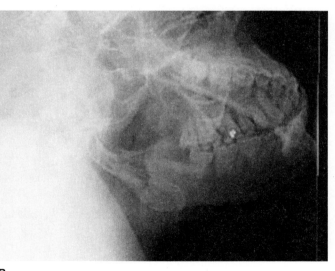
B

Figure 6–67. **(A)** PA mandible. **(B)** Axiolateral mandible, projects body, and ramus for visualization. (Courtesy of Stamford Hospital, Department of Radiology.)

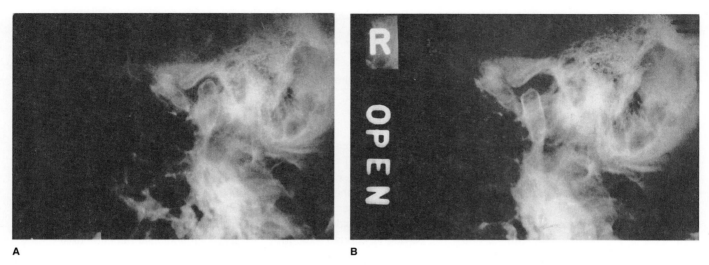

A   B

Figure 6–68. (A) Radiograph demonstrates the oblique lateral projection of the TMJ in the closed-mouth position. **(B)** The open-mouth position. (Courtesy of Stamford Hospital, Department of Radiology.)

TABLE 6–41. The Temperomandibular Joint (TMJ)

TMJ	Position of Part	Central Ray Directed	Structures Included/Best Seen
AP axial (*Towne*)	Patient AP, MSP ⊥ mid-IR, OML ⊥ table	30 degree caudad, enters ≈3″ above nasion	AP axial proj of condyloid processes and their articulations; *unless contraindicated*, another exposure is made with the *mouth open* (Fig. 6–68)
Lateral (*Schüller*)	Patient PA oblique w/ skull MSP ∥ grid, interpupillary line vertical, IOML ∥ transverse axis of IR	25 degree caudad, exiting lower-most TMJ	Axiolateral TMJ *unless contraindicated, a second exposure is made with the mouth open*
Axiolateral (*Law*)	Patient PA oblique w/ IOML ∥ IR and MSP ∥ Rotate MSP down 15 degree *toward* grid	15 degree caudad, enters 1¹⁄₂″ superior to uppermost EAM, exiting lowermost TMJ	Axiolateral TMJ of side down; *unless contraindicated, a second exposure is made with the mouth open*

Paranasal Sinuses. There are four paired *paranasal sinuses: frontal, ethmoidal, maxillary,* and *sphenoidal* (Fig. 6–69); they vary greatly in their size and shape. The left and right frontal sinuses are usually asymmetrical. They are located behind the glabella and superciliary arches of the frontal bone. The frontal sinuses are not present in young children and reach their adult size in the 15th or 16th year. The ethmoidal sinuses are composed of 6 to 18 thin-walled air cells that occupy the bony labyrinth of the ethmoid bone. The ethmoidal sinuses of children are very small and do not fully develop until after the 14th year. The maxillary sinuses (maxillary antra/antra of Highmore) are the largest of the paranasal sinuses and are located in the body of the maxillae. The *maxillary* antra are particularly prone to infection and collections of stagnant mucus. The maxillary antra reach their adult size around the 12th year. The sphenoidal sinuses are located in the body of the sphenoid

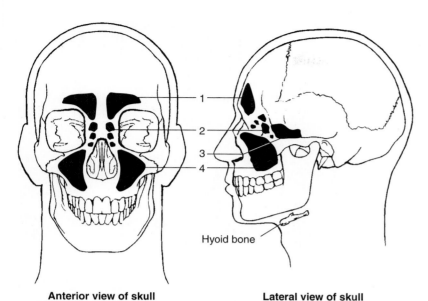

Anterior view of skull   **Lateral view of skull**

Figure 6–69. The paranasal sinuses, AP and lateral views. Frontal sinuses (1), Ethmoid sinuses (2), Sphenoid sinuses (3), Maxillary sinuses (4).

bone and are usually asymmetrical. They generally reach adult size by the 14th year.

Radiography of the paranasal sinuses must be performed in the erect position so that any *fluid levels* may be demonstrated and to distinguish between fluid and other pathology such as *polyps*.

To demonstrate air/fluid levels, *the CR must always be directed parallel to the floor*, even if the patient is not completely erect (just as in chest radiography). If the CR is angled to parallel the plane of the body, any fluid levels will be distorted or actually obliterated (see Table 6–42).

TABLE 6–42. The Paranasal Sinuses

Paranasal Sinuses	Position of Part	Central Ray Directed	Structures Included/Best Seen
PA axial (*Caldwell*)	Patient PA, skull MSP centered to grid, elevate chin to place OML 15 degree w/ horizontal	⊥ to nasion	PA axial of *frontal* and *anterior ethmoid* sinuses, petrous pyramids are seen in the *lower one-third of the orbits* (see Fig. 6–70)
Parietoa-canthial (*Waters*)	Patient PA, skull MSP centered to grid, OML 37 degree to IR centered to acanthion	⊥ enters parietal region and exits acanthion	Parietoacanthial proj of *maxillary* sinuses projected *above petrous pyramids* (see Fig. 6–71)

Note: Insufficient neck extension results in petrosae superimposed on floor of maxillary sinus; distorted projection of frontal and ethmoid.

A modification of the parietoacanthiasl projection made with the ***mouth open*** will demonstrate the *sphenoid sinuses* through the open mouth.

Lateral	Patient PA obl, skull MSP ∥ to IR centered 1″ posterior to outer canthus, interpupillary line vertical	⊥ mid-IR, enters 1″ posterior to outer canthus	Lat proj of all paranasal sinuses (see Fig. 6–72)
SMV (*full basal*)	AP erect, neck hyperextended to place IOML ∥ IR and CR, MSP ⊥ IR ⊥	⊥ IOML and IR, enters MSP at level of sella	Basal proj of sphenoid and ethmoid sinuses; mandibular symphysis should be super-imposed on frontal bone (see Fig. 6–73)

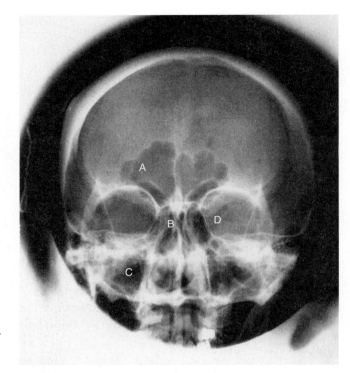

Figure 6–70. PA axial projection (Caldwell position) of the frontal and anterior ethmoid sinuses. The caudal angulation is somewhat excessive because the petrous pyramids are seen at the lowermost portion of the orbits. Correct angulation places the petrous pyramids in the lower one-third of the orbits. A, frontal sinuses; B, ethmoid air cells/sinuses; C, maxillary sinus; D, superior orbital fissure. (Courtesy of Stamford Hospital, Department of Radiology.)

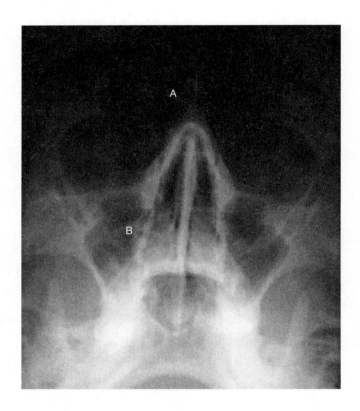

Figure 6–71. Parietoacanthial projection (Water method). The sinuses are centered to the image receptor. The chin is adequately extended and the petrous pyramids are seen below the floor of the maxillary sinuses. The parietoacanthial projection provides a fore-shortened view of the frontal and ethmoid sinuses. In a modification of this projection, the sphenoid sinuses would be seen through the open mouth. A, frontal sinuses; B, maxillary sinus. (Courtesy of Stamford Hospital, Department of Radiology.)

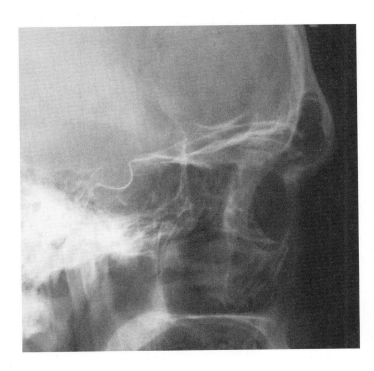

Figure 6–72. Lateral projection of the paranasal sinuses. All paranasal sinuses are demonstrated on the lateral projection. (Courtesy of Stamford Hospital, Department of Radiology.)

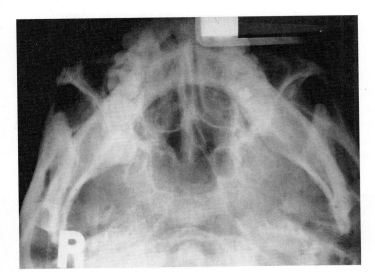

Figure 6–73. SMV projection of paranasal sinuses. Sphenoid and posterior ethmoid are demonstrated.

Soft Tissue Neck. The *upper airway* (Fig. 6–74 and Table 6–43) can be examined in the *AP* and *lateral* positions. These projections are used to demonstrate hypertrophy of the pharyngeal tonsils or adenoids. It is desired to see the nasopharynx *filled with air* to provide adequate contrast; therefore, the exposure must be made on *slow nasal inspiration.*

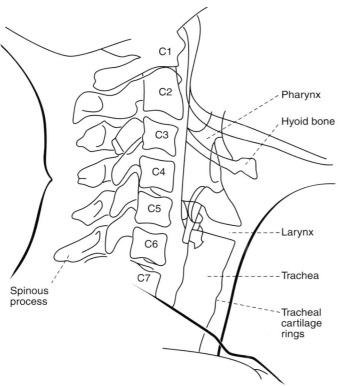

Figure 6–74. Anatomy of the neck, especially structures demonstrated in soft tissue study.

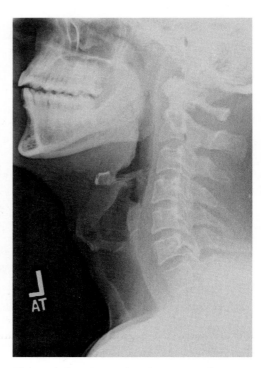

Figure 6–75. Lateral projection, soft tissue neck study (see Table 6–43).

TABLE 6–43. The Upper Airway

Upper Airway	Position of Part	Central Ray Directed	Structures Included/Best Seen
AP	Patient AP supine or erect, MSP ⊥ IR	⊥ to IR at level of EAM; expose on slow nasal inspiration	Air-filled nasopharynx/upper airway
Lateral	Patient lateral, preferably erect, MSP ∥ IR	⊥ to IR at level of EAM; expose on slow nasal inspiration	Air-filled nasopharynx/upper airway (Fig. 6–75)

COMPREHENSION CHECK

Congratulations! You have completed a large portion of this chapter. If you are able to answer the following group of very comprehensive questions, you should feel confident that you have really mastered this section. You can refer back to the indicated pages to check your answers and/or review the subject matter.

1. Identify the bony structures comprising the axial skeleton (p. 133-136).

2. Describe the (a) method of positioning, (b) direction and point of entry of the CR, (c) principal structures visualized, and (d) pertinent traumatic and pathologic conditions and any technical adjust-

ments they may necessitate relative to the axial skeleton, to include routine and special views of the

A. Cervical spine (p. 137, 138).

B. Thoracic spine (p. 139, 140).

C. Lumbar spine (p. 140-143).

D. Sacrum, coccyx (p. 143-145).

E. Scoliosis series (p. 145).

F. Sternum and ribs (p. 146-148).

G. Cranial and facial bones (p. 156-162).

H. Paranasal sinuses; upper airway (p. 162-166).

BODY SYSTEMS

Respiratory System

Introduction. The respiratory system includes the nose, pharynx ("throat"), larynx ("voice box"), trachea ("windpipe"), bronchi, and lungs. The nose, pharynx, and larynx make up the *upper respiratory system*, while the trachea, bronchi, and lungs make up the *lower respiratory system*. The functions of the respiratory system include supplying oxygen to the blood and relieving the body of carbon dioxide (Fig. 6–76). Pulmonary function depends on the processes of *ventilation* and *alveolar gas exchange.*

The external openings of the *nose* are the nostrils, or *nares*; its internal/posterior openings are the *choanae* or *internal nares*. The external visible portion of the nose consists of hyaline cartilage, muscle, and skin—while its inner surface is lined with mucous membrane and receives olfactory nerve endings for the sense of smell. The internal nose structures function to warm, moisten, and filter incoming air and to detect smell.

The *pharynx* is divided into three portions: the *nasopharynx*, the *oropharynx*, and the *laryngopharynx*. The pharynx is just posterior to the oral cavity; it begins at the choanae and terminates at the level of the cricoid cartilage. The pharynx functions as part of the digestive system, as well as the respiratory system, because it serves as passageway for both food and air. As part of the digestive system, the pharynx aids in *deglutition* (swallowing); it also houses the pharyngeal *tonsils,* which have immunological functions.

The auditory tubes open into the nasopharynx; the oropharynx and laryngopharynx are the pharyngeal portions common to both the respiratory and digestive systems; the laryngopharynx opens into the larynx anteriorly and the esophagus posteriorly.

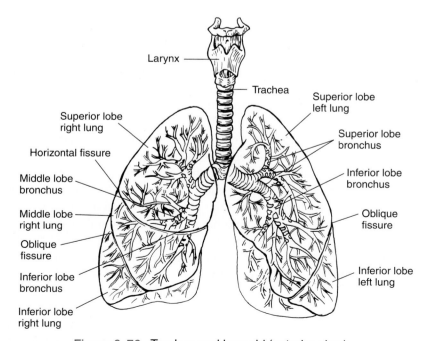

Figure 6–76. Trachea and bronchi (anterior view).

The *larynx* lies in the anterior neck at about the level of C4 to C6; it connects the laryngopharynx and trachea. The laryngeal walls are composed of nine cartilages. Three of the cartilages are *single/unpaired*; they are the *thyroid* cartilage, the *epiglottis*, and the *cricoid* cartilage. Three of the cartilages are *paired*: the *arytenoid*, the *cuneiform*, and the *corniculate* cartilages. The paired cartilages are principally concerned with speech.

The thyroid cartilage, also referred to as the laryngeal prominence or Adam's Apple, is the most superior cartilage and forms the anterior laryngeal wall. The epiglottis is a leaf-shaped (elastic) cartilage that covers the glottis (vocal folds) during deglutition. The cricoid (hyaline) cartilage is the most inferior of the nine cartilages; incision for emergency tracheotomy is made just below the cricoid cartilage.

The *trachea* ("windpipe") is a cylindrical cartilaginous tube, approximately $4\frac{1}{2}$ in. in length, extending from the larynx (approximately C6) to the primary bronchi (approximately T5). Its ciliated mucosa functions to protect against mucus, dust, and pathogens. The trachea is formed by *16 to 20 C-shaped* cartilaginous (hyaline) rings that can be palpated through the skin of the anterior neck.

At about the level of T5, the trachea divides into the right and left *mainstem*, or primary, *bronchi*; at the bifurcation is a ridge called the *carina*, which separates the openings of the primary bronchi. The right main bronchus is wider and more vertical; therefore, aspirated foreign bodies are more likely to enter it than the left main bronchus, which is narrower and angles more sharply from the trachea. Each mainstem bronchus opens into the *hilum* of the corresponding lung.

The right lung is shorter because the liver is below it; the left lung is narrower because the heart occupies a portion of the lung's left side. The lungs have a somewhat conical shape; their narrow upper portion is called the *apex*, and their wide *base* is defined by the *diaphragmatic surface*. Structures such as the mainstem bronchi and pulmonary artery and veins enter and leave the lungs at the *hilum*. The *right lung* has *three lobes*; the upper and middle lobes are separated by the *horizontal fissure*, and the middle and lower lobes are separated by the *oblique fissure*. The *left lung* has *two lobes*; the upper and lower lobes are separated by the *oblique fissure* (Fig. 6–76).

The lungs are enclosed in a serous membrane, the *parietal pleura*. The *visceral pleura* lines the inner thoracic wall and covers the superior surface of the diaphragm; the potential space between the two layers of pleura is the *pleural cavity*.

Pneumothorax is the presence of air in the pleural cavity. A large pneumothorax is usually accompanied by a partial or complete collapse of the lung (atelectasis). Radiographic indications of atelectasis include *elevation of the hemidiaphragm of the affected side* and an *increase in tissue* density of the collapsed lung. *Thoracentesis* is the procedure required to remove significant amounts of air, blood, or other fluids in the pleural cavity.

One of the most diagnostically useful and frequently performed radiographic examinations is the chest x-ray examination. During the course of their illness and recovery, patients often need successive chest examinations to monitor their progress, and reproduction of quality images is an important part of quality control. Accurate positioning and selection of technical factors is critical to the diagnostic value of the radiographic images. *Even slight rotation or leaning can cause significant*

Divisions of Pharynx:

- Nasopharynx
- Oropharynx
- Laryngopharynx

Laryngeal Cartilages (9):

Three single/unpaired:
- Thyroid
- Epiglottis
- Cricoid

Three paired:
- Arytenoid
- Cuneiform
- Corniculate

distortion of the size and shape of the heart. Consistent and accurate positioning is essential to radiographic quality.

The radiographer must take careful note of each patient's apparel, body type, and clinical information. Important considerations include removal of any radiopaque clothing and accessories, placing the IR transversely for broad-chested individuals (in order to include the *costophrenic angles*—blunting of the costophrenic angles is often a result of pleural effusion), instructing female patients with large breasts to move them up and laterally for the PA projection, exposing on the second inspiration for hypersthenic individuals, and adjusting exposure factors for various pathologic conditions. Appropriate radiation protection measures must always be provided.

Mobile chest radiography often brings the radiographer into contact with seriously ill patients. The radiographer must be very cautious when positioning these patients for there are often numerous tubes (e.g., chest tubes, endotracheal tubes, electrocardiographic [ECG] leads, Swan–Ganz lines, urinary catheters) associated with maintaining the patient's airway or reinflating a collapsed lung, removing fluid or air from the pleural cavity, administering medications, measuring central venous pressure, or measuring urine output (Fig. 6–77). The variety of wires and/or tubes can interfere with visualization of anatomic structures needed for optimum diagnostic value. Whenever possible, and with appropriate knowledge and caution, it is helpful to have these moved away from areas of interest.

Tables 6–44 and 6–45 provide a summary of routine projections and frequently performed special projections.

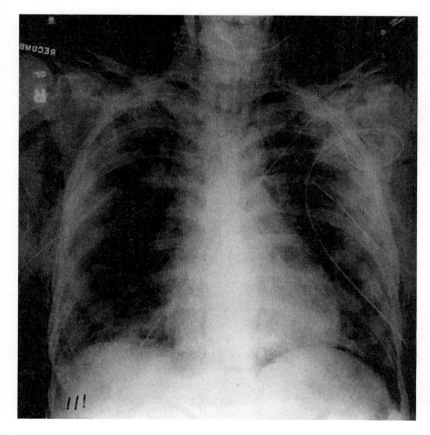

Figure 6–77. Mobile AP chest radiograph. Observe an endotracheal tube and ECG leads, one chest tube on the right and two on the left. The patient has extensive soft-tissue emphysema. Radiographers must exercise particular care when working around various patient tubes. (From the American College of Radiology Learning File. Courtesy of the ACR.)

Chest: PA, Lateral, and Oblique

TABLE 6–44. The Chest: PA and Lateral

Chest	Position of Part	Central Ray Directed	Structures Included/Best Seen
PA	Patient erect PA, MSP exactly ⊥ IR, shoulders depressed and rolled forward w/ back of hands on hips, top of IR 1.5–2″ above shoulders	⊥ T7	PA proj of thoracic viscera and skeletal anatomy; *inspiration* demonstrates air-filled trachea and lungs, 10 posterior ribs; *expiration* shows pulmonary vascular markings; *inspiration and expiration* are done for pneumothorax, foreign body, diaphragm excursion, and atelectasis (Fig. 6–78A)

Note: Chest radiography is performed *erect* whenever possible to demonstrate air/fluid levels. The MSP must be exactly vertical; any *rotation can cause significant distortion* and misrepresentation of the visceral structures (see Fig. 6–79A). *Rotation is detected on the PA radiograph by asymmetrical distance between the sternal ends of the clavicles and the lateral border of the thoracic vertebrae.* The shoulders are rolled forward to remove the scapulae from super-imposition on the lung fields. Superiorly, the *pulmonary apices* must be seen; inferiorly the *costophrenic angles* must be seen in their entirety. *Inspiration must be adequate to demonstrate 10 posterior ribs.* A 72 SID is recommended to decrease *magnification* of the heart. *Oblique* projections of the chest are occasionally performed as supplemental views. The *LAO and RAO* positions are performed with the MSP at 45 degree to the IR.

| Lateral | Patient erect L lat, MSP IR, arms over head, top of IR 1.5–2 above shoulders | ⊥ IR, enters at level of T7 | Lat proj of chest particularly useful for heart, aorta, L lung and its fissures, and other left-sided structures/pathology; L lat usually done to place heart closer to IR (Fig. 6–78B) |

Note: The MSP must be *exactly vertical;* any lateral leaning can cause significant distortion and misrepresentation of the visceral structures. *Rotation* is detected on the lateral radiograph by superimposition of ribs on sternum or vertebrae. Pulmonary apices and angles must be visualized (see Fig. 6–79B).

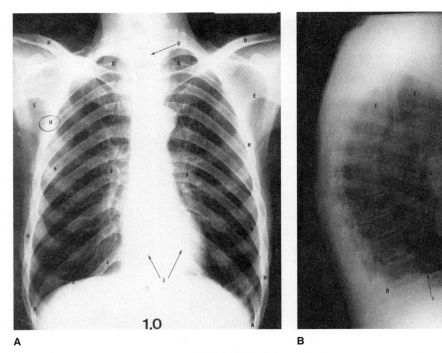

A   **B**

Figure 6–78. **(A)** PA projection of the chest. Identify the lettered structures. A, costophrenic angle; B, clavicle; C, diaphragmatic domes; D, pulmonary apices; E, scapula; F, rib—8th posterior; G, air-filled trachea; H, 4th rib—axillary portion; I, heart; a, 6th rib; b, axillary portion—8th rib; c, vertebral/floating rib. **(B)** Lateral projection of the chest. A, sternum; B, intervertebral foramen; C, apex of heart; D, heart; E, thoracic vertebra; F, pulmonary apices; G, hilar region; H, air-filled trachea; I and J, L and R hemidiaphragms. (Courtesy of Bob Wong, RT.)

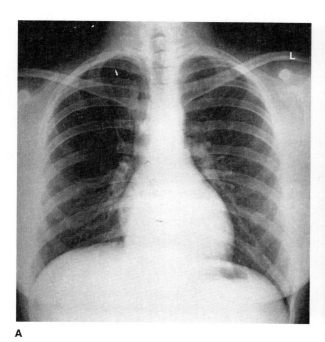
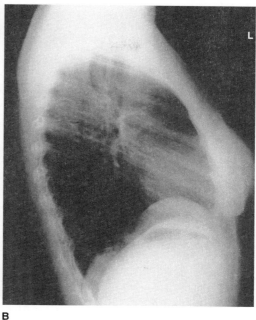

A   B

Figure 6–79. **(A)** PA projection of the chest of a normal, healthy adult *demonstrating the importance of positioning accuracy.* Slight rotation has made the manubrium visible at the site of the right sternoclavicular joint, *providing a density very similar to that created by a paraspinous or mediastinal mass.* **(B)** Lateral projection of the same chest and without rotation. The sternum is seen free of superimposed ribs; the thoracic and lumbar vertebral spinous processes are seen. (From the American College of Radiology Learning File. Courtesy of the ACR.)

Chest: Axial and Decubitus

TABLE 6–45. The Chest: Axial and Decubitus

Chest	Position of Part	Central Ray Directed	Structures Included/Best Seen
AP axial (*lordotic*)	Patient erect AP, MSP ⊥ mid-IR at level of T2	15–20 degree cephalad to T2	AP axial (lordotic) proj of pulmonary apices projected below clavicles (can also be done with patient leaning back and CR ⊥ IR)
Decubitus (*L and R lat*)	Patient recumbent lat on affected or unaffected side as indicated by hx; anterior or posterior surface adjacent to IR. MSP ⊥ mid-IR w/ top of IR 1.5 above shoulders	⊥ mid-IR	Frontal (AP or PA) proj of the chest useful for demonstration of air or fluid levels

Note: If free *air* is suspected, the affected side must be *up*; if *fluid* is suspected, the affected side must be placed *down*.

Airway. AP and lateral projections of the airway and larynx are occasionally required to rule out *foreign body, polyps, tumors,* or any other condition suspected of causing some airway obstruction.

The AP is positioned as for an AP cervical spine with the CR perpendicular to the *laryngeal prominence.* The lateral is positioned as for a lateral cervical spine and centered to the coronal plane passing through the trachea (anterior to the cervical spine) at the level of the laryngeal prominence. *Exposures are made on slow inspiration* to visualize air-filled structures.

Depending on the structure(s) of interest being examined, these positions may be performed with barium and/or during performance of the *Valsalva/modified Valsalva maneuver.* Phonation of vowel sounds can help demonstrate more superior structures such as the larynx and/or vocal cords.

Terminology and Pathology. The following is a list of radiographically significant conditions and devices with which the student radiographer should be familiar:

- Asthma
- Atelectasis
- Bronchiectasis
- Bronchitis
- Central venous pressure line
- Chest tube (see Fig. 6–77)
- Chronic obstructive pulmonary disease
- Cystic fibrosis
- Dextrocardia (see Fig. 6–81)
- Emphysema (see Figs. 6–77 and 6–80)
- Empyema
- Endotracheal tube (see Fig. 6–77)
- Hemothorax
- Hickman catheter
- Pneumoconiosis
- Pneumonia Pneumothorax
- Swan–Ganz catheter
- Thoracentesis
- Tuberculosis

Biliary System

Introduction. The biliary tree consists of the left and right hepatic ducts, common hepatic duct, cystic duct, common bile duct, and the gallbladder

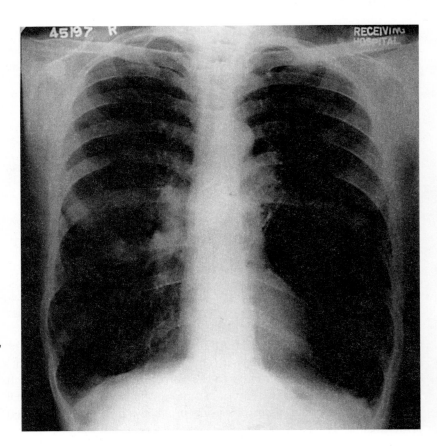

Figure 6–80. PA chest radiograph demonstrates the characteristic irreversible trapping of air found in emphysema, which gradually increases and overexpands the lungs, thus producing the *characteristic flattening of the diaphragm* and *widening of the intercostal spaces.* The increased air content of the lungs requires a compensating decrease in technical factors. (From the American College of Radiology Learning File. Courtesy of the ACR.)

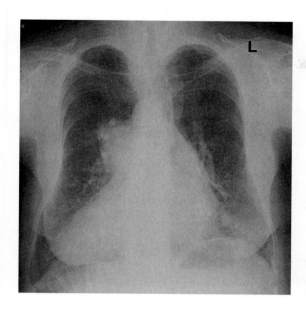

Figure 6–81. PA chest demonstrating dextrocardia. Dextrocardia is often associated with other heart defects. (Courtesy of Stamford Hospital, Department of Radiology.)

(GB) (Fig. 6–82). The hepatic ducts leave the liver and join to form the *common hepatic duct*. The short *cystic duct* continues to the GB. The common hepatic and cystic ducts unite to form the long *common bile duct*, which joints with the pancreatic duct to form the short *hepatopancreatic ampulla (of Vater)*. The ampulla opens into the descending duodenum through the *duodenal papilla*, that is surrounded by the *hepatopancreatic sphincter (of Oddi)*.

The *gallbladder* is located in a shallow fossa on the inferior surface of the liver between its right and quadrate lobes. Small gallstones are able to pass out the GB through the cystic duct; those that are too large irritate the GB mucosa, resulting in *cholecystitis*. *Gallstones* can also lodge in ducts. If a stone lodges in the cystic duct, cholecystitis without *jaundice* is the result, because bile can still drain into the duodenum. A stone lodged in the common bile duct will result in jaundice as well as cholecystitis. A "gallbladder attack" is the painful result of fatty chyme stimulating the release of *cholecystokinin*, which elevates pressure within the stone-laden GB.

Radiographic examinations of the biliary system include *oral cholecystography*, *operative cholangiography*, *T-tube cholangiography*, and *endoscopic retrograde cholangiopancreatography (ERCP)*. Each of these examinations requires the use of a contrast agent. With the exception of the ERCP, few of these examinations are performed today, but rather are imaged via *sonography* (Fig. 6–83).

Patient Preparation. For *oral cholecystograms* (OCG), iodinated tablets are taken the evening before the examination. The GB stores and concentrates the contrast-laden bile, rendering the GB radiopaque. The evening meal must be fat-free to prevent GB contraction and subsequent release of the radiopaque bile. Oral cholecystography is used to evaluate the function of the biliary system as well as demonstrate the structure and contents of the GB.

Operative cholangiography is used to examine the bile ducts and frequently follows a *cholecystectomy*. An iodinated contrast agent is introduced into the common bile duct to evaluate biliary patency and

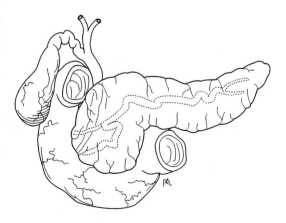

Figure 6–82. This illustrates the main hepatic and biliary ducts, gallbladder, and pancreas within the duodenal loop.

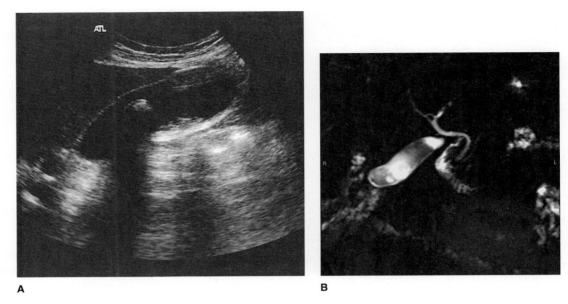

Figure 6–83. **(A)** A sonogram of the gallbladder demonstrating the presence of gallstones. (Courtesy of Stamford Hospital, Department of Radiology.) **(B)** MR image (Coronal T2) of biliary system. (Courtesy of Conrad P. Ehrlich, MD)

that of the hepatopancreatic ampulla. Any calculi can be detected and removed before completion of surgery.

Occasionally, a T-shaped tube is left in the common bile duct for postsurgical drainage. T-tube cholangiography is performed by injecting a contrast agent through the tube to detect any remaining calculi and evaluate the biliary tree patency.

ERCP is a specialized procedure used to evaluate suspected biliary and/or pancreatic conditions. An *endoscope* is passed through the mouth, esophagus, and stomach, and into the descending duodenum to the orifice of the hepatopancreatic ampulla. Contrast material is injected into the common bile duct for evaluation of the biliary system.

Tables 6–46 (OCG) and 6–47 (Surgical and T-tube) provide a summary of routine positions/projections for biliary system imaging.

Gallbladder. An oral cholecystogram frequently begins with a prone 14 × 17-inch image of the abdomen to check *opacification* and location of the GB as well as patient preparation and technical factors. Collimated recumbent PA and oblique, and erect or decubitus radiographs follow. In the absence of gallstones, a fatty meal may then be given to the patient and another similar series of images taken 20 to 30 minutes later. The fatty meal is used to check GB function: in the presence of fat, the GB should contract and evacuate its bile. Fluoroscopic images may be taken in addition to, or in place of, the postfat radiographs.

The gallbladder of the average-build patient is located between the 10th and 12th ribs on the right, midway between the vertebral column and lateral border of the body. *Hypersthenic* individuals usually require centering approximately 2 in. higher and more laterally, while centering for *asthenic* individuals is usually 2 in. lower and more midline. In the *erect* position, the GB of an asthenic patient can be as low as the iliac fossa.

TABLE 6–46. The OCG

OCG	Position of Part	Central Ray Directed	Structures Included/Best Seen
PA	Prone or PA erect, sagittal plane passing m/w b/w spine and R lat border of body, at level of 9th rib centered to grid (CR lower when done erect)	⊥ center of IR	PA recumbent or erect proj of GB. *The erect position will demonstrate layering of any gallstones* (Fig. 6–84A)
Oblique (*LAO*)	Recumbent LAO, sagittal plane passing m/w b/w spine and R lat border of body centered to grid at level of 9th rib	⊥ center of IR	Obl GB, with less foreshortening and self-superimposition than in PA. *Greater obliquity (40 degree) for asthenic patients* than for hypersthenic (15 degree) (Fig. 6–84B)
R Lateral Decubitus	Patient recumbent R ⊥ lat, posterior surface adjacent to upright grid and centered to level of gallbladder	⊥ center of IR	R lat decubitus of gallbladder useful for *stratification* (layering) of gallstones (Fig. 6–84) and the GB free of super-imposed bowel loops

Cholangiography: Surgical and T-Tube (Table 6–47)

TABLE 6–47. Surgical and T-Tube Imaging

Surgical/ T-Tube	Position of Part	Central Ray Directed	Structures Included/Best Seen
AP	Patient supine	⊥ center of IR	AP of biliary tree and gallbladder area; to evaluate the hepatopancreatic ampulla and biliary tree for calculi or other pathology (following injection of contrast into common bile duct) (Fig. 6–84C)

Note: Can be performed RPO with L side elevated 15 degree to 20 degree and R upper quadrant centered to grid.

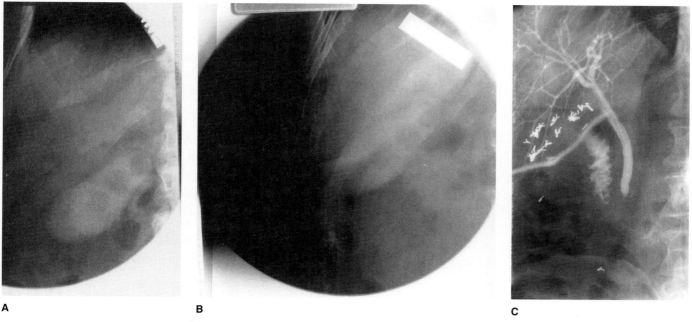

A   B   C

Figure 6–84. (A) PA projection of GB (with gallstones). (B) LAO of same GB. Oblique position moves GB away from verte-brae. (C) T-tube cholangiogram. (Courtesy of Stamford Hospital, Department of Radiology.)

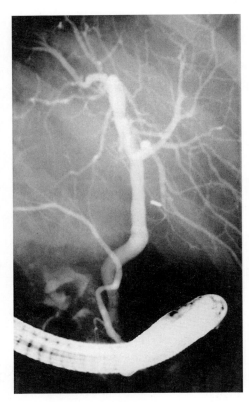

Figure 6–85. Fluoroscopic image of a normal ERCP. The pancreatic and common bile ducts are clearly delineated. (Courtesy of Stamford Hospital, Department of Radiology.)

ERCP. Following *canalization* of the hepatopancreatic ampulla, fluoroscopic images are made in the AP (RPO) or PA (LAO) position. Imaging procedure should immediately follow injection, since, under normal conditions, contrast will empty from the biliary ducts in approximately 5 minutes (Fig. 6–85).

Terminology and Pathology. The following is a list of radiographically significant conditions with which the student radiographer should be familiar:

- Cholecystitis
- Cholelithiasis
- Cirrhosis
- Hepatitis
- Jaundice
- Pancreatitis

Digestive System

Introduction. The major portion of the GI tract lies within the abdominopelvic cavity. Its principal functions are the chemical breakdown and absorption of nutrients. The digestive system (Fig. 6–86 A and B) consists of the *gastrointestinal (GI) tract* and *accessory organs*. The *gastrointestinal tract*, or *alimentary canal*, is a continuous tube of varying dimensions consisting of the esophagus, stomach, and small and large intestines. The teeth, tongue, salivary glands, liver, gallbladder, and pancreas are *accessory organs* that aid in the mechanical and chemical breakdown of food.

The lobulated salivary glands encircle the entrance to the oropharynx. The largest of the salivary glands is the *parotid* gland. The parotid is located just anterior to the ear and above the mandibular angle and is emptied by Stenson duct. The *submandibular* glands are located near the inner surface of the mandibular body and empty their digestive juices into the mouth via Wharton duct. The *sublingual* gland is located in the floor of the mouth and opens into the mouth by way of multiple ducts of Rivinas—the largest of these is Bartholins duct.

Salivary glands can be investigated radiographically (termed *sialography*) via injection of contrast material for demonstration of glandular disorders such as tumors, calculi, or fistula formation following trauma to the area. Sialography involves cannulation of the ostium of the parotid duct (Stenson) or the submandibular duct (Wharton). Figure 6–87 illustrates submandibular sialography.

The *esophagus* functions to propel a food bolus toward the stomach through *peristaltic* motion. The *cardiac sphincter* is located at the distal end of the esophagus. "Heartburn" is an inflammation of the esophageal *mucosa* as a result of gastric *reflux* of acidic material into the esophagus. *Esophageal varices* are dilated, *tortuous* veins directly beneath the esophageal mucosa. A hiatal hernia is a herniation of the stomach through the esophageal hiatus of the diaphragm, producing a sac-like dilatation above the diaphragm (Fig. 6–88A and B). The presence of reflux, varices, or herniation can be detected radiographically with the use of barium sulfate.

From the lower esophagus through the anal canal, the GI tract has the same four tissue layers. The innermost lining layer is the *mucosa*; mucous membranes line cavities that directly open to the exterior. This mucous membrane is composed of a layer of epithelium, whose cells

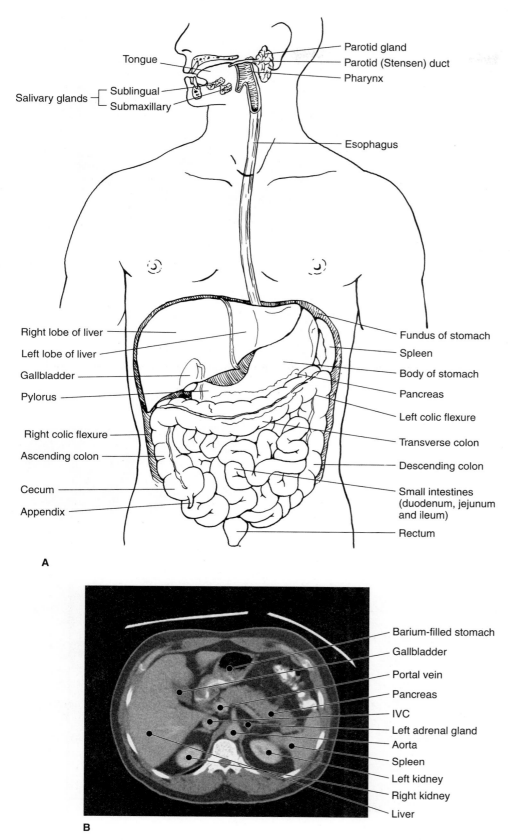

Tongue

Salivary glands
- Sublingual
- Submaxillary

Parotid gland
Parotid (Stensen) duct
Pharynx

Esophagus

Right lobe of liver
Left lobe of liver
Gallbladder
Pylorus

Right colic flexure
Ascending colon

Cecum
Appendix

Fundus of stomach
Spleen
Body of stomach
Pancreas
Left colic flexure

Transverse colon

Descending colon

Small intestines
(duodenum, jejunum
and ileum)

Rectum

A

Barium-filled stomach
Gallbladder
Portal vein
Pancreas
IVC
Left adrenal gland
Aorta
Spleen
Left kidney
Right kidney
Liver

B

Figure 6–86.   **(A)** The Digestive System **(B)** Axial CT image of the abdomen demonstrating many Digestive and Circulatory structures.

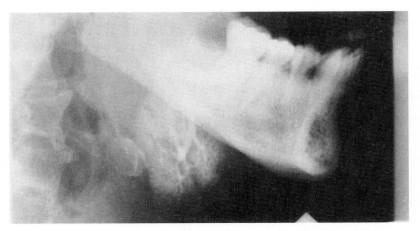

Figure 6–87. Submandibular sialogram (Courtesy of Stamford Hospital, Department of Radiology.)

are shed and are replaced every five to seven days. The two other layers of the mucosa are the lamina propria and a thin muscular layer. They assist, respectively, in immunity and in forming gastric folds (rugae).

The *submucosa* is highly vascular (blood and lymphatic vessels), contains a broad complex of neurons, and can also include glands and lymphatic tissue.

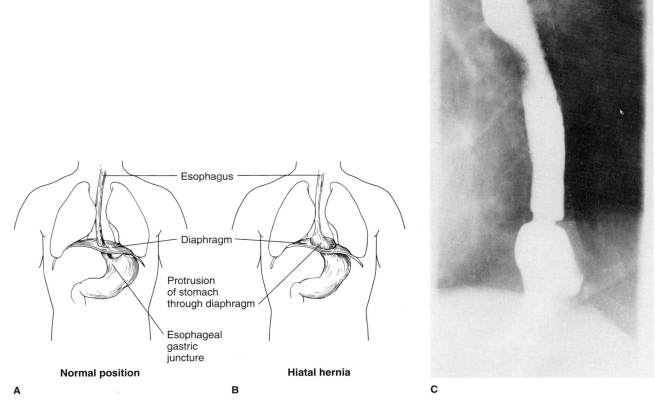

Figure 6–88. (A) Normal position of the stomach. (B) Note protrusion of stomach through esophageal hiatus (hiatal hernia). (C) Esophagram demonstrating hiatal hernia (with Schatzki ring). (Courtesy of Stamford Hospital, Department of Radiology.)

The *muscular* layer of structures through the esophagus consists of skeletal muscle, which permits the voluntary muscular actions of chewing and swallowing. Skeletal muscle is also found at the anal sphincter, permitting defecation. The remainder of the GI tract muscular layer is smooth/involuntary muscle that functions to mix and propel digestive secretions and food content.

The *serosa*/serous membrane is the outermost layer of the GI tract. Serous membranes line body cavities and covers organs that do not directly open to the exterior. Serous membranes produce a lubricating serous fluid that allows organs to glide over one another without friction. The serous membrane of the thoracic cavity is the double-walled pleura; the serous membrane of the abdominal cavity is the double-walled *peritoneum.*

The peritoneum has an outer parietal layer that lines the abdominal cavity. Its inner visceral layer is reflected over and between the abdominal organs forming large folds between the viscera; these folds attach the organs to the abdominal cavity and to each other. These folds also house nerves, and blood and lymphatic vessels. There are five major peritoneal folds: the greater omentum, the lesser omentum, the mesentery, the falciform ligament, and the mesocolon.

The *stomach* is the dilated, sac-like portion of the GI tract. When the stomach is empty, its mucosal lining forms soft folds called *rugae* (Fig. 6–89A). *Gastritis* is an inflammation of the gastric mucosa that can be caused by excessive secretion of acids or by ingestion of irritants such as aspirin or corticosteroids. Exteriorly, it presents a *greater curvature* on its lateral surface and a *lesser curvature* on its medial surface. The proximal opening of the stomach, at the *gastroesophageal junction* (GEJ), is the *cardiac sphincter*; the *pyloric sphincter* is located at its distal end. The portion of the stomach around the distal esophagus is called the *cardia*; that portion superior to the esophageal juncture is the *fundus.* The sharp angle between the esophagus and fundus is the *cardiac notch.* The major portion of the stomach is the *body*; the distal portion is the *pylorus.* The *incisura angularis* is located on the lesser curvature and marks the beginning of the pylorus. The distal portion of the pylorus is marked by the *pyloric sphincter.*

The *small intestine* is composed of the duodenum, jejunum, and ileum. The *duodenum* is the shortest portion. It begins just beyond the pyloric sphincter and is divided into four portions: the duodenal cap or bulb, descending duodenum, transverse duodenum, and ascending duodenum. These portions form a C-shaped loop (*duodenal loop*) that is occupied by the head of the pancreas (Fig. 6–89B). The descending portion receives the hepatopancreatic ampulla and duodenal papilla (see "Biliary System" section). The ascending portion terminates at the duodenojejunal flexure (angle of Treitz). While the position of the short (9 in.) duodenum is fixed, the *jejunum* (9 ft.) and *ileum* (13 ft.) are very mobile. Twisting of the small intestine is called *volvulus* and can cause compression of blood vessels, leading to loss of blood supply, *ischemia,* and *infarct* of the affected area. The small intestine terminates at the *ileocecal valve.*

The approximately 5-ft-long *large intestine (colon)* (Fig. 6–90A) functions in the formation, transport, and evacuation of feces. The colon begins at the terminus of the small intestine; its first portion is the

GI Tract Tissue Layers

Inner to Outer:
- Mucosa
- Submucosa
- Muscular
- Serosa

Five Major Peritoneal Folds

- *Greater Omentum:* an apron of fat over transverse colon and small bowel
- *Lesser Omentum:* suspends stomach and duodenum from liver; contains some biliary vessels
- *Mesentery:* binds jejunum and ileum to posterior abdominal wall; fan-shaped
- *Mesocolon:* binds transverse and sigmoid colon to posterior abdominal wall

Salivary Glands and their Ducts

- Parotid: *Stenson Duct*
- Submandibular: *Wharton Duct*
- Sublingual: *Bartholin Duct*

Stomach

- Fundus
- Body
- Pylorus

Small Intestine

- Duodenum (approximately 9–12 in.)
- Jejunum (approximately 9 ft.)
- Ileum (approximately 13 ft.)

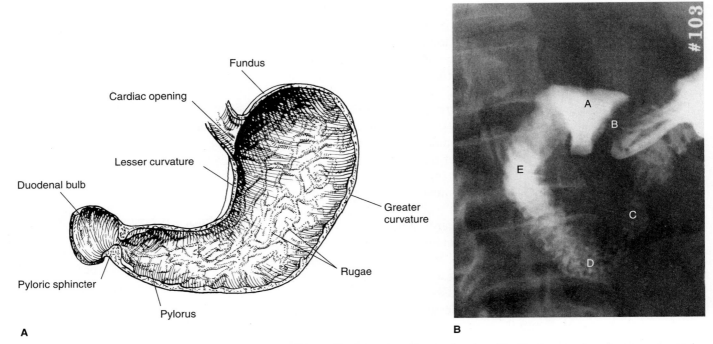

Figure 6–89. **(A)** Stomach (internal aspect). **(B)** Barium-filled duodenal loop; duodenal bulb, descending, transverse, and ascending duodenum are well demonstrated. A, duodenal bulb; B, pyloric valve; C, ascending duodenum; D, transverse duodenum; E, descending duodenum. (Courtesy of Stamford Hospital, Department of Radiology.)

dilated sac-like *cecum*, located inferior to the ileocecal valve (Fig. 6–90A and B). Projecting posteromedially from the cecum is the short (approximately 3.5 in.) *vermiform appendix*. Its lumen is particularly narrow in adolescents and young adults and may become occluded by a fecalith and result in inflammation (appendicitis).

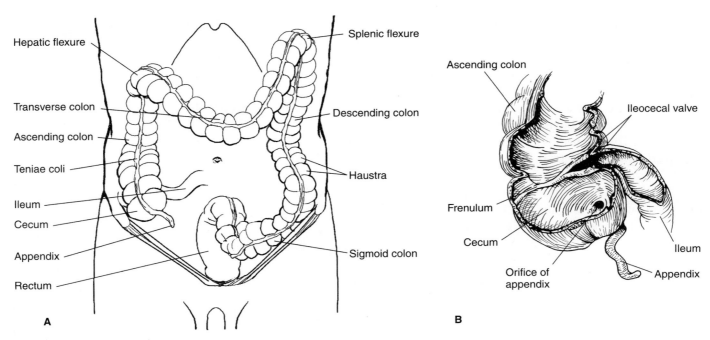

Figure 6–90. **(A)** The colon. **(B)** The ileocecal valve.

The *ascending colon* is continuous with the cecum and is located along the right side of the abdominal cavity. It bends medially and anteriorly in the right hypochondrium, forming the *right colic (hepatic) flexure*. The colon traverses the abdomen as the *transverse colon* and bends posteriorly and inferiorly in the left hypochondrium, forming the *left colic (splenic) flexure*. The *descending colon* continues down the left side of the abdominal cavity and, at about the level of the pelvic brim, the colon moves medially to form the S-shaped *sigmoid colon*. The *rectum* is that part of the large intestine, approximately 5 in. in length, between the sigmoid and the anal canal.

Diverticula are small saccular protrusions of intestinal mucosa through the intestinal wall. They are most commonly associated with the sigmoid colon and can become occluded by fecaliths and subsequently inflamed (diverticulitis). If an inflamed diverticulum perforates, it can result in severe bleeding and peritonitis.

Patient Preparation. Preliminary patient preparation is generally required of patients undergoing radiographic examinations of various portions of the digestive system. The upper GI tract (stomach and small intestine) must be empty and the lower tract (large intestine) must be cleansed of any gas and fecal material. Patients should be questioned about their preparation and a preliminary "scout" image taken to check abdominal contents and for any radiopaque (e.g., gallstones, residual barium) material.

To make up for the lack of subject contrast, radiography of the digestive system most often requires the use of artificial contrast media in the form of barium sulfate suspension or water-soluble iodine and, frequently, air. *Double-contrast studies* of the stomach and large intestine are frequently performed. Barium sulfate functions to coat the organ with radiopaque material, while air inflates the structure. This permits visualization of the shape of the structure as well as *visualization of pathology within its lumen*. Thus, conditions such as *polyps* can be seen projecting within the air-filled lumen. A barium-filled *lumen* would make visualization of anything but the organ shape virtually impossible.

The speed with which barium sulfate passes through the alimentary canal depends on patient habitus (hypersthenic usually fastest) and the concentration of the barium suspension.

When performing examinations on patients suspected or known to have stomach or intestinal perforation, *water-soluble* iodinated contrast media should be used instead of barium sulfate. If the water-soluble medium leaks through a perforation into the peritoneal cavity, it will simply be absorbed and excreted by the kidneys. Water-soluble contrast media are excreted more rapidly than are barium sulfate preparations.

These studies are far from pleasant for patients and the radiographer should make every effort to fully explain the procedure while endeavoring to expedite the examination and make the patient as comfortable as possible.

With the increased use of digital fluoroscopy, fewer "overhead" radiographs are done today. Tables 6–48 through 6–51 provide a summary of the most frequently performed positions/projections of the upper and lower GI tract.

Large Intestine (approximately 6 ft.)

- Cecum
- Ascending colon
- Transverse colon
- Descending colon
- Sigmoid colon
- Rectum

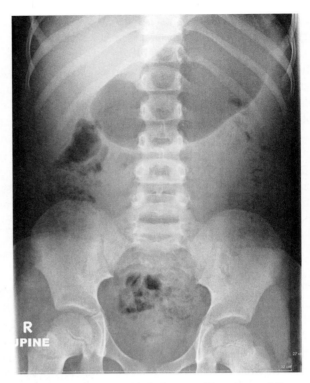

Figure 6–91. AP projection of the abdomen. (Courtesy of Conrad P. Ehrlich, MD)

Abdomen

A *three-way abdomen* study is often performed to evaluate possible obstruction (Fig. 6–93) or free air and fluid within the abdomen and usually consists of AP recumbent, AP erect, and L lateral decubitus projections of the abdomen (see Table 6–48).

TABLE 6–48. The Abdomen

Abdomen	Position of Part	Central Ray Directed	Structures Included/Best Seen
AP	Supine, MSP centered to grid, IR centered to iliac crest (see Fig. 6–91)	⊥ to midline at level of crest	AP proj often used as "scout" image preliminary to contrast studies; shows size and shape of kidneys, liver, and spleen, psoas muscles, as well as any calcifications or masses
Erect	AP erect, MSP centered to grid, IR centered ≈2″ above iliac crest	⊥ to mid-IR	AP erect proj used to demonstrate air/fluid levels; both hemidiaphragms should be included (see Fig. 6–92)
Lateral Decubitus	Patient lat recumbent (AP or PA) MSP ⊥ and centered to upright grid, cassette centered ≈2″ above iliac crest	Horizontal and ⊥ mid-IR	Usually, *left* lat decubitus of abdomen to demonstrate air/fluid levels in patients unable to assume the erect position; both hemidiaphragms should be included

Note: A *dorsal decubitus* can also be a valuable supplement to show air/fluid levels. The patient is placed in the dorsal decubitus (supine) position and a horizontal x-ray beam is used.

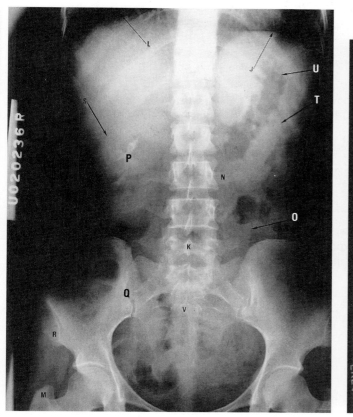

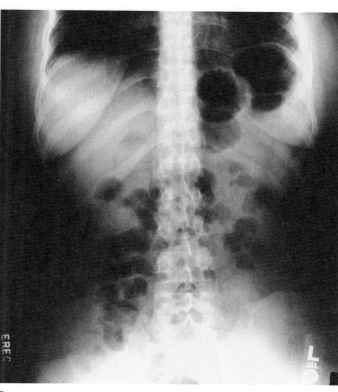

A   B

Figure 6–92. Observe the differences between these two x-ray images. **(A)** Part of an intravenous urogram (IVU) examination made in the recumbent position. J, left hemidiaphragm; K, spinous process L4; L, right hemidiaphragm; M, transverse process L3; O, border of psoas muscle; P, renal calyces; Q, sacroiliac joint; R, anterior inferior iliac spine; S, renal capsule/shadow; T, 11th rib; U, air in stomach; V, sacrum. (Courtesy of Bob Wong, RT.) **(B)** Part of an abdominal survey made in the erect position. Observe the change in appearance and radiographic density, especially of the lower abdomen, as the patient is moved erect and the abdominal viscera assume a lower position; the lower abdomen essentially becomes "thicker" and radiographic density decreases. Each hemidiaphragm must be observed on the erect abdomen. (From the American College of Radiology Learning File. Courtesy of the ACR.)

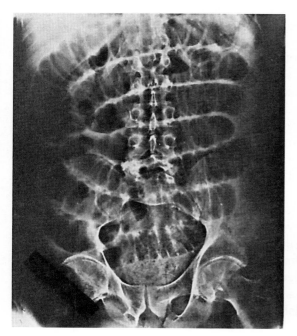

Figure 6–93. Small-bowel obstruction indicated by the dilated bowel loops having a ladder-like pattern. Patient is recumbent; therefore, air/fluid levels are not demonstrated. (Reproduced with permission, from Doherty GM, ed. *Current Surgical Diagnosis & Treatment*, 12th ed. New York: McGraw-Hill, 2006:666.)

Esophagus (Table 6–49)
TABLE 6–49. The Esophagus

Esophagus	Position of Part	Central Ray Directed	Structures Included/Best Seen
AP	Supine, MSP centered and ⊥ table, IR top 1–2″ above shoulders, patient swallowing barium during <0.1 s)	⊥ mid-IR, ≈T6–T7	Barium-filled esophagus in AP proj
RAO	Prone obl, 35–40 degree RAO, IR top 1–2″ above shoulders, patient swallowing barium during exposure	⊥ mid-IR, ≈T6–T7	Barium-filled esophagus in RAO proj, demonstrated b/w vertebrae and heart; best single proj of barium-filled esophagus (see Fig. 6–94)
Lateral (L or R)	Recumbent lat, MCP centered to grid, top of IR just above shoulders, patient swallowing during exposure	⊥ mid-IR	Barium-filled esophagus in lat proj

Note: Esophagus for demonstration of *varices* must be performed in the *recumbent* position; table slightly Trendelenburg and/or performance of the Valsalva maneuver is also helpful. Exposure times of 0.1 second or less should be used to avoid motion; however, respiration normally stops during and shortly after the act of swallowing, so that patients need not be instructed to stop breathing.

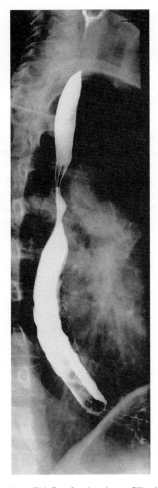

Figure 6–94. RAO of a barium-filled esophagus. The esophagus has three normal constrictions at the levels of the cricoid cartilage, the left bronchus, and the esophageal hiatus of the diaphragm. (Courtesy of Stamford Hospital, Department of Radiology.)

Stomach and Small Intestine. Radiologic examination of the stomach and/or small bowel generally begins with fluoroscopic examination. The fluoroscopist observes the swallowing mechanism, mucosal lining (rugae) of the stomach, and the filling and emptying mechanisms of the stomach and proximal small bowel in various positions. The patient is turned and rotated in various positions so that all aspects of the stomach and any abnormalities such as hiatal hernia (see Fig. 6–88C) can be visualized. Double-contrast examinations of the upper GI system are performed frequently. Occasionally, glucagon or another similar drug will be given to the patient (IV or IM) prior to the examination to relax the GI tract and permit more complete filling. Various images will be made by the fluoroscopist and the radiographer may take supplemental "overhead" projections. *Small-bowel series* examinations require that successive images be made of the abdomen at specified intervals; an additional fluoroscopic image is made when barium reaches the *ileocecal valve.*

Contrast material (usually water soluble) may occasionally be instilled through a gastrointestinal (GI) tube for visualization of the GI tract. GI tubes can be used therapeutically to siphon gas and fluid from the GI tract or diagnostically, using contrast agent, to locate the site of obstruction or pathology (see Table 6–50).

TALE 6–50. **The Stomach**

Stomach	Position of Part	Central Ray Directed	Structures Included/Best Seen
LPO	Supine, obliqued ≈40 degree to left, centered midway b/w vertebrae and L abdominal wall at level of L1	⊥ mid-IR (at level of L1)	Barium-filled fundus good position for *double contrast* of body, pylorus, and duodenal bulb (see Fig. 6–95)
Note: As the fundus is the most *posterior* portion of stomach, it readily fills w/ barium in AP position and moves more superiorly.			
Lateral	Recumbent lateral (usually R), center m/w b/w MCP and anterior abdominal wall to IR at level of L2	⊥ mid-IR (at level of L2)	Lat stomach and prox small bowel demonstrating anterior and posterior aspects of stomach, retrogastric space, pyloric canal, and duodenal loop (see Fig. 6–96)
Note: This projection provides the best visualization of the pyloric canal and duodenal bulb in the hypersthenic patient.			
RAO	Recumbent PA obliqued 40–70 degree, centered m/w b/w vertebrae and lateral abdominal wall at level of L2	⊥ mid-IR (at level of L2)	Right PA obl proj of stomach barium-filled pyloric canal and duodenal loop; demonstrates stomach's emptying mechanism, because *peristaltic activity is greatest in this position*
PA	Prone, MSP centered to IR, at level of L2	⊥ mid-IR (at level of L2)	PA proj of transversely spread stomach, demonstrating contours, greater and lesser curvatures (Fig. 6–97)
Note: Hypersthenic patients frequently have high, transverse stomachs with indistinguishable curvatures. The adult hypersthenic stomach can be "opened" and its *contours* made readily visible by angling the CR 35–45 degree cephalad. The top edge of a lengthwise 14″ × 17″ IR is placed level with the patient's chin and the CR directed to mid-IR.			
AP/PA small bowel	Patient supine, MSP centered to grid, IR centered to level of L2	⊥ mid-IR	AP proj of dist esophagus area, stomach, and proximal small bowel; demonstrates hiatal hernias w/ patient in Trendelenburg position
Note: This position is used to record progress of the barium column in *small bowel* examinations. The first radiograph is usually made 15 minutes after ingestion of the barium drink and centered at level of L2. Subsequent radiographs are made at 15- to 30-minute intervals (and centered at level of crest), according to the individual patient and how quickly or slowly the barium progresses. Spot images are usually taken when the barium column reaches the ileocecal valve.			

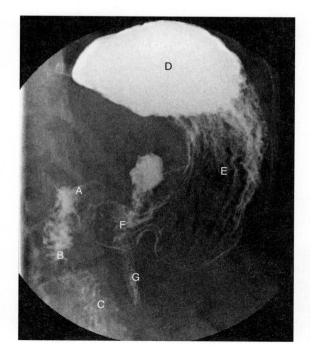

Figure 6–95. LPO of the stomach. In this position, air replaces the barium that drains from the duodenal bulb and pylorus, thus providing double-contrast visualization of these structures. A, duodenal bulb; B, descending duodenum; C, transverse duodenum; D, fundus; E, body/gastric mucosa; F, pylorus; G, ascending duodenum. (Courtesy of Stamford Hospital, Department of Radiology.)

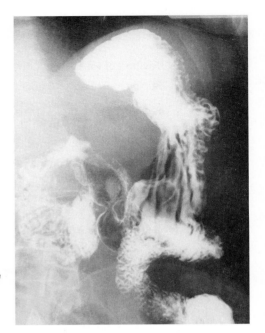

Figure 6–96. Lateral projection demonstrates the anterior and posterior stomach surfaces and the retrogastric space. (Courtesy of Stamford Hospital, Department of Radiology.)

Barium sulfate is *contraindicated* if a *perforation* is suspected somewhere along the course of the GI tract (e.g., a perforated diverticulum or gastric ulcer); a water-soluble (absorbable) iodinated contrast medium is generally used instead. A patient with a nasogastric (NG)

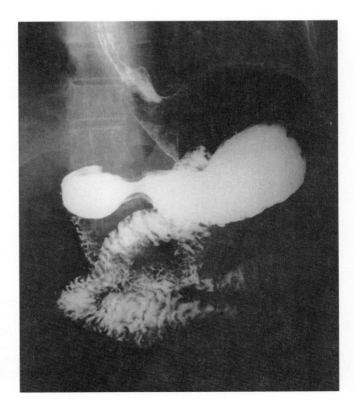

Figure 6–97. PA projection of the stomach. Note barium in body and pylorus. (Courtesy of Stamford Hospital, Department of Radiology.)

tube can have the contrast medium administered through it for the purpose of locating and studying any site of obstruction. This procedure is called *enteroclysis*.

Large Intestine. The lower GI tract is most often examined by *retrograde* filling with barium sulfate and, frequently, air. The fluoroscopist observes filling of the large bowel in various positions and makes images as indicated. Much of the barium is then drained from the intestine, and air is introduced. The objective is to coat the bowel with barium, then distend its lumen with air. The double-contrast method is ideal for demonstration of intraluminal lesions, such as polyps.

The success of the barium enema examination depends on several factors, but without proper patient preparation, a diagnostic examination is often impossible. *Poor preparation resulting in retained fecal material in the colon can mimic or conceal pathologic conditions.*

The barium enema is most easily tolerated and retained by the patient if it is cool or actually cold ($\approx$40–45 degree F). There is probably no radiographic examination that causes more embarrassment and anxiety than the barium-enema and air-contrast procedure. The radiographer must be sensitive to the concerns and needs of the patient by providing a complete explanation of the procedure and by providing for the patient's modesty as much as possible.

Table 6–51 summarizes frequently performed BE projections taken following the fluoroscopic procedure.

TABLE 6–51. The Large Intestine

BE	Position of Part	Central Ray Directed	Structures Included/Best Seen
AP	Supine, MSP centered to IR at level of iliac crest	$\perp$ mid-IR	AP proj of entire contrast-filled large intestine
Note: The large intestine of hypersthenic patients is high and around the periphery of the abdomen; hence, they may require that the AP and PA be done on (2) 14"× 17", IRs placed crosswise in the Bucky tray. In contrast, the colon of the asthenic patient is low, redundant, and more midline.			
PA	Prone, MSP centered to IR at level of iliac	$\perp$ mid-IR	PA proj of entire contrast-filled large intestine; AP or PA erect may be used to demonstrate double-contrast *flexures*
PA axial	Prone, MSP centered to IR at level of pubic symphysis	35 degree caudad to midline at level of ASIS	PA axial proj of *sigmoid colon*; angulation opens the length of the S-shaped colon (see Fig. 6–98)
Note: AP axial may be performed to show similar structures; CR is directed 35 degree cephalad.			
RAO	PA, obl $\approx$40 degree, centered to midline, cassette centered to level of iliac crest	$\perp$ mid-IR	Right PA obl proj of the colon, demonstrates *ascending colon and hepatic flexure* (see Fig. 6–99)

(continued)

TABLE 6–51. (*continued*)

Be	Position of Part	Central Ray Directed	Structures Included/Best Seen
LAO	PA obl ≈40 degree, centered to midline, cassette centered to level of iliac crest	⊥ mid-IR	Left PA obl proj of the colon, demonstrates *descending colon and splenic flexure*

Note: RPO will demonstrate descending colon and splenic flexure; LPO will demonstrate ascending colon and hepatic flexure.

Lateral	Lat recumbent, MCP centered to grid, IR centered at level of ASIS	⊥ mid-IR	L or R lat proj, especially for *rectum* and *rectosigmoid* area
Lateral Decubitus (R and L)	Lat recumbent, (AP or PA), MSP ⊥ and centered to upright grid at level of iliac crest	Horizontal and ⊥ mid-IR	Air rises to provide double-contrast delineation of lat walls of colon; both decubitus are routinely performed (see Fig. 6–100)

Note: A postevacuation PA or AP projection is usually performed to demonstrate large bowel mucosa.

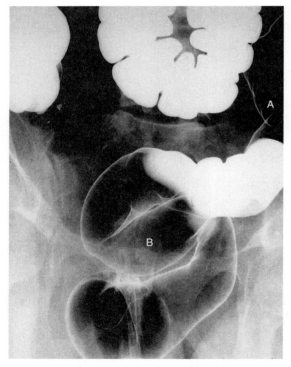

Figure 6–98. Double-contrast PA axial projection of the rectum and sigmoid. The caudal tube angulation serves to "open" the redundant S-shaped sigmoid colon. Similar results may be obtained in the AP position with a cephalad tube angle. A, descending colon; B, sigmoid colon. (Courtesy of Stamford Hospital, Department of Radiology.)

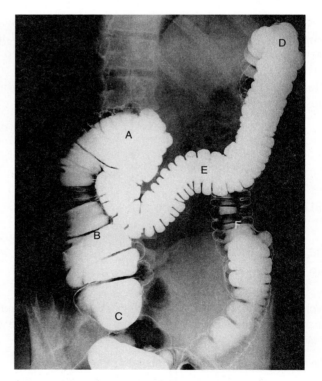

Figure 6–99. RAO of the barium and air-filled large bowel. Note that the hepatic flexure is "opened" for better visualization. An LPO would provide similar results. The opposite obliques (LAO, RPO) are used to demonstrate the splenic flexure and descending colon. A, right colic/hepatic flexure; B, ascending colon; C, cecum; D, left colic/splenic flexure; E, transverse colon; F, descending colon. (Courtesy of Stamford Hospital, Department of Radiology.)

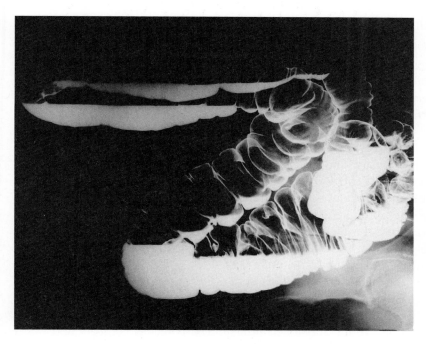

Figure 6-100. Right lateral decubitus view of the air- and barium-filled colon. The heavier barium sulfate moves toward the dependent side, while air rises to fill the remainder of the barium-coated lumen. Thus, the *right lateral decubitus demonstrates double contrast of the "left-sided walls" of the ascending and descending colons* (i.e., lateral side of descending colon and medial side of ascending colon). (Courtesy of Stamford Hospital, Department of Radiology.)

Terminology and Pathology. The following is a list of radiographically significant abdominal and digestive conditions and devices with which the student radiographer should be familiar:

- Achalasia
- Appendicitis
- Ascites
- Colostomy
- Crohn disease
- Diverticulitis
- Diverticulosis
- Dysphagia
- Enteritis
- Esophageal reflux
- Esophageal varices
- Gastroenteritis
- Hiatal hernia (see Fig. 6–88)
- Ileostomy
- Intussusception
- Irritable-bowel syndrome
- Peptic ulcer
- Peritonitis
- Polyp
- Pyloric stenosis
- Ulcerative colitis
- Volvulus

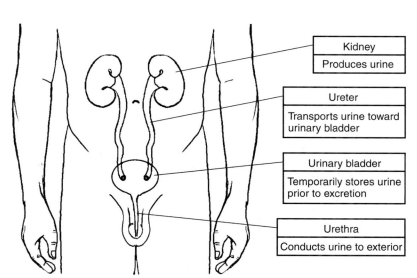

Kidney
Produces urine

Ureter
Transports urine toward urinary bladder

Urinary bladder
Temporarily stores urine prior to excretion

Urethra
Conducts urine to exterior

Figure 6-101. Components of the urinary system.

Urinary System

Introduction. Two of the functions of the urinary system (Fig. 6–101) are to *remove wastes from the blood* and *eliminate it in the form of urine.* The tiny units within the renal substance that perform these functions are called *nephrons.* The major components of the urinary system are the *kidneys, ureters,* and *bladder.*

The paired *kidneys* are *retroperitoneal* and embedded in adipose tissue between the vertebral levels of T12 and L3. The right kidney is usually 1 to 2 in. lower than the left because of the presence of the liver on the right. The kidneys move inferiorly 1 to 3 in. when the body assumes an erect position; they move inferiorly and superiorly during respiration. The slit-like opening on the medial concave surface of each kidney is the *hilum*, which opens into a space called the *renal sinus* (Fig. 6–102). The renal artery and vein, lymphatic vessels, and nerves pass through the hilum. The upper, expanded portion of the ureter is called the *renal pelvis*, or *infundibulum*, and also passes through the hilum; it is continuous with the major and minor *calyces* within the kidney.

Within each kidney, the renal *parenchyma* is divided into two parts: the outer *cortex* and inner *medulla.* The cortex is compact and has a grainy appearance as a result of the many *glomeruli* within its tissues. The medulla contains 10 to 14 *renal pyramids* with a characteristic striated appearance that is due to the *collecting tubules* within (see Fig. 6–102).

The proximal portion of each *ureter* is at the renal pelvis. As the ureter passes inferiorly, three normal constrictions can be observed: at the ureteropelvic junction, at the pelvic brim, and at the ureterovesicular junction. The ureters lie in a plane anterior to the kidneys, ureteral filling with contrast media is best achieved using the PA projection. Urine is carried through the ureters by peristaltic activity. If a ureter is obstructed by a kidney stone, *hydronephrosis* occurs. The ureters enter the *urinary bladder* posteroinferiorly (Fig. 6–103). The base of the bladder rests on the pelvic floor. The triangular-shaped area formed by the *ureteral* and *urethral orifices* is called the *trigone.* Micturition is the

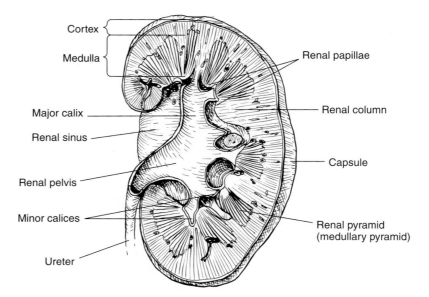

Figure 6–102. Section through the left renal pelvis.

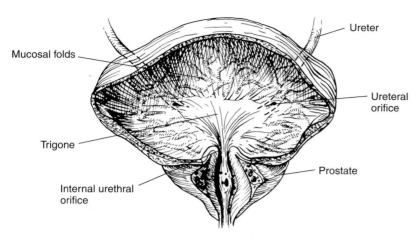

Figure 6–103. Bladder trigone (anterior portion of bladder removed).

process of emptying the urinary bladder of its contents through the *urethra.* The male urethra is approximately 7 to 8 in. long and is divided into prostatic, membranous, and penile portions. The female urethra is approximately 1.5 in. in length.

A common complication of regional enteritis or diverticular disease is the formation of a *fistula* between the urinary bladder and small or large intestine. Fistulous tracts may often be evaluated radiographically with contrast media.

Routine radiographic procedures of the urinary system are generally performed via the IV route. When performed in the retrograde manner, *cystoscopy* is required.

Though the numbers of urinary system x-ray examinations have been steadily decreasing, and are infrequently performed in many institutions today, a review of these examinations follows.

Patient Preparation and Procedure. Investigation of the urinary tract requires patient preparation sufficient to rid the intestinal tract of gas and fecal material. Typical preparation usually begins the evening before the examination with a light dinner, a gentle laxative, and nothing to eat or drink (NPO; non per os [nothing by mouth]) after midnight. Immediately before beginning the IVU, the patient must be instructed to empty his or her bladder; this prevents dilution of opacified urine in the bladder. If the patient has a urinary catheter, it is generally clamped just before the injection and unclamped before the postvoid image. The IVU is preceded by a preliminary scout image of the abdomen to evaluate patient preparation and reveal any calcifications (renal or gallstones), position of kidneys, and accuracy of technical factor selection (Fig. 6–104).

Because the urinary structures have so little subject contrast, artificial contrast material must be employed for better visualization of these structures. Contrast agents used for urographic procedures can have unpleasant and (rarely) even lethal side effects. Intravenous injection of contrast frequently produces a warm, flushed feeling, a bitter or metallic taste, or mild nausea. These side effects are of short duration and usually pass as quickly as they come. More serious side effects include *urticaria,* respiratory discomfort and distress, and, rarely, *anaphylaxis.* An *antihistamine* is appropriate treatment for simple side effects, but the radiographer

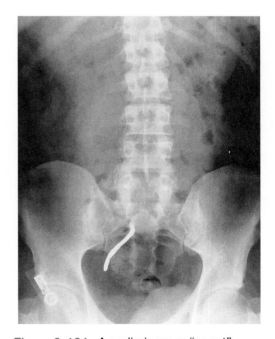

Figure 6–104. A preliminary or "scout" image of the abdomen is taken before the start of an IVU. The radiograph is checked for residual barium from previous contrast studies, patient preparation (including barium from previous studies; note residual barium in patient's appendix), location of kidneys, technical factors, and any calcifications. (Courtesy of Stamford Hospital, Department of Radiology.)

must always be prepared to deal quickly and efficiently with patients experiencing more serious reactions. *Nonionic* contrast agents are far less likely to produce side effects. Contrast agents and their side effects are more thoroughly discussed in Chapter 1.

The selected contrast agent is injected intravenously and successive radiographs are made at specified intervals. A time-interval marker must be included on each image to indicate the elapsed postinjection time. Injection and postinjection protocol varies with the institution, radiologist, patient condition, and diagnosis. The contrast may be rapidly injected in a *bolus* to obtain a 30-second *nephrogram*.

Compression over the distal ureters (delaying contrast or urine travel to bladder) may be required to more completely fill the kidneys with contrast medium or to visualize the contrast-filled kidneys for a longer period of time (Fig. 6–105). Maximum concentration of the contrast material usually occurs at 15 to 20 minutes after injection, but varies with degree of patient hydration.

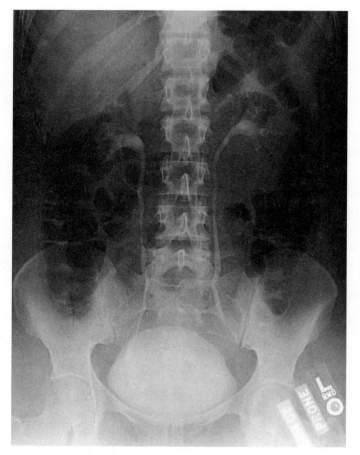

Figure 6–105. PA projection of IVU, demonstrating contrast-filled ureters. Since the ureters lie in a plane that is anterior to that of the kidneys, they are best demonstrated as contrast-filled structures in the *PA position.* The contrast material, which is heavier than urine, gravitates to fill the anterior ureters. (Courtesy of Stamford Hospital, Department of Radiology.)

Radiographs collimated to the kidneys (11 × 14 in. crosswise) may be required at 1, 3, and 5 minutes to evaluate a diagnosis of renal hypertension. Both obliques may be required to evaluate a suspected tumor or lesion. AP and oblique kidney, ureter, and bladder images (KUBs) are usually required at 10 to 15 minutes after injection. A prone KUB is frequently requested at 20 minutes. Because the ureters lie in a plane anterior to the kidneys, *ureteral filling* with contrast media is best achieved using the PA projection (see Fig. 6–107).

Types of Examinations. Routine IV procedures are most correctly referred to as *intravenous urography* (IVU), or *excretory urography*, although they are still commonly referred to as intravenous *pyelography* (IVP) (*pyel* refers only to renal *pelvis*). Intravenous procedures demonstrate *function* of the urinary system. Retrograde studies demonstrate only the *structure* of the part and are generally performed to evaluate the lower urinary tract (lower ureters, bladder, and urethra).

Retrograde urograms (Fig. 6–106) require catheterization of the ureter(s). Radiographs that include the kidney(s) and ureter(s) in their entirety are made after retrograde filling of the structures. A cystogram or (voiding) *cystourethrogram* requires urethral catheterization only.

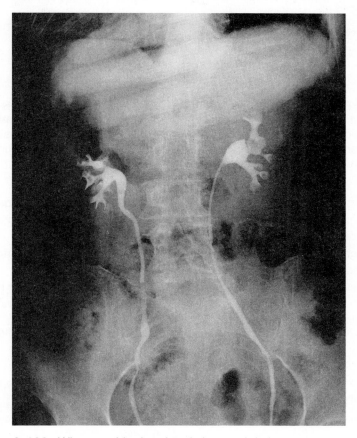

Figure 6–106. When positioning the abdomen, it is important to position the patient's hands at his or her side or resting high on the chest. Note the position of the patient's right hand in this retrograde urogram. (From the American College of Radiology Learning File. Courtesy of the ACR.)

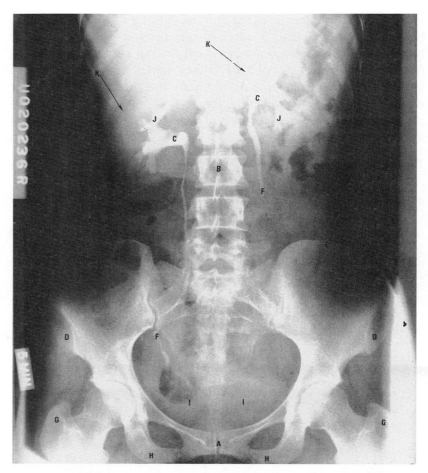

Figure 6–107. This KUB is a 5-minute IVU image. Good collimation is evident and the kidneys, ureters, and bladder are included in their entirety. A, pubic symphysis; B, body, L3; C, renal pelvis; D, ASIS; E, iliac crest; F, ureter; G, greater trochanter; H, ischium; I, bladder; J, renal collecting system/calyces; K, renal cortex. (Courtesy of Bob Wong, RT.)

Radiographs are made of the contrast-filled bladder and frequently of the contrast-filled urethra during voiding. *Cystoscopy* is required for location and catheterization of the vesicoureteral orifices.

Excretory and retrograde urography involve accurate positioning of the abdomen to include the kidneys, ureters, and bladder. If these structures cannot fit on a single image, a second radiograph is generally taken for the bladder. Tables 6–52 and 6–53 provide a review of abdomen/KUB and bladder positioning for IVU examinations.

TABLE 6–52. The Kidney, Ureters, and Bladder (KUB)

KUB	Position of Part	Central Ray Directed	Structures Included/Best Seen
	Patient supine, MSP ⊥ centered to grid, IR centered to iliac crest	⊥ to midline at level of crest	AP proj of abdomen shows size and shape of kidneys, liver, spleen, psoas muscles, and any calcifications or masses

Note: AP abdomen should include from top of kidneys through symphysis pubis (see Fig. 6–107); obliques are performed at 30 degree.

KUB (Kidneys, Ureters, and Bladder)

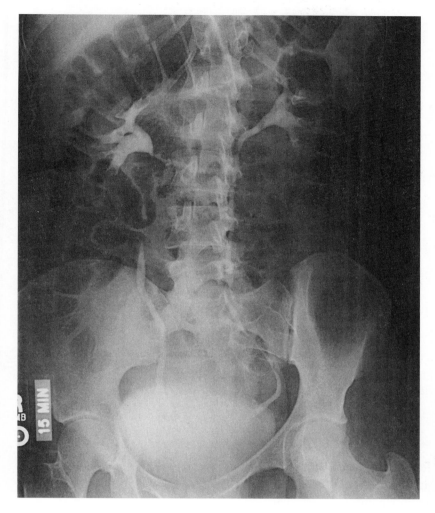

Figure 6–108. Fifteen-minute RPO during IVU, demonstrating the left kidney and right ureter parallel to the image receptor. The 30 degree oblique KUB places the *kidney* of the *up* side *parallel* to the image receptor, and the *ureter* of the side *down* parallel to the image receptor. (Courtesy of Stamford Hospital, Department of Radiology.)

The PA projection will best demonstrate *contrast-filled ureters* (see Fig. 6–106).

The 30 degree oblique KUB places the kidney of the *up* side *parallel* to the image receptor; the ureter of the side *down* parallel to the image receptor. Figure 6–108 is an RPO that places the left kidney and right ureter parallel to the image receptor.

TABLE 6–53. The Bladder

KUB	Position of Part	Central Ray Directed	Structures Included/Best Seen
AP	Patient supine, ⊥ MSP ⊥ centered to grid, lower edge of IR just below pubic symphysis	⊥ to center of IR	AP proj shows contrast-filled or postvoid bladder
AP (Voiding Studies)	Patient supine, ⊥ MSP ⊥ centered to grid, IR centered to pubic symphysis	⊥ to midline at level of pubic symphysis	AP projection of bladder and proximal urethra; used for voiding cystourethrograms (see Fig. 6–109); a 5 degree ∠caudad can be used for the female to place bladder neck and urethra below pubis

Note: Oblique projections are obtained at 40–60 degree for the female and at 30 degree for the male.

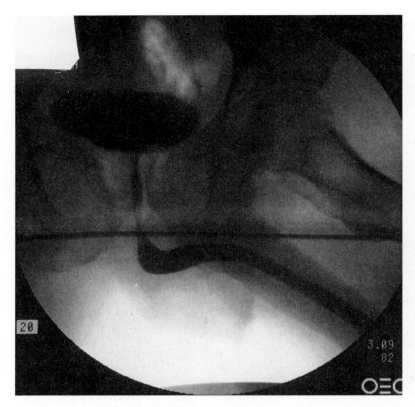

Figure 6–109. Voiding cystourethogram. (From the American College of Radiology Learning File. Courtesy of the ACR.)

Terminology and Pathology. The following is a list of radiographically significant urinary conditions and devices with which the student radiographer should be familiar:

- Cystitis
- Double-collecting system
- Double ureter
- Fistula
- Foley catheter
- Horseshoe kidney
- Hydronephrosis
- Hydroureter
- Incontinence
- Nephroptosis
- Nephrostomy tube
- Pelvic kidney
- Polycystic kidney
- Prostatic hypertrophy
- Pyelonephritis
- Renal calculi
- Renal hypotension
- Staghorn calculus (see Fig. 6–110)
- Supernumerary kidney
- Uremia
- Ureteral stent
- Ureterocele
- Vesicoureteral reflux

Female Reproductive System

Introduction. The female reproductive system consists of the ovaries, oviducts, and uterus. The broad, suspensory, round, and ovarian ligaments are all associated with support of the reproductive organs.

The *ovaries* are the female gonads that function to release ova (female reproductive cells) during ovulation and produce various

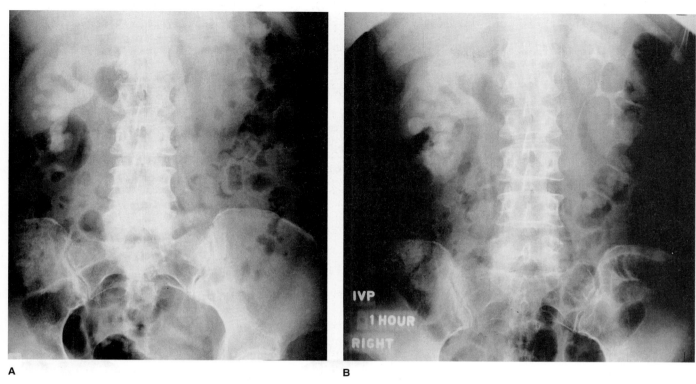

Figure 6–110. Although radiograph (**A**) may appear to be part of an IVU examination, no contrast agent is associated with the opaque right kidney; the opaque area is due to formation of a *staghorn calculus*. Radiograph (**B**) is a 1-hour IVU demonstrating both collecting systems. Staghorn calculi are usually associated with chronic infection and alkaline urine. They may be associated with a single calyx or an entire renal pelvis and may be unilateral or bilateral. Whenever possible, staghorn (named for their shape, resembling a stag's antlers) calculi are removed because they can cause partial obstruction of the calyces and/or ureteropelvic junction. (From the American College of Radiology Learning File. Courtesy of the ACR.)

female hormones, including estrogen and progesterone. The *oviducts*, or Fallopian tubes, are 3 to 5 in. long, arise from the uterine cornua (angles), and extend laterally to arch over each ovary. The oviduct lateral extremities are broader than their medial ends and are bordered by motile *fimbriae* (see Figs. 6–111 and 6–112). The fimbriae sweep over the ovary and function to collect the liberated ovum. *Fertilization* of the ovum usually occurs in the outer portion of the oviducts. Ova are propelled through the oviduct by peristaltic motion. *Salpingitis* is possibly the most common cause of female sterility; if fertilization does occur, the zygote is unable to traverse the oviduct due to its scarred or narrowed condition. Occasionally, a fertilized ovum will become implanted in the oviduct, a condition known as ectopic, or tubal, pregnancy. This condition is a gynecologic emergency because, if left untreated, the patient can die from internal hemorrhage.

The most superior, arched, portion of the *uterus* is the fundus. The angle on each side is the cornu and marks the point of entry of the oviducts. The *body* is the large central region and the narrow inferior portion is the *cervix*.

Hysterosalpingogram. The most commonly performed radiologic examination of the reproductive system is hysterosalpingography, which is

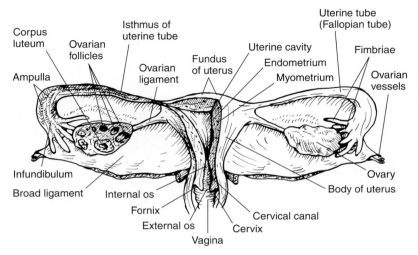

Figure 6–111. Uterus, uterine tubes (oviducts), and ovaries.

employed for evaluation of the uterus, oviducts, and ovaries of the female reproductive system. The procedure serves to delineate the position, size, and shape of the structures, and demonstrates pathology such as *polyps, tumors,* and *fistulas.* However, it is most often used to demonstrate *patency* of the oviducts in cases of *infertility,* and is sometimes therapeutic in terms of opening a blocked oviduct.

Hysterosalpingograms should be *scheduled* approximately 10 days after the start of menstruation. This is the time just *before* ovulation,

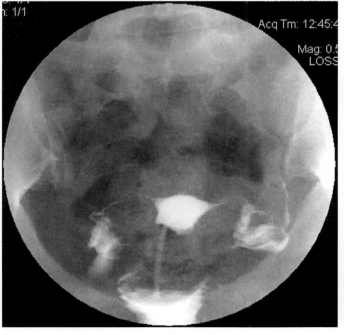

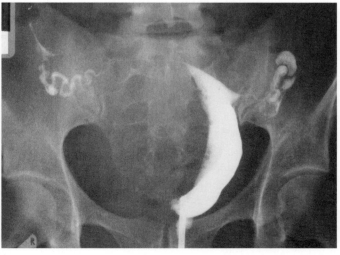

A **B**

Figure 6–112. (A) AP projection of hysterosalpingogram study. Contrast-filled uterus and oviducts are shown, with spillage into pelvic cavity. (Courtesy of Stamford Hospital, Department of Radiology.) **(B)** Large mass distorting uterus.

when there should be little chance of irradiating a newly fertilized ovum.

After the cervical canal is cannulated, an iodinated contrast agent is injected via the cannula into the uterine cavity. If the oviducts are patent, contrast will flow through them and into the peritoneal cavity. Fluoroscopy is performed during injection and spot images are taken. Overhead radiographs may be performed following the fluoroscopic procedure. Table 6-53 addresses positioning for hysterosalpingography.

TABLE 6–53. Hysterosalpingogram

	Position of Part	Central Ray Directed	Structures Included/Best Seen
AP	Patient supine, MSP centered to grid, and a point 2″ above the pubic symphysis centered to the IR	⊥ mid-IR	AP proj of uterus and oviducts; 30 degree obliques may be taken as required (see Fig. 6–112A and B)

Terminology and Pathology. The following is a list of radiographically significant reproductive conditions with which the student radiographer should be familiar:

- Bicornuate uterus
- Ectopic pregnancy
- Endometriosis
- Infertility
- Leiomyoma
- Pelvic inflammatory disease
- Placenta previa
- Salpingitis

Central Nervous System

Introduction. The central nervous system (CNS) is composed of the *brain* and *spinal cord* (Fig. 6–113), enclosed within the bony skull and vertebral column. The brain consists of the cerebrum (largest part), *cerebellum, pons varolii,* and *medulla oblongata*. The *gray matter* of the brain consists of neuron cell bodies; the *white matter* consists of tracts (pathways) of axons. In transverse section, the spinal cord is seen to have an H-shaped configuration of gray matter internally, surrounded by white matter (Fig. 6–114). The brain and spinal cord work together in the perception of sensory stimuli, in integration and correlation of stimuli with memory, and in neural actions resulting in coordinated motor responses to stimuli.

The CNS is enclosed within three tissue membranes, the *meninges*. The *pia mater* is the innermost vascular membrane, which is closely attached to the brain and spinal cord. The *arachnoid mater* is a thin layer outside the pia mater and attached to it by web-like fibers. The *subarachnoid space* is between the pia and arachnoid mater and is filled with cerebrospinal fluid (CSF). The brain and spinal cord float in CSF, which acts as a shock absorber.

Cerebral artery hemorrhage will leak blood into the CSF. *Lumbar puncture* is performed (between L3 and L4 or L4 and L5) to remove small quantities of CSF for testing and to introduce contrast medium during myelography. The *dura mater* is a double-layered fibrous mem-

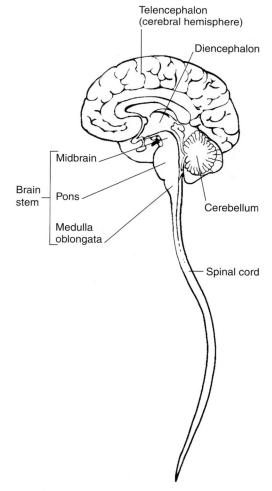

Figure 6–113. The CNS: brain and spinal cord.

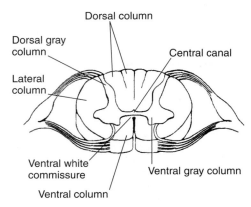

Figure 6–114. Cross section of the spinal cord.

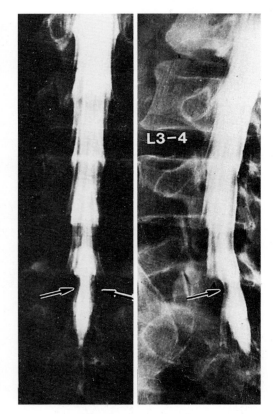

Figure 6–115. Myelograms demonstrating herniated L4–L5 disk. (Reproduced, with permission, from deGroot J. *Correlative Neuroanatomy*, 21st ed. East Norwalk, CT: Appleton & Lange, 1991.)

brane outside the arachnoid mater. The *subdural space* is located between the arachnoid and dura mater; it does not contain CSF. The *epidural space* is located between the two layers of dura mater.

The cylindrical spinal cord is a continuation of the medulla oblongata, extending through the foramen magnum and spinal canal to its termination at the *conus medullaris* (about the level of L1). The lumbar and sacral nerves have long roots that extend from the spinal cord as the *cauda equina* (horse's tail).

Procedures. Routine radiographic examination of the bony components of the CNS includes studies of the skull and vertebral column. Computerized tomography (CT) and magnetic resonance imaging (MRI) procedures have replaced many plain radiographic procedures in the diagnosis and management of traumatic injuries and pathologic processes of the brain and spinal cord.

Myelogram. Nevertheless, *myelography* remains a valuable diagnostic tool to demonstrate the site and extent of *spinal cord tumors* and *herniated intervertebral disks*. The intervertebral disk can rupture due to trauma or degeneration. The *nucleus pulposus* protrudes posteriorly through a tear in the *annulus fibrosus* and impinges on nerve roots (Fig. 6–115). More than 90% of disk ruptures occur at the L4–L5 and L5–S1 interspaces. Narrowing of the affected disk space may often be detected radiographically and the defects caused by the rupture can generally be demonstrated through myelography, CT, or MRI.

Water-soluble nonionic iodinated contrast agents are the most widely used contrast media for myelography. Advantages of water-soluble contrast agents (over non–water-soluble) include better visualization of the nerve roots (see Fig. 6–116) and absorption properties that allow it to be left in the subarachnoid space after the examination (because it is easily absorbed by the body). However, the use of water-soluble contrast agents for myelography does require that radiographs be made accurately and without delay, because it is absorbed fairly quickly.

Foot and shoulder supports must be securely attached to the x-ray table. The patient should receive a complete explanation of the examination and must be instructed about the importance of keeping his or her chin extended when the table is lowered into the Trendelenburg position.

A lumbar puncture is performed (usually at the fourth intervertebral space with the patient in the prone or flexed lateral position), a small quantity of CSF is removed from the subarachnoid space and sent to the laboratory for testing, and an equal amount of contrast agent is injected intrathecally (i.e., into the subarachnoid space of the spinal canal). The position of the contrast column will change according to gravitational forces, and its movement is observed fluoroscopically as the x-ray table is angled to varying degrees of Trendelenburg position and Fowler position. Fluoroscopic spot images are taken as needed, followed by overhead radiographs. Routine protocol generally includes an AP or PA and a horizontal beam (cross-table) lateral view of the vertebral area examined.

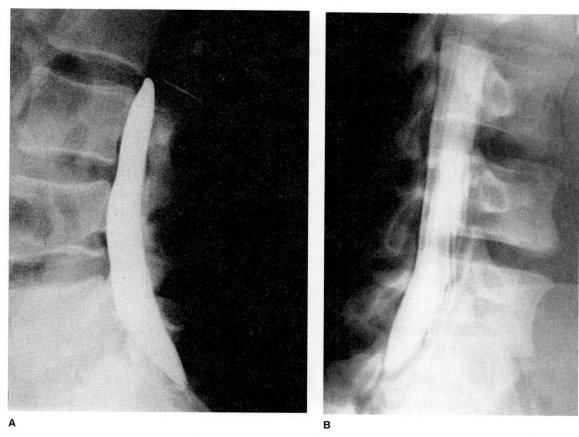

A   **B**

Figure 6–116. **(A)** Non–water-soluble contrast (Pantopaque) myelography. (Courtesy of Stamford Hospital, Department of Radiology.) **(B)** Water-soluble contrast myelography; observe improved visualization of nerve roots seen at the level of each pedicle as linear radiolucencies within the small inferolateral extensions of the contrast agent. (From the American College of Radiology Learning File. Courtesy of the ACR.)

Terminology and Pathology. The following is a list of radiographically significant CNS conditions with which the student radiographer should be familiar:

- Degenerative disk disease
- Herniated nucleus pulposus
- Hydrocephalus
- Meningioma
- Parkinson disease
- Meningitis
- Meningomyelocele
- Spondylosis

Circulatory System

Introduction. The circulatory system consists of the *heart* and vessels (arteries, capillaries, veins) that distribute blood throughout the body (see Fig. 6–117). The heart is the muscular pump, and the *arteries* conduct oxygenated blood throughout the body. The *capillaries* are responsible for diffusion of gases and exchange of nutrients and wastes. The *veins* collect deoxygenated blood and return it to the heart and lungs.

Contraction of the heart muscle as it pumps blood is called *systole*; relaxation is called *diastole*; these values are measured with a *sphygmomanometer*. Accompanying the contraction and expansion of the heart is contraction and expansion of arterial walls, called *pulse*.

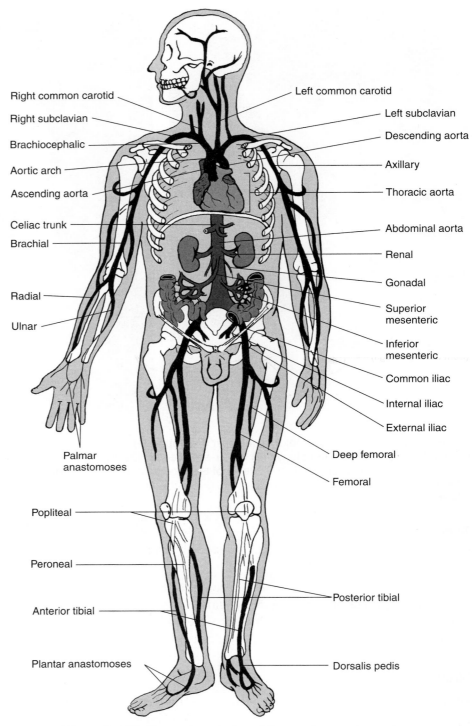

Figure 6–117. The major arteries of the cardiovascular system.

The heart wall is made up of the external *epicardium*, the middle *myocardium*, and the internal *endocardium*. The *pericardium* is the fibroserous sac enclosing the heart and roots of the great vessels. The heart has four chambers. The two upper chambers are the *atria* and the two lower chambers are the *ventricles*. The apex of the heart is the tip of the left ventricle.

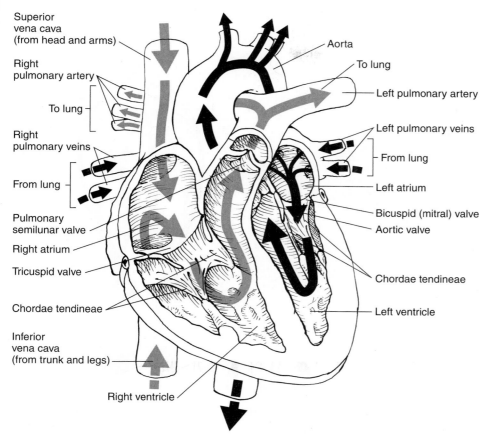

Figure 6–118. The four chambers of the heart and the major blood vessels. Directions of blood flow are indicated.

Venous blood is returned to the right atrium of the heart via the *superior* (from the upper part of the body) and *inferior* (from the lower body) *vena cavae* and the *coronary sinus* (from the heart substance; see Fig. 6–118). Upon atrial systole, the blood passes through the *tricuspid valve* into the right ventricle. During ventricular systole, the blood is pumped through the *pulmonary semilunar valve* into the *pulmonary artery* (the only artery to carry deoxygenated blood) to the lungs for oxygenation.

Blood is returned via the *pulmonary veins* (the only veins to carry oxygenated blood) to the left atrium. During atrial systole, blood passes through the *mitral (bicuspid) valve* into the left ventricle. During ventricular systole, the oxygenated blood is pumped through the *aortic semilunar valve* into the aorta. When blood pressure is reported, as for example "130 over 85," the top number (130) represents the systolic pressure and the lower number (85) represents the diastolic pressure.

The *aorta* is the trunk artery of the body; it is divided into the ascending aorta, aortic arch (see Fig. 6–119), descending thoracic aorta, and abdominal aorta. Many arteries arise from the aorta to supply destinations throughout the body. The *superior* and *inferior vena cavae* and the *coronary sinus* are the major veins, collecting venous blood from the upper and lower body areas and heart substance, respectively. The formation of sclerotic plaques (as in *atherosclerosis*)

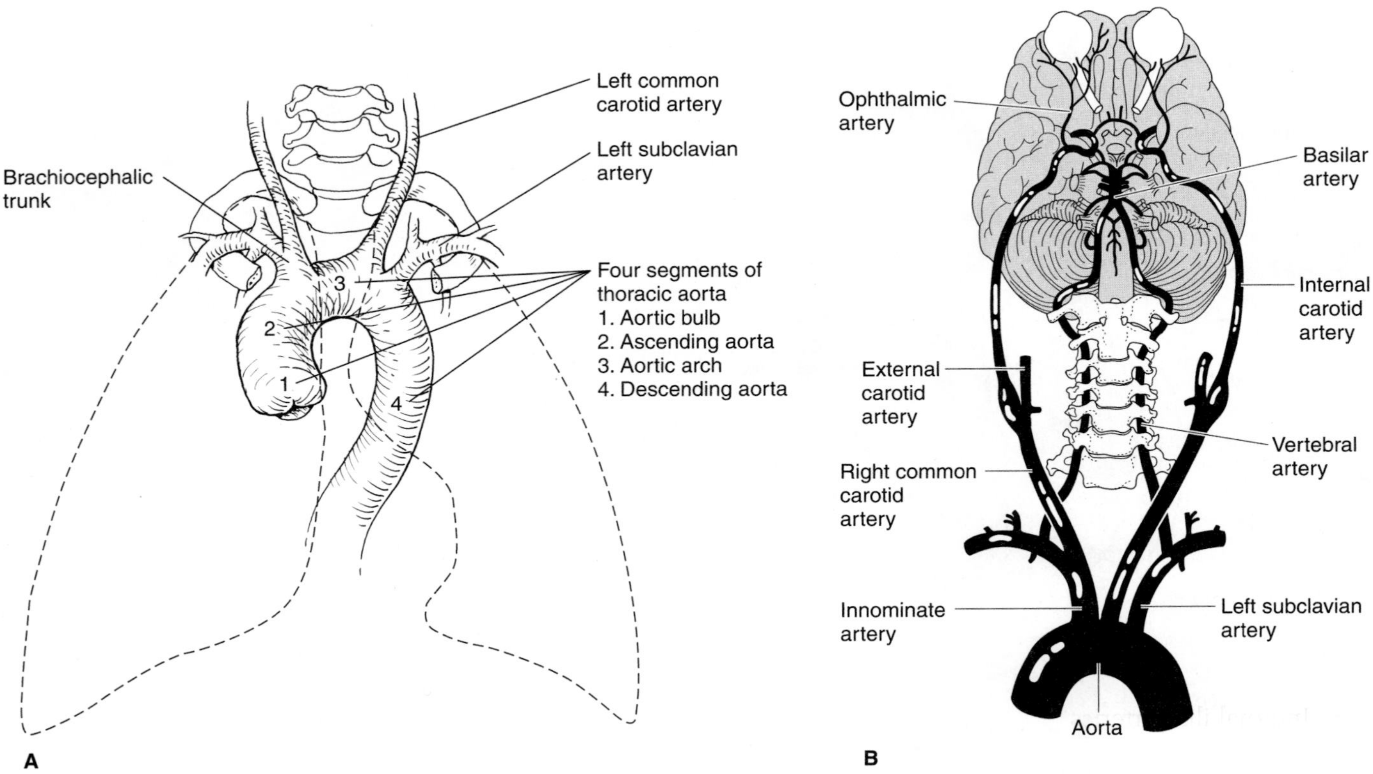

Figure 6–119. **(A)** Thoracic aorta illustrating major branches of aortic arch. **(B)** Blood supply to the brain. (Reproduced, with permission, from Doherty GM, ed. *Current Surgical Diagnosis & Treatment*, 12th ed. New York: McGraw-Hill, 2006:824.)

and other conditions that impair the flow of blood can lead to *ischemia* and tissue *infarction*. Atherosclerosis of the coronary arteries can cause *angina pectoris* and *myocardial infarction*.

The *four divisions* of the aorta and *their major branches* are as follows:

Ascending Aorta

- L and R coronary arteries

Aortic Arch (Fig. 6–119A and B)

- Brachiocephalic (Innominate) artery
  - R common carotid artery
  - R subclavian artery
- L common carotid artery
- L subclavian artery

Blood Supply to the Brain:

- Internal carotid arteries (Fig. 6–119A and B)
  - branch from common carotid arteries
  - supply anterior brain
- Vertebral arteries
  - branch from subclavian arteries
  - supply posterior brain

Pulmonary Circulation

- Unoxygenated blood from the right side of the heart is directed to the lungs for oxygenation, then to the left side of the heart

Systemic Circulation

- Oxygenated blood from the left side of the heart is pumped to the body tissues then back to the right side of the heart

Thoracic Aorta

- Intercostal arteries
- Superior phrenic arteries
- Bronchial arteries
- Esophageal arteries

Abdominal Aorta

- Inferior phrenic arteries
- Celiac (axis) artery/trunk gives rise to:
  - Common hepatic artery
  - L Gastric artery
  - Splenic artery
- Superior mesenteric artery
- Suprarenal arteries
- Renal arteries
- Gonadal arteries (testicular or ovarian)
- Inferior mesenteric artery
- Common Iliac arteries give rise to:
  - Internal iliac arteries
  - External iliac (Hypogastric) arteries

Arteries of the Lower Extremity

- Internal iliac arteries
- External iliac arteries
- Femoral arteries
- Popliteal arteries
- Anterior tibial arteries and posterior tibial arteries
- Dorsalis pedis, peroneal/fibular, medial, and lateral plantar arteries

The majority of peripheral and visceral angiographic procedures are performed in a specially equipped angiographic suite by cardiovascular–interventional technologists (Figs. 6–120 and 6–121). Many cardiovascular suites today use digital subtraction angiography (DSA). *Subtraction* is a technique that removes unnecessary structures such as bone from superimposition on contrast-filled blood vessels. DSA is subtraction achieved by means of a computer, which can also permit manipulation of contrast and other image characteristics by the technologist. The student radiographer, while not performing most of these examinations, should be familiar with the names of the most common procedures and the conditions and disorders for which they are performed.

Venogram. The one vascular procedure that might still be performed in general radiography is the lower extremity *venogram* (Fig. 6–122). This examination is generally performed to confirm a suspected deep vein thrombosis in an effort to avoid the complications of a pulmonary embolism.

The patient should be examined on a radiographic table that can be tilted to a semierect position of at least 45 degree. Tourniquets are used to

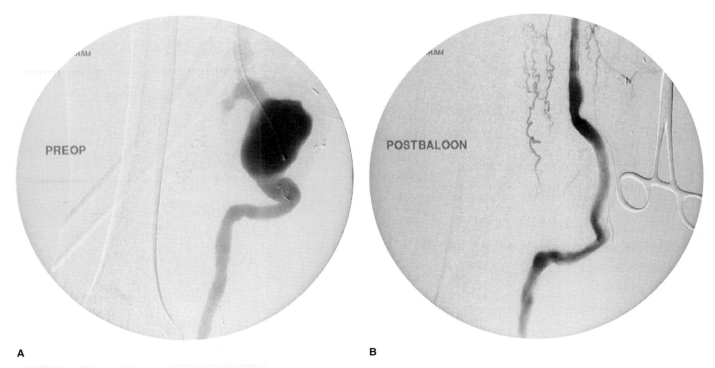

A
B

Figure 6–120. Lower extremity arteriogram subtraction demonstrating *aneurysm*, *before* **(A)** and *after* **(B)** repair. (Courtesy of Stamford Hospital, Department of Radiology.)

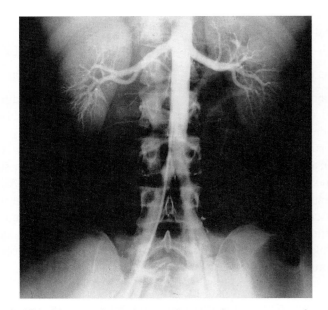

Figure 6–121. The renal arteriogram is one of many types of procedures performed by specially trained teams of health care professionals. (From the American College of Radiology Learning File. Courtesy of the ACR.)

force contrast medium into the deep veins. Sterile technique must be rigorously maintained. An injection of 50 to 100 mL at 1 to 2 mL/second is usually made through a superficial vein in the foot. Images are made at approximately 5- to 10-second intervals of the lower leg, thigh, and pelvis.

Terminology and Pathology. The following is a list of radiographically significant circulatory conditions with which the student radiographer should be familiar:

- Aneurysm
- Angina pectoris
- Atherosclerosis
- Atrial septal defect
- CVA (cerebrovascular accident)
- Coarctation of aorta
- Congestive heart failure
- Coronary artery disease

- Hypertension
- Myocardial infarction
- Phlebitis
- Pulmonary edema
- Pulmonary embolism
- Rheumatic heart disease
- Thrombophlebitis
- Ventricular septal defect

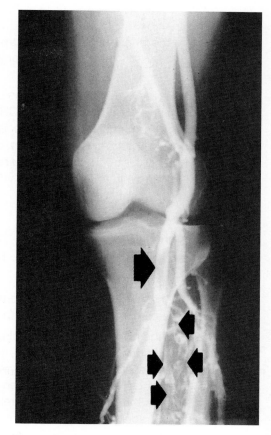

Figure 6–122. AP projection of a lower extremity venogram demonstrating multiple intraluminal filling defects. (Reproduced with permission from Way LW, ed. *Current Surgical Diagnosis & Treatment*, 10th ed. East Norwalk, CT: Appleton & Lange, 1994.)

COMPREHENSION CHECK

Congratulations! You have completed the last section of this chapter. If you are able to answer the following group of very comprehensive questions, you should feel confident that you have really mastered this section. You can refer back to the indicated pages to check your answers and/or review the subject matter.

1. Identify the principal structures comprising the respiratory system and their function(s) (p. 167-169).

2. Describe the (a) method of positioning, (b) direction and point of entry of the CR, (c) principal structures visualized, and (d) pertinent traumatic and pathologic conditions and any technical adjustments that may be required relative to the routine and special views of the chest

(PA, lateral, obl, lordotic, decubitus) and airway (p. 170-172).

3. Identify the principal structures comprising the biliary system and their function(s) (p. 172-174).

4. Describe the (a) method of positioning, (b) direction and point of entry of the CR, (c) principal structures visualized, and (d) pertinent traumatic and pathologic conditions and any technical adjustments that may be required relative to the routine and special views of the biliary system, including

A. OCG (p. 175).

B. Surgical and T-tube cholangiograms (p. 175).

C. ERCP (p. 176).

5. Identify the principal structures comprising the digestive system and their function(s) (p. 176-181).

6. Describe the (a) method of positioning, (b) direction and point of entry of the CR, (c) principal structures visualized, and (d) pertinent traumatic and pathologic conditions and any technical adjustments that may be required relative to the routine and special views of the digestive system, to include

   A. Abdomen (p. 182).

   B. Esophagus (p. 184).

   C. Stomach and small intestine (p. 184-186).

   D. Large intestine (p. 187-189).

7. Identify the principal structures comprising the urinary system and their function(s) (p. 190-191).

8. Describe the (a) method of positioning, (b) direction and point of entry of the CR, (c) principal structures visualized, and (d) pertinent traumatic and pathologic conditions and any technical adjustments that may be required relative to the routine and special views of the urinary system, to include

   A. KUB (p. 194).

   B. Retrograde examinations (p. 193).

   C. Voiding examinations: male versus female (p. 193-196).

D. Compression (p. 192, 194).

E. Bladder (p. 190, 191, 195).

9. Identify the principal structures comprising the female reproductive system and their function(s) (p. 196, 197).

10. Describe the (a) method of positioning, (b) direction and point of entry of the CR, (c) principal structures visualized, and (d) pertinent traumatic and pathologic conditions and any technical adjustments that may be required in hysterosalpingography (p. 197-199).

11. Identify the principal structures comprising the CNS and their function(s) (p. 199, 200).

12. Describe the (a) method of positioning, (b) direction and point of entry of the CR, (c) principal structures visualized, and (d) pertinent traumatic and pathologic conditions and any technical adjustments that may be required in myelography (p. 200, 201).

13. Identify the principal structures comprising the circulatory system and their function(s) (p. 201-205).

14. List the kinds of specialized examinations that might be performed to demonstrate various traumatic and pathologic conditions of the circulatory system (p. 205-207).

CHAPTER REVIEW QUESTIONS

Congratulations! You have completed this chapter. You may go on to the "Registry-type" multiple-choice questions that follow. For greatest success, be sure to also complete the short-answer questions found at the end of each section of this chapter.

Questions 1 through 10 refer to the Appendicular Skeleton section

1. In the AP projection of the knee, the
   1. Femoral condyles are superimposed
   2. CR is directed ½ in. distal to the patellar apex
   3. Patella is visualized through the femur
   (A) 1 only
   (B) 1 and 2 only
   (C) 2 and 3 only
   (D) 1, 2, and 3

2. A Colles fracture usually involves the following:
   1. Transverse fracture of the distal radius
   2. Posterior and outward displacement of the hand
   3. Chip fracture of the ulnar styloid process
   (A) 1 only
   (B) 1 and 2 only
   (C) 2 and 3 only
   (D) 1, 2, and 3

3. Which of the following projections require(s) that the humeral epicondyles be superimposed?
   1. Lateral thumb
   2. Lateral wrist
   3. Lateral humerus
   (A) 1 only
   (B) 1 and 2 only
   (C) 2 and 3 only
   (D) 1, 2, and 3

4. An axial projection of the clavicle is often helpful in demonstrating a fracture not visualized using a perpendicular central ray. When examining the clavicle in the AP axial projection, how should the central ray be directed?
   (A) Cephalad
   (B) Caudad
   (C) Medially
   (D) Laterally

5. The following projection(s) should not be performed until a transverse fracture of the patella has been ruled out:
   1. AP knee
   2. Lateral knee
   3. Axial/tangential patella
   (A) 1 only
   (B) 1 and 2 only
   (C) 2 and 3 only
   (D) 1, 2, and 3

6. Which of the following best demonstrates the cuboid, sinus tarsi, and tuberosity of the fifth metatarsal?
   (A) Lateral foot
   (B) Lateral oblique foot
   (C) Medial oblique foot
   (D) Weight-bearing foot

7. The right sacroiliac joint is placed perpendicular to the IR when the patient is placed in a
   (A) Right lateral position
   (B) 25–30 degree RAO position
   (C) 25–30 degree RPO position
   (D) 30–40 degree RPO position

8. The proximal tibiofibular articulation is best demonstrated in which of the following positions?
   (A) Medial oblique
   (B) Lateral oblique
   (C) AP
   (D) Lateral

9. In the 15–20 degree mortise oblique position of the ankle, the
   1. Talofibular joint is visualized
   2. Talotibial joint is visualized
   3. Plantar surface should be vertical
   (A) 1 only
   (B) 1 and 3 only
   (C) 2 and 3 only
   (D) 1, 2, and 3

10. The scapular Y projection of the shoulder demonstrates
    1. An oblique projection of the shoulder
    2. Anterior or posterior dislocation
    3. A lateral projection of the shoulder
    (A) 1 only
    (B) 1 and 2 only
    (C) 1 and 3 only
    (D) 1, 2, and 3

Questions 11 through 20 refer to the Axial Skeleton section

11. In the AP axial projection (Towne method) of the skull, with the central ray directed 30 degree caudad to the OML and passing midway between the external auditory meati, which of the following is best demonstrated?
    (A) Facial bones
    (B) Frontal bone
    (C) Occipital bone
    (D) Basal foramina

12. All of the following statements regarding the PA projection of the skull, with central ray perpendicular to the IR are true, *except*
    (A) Orbitomeatal line is perpendicular to the IR
    (B) Petrous pyramids fill the orbits
    (C) Midsagittal plane (MSP) is parallel to the IR
    (D) Central ray exits at the nasion

13. The AP projection of the coccyx requires that the central ray be directed
    1. 15 degree cephalad
    2. 2″ above the pubic symphysis
    3. Midline at the level of the lesser trochanter
    (A) 1 only
    (B) 2 only
    (C) 1 and 2 only
    (D) 1 and 3 only

14. Which of the following is (are) demonstrated in the oblique projection of the thoracic spine?
    1. Intervertebral joints
    2. Apophyseal joints
    3. Intervertebral foramina
    (A) 1 only
    (B) 2 only
    (C) 1 and 2 only
    (D) 1 and 3 only

15. The thoracic vertebrae are unique in that they participate in the following articulations:
    1. Costovertebral
    2. Costotransverse
    3. Costochondral
    (A) 1 only
    (B) 1 and 2 only
    (C) 2 and 3 only
    (D) 1, 2, and 3

16. In order to demonstrate undistorted air/fluid levels, the CR must always be directed
    (A) Parallel with the long axis of the body/part
    (B) Parallel with the floor
    (C) Perpendicular to the long axis of the body/part
    (D) Perpendicular to the floor

17. Which of the following is a functional study used to demonstrate the degree of AP motion present in the cervical spine?
    (A) Open-mount projection
    (B) Moving mandible AP
    (C) Flexion and extension laterals
    (D) Right and left bending

18. Which of the paranasal sinuses is composed of many thin-walled air cells?
    (A) Frontal
    (B) Sphenoid
    (C) Ethmoid
    (D) Maxillary

19. The intervertebral foramina of the thoracic spine are demonstrated with the
    (A) Coronal plane 45 degree to the IR
    (B) Midsagittal plane 45 degree to the IR
    (C) Coronal plane 70 degree to the IR
    (D) Midsagittal plane parallel to the IR

20. Which of the following structures is subject to blowout fracture?
    (A) Ethmoid sinuses
    (B) Zygomatic arch
    (C) Mandibular condyle
    (D) Orbital floor

Questions 21 through 60 refer to the Body Systems section

21. Aspirated foreign bodies in older children and adults are most likely to lodge in the
    (A) Right main bronchus
    (B) Left main bronchus
    (C) Esophagus
    (D) Proximal stomach

22. Which of the following is (are) important when positioning the patient for a PA projection of the chest?
    1. The patient should be examined erect
    2. Clavicles should be brought above the apices
    3. Scapulae should be brought lateral to the lung fields
    (A) 1 only
    (B) 1 and 2 only
    (C) 1 and 3 only
    (D) 1, 2, and 3

23. Chest radiography should be performed using 72 in. SID whenever possible in order to
    1. Maximize magnification of the heart
    2. Obtain better lung detail
    3. Visualize vascular markings
    (A) 1 only
    (B) 1 and 2 only
    (C) 2 and 3 only
    (D) 1, 2, and 3

24. Blunting of the costophrenic angles seen on a PA projection of the chest can be an indication of
    (A) Pleural effusion
    (B) Ascites
    (C) Bronchitis
    (D) Emphysema

25. Which of the following conditions is characterized by widening of the intercostal spaces?
    (A) Emphysema
    (B) Empyema
    (C) Atelectasis
    (D) Pneumonia

26. Inspiration and expiration projections of the chest may be performed to demonstrate
    1. Pneumothorax
    2. Diaphragm excursion
    3. Bronchitis
    (A) 1 only
    (B) 1 and 2 only
    (C) 1 and 3 only
    (D) 1, 2, and 3

27. Which of the following criteria are used to evaluate a good PA projection of the chest?
    1. 10 posterior ribs should be visualized
    2. Sternoclavicular joints should be symmetrical
    3. Scapulae should be outside the lung fields
    (A) 1 and 2 only
    (B) 1 and 3 only
    (C) 2 and 3 only
    (D) 1, 2, and 3

28. All of the following statements regarding respiratory structures are true, *except*
    (A) The right lung has three lobes
    (B) The uppermost portion of a lung is its apex
    (C) The lobes of the left lung are separated by the horizontal fissure
    (D) The trachea bifurcates into mainstem bronchi

29. To demonstrate the pulmonary apices below the level of the clavicles in the AP position, the CR should be directed
    (A) Perpendicular
    (B) 15 degree to 20 degree caudad
    (C) 15 degree to 20 degree cephalad
    (D) 40 degree cephalad

30. Radiographic indications of atelectasis include(s)
    1. Decreased radiographic density/increased brightness of the affected side
    2. Elevation of the hemidiaphragm of the affected side
    3. Flattening of the hemidiaphragm of the affected side
    (A) 1 only
    (B) 3 only
    (C) 1 and 2 only
    (D) 1 and 3 only

31. During a gastrointestinal examination, the AP recumbent projection of a stomach of average size and shape will usually demonstrate
    1. Barium-filled fundus
    2. Double contrast of distal stomach portions
    3. Barium-filled duodenum and pylorus
    (A) 1 only
    (B) 1 and 2 only
    (C) 1 and 3 only
    (D) 1, 2, and 3

32. During a GI examination, the lateral recumbent projection of a stomach of average shape will demonstrate
    1. Anterior and posterior aspects of the stomach
    2. Medial and lateral aspects of the stomach
    3. Double-contrast body and antral portions
    (A) 1 only
    (B) 1 and 2 only
    (C) 2 and 3 only
    (D) 1, 2, and 3

33. Which of the following projections of the abdomen could be used to demonstrate air or fluid levels when the erect position cannot be obtained?
    1. AP Trendelenburg
    2. Dorsal decubitus
    3. Lateral decubitus
    (A) 1 only
    (B) 1 and 2 only
    (C) 2 and 3 only
    (D) 1, 2, and 3

34. Which of the following best describes the relationship between the esophagus and trachea?
    (A) Esophagus is posterior to the trachea
    (B) Trachea is posterior to the esophagus
    (C) Esophagus is lateral to the trachea
    (D) Trachea is lateral to the esophagus

35. To demonstrate esophageal varices, the patient must be examined in the
    (A) Recumbent position
    (B) Erect position
    (C) Anatomic position
    (D) Fowler position

36. The usual preparation for an upper GI series is
    (A) Clear fluids 8 hours prior to examination
    (B) NPO after midnight
    (C) Enemas until clear before examination
    (D) Light breakfast day of the examination

37. Which of the following positions would best demonstrate a double contrast of the left and right colic flexures?

    (A) Left lateral decubitus

    (B) AP recumbent

    (C) Right lateral decubitus

    (D) AP erect

38. In which of the following positions are a barium-filled pyloric canal and duodenal bulb best demonstrated during a GI series?

    (A) RAO

    (B) Left lateral

    (C) Recumbent PA

    (D) Recumbent AP

39. What position is frequently used to project the GB away from the vertebrae in the asthenic patient?

    (A) RAO

    (B) LAO

    (C) Left lateral decubitus

    (D) PA erect

40. Which of the following barium-/air-filled anatomic structures is best demonstrated in the RAO position?

    (A) Splenic flexure

    (B) Hepatic flexure

    (C) Sigmoid colon

    (D) Ileocecal valve

41. In what order should the following studies be performed?

    1. Barium enema

    2. Intravenous urogram

    3. Upper GI

    (A) 3, 1, 2

    (B) 1, 3, 2

    (C) 2, 1, 3

    (D) 2, 3, 1

42. All of the following statements regarding the urinary system are true, *except*

    (A) The left kidney is usually higher than the right

    (B) The kidneys move inferiorly in the erect position

    (C) The upper, expanded part of the ureter is the hilum

    (D) Vessels, nerves, and lymphatics pass through the renal hilum

43. Which of the following examinations require(s) restriction of the patient's diet?

    1. GI series

    2. Abdominal survey

    3. Urogram

    (A) 1 only

    (B) 1 and 2 only

    (C) 1 and 3 only

    (D) 1, 2, and 3

44. During IV urography, the prone position is generally recommended to demonstrate

    1. Filling of obstructed ureters

    2. The renal pelvis

    3. The superior calyces

    (A) 1 only

    (B) 1 and 2 only

    (C) 1 and 3 only

    (D) 1, 2, and 3

45. Which of the following examinations require(s) catheterization of the ureters?

    1. Retrograde urogram

    2. Cystogram

    3. Voiding cystogram

    (A) 1 only

    (B) 1 and 2 only

    (C) 2 and 3 only

    (D) 1, 2, and 3

46. Some common mild side effects of intravenous administration of water-soluble iodinated contrast agents include
    1. Flushed feeling
    2. Bitter taste
    3. Urticaria
    (A) 1 only
    (B) 1 and 2 only
    (C) 1 and 3 only
    (D) 1, 2, and 3

47. Hysterosalpingograms may be performed for the following reason(s):
    1. Demonstration of fistulous tracts
    2. Investigation of infertility
    3. Demonstration of tubal patency
    (A) 1 only
    (B) 1 and 2 only
    (C) 1 and 3 only
    (D) 1, 2, and 3

48. A postvoid image of the urinary bladder is usually requested at the completion of an IVU and may be helpful in demonstrating
    1. Residual urine
    2. Prostate enlargement
    3. Ureteral tortuosity
    (A) 1 only
    (B) 1 and 2 only
    (C) 1 and 3 only
    (D) 1, 2, and 3

49. During routine intravenous urography, the oblique position demonstrates the
    (A) Kidney of the side up parallel to the IR
    (B) Kidney of the side up perpendicular to the IR
    (C) Urinary bladder parallel to the IR
    (D) Urinary bladder perpendicular to the IR

50. To better demonstrate contrast-filled distal ureters during intravenous urography, it is helpful to
    1. Use a 15 degree AP Trendelenburg position
    2. Apply compression to the proximal ureters
    3. Apply compression to the distal ureters
    (A) 1 only
    (B) 2 only
    (C) 1 and 2 only
    (D) 1 and 3 only

51. The space located between the arachnoid mater and dura mater is the
    (A) Subarachnoid space
    (B) Subdural space
    (C) Epidural space
    (D) Epiarachnoid space

52. The contraction and expansion of arterial walls in accordance with forceful contraction and relaxation of the heart is called
    (A) Hypertension
    (B) Elasticity
    (C) Pulse
    (D) Pressure

53. The method by which contrast-filled vascular images are removed from superimposition upon bone is called
    (A) Positive masking
    (B) Reversal
    (C) Subtraction
    (D) Registration

54. Indicate the correct sequence of oxygenated blood as it returns from the lungs to the heart
    (A) Pulmonary veins, left atrium, left ventricle, aortic valve
    (B) Pulmonary artery, left atrium, left ventricle, aortic valve
    (C) Pulmonary veins, right atrium, right ventricle, pulmonary semilunar valve
    (D) Pulmonary artery, right atrium, right ventricle, pulmonary semilunar valve

55. In myelography, the contrast medium is generally injected into the
    (A) Cisterna magna
    (B) Individual intervertebral disks
    (C) Subarachnoid space between the first and second lumbar vertebrae
    (D) Subarachnoid space between the third and fourth lumbar vertebrae

56. The upper chambers of the heart are the
    (A) Ventricles
    (B) Atria
    (C) Pericardia
    (D) Myocardia

57. Myelography is a diagnostic examination used to demonstrate
    1. Posterior protrusion of herniated intervertebral disk
    2. Anterior protrusion of herniated intervertebral disk
    3. Internal disk lesions
    (A) 1 only
    (B) 2 only
    (C) 1 and 2 only
    (D) 1 and 3 only

58. The four major arteries supplying the brain include the
    1. Brachiocephalic artery
    2. Common carotid arteries
    3. Vertebral arteries
    (A) 1 and 2 only
    (B) 1 and 3 only
    (C) 2 and 3 only
    (D) 1, 2, and 3

59. Venous, or deoxygenated, blood is returned to the heart via the:
    1. Inferior vena cava
    2. Superior vena cava
    3. Coronary sinus
    (A) 1 only
    (B) 2 only
    (C) 1 and 2 only
    (D) 1, 2, and 3

60. The apex of the heart is formed by the
    (A) Left atrium
    (B) Right atrium
    (C) Left ventricle
    (D) Right ventricle

Answers and Explanations

1. (C) The AP projection of the knee requires the knee to be extended. There should be no pelvic rotation although the leg may be rotated 3–5 degree internally. The central ray is directed to 1/2″ below patellar apex (location of knee joint). The direction of the CR depends on the distance between the ASIS and the tabletop; that is up to 19 cm (thin pelvis) angle 3 degree to 5 degree caudad; 19 to 24 cm 0 degree (perpendicular) CR; greater than 24 cm (thick pelvis) 3 to 5 degree cephalad. This projection demonstrates an AP of the knee joint, distal femur, and proximal tibia/fibula. The patella is seen through the femur. The femoral condyles are superimposed in the lateral projection of the knee.

2. (D) A Colles fracture is often caused by a fall onto an outstretched hand, in order to "brake" the fall. As a result, the wrist suffers an impacted transverse fracture of the distal inch of the radius, with displacement of the hand posteriorly (i.e., backward, approximately 30 degree) and outward, causing the characteristic "dinnerfork" deformity seen on x-ray examination. This injury is usually accompanied by a chip fracture of the ulnar styloid process.

3. (C) For the lateral projections of the hand, wrist, forearm, and elbow, the elbow must be flexed 90 degree to superimpose the distal radius and ulna and humeral epicondyles. Although a lateral humerus can be performed with the elbow flexed, if flexion is not possible, the elbow may remain in the anteroposterior (AP) position and a transthoracic lateral projection of the upper one-half to two-thirds of the humerus may be obtained. Because a coronal plane passing through the epicondyles is perpendicular to the IR in this position, the epicondyles will be superimposed. To obtain a lateral projection of the thumb (first digit), the patient's wrist must be somewhat internally rotated. Remember that an oblique projection of the thumb is obtained in a PA projection of the hand.

4. (A) With the patient positioned for an AP axial projection, the central ray is directed cephalad. The reverse is true when examining the clavicle in the prone position. This serves to project the pulmonary apices away from the clavicle. Patients having clavicular pain are more comfortably examined using the PA erect or AP recumbent projections/positions.

5. (C) If a transverse fracture of the patella is present and the knee is *flexed*, there is a danger of *separation* of the fractured segments. Because both a lateral knee and axial patella require knee flexion, they should be avoided until a transverse fracture is ruled out. When present, a transverse fracture may be seen through the femur on the AP projection. The axial ("sunrise") projection of the patella is generally used for demonstrating *vertical* patellar fractures.

6. (C) To demonstrate many of the tarsals and intertarsal spaces, including the cuboid, third (lateral) cuneiform, sinus tarsi, and tuberosity of the fifth metatarsal, a *medial oblique* is required (plantar surface and IR form a 30 degree angle). The *lateral* oblique projection of the foot demonstrates the navicular and first (medial) and second (intermediate) cuneiforms. Weight-bearing lateral feet are used to demonstrate the longitudinal arches.

7. (B) Sacroiliac joints lie obliquely in the pelvis and open anteriorly at an angle of 25 to 30 degree to the MSP. A 25 to 30 degree Oblique position places the joints perpendicular to the IR. The right sacroiliac joint is demonstrated in the RAO and LPO positions with little difference in magnification.

8. (A) With the femoral condyles of the affected side rotated *medially/internally* to form a 45 degree angle with the IR, the *proximal* tibiofibular articulation is placed parallel with the IR and the fibula is free of superimposition with the tibia. The lateral oblique completely superimposes the tibia and fibula. The AP and lateral projections superimpose enough of the tibia and fibula so that the tibiofibular articulation is "closed."

9. (D) The medial oblique projection (15–20 degree mortise view) of the ankle is valuable because it demonstrates the tibiofibular joint as well as the talotibial joint, thereby visualizing all the major articulating surfaces of the ankle joint. To demonstrate maximum joint volume, it is recommended that the plantar surface be vertical.

10. (B) The scapular Y projection requires that the coronal plane be approximately 60 degree to the IR, thus resulting in an oblique projection of the shoulder. The vertebral and axillary borders of the scapula are superimposed on the humeral shaft and the resulting relationship between the glenoid fossa and humeral head will demonstrate anterior or posterior dislocation. Lateral or medial dislocation is evaluated on the AP projection.

11. (C) The AP axial position projects the anterior structures (frontal and facial bones) downward, thus permitting visualization of the *occipital bone* without superimposition (Towne method). The dorsum sella and posterior clinoid processes of the sphenoid bone should be visualized within the foramen magnum. This projection may also be obtained by angling the central ray 30 degree caudad to the OML (Fig. 6–63A). The *frontal bone* is best shown with the patient PA and a perpendicular central ray. The parietoacanthial projection is the single best position for *facial bones. Basal foramina* are well demonstrated in the submentovertical projection.

12. (C) In the exact PA projection of the skull, the central ray is perpendicular and exits the nasion. The petrous pyramids should *fill* the orbits. If the central ray (CR) is angled caudally, the petrous pyramids are projected lower in the orbits; at approximately 25 to 30 degree caudal angle, they are projected *below* the orbits. In the PA projection, the orbitomeatal line (OML) must be perpendicular to the image receptor, or the petrous pyramids will not fill the orbits. The midsagittal plane (MSP) must be perpendicular to the image receptor or the skull will be rotated and anatomic details will lose L–R symmetry. The MSP is parallel to the IR in the lateral projection of the skull.

13. (B) The AP projection of the *coccyx* requires that the CR be directed 10 caudally and centered to a point 2 in. above the pubic symphysis. The AP projection of the *sacrum* requires a 15 cephalad angle of the CR, centered to a point midway between the pubic symphysis and the ASIS.

14. (B) Intervertebral joints are well visualized in the *lateral* projection of all the vertebral groups. Thoracic and lumbar intervertebral foramina are well demonstrated in the *lateral* projection. Thoracic and lumbar *apophyseal joints* are demonstrated in an *oblique* position—thoracic requires a 70° oblique and lumbar requires a 45° oblique. Cervical articular facets (forming apophyseal joints) are 90° to the midsagittal plane (MSP) and are therefore well demonstrated in the lateral projection. The cervical intervertebral foramina lie 45° to the MSP (and 15–20° to a transverse plane) and are therefore demonstrated in the oblique position.

15. (B) There are 12 thoracic vertebrae, which are larger in size than cervical vertebrae and which increase in size as they progress inferiorly toward the lumbar region. Thoracic spinous processes are fairly long and are sharply angled caudally. The bodies and transverse processes have *articular facets* for the *diarthrotic* rib articulations (*see Fig. 6–48*). These structures form the *costovertebral* (head of rib with body of vertebra) and *costotransverse* (tubercle of rib with transverse process of vertebra) articulations. The *costochondral* articulation describes where the anterior end of the rib articulates with its costal cartilage.

16. (B) Radiography of the paranasal sinuses, and other structures such as the chest, must be performed in the erect position so that any *air/fluid levels* may be demonstrated. In the paranasal sinuses, the erect position helps to distinguish between fluid and other pathology such as *polyps*.

To demonstrate air/fluid levels, *the CR must always be directed parallel to the floor*, even if the patient is not completely erect (just as in chest radiography). If the CR is angled to parallel the plane of the body, any fluid levels will be distorted or indeed obliterated.

17. (C) The degree of anterior and posterior motion is occasionally diminished with a "whiplash"-type injury. Anterior (forward, flexion) and posterior (backward, extension) motion is evaluated in the lateral position with the patient assuming flexion and extension as best as possible. Left and right bending images of the vertebral column are frequently obtained to evaluate scoliosis.

18. (C) There are four paired paranasal sinuses: *frontal, ethmoidal, maxillary*, and *sphenoidal* (see Fig. 6–69). They vary greatly in their size and shape. The left and right *frontal* sinuses are usually asymmetrical. They are located behind the glabella and superciliary arches of the frontal bone. The *frontal* sinuses are not present in young children and generally reach their adult size in the 15th or 16th year. The *ethmoid* sinuses are composed of 6 to 18 *thin-walled air cells* that occupy the bony labyrinth of the ethmoid bone. The ethmoidal sinuses of children are very small and do not fully develop until after the 14th year. The *maxillary* sinuses (maxillary antra/antra of Highmore) are the largest of the paranasal sinuses and are located in the body of the maxillae. The maxillary antra are particularly prone to infection and collections of stagnant mucus. The maxillary antra reach their adult size around the 12th year. The *sphenoid* sinuses are located in the body of the sphenoid bone and are usually asymmetrical. They generally reach adult size by the 14th year.

19. (D) Intervertebral joints are well visualized in the *lateral* projection of all the vertebral groups. Thoracic and lumbar intervertebral foramina are well demonstrated in the *lateral* projection. Thoracic and lumbar *apophyseal joints* are demonstrated in an *oblique* position—thoracic requires a 70° oblique and lumbar requires a 45° oblique. Cervical articular facets (forming apophyseal joints) are 90° to the midsagittal plane (MSP) and are therefore well demonstrated in the lateral projection. The cervical intervertebral foramina lie 45° to the MSP (and 15–20° to a transverse plane) and are therefore demonstrated in the oblique position.

20. (D) The orbital cavities are formed by seven bones (frontal, sphenoid, ethmoid, maxilla, palatine, zygoma/malar, and lacrimal). The orbital walls are fragile and the orbital floor is subject to traumatic *blowout* fractures—the second most common facial fracture (nasal fractures being number one). Orbital fractures can be accompanied by injury to adjacent structures—bone, muscle, and other soft tissues. Leakage of air from the adjacent maxillary sinuses can cause orbital edema. *Orbital floor* fractures can be demonstrated using the *parietoacanthial (Waters)* projection; CT is often indicated for further evaluation.

21. (A) Because the right main bronchus is wider and more vertical, aspirated foreign bodies are more likely to enter it than the left main bronchus, which is narrower and angles more sharply from the trachea. An aspirated foreign body does not enter the esophagus or stomach, as they are digestive, not respiratory, structures.

22. (C) The chest should be examined in the *erect* position whenever possible to demonstrate any air or fluid levels. The shoulders should be relaxed and depressed to move the clavicles *below* the lung apices. The shoulders should be rolled forward to move the *scapulae* out of the lung fields.

23. (C) Chest radiographs are performed in the erect position at 72 in. SID whenever possible. The long source-to-image receptor distance (SID) is easily achieved with a minimum patient exposure due to the low tissue densities being examined (ribs and lungs). The longer SID *minimizes* magnification of the heart and provides better visualization of pulmonary vascular markings.

24. (A) Fluid in the thoracic cavity between the visceral and parietal pleura is called *pleural effusion.* In the erect position, fluid gravitates to the lowest point, settling in, and "blunting," the costophrenic angles. *Ascites* is an accumulation of serous fluid in the peritoneal cavity. *Bronchitis* is an inflammation of the bronchial tubes. Pulmonary *emphysema* is a chronic pulmonary disease characterized by increase beyond the normal in the size of air spaces distal to the terminal bronchiole and with destructive changes in the walls of the bronchioles.

25. (A) *Emphysema* is characterized by irreversible trapping of air, which gradually increases and overexpands the lungs, thus producing the characteristic *flattening of the diaphragm* and *widening of the intercostal spaces* (see Fig. 6–80). The increased air content of the lungs requires a compensating *decrease in technical factors. Empyema* describes pus in the pleural cavity as a result of an infection of the lungs. *Atelectasis* is a collapsed or airless lung. *Pneumonia* is an inflammation of the lung; there are more than 50 causes of pneumonia.

26. (B) Phase of respiration is exceedingly important in thoracic radiography; lung expansion and the position of the diaphragm strongly influence the appearance of the finished radiograph. Inspiration and expiration radiographs of the chest are taken to demonstrate air in the pleural cavity (pneumothorax), to demonstrate degree of diaphragm excursion, or to detect the presence of foreign body. The expiration image will require a somewhat greater exposure (6–8 kV or more) to compensate for the diminished quantity of air in the lungs.

27. (D) To evaluate sufficient inspiration and lung expansion, 10 posterior ribs should be visualized. Sternoclavicular joints should be symmetrical; any loss of symmetry indicates rotation. Accurate positioning and selection of technical factors is critical to the diagnostic value of the radiographic images. Even slight rotation or leaning can cause significant distortion of the heart size and shape. To visualize maximum lung area, the shoulders are rolled forward to remove the scapulae from the lung fields.

28. (C) The trachea (windpipe) bifurcates into left and right mainstem bronchi, each entering its respective lung hilum. The left bronchus divides into two parts, one for each lobe of the left lung; the right bronchus divides into three parts, one for each lobe of the right lung. The lungs have a somewhat conical shape; their narrow upper portion is called the *apex*, and their wide lower portion is the *base*. Structures such as the mainstem bronchi and pulmonary artery and veins enter and leave the lungs at the *hilum*. The *right* lung has *three* lobes; the upper and middle lobes are separated by the horizontal fissure, and the middle and lower lobes are separated by the oblique fissure. The *left lung* has *two lobes*; the upper and lower lobes are separated by the *oblique fissure* (see Fig. 6–76).

29. **(C)** When the shoulders are relaxed, the clavicles are usually carried below the pulmonary apices. To examine the portions of lungs lying behind the clavicles, the CR is directed cephalad 15 to 20 degree to project the *clavicles above the apices*, when the patient is examined in the AP position.

30. **(C)** Pneumothorax is the presence of air in the pleural cavity. A large pneumothorax is usually accompanied by a partial or complete *atelectasis* (collapse of the lung). Radiographic indications of atelectasis include an increase in *tissue* density of the collapsed lung (therefore *decreased image density/increased brightness*), and elevation of the hemidiaphragm of the *affected* side. The procedure required to remove significant amounts of air, blood, or other fluids in the pleural cavity is thoracentesis.

31. **(B)** With the body in the anteroposterior (AP) recumbent position, barium flows easily into the fundus of the stomach, displacing it somewhat superiorly. The fundus, then, is filled with barium, while the air that had been in the fundus is displaced into the gastric body, pylorus, and duodenum, illustrating them in double-contrast fashion. Air-contrast delineation of these structures allows us to see through the stomach to retrogastric areas and structures. Barium-filled duodenum and pylorus is best demonstrated in the right anterior oblique (RAO) position.

32. **(A)** *Anterior and posterior aspects* of the stomach are visualized in the *lateral* position; medial and lateral aspects of the stomach are visualized in the AP projection. With the body in the AP recumbent position, *barium* flows easily into the *fundus* of the stomach, displacing the stomach somewhat superiorly. The fundus, then, is filled with barium, while *air* is displaced into the *gastric body, pylorus,* and *duodenum,* demonstrating them as double-contrast. Air-contrast delineation of these structures allows us to see through the stomach to the retrogastric areas and structures.

33. **(C)** Air or fluid levels will be clearly demonstrated only if the central ray is directed parallel to them. Therefore, to demonstrate air or fluid levels, erect or decubitus positions should be used. A "three-way abdomen" study is often performed to evaluate

possible obstruction or free air or fluid within the abdomen and usually consists of anteroposterior (AP) recumbent, AP erect, and left lateral decubitus projections of the abdomen.

34. **(A)** The trachea (windpipe) is a tube-like passageway for air that is supported by C-shaped cartilaginous rings. The trachea is part of the respiratory system and is continuous with the main stem bronchi. The esophagus, part of the alimentary canal, is a hollow tube-like structure connecting the mouth and stomach, and lies posterior to the trachea. If one inadvertently aspirates food or drink into the trachea, choking occurs.

35. **(A)** Esophageal varices are tortuous dilatations of the esophageal veins. They are much less pronounced in the erect position and must always be examined with the patient recumbent. The recumbent position affords more complete filling of the veins, as blood flows against gravity.

36. **(B)** The upper gastrointestinal (GI) tract must be empty for best x-ray evaluation. Any food or liquid mixed with the barium sulfate suspension can simulate pathology. Preparation therefore is to withhold food and fluids for 8 to 9 hours before the examination, typically after midnight, as fasting examinations are usually performed first thing in the morning.

37. **(D)** To demonstrate structures via double contrast, the barium must be moved away from the area and replaced with air. The *anteroposterior (AP) erect position* will accomplish that for both the colic flexures. The erect position allows barium to move downward, while air rises to fill the flexures. The decubitus positions are useful to demonstrate the lateral and medial walls of the ascending and descending colon.

38. **(A)** The right anterior oblique (RAO) position affords a good view of the pyloric canal and duodenal bulb. It is also a good position for the barium-filled esophagus, projecting it between the vertebrae and heart. The left lateral projection of the stomach demonstrates the left retrogastric space; the recumbent posteroanterior (PA) is used as a general survey of the gastric surfaces, and the recumbent anteroposterior (AP) with a slight left oblique affords a double contrast of the pylorus and duodenum.

39. **(B)** There are four types of body habitus. Listed from largest to smallest, they are hypersthenic, sthenic, hyposthenic, and asthenic. The position, shape, and motility of various organs can differ greatly from one body type to another. The typical asthenic gallbladder

(GB) is situated low and medial, often very close to the midline. To move the GB away from the midline, left anterior oblique (LAO) position is used. The GB of hypersthenic individuals occupies a high lateral and transverse position.

40. **(B)** In the prone oblique positions (right/left anterior oblique [RAO/LAO]), the flexure disclosed is the one closer to the IR. Therefore, the RAO position will open up the hepatic flexure. The anteroposterior (AP) oblique positions (right/left posterior oblique [RPO/LPO]) demonstrate the side away from the IR.

41. **(C)** When scheduling patient examinations, it is important to avoid the possibility of residual contrast medium covering areas of interest on later examinations. The intravenous urogram (IVU) should be scheduled first because the contrast medium used is excreted rapidly. The barium enema (BE) should be scheduled next. The gastrointestinal (GI) series is scheduled last. Any barium remaining from the previous BE should not be enough to interfere with the stomach or duodenum, although a preliminary scout image should be taken in each case.

42. **(C)** The major components of the urinary system are the *kidneys*, *ureters*, and *bladder*. The tiny functional units within the renal substance are *nephrons*.

The kidneys are retroperitoneal structures held in position by adipose tissue. They are located between the vertebral levels of T12 and L3. The right kidney is usually 1 to 2 in. lower than the left because of the presence of the liver on the right. The kidneys move inferiorly 1 to 3 in. when the body assumes an erect position; they move inferiorly and superiorly during respiration. The slit-like opening on the medial concave surface of each kidney is the *hilum*, which opens into a space called the renal sinus (see Fig. 6–102). The renal artery and vein, lymphatic vessels, and nerves pass through the hilum. The upper, expanded portion of the ureter is called the *renal pelvis*, or *infundibulum*, and also passes through the hilum; it is continuous with the major and minor *calyces* within the kidney.

43. **(C)** A patient having a gastrointestinal (GI) series is required to be NPO (nothing by mouth) for at least 8 hours prior to the examination; food or drink in the stomach can simulate disease. A patient scheduled for a urogram must have the preceding meal withheld so as to avoid the possibility of aspirating vomitus in case of allergic reaction. An abdominal survey does not require the use of contrast medium and no patient preparation is required.

44. **(B)** The kidneys lie obliquely in the posterior portion of the trunk, with their superior portions angled posteriorly and their inferior portions and ureters angled anteriorly. Therefore, to facilitate filling of the most anteriorly placed structures, the patient is examined in the prone position. Opacified urine then flows to the most dependent part of the kidney and ureter—the ureteropelvic region, inferior calyces, and ureters.

45. **(A)** Retrograde urograms require catheterization of the urethra and/or ureter(s). Radiographs that include the kidney(s) and ureter(s) in their entirety are made after retrograde filling of the structures. A cystogram or (voiding) cystourethrogram requires *urethral* catheterization only. Radiographs are made of the contrast-filled bladder and frequently of the contrast-filled urethra during voiding. Cystoscopy is required for location and catheterization of the vesicoureteral orifices.

46. **(B)** Because the urinary structures have so little subject contrast, artificial contrast material must be employed for better visualization of these structures. Contrast agents used for urographic procedures can have unpleasant, and (rarely) even lethal, side effects. Intravenous injection of contrast frequently produces a warm, flushed feeling, a bitter or metallic taste, or mild nausea. These side effects are of short duration and usually pass as quickly as they come. More serious side effects include urticaria, respiratory discomfort/distress, and, rarely, anaphylaxis. An antihistamine is appropriate treatment for simple side effects, but the radiographer must always be prepared to deal quickly and efficiently with patients experiencing more serious reactions. Nonionic contrast agents are far less likely to produce side effects.

47. **(D)** The most commonly performed radiologic examination of the reproductive system is hysterosalpingography, which is employed for evaluation of the uterus, oviducts, and ovaries of the female reproductive system. The procedure serves to delineate the position, size, and shape of the structures, and demonstrate pathology such as polyps, tumors, and fistulas. However, it is most often used to demonstrate *patency* of the oviducts in cases of *infertility* and is sometimes therapeutic in terms of opening a blocked oviduct.

48. (B) An anteroposterior (AP) postvoid bladder image is usually required to detect any *residual urine* in the evaluation of *tumor masses* or *enlarged prostate glands*. An erect image is occasionally requested to demonstrate renal mobility and ureteral tortuosity.

49. (A) During intravenous urography, both oblique positions are generally obtained. The 30 degree oblique KUB (kidney, ureters, bladder) places the kidney of the side *away* from the x-ray table *parallel* to the IR. The kidney closer to the x-ray table is placed perpendicular to the IR. The oblique positions provide an oblique projection of the urinary bladder.

50. (A) A 15 to 20 degree anteroposterior (AP) Trendelenburg position during intravenous (IV) urography is often helpful in demonstrating filling of the distal ureters and the area of the vesicoureteral orifices. In this position, the contrast-filled urinary bladder moves superiorly, encouraging filling of the distal ureters and superior bladder, and provides better delineation of these areas. The central ray should be directed perpendicular to the IR. Compression of the *distal* ureters is used to prolong filling of the renal pelvis and calyces. Compression of the *proximal* ureters is not advocated.

51. (B) The CNS is enclosed within three tissue membranes, the *meninges*. The pia mater is the innermost vascular membrane, which is closely attached to the brain and spinal cord. The arachnoid mater is a thin layer outside the pia mater and attached to it by weblike fibers. The *subarachnoid space* is between the pia and arachnoid mater and is filled with cerebrospinal fluid (CSF). The brain and spinal cord float in CSF, which acts as a shock absorber. The dura mater is a double-layered fibrous membrane outside the arachnoid mater. The *subdural space* is located between the arachnoid and dura mater; it does not contain CSF. The *epidural space* is located between the two layers of dura mater.

52. (C) As the heart contracts and relaxes while functioning to pump blood from the heart, those arteries that are large and those in closest proximity to the heart will feel the effect of the heart's forceful contractions in their walls. The arterial walls pulsate in unison with the heart's contractions. This movement may be detected with the fingers in various parts of the body and is referred to as the *pulse*.

53. (C) Superimposition of bony details frequently makes angiographic demonstration of blood vessels less than optimal. The method used to remove these superimposed bony details is called *subtraction*. *Digital* subtraction can accomplish this through the use of a computer, but *photographic* subtraction may also be performed using images from an angiographic series. *Registration* is the process of matching one series image exactly over another. A reversal image, or positive mask, is a reverse of the black and white radiographic tones.

54. (A) Deoxygenated blood is returned by way of the inferior and superior vena cava to the right side of the heart. The blood is emptied into the right atrium, passes through the tricuspid valve, and enters the right ventricle. It is forced through the pulmonary semilunar valve into the pulmonary artery (by contraction of the right ventricle) and passes to the lungs for reoxygenation. From the lungs, it is collected by the *pulmonary* veins, which carry the oxygenated blood to the left atrium, where it travels through the mitral valve into the *left ventricle*. Upon contraction of the left ventricle, blood passes through the *aortic valve* into the aorta and to all parts of the body.

55. (D) Generally, contrast medium is injected into the subarachnoid space between the third and fourth lumbar vertebrae. Because the spinal cord ends at the level of the first or second lumbar vertebrae, this is considered to be a relatively safe injection site. The cisterna magna can be used, but the risk of contrast entering and causing side effects increases.

56. (B) The heart wall is made up of the external epicardium, the middle myocardium, and the internal endocardium. The pericardium is the fibroserous sac enclosing the heart and roots of the great vessels. The heart has four chambers. The two *upper* chambers are the *atria* and the two *lower* chambers are the *ventricles*. The apex of the heart is the tip of the left ventricle.

57. (A) An intervertebral disk can rupture due to trauma or degeneration. The nucleus pulposus protrudes *posteriorly* through a tear in the annulus fibrosus and impinges on nerve roots and can be demonstrated by placing positive or negative contrast media into the subarachnoid space. Internal disk lesions can be demonstrated only by injecting contrast into the individual disks (this procedure is termed *diskography*). Anterior protrusion of a herniated intervertebral disk does not impinge on the spinal cord and is not demonstrated in myelography.

58. (C) Major branches of the common carotid arteries (internal carotids) function to supply the anterior brain, while the posterior brain is supplied by the vertebral arteries (branches of the subclavian arteries). The brachiocephalic (innominate) artery is unpaired and is one of three branches of the aortic arch, from which the right common carotid artery is derived. The left common carotid artery comes directly off the aortic arch.

59. (D) Venous blood is returned to the right atrium of the heart via the *superior* (from upper body) and *inferior* (from lower body) *vena cavae* and the *coronary sinus* (from the heart substance; see Fig. 6–118). Upon atrial systole, the blood passes through the *tricuspid* valve into the right ventricle. During ventricular systole, the blood is pumped through the pulmonary semilunar valve into the pulmonary artery to the lungs for oxygenation. Blood is returned via the pulmonary veins to the left atrium. During atrial systole, blood passes through the mitral (bicuspid) valve into the left ventricle. During ventricular systole, the oxygenated blood is pumped through the aortic semilunar valve into the aorta.

60. (C) The heart wall is made up of the external epicardium, the middle myocardium, and the internal endocardium. The pericardium is the fibroserous sac enclosing the heart and roots of the great vessels. The heart has four chambers. The two upper chambers are the atria, and the two lower chambers are the ventricles. The *apex* of the heart is the tip of the left ventricle.

IONIZING EFFECTS OF X-RADIATION

Electromagnetic Radiation

A review of electromagnetic radiation and energy is essential to the study of x-rays and other forms of ionizing radiation. *Electromagnetic radiation* can be described as wave-like fluctuations of electric and magnetic fields. There are many kinds of electromagnetic radiation. Figure 7–1 illustrates that visible light, microwaves, and radio waves, as well as x-ray and gamma rays, are all part of the *electromagnetic spectrum*. All the electromagnetic radiations have the same *velocity*, that is, 3×10^8 m/s (1,86,000 miles per second); however, they differ greatly in *wavelength* and *frequency*.

Wavelength refers to the distance between two consecutive wave crests (Fig. 7–2). *Frequency* refers to the number of cycles per second; its unit of measurement is *hertz* (Hz), which is equal to 1 cycle per second.

Frequency and wavelength are closely associated with the relative *energy* of electromagnetic radiations. More energetic radiations have shorter wavelength and higher frequency. The relationship among frequency, wavelength, and energy is graphically illustrated in the electromagnetic spectrum (Fig. 7–1).

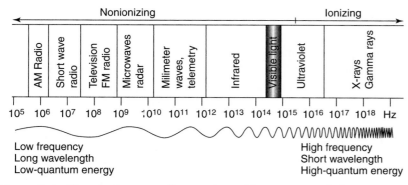

Figure 7–1. The electromagnetic spectrum. Frequency and photon energy are *directly* related; frequency and photon energy are *inversely* related to wavelength.

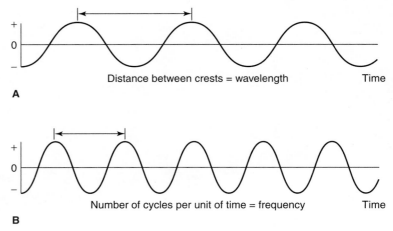

A

Distance between crests = wavelength   Time

B

Number of cycles per unit of time = frequency   Time

Figure 7–2. Wavelength versus frequency. *Wavelength* is described as the distance between successive crests. The shorter the wavelength, the more crests or cycles per unit of time (e.g., per second). Therefore, the shorter the wavelength the greater the *frequency* (number of cycles/s). Wavelength and frequency are *inversely* related.

Some radiations are energetic enough to rearrange atoms in materials through which they pass, and they can therefore be hazardous to living tissue. These radiations are called *ionizing radiation* because they have the energetic potential to break apart electrically neutral atoms, resulting in the production of negative and/or positive *ions*. X-ray photons, having the dual nature of both particles and electromagnetic waves, are highly energetic ionizing radiation. Diagnostic x-rays are extremely short, between 10^{-8} and 10^{-12} m in wavelength. The unit formerly used for such small dimensions is the angstrom (Å); $1\ \text{Å} = 10^{-10}$ m.

Humans are exposed to ionizing radiation from both natural and manmade sources (see Fig. 7–3). High doses of (manmade) ionizing radiation can cause tissue damage that can manifest within days after exposure. Late effects such as cancer, which can occur after more ordinary doses, may take many years to develop.

Humans have always been exposed to ionizing radiation. Some ionizing radiations (such as those emitted by uranium) occur naturally in the earth's crust and in its atmosphere (from the sun and cosmic reactions in space). These radiations are present in the structures in which we live and in the food we consume; radioactive gas is present in the air that we breathe, and there are traces of radioactive materials in our bodies. These radiations are referred to as *natural background* (environmental) *radiation*. The levels of natural background radiation vary greatly from one geographic location to another. *The greatest portion of our exposure to background radiation comes from naturally occurring sources such as these.*

In addition to natural background radiation, we are also exposed to sources of radiation created by humans. Various types of *artificial* or *manmade* radiation contribute to the dose received by the U.S. population. According to the BEIR VII report, medical and dental x-rays and nuclear medicine studies account for approximately 79% of the manmade radiation exposure in the United States.

Substances in consumer products such as tobacco, the domestic water supply, building materials, and to a lesser extent, smoke detectors, televisions, and computer screens, account for another 16%. Occupational exposures, fallout, and the nuclear fuel cycle comprise approximately 5%

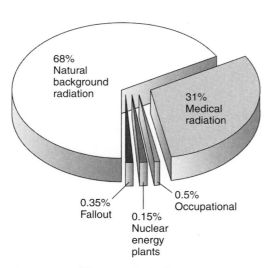

68%
Natural background radiation

31%
Medical radiation

0.35%
Fallout

0.15%
Nuclear energy plants

0.5%
Occupational

Figure 7–3. The population's exposure to various sources of ionizing radiation. Natural background radiations (the earth, the sun, building materials) compose the majority of our exposure. Medical irradiation is the largest portion of our exposure to artificial sources of radiation. *Occupational radiation, nuclear energy, and fallout are responsible for only a minute portion of our total exposure.*

of the manmade component. Figure 7–3 illustrates the approximate quantity of ionizing radiation received from natural and artificial sources.

X-ray *photons* are infinitesimal bundles of energy that deposit some of their energy into matter as they travel through it. This deposition of energy and subsequent *ionization* has the potential to cause chemical and biologic damage.

The process of ionization in living material necessarily changes atoms/molecules at least briefly and, consequently, can damage cells. If cell damage does occur and is not effectively repaired, the cell may not (1) survive (2) reproduce, or (3) perform its normal function. Alternatively, it can result in a working but *modified* cell, which could eventually become cancerous if it is a *somatic* cell, or lead to inherited/genetic disease if it is a *germ* cell.

Production of X-Rays at the Tungsten Target

Diagnostic x-rays are produced within the x-ray tube as high-speed *electrons* are suddenly decelerated by the tungsten target. The *source* of electrons is the heated cathode filament; the electrons are driven across to the anode's focal spot when thousands of volts (kilovolts) are applied. When the high-speed electrons are suddenly stopped at the focal spot, they interact with tungsten atoms, and their kinetic energy is converted to x-ray photon energy. This happens in the following two ways.

Bremsstrahlung (Brems) or "Braking" Radiation. A high-speed electron is accelerated toward a tungsten atom within the anode focal track. The negative electron is attracted by the positively charged nucleus of the tungsten atom and, as a result, pulled off course and redirected toward the nucleus. The electron's deflection from its original course caused by the "braking" (slowing down) results in a loss of energy. *This energy loss is given up in the form of an x-ray photon: Brems or braking radiation* (Fig. 7–4). The electron might not give up all its kinetic energy in one such interaction; it might go on to have several more interactions deeper in the target, each time giving up an x-ray photon having less and less energy. This is one reason the x-ray beam is heterogeneous (polyenergetic), that is, has a spectrum of energies. *Brems radiation comprises 70%–90% of the x-ray beam.*

Characteristic Radiation. In this case, a high-speed electron encounters a tungsten atom in the anode's focal track and ejects a K-shell electron (Fig. 7–5A), thereby leaving a vacancy in the K shell (Fig. 7–5B). An electron from a higher energy level shell (e.g., the L shell) fills the vacancy. In doing so, because of the difference in energy level between the K and L shell, a K-*characteristic primary ray* is emitted (Fig. 7–5C). The *energy of the characteristic ray* is equal to the difference in energy between the K and L shells. K-characteristic primary x rays from a tungsten target x-ray tube have 69 keV energy. Characteristic radiation comprises very little of the x-ray beam (10%–30%).

Interactions Between X-Ray Photons and Matter

The gradual decrease in exposure rate as ionizing radiation passes through tissues is called *attenuation*. Attenuation is principally attributable to the following two major types of interactions that occur between x-ray photons and tissue in the diagnostic x-ray range of energies.

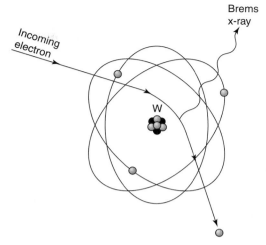

Figure 7–4. Production of Bremsstrahlung (Brems) radiation. A high-speed electron is deflected from its path and the loss of kinetic energy is emitted in the form of an x-ray photon.

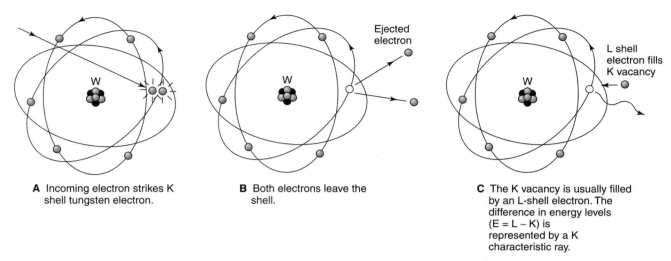

A Incoming electron strikes K shell tungsten electron.

B Both electrons leave the shell.

C The K vacancy is usually filled by an L-shell electron. The difference in energy levels (E = L − K) is represented by a K characteristic ray.

Figure 7–5. Production of characteristic radiation. A high-speed electron (**A**) ejects a tungsten K-shell electron, leaving a K-shell vacancy (**B**). An electron from the L shell fills the vacancy and emits a K-characteristic ray (**C**).

Photoelectric Effect. In the *photoelectric effect*, a relatively *low*-energy (low kV) x-ray photon interacts with tissue and uses all its energy (true/total absorption) to eject an *inner shell* electron. This leaves an inner shell orbital vacancy. An electron from the shell above drops down to fill the vacancy and, in doing so, gives up energy in the form of a *characteristic ray* (Fig. 7–6).

The photoelectric effect is more likely to occur in absorbers having *high atomic number* (e.g., bone, positive contrast media) and with *low-energy photons*. The photoelectric effect contributes significantly to patient dose, as all the x-ray photon energy is absorbed by the tissue (and, therefore, is responsible for the production of short-scale contrast). Its probability is Z^3/E^3 in the diagnostic energy range.

Compton Scatter. In *Compton scatter*, a fairly *high*-energy (high kV) x-ray photon interacts with tissue and ejects an *outer shell* electron (Fig. 7–7). The ejected electron is called a *recoil electron*. The scattered x-ray photon is deflected with somewhat reduced energy ("modified scatter"). However, it retains most of its original energy and exits the body as an energetic scattered photon.

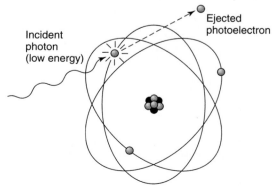

Incident photon (low energy)

Ejected photoelectron

Figure 7–6. In the photoelectric effect, the incoming (low energy) photon releases *all* its energy as it ejects an inner shell electron from orbit.

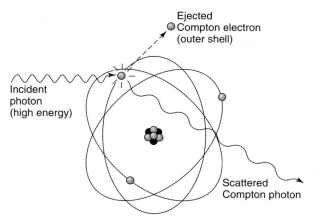

Figure 7–7. In Compton scatter, the incoming (high energy) photon uses *part* of its energy to eject an outer shell electron; in doing so, the photon changes direction (scatters) but retains much of its original energy.

Because the scattered photon exits the body, it does not pose a radiation hazard to the patient. It can, however, contribute to *image fog* and pose a *radiation hazard to personnel* (as in fluoroscopic procedures).

Summary

- The radiations of the electromagnetic spectrum all travel at the same velocity, 186,000 miles/s, but differ in wavelength and frequency.
- Wavelength is the distance between two consecutive wave crests. The number of cycles and crests per second is frequency; its unit of measurement is hertz.
- Wavelength and frequency are inversely related.
- Speed of light = frequency × wavelength ($c = f\lambda$)
- The two kinds of background radiation sources are natural background radiation and artificial/manmade background radiation; natural sources account for the largest human exposure to ionizing radiation.
- Medical radiation exposure is the largest source of artificial/manmade ionizing radiation exposure to humans.
- Ionization is caused by high-energy, short-wavelength electromagnetic radiations that break apart electrically neutral atoms.
- Two types of x-radiation are produced at the anode through energy conversion processes: Brems radiation and characteristic radiation; Brems radiation predominates.
- X rays can interact with tissue cells and cause ionization; the interactions between x-rays and tissue cells that occur most often are Compton scatter and the photoelectric effect.
- Characteristics of photoelectric effect:
  - Low-energy x-ray photon gives up all its energy ejecting an inner-shell electron.
  - Produces a characteristic ray.
  - Is a major contributor to patient dose.

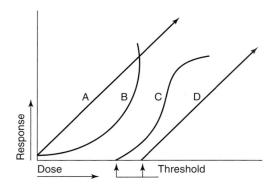

Figure 7–8. Dose–effect curves. **(A)** Linear, nonthreshold. **(B)** Nonlinear, nonthreshold. **(C)** Nonlinear, threshold. **(D)** Linear, threshold.

- Occurs in absorbers having high atomic number.
- Produces short-scale contrast.
- Characteristics of Compton scatter:
  - The interaction that predominates in the diagnostic x-ray range.
  - High-energy x-ray photon uses a portion of its energy to eject an outer shell electron.
  - Is responsible for scattered radiation fog to the image.
  - Poses radiation hazard to personnel.
- Exposure dose depends on beam attenuation and on which type of interaction occurs between x-ray photons and tissue. Exposure dose is, therefore, affected by radiation quality (kV) and the subject being irradiated (i.e., thickness and nature of part; atomic number of part).

DOSE–RESPONSE RELATIONSHIPS

Dose–Response Curves

The association between a dose of ionizing radiation and the magnitude of the resulting response or effect is referred to as a *dose–response, or dose–effect, relationship.*

Dose–response curves are used to illustrate the relationship between exposure to ionizing radiation and possible resultant biologic responses (Fig. 7–8). *Linear* (straight line) relationships are those in which the response is directly related to the dose received; that is, if the dose is increased, the biologic response is increased. In *nonlinear* relationships, the effects are not proportional to the dose. The term *threshold* refers to the dose below which no harmful effects are likely to occur, or, the point/dose at which a response first begins. The two most frequently used dose–response curves in radiation protection are the *linear, nonthreshold*, and the *nonlinear, threshold*. The Committee on Biologic Effects of Ionizing Radiation (BEIR) reports on the most current and comprehensive risk estimates for cancer and other health effects from exposure to low-level ionizing radiation. The BEIR VII report not only supports previously reported risk estimates for cancer and leukemia; but newer and broader data also has *reinforced* confidence in these risk estimates. The BEIR VII report states that "a comprehensive review of available biologic and biophysical data supports a 'linear-no-threshold' (LNT) risk model—that the risk of cancer proceeds in a linear fashion at lower doses without a threshold and that the smallest dose has the potential to cause a small increase in risk to humans."

Most sources of ionizing radiation have a mixture of high- and low-LET radiations. Low LET radiations deposit less energy in cells/tissues along their path, than high-LET radiations, and is considered less destructive as it traverses tissues. The BEIR VII report identifies *low dose* as near zero to approximately 100 mSv (0.1 Sv) of low-LET radiation. The U.S. population is exposed to average annual background radiation levels of approximately 3 mSv; exposure from a chest x-ray is approximately 0.10 mSv and exposure from a whole-body computerized tomography (CT) scan is approximately 10.0 mSv.

Average U.S. Doses

- Annual background dose = approximately 3 mSv (300 mrem)
- Average chest x-ray = approximately 0.10 mSv (10 mrem)
- Average whole body CT = approximately 10.0 mSv (1000 mrem)

Linear: Threshold and Nonthreshold

The *linear threshold* curve is shown in Figure 7–8D and illustrates responses that are proportional to the radiation dose received only after some particular dose is received—below this "threshold" dose, no response–effect is likely to occur. The *linear nonthreshold* curve (Fig. 7–8A) is used to illustrate responses such as radiation-induced leukemia, cancer, and genetic effects. These are sometimes referred to as *stochastic effects*. Stochastic effects occur randomly and are "all or nothing" type effects; that is, they do not occur with degrees of severity. It must be noted that *in a nonthreshold curve there is no safe dose*, that is, no dose below which there will definitely be no biologic response—any dose can cause a biologic effect. Theoretically, even one x-ray photon can cause a biologic response. This is the curve of choice to predict effects of low-level (e.g., medical and occupational) exposure to ionizing radiation.

Nonlinear: Threshold and Nonthreshold

In *nonlinear* curves, the effects of radiation are not proportional to the dose received. Figures 7–8B and 7–8C illustrate nonlinear dose–response curves. In nonlinear curves, a considerable dose could be required before effects occur, and then effects might increase significantly with only a little more increase in dose. Response could level off at some point and further doses might have much less effect. Thus, the term *nonlinear*. Nonlinear curves can be threshold or nonthreshold. A familiar nonlinear curve is the *S*, or *sigmoid*, type seen in Figure 7–8C. The *nonlinear (sigmoid) threshold* curve is used to illustrate certain radiation-induced somatic conditions such as skin *erythema*. These responses are *predictable* and sometimes referred to as *nonstochastic effects*.

Late Effects

The Committee on the BEIR in 1990 reported in their revised risk estimates that effects of ionizing radiation exposure are approximately *three to four times more than reported in the previous statement*. The more recent (2005) BEIR VII report not only supports previously reported risk estimates for cancer and leukemia; but newer and broader data has *reinforced* confidence in these risk estimates.

Occupationally exposed individuals are concerned principally with *late* (i.e., *long-term* or *delayed*) effects of ionizing radiation such as radiation-induced *genetic effects*, *leukemia*, *cancers* (bone, lung, thyroid, breast), and *local effects* such as skin erythema, infertility, and cataracts—these can occur many years following initial exposure to low levels of ionizing radiation. These long-term/delayed effects are usually *chronic* and many are represented by the linear, nonthreshold dose–response curve.

History provides us with many examples of the delayed effects of ionizing radiation: many of the early radiologists and radiation scientists, A-bomb survivors of Hiroshima and Nagasaki, and patients with ankylosing spondylitis in Great Britain in the 1940s developed leukemia and other *lifespan–shortening* diseases as a result of exposure to varying quantities of ionizing radiation over a period of time. Some children irradiated in the 1940s for enlarged thymus glands developed thyroid cancer as adults 20 years later. Radium watch-dial

---

Dose–Response Terminology

- *Linear:*
  Response is *proportional* to dose
- *Nonlinear:*
  Response is *not proportional* to dose
- *Threshold:*
  A *dose* must be received before a response can occur
- *Nonthreshold:*
  No safe dose—even *one photon* can cause a response

Early Effects:

- Appear a short time after exposure
- Usually as a result of high dose in short period of time
- Should not be seen in diagnostic radiology

Late Effects:

Can appear years after exposure:
- Carcinogenesis
- Cataractogenesis
- Embryologic effect
- Lifespan shortening

painters in the 1920s developed a variety of bone cancers following a latent period of 20 to 30 years. These are all delayed effects of radiation and are represented by the linear, nonthreshold dose–response curve.

Cataractogenesis is another late effect of exposure to ionizing radiation, but it is represented by the *nonlinear, threshold* dose–response curve. An acute dose of approximately 200 rad is required to cause radiogenic cataracts. A far greater occupational or otherwise fractionated dose of approximately 1,000 rad is required to induce cataracts.

Early, or short-term, effects of radiation are those responses that occur very soon after exposure to ionizing radiation. Short-term effects are usually *acute effects* and occur only after exposure to a very large amount of radiation all at one time (and perhaps to the whole body) and therefore should not occur in diagnostic radiology.

Types of Risk

Risks associated with exposure to ionizing radiation can be divided into two categories: *Deterministic* and *Stochastic*.

Deterministic risks are characterized by nonlinear dose responses and are associated with a threshold (safe) dose below which no effect is observed. Deterministic effects are believed to result from radiation-induced death of large groups of tissue cells, resulting in serious functional impairment. The severity of any injury increases with increasing ionizing radiation dose. Examples include radiation-induced skin injury, hypothyroidism, cataract formation, hair loss, temporary infertility, and sterility.

Although deterministic effects generally arise within days or weeks after exposure, some of the induced skin injuries, cataracts, and hypothyroidism have long latency periods.

"In recent years, there has been a marked increase in the number of patient skin injuries due to the increasing number and duration of fluoroscopically guided medical procedures." (*T. Shope, Radiographics, 16, 1996*).

Stochastic effects include heritable genetic effects and some somatic effects (cancer). Stochastic effects are the foremost late effects that are expected to occur in populations exposed to ionizing radiation, somatic effects (i.e. radiation-induced cancer) is the leading health detriment.

For both somatic and genetic effects, the probability of their occurrence—but not their severity—is dependent on the radiation dose. However, for most stochastic effects it is generally accepted that there is *no threshold*, that is, *no safe dose*. Radiation-induced cancers and genetic effects cannot be distinguished from those that appear spontaneously.

Types of Risks

Deterministic:
- Threshold
- Non-linear
- Includes all early effects
- Includes some later effects

Stochastic:
- No threshold
- Linear
- Genetic effects
- Cancer
- Includes most late effects

Summary

- Ionization of living tissue can cause chemical and biologic damage to somatic and/or genetic cells.

- A nonthreshold dose–response relationship indicates that there is no safe dose of radiation; any dose can cause a biologic effect.

- The linear nonthreshold dose–response relationship illustrates stochastic responses (cancer, genetic effects) and is the curve of choice for occupational exposure.

- Occupationally exposed workers are concerned with late (i.e., long-term or delayed) effects of ionizing radiation such as radiation-induced genetic effects, leukemia, and cancers (bone, lung, thyroid, breast).
- Risks associated with exposure to ionizing radiation can be divided into two categories: *deterministic* and *stochastic.*

BIOLOGIC EFFECTS OF IONIZING RADIATION

Law of Bergonié and Tribondeau

Before beginning our review of somatic and genetic effects of ionizing radiation, a brief review of *radiobiology* is in order. Radiobiology is the study of the effects of ionizing radiation on biologic material at the cellular level.

In 1906, two scientists, Bergonié and Tribondeau, proposed that certain cellular qualities made tissues more or less radiosensitive. The Law of Bergonié and Tribondeau addresses relative tissue sensitivity and states that the following are particularly radiosensitive:

1. Stem (undifferentiated, or precursor) cells
2. Young, immature tissues
3. Highly mitotic cells

Thus, very young cells, undifferentiated cells (nonspecialized in structure and function), and cells having the most reproductive activity are highly *radiosensitive*. Examples of highly radiosensitive tissues are intestinal epithelial cells and cells of the rapidly developing embryo and fetus.

Radiation Weighting and Tissue Weighting Factors

Ionization causes the removal of electrons from some atoms and the addition of electrons to other atoms. Thus, the stage is set for biologic effects; as a result of the ionization, appropriate chemical bonds cannot be maintained.

Similar absorbed doses of *different kinds* of radiation can cause different biologic effects to *tissues of differing radiosensitivity*. A *radiation weighting factor* (W_r) is a number assigned to different types of ionizing radiations so that their effect(s) may be better determined (e.g., x-ray vs. alpha particles). The W_r of different ionizing radiations is dependent on the linear energy transfer (LET) of that particular radiation. A *tissue weighting factor* (W_t) represents the relative tissue radiosensitivity of the irradiated material (e.g., muscle vs. intestinal epithelium vs. bone, etc.).

The term *equivalent dose* (EqD) refers simply to the product of the absorbed dose (rad/Gy) and its radiation weighting factor (W_r). The W_t is not considered in EqD. The term *effective dose equivalent* refers to the dose from radiation sources internal and/or external to the body and is expressed in units of rem.

To determine effective dose (*EfD*), the following formula is used:

Radiation Type/Energy	W_r
X or gamma	1
Protons	2
Neutrons: 10–100 keV	10
Neutrons: 100 keV–2 MeV	20
Alpha particles	20

Effective dose (*EfD*) = Radiation weighting factor (W_r)

× Tissue weighting factor (W_t)

× Absorbed dose (*D*)

Organ/Tissue	W_t
Skin	0.01
Thyroid	0.05
Breast	0.05
Red bone marrow	0.12
Lung	0.12
Stomach	0.12
Gonads	0.20

Linear Energy Transfer and Relative Biologic Effectiveness Versus Biologic Damage

Radiation deposits energy as it passes through tissue. The rate at which this occurs is described as *linear energy transfer.* LET is another means of expressing radiation quality and determining the W_r. It expresses the ability of radiation to do damage. As the LET of radiation increases, the radiation's ability to produce biologic damage also increases. This is described quantitatively by *relative biologic effectiveness (RBE);* LET and RBE are directly related.

Because of the relative high effective atomic number (Z*eff*) and mass density of biologic material, low-energy x-ray photons are more readily absorbed in biologic material than are high-energy photons.

Diagnostic x-rays are considered low LET radiation; the approximate LET of diagnostic x-rays is expressed in keV/μm. Energy transferred to tissue can cause molecular damage. Any manifestation of that damage will depend on the extent of molecular disruption and the type of tissue affected.

Molecular Effects of Ionizing Radiation

The principal interactions that occur between x-ray photons and body tissues in the diagnostic x-ray range, the *photoelectric effect* and *Compton scatter*, are ionization processes producing photoelectrons and recoil electrons that traverse tissue and subsequently ionize molecules. These interactions occur randomly but can lead to molecular damage in the form of *impaired function* or *cell death.* The *target theory* specifies that deoxyribonucleic acid (DNA) molecules are the targets of greatest importance and sensitivity; that is, DNA is the key sensitive molecule. However, because 65%–80% of the body is composed of water, most interactions between ionizing radiation and body cells will involve radiolysis of water rather than direct interaction with DNA. The two major types of effects that occur are the *direct effect* and the *indirect effect.*

Direct Effect. The direct effect occurs when the ionizing particle (e.g., an electron) interacts directly with the *key molecule* (DNA) or another critical enzyme or protein (i.e., RNA). Chemical damage can occur as chemical bonds are broken and chemical structure is changed. This can result in impaired function or cell death. Direct effect usually occurs with high LET radiations (e.g., alpha particles and neutrons) and when ionization occurs at the DNA molecule itself.

Indirect Effect. The indirect effect, which *occurs most frequently,* happens when ionization takes place away from the DNA molecule, in cellular water. Ionization of water molecules in the body (i.e., *radiolysis of cellular water*) breaks water molecules into smaller molecules, often producing one or more atoms having unpaired electrons ("*free radicals*"). A free radical is very short lived but highly reactive; it can break chemical bonds in an effort to pair with another electron, and can even travel a considerable distance from its source. The indirect effect is predominant with low LET radiation (e.g., x- and gamma rays).

DNA is the primary target for cell damage from ionizing radiation. Possible types of damage to the DNA molecule are diverse. A single main chain/side rail scission (break) on the DNA molecule is *repairable*. A double main chain/side rail scission may repair with difficulty or may result in *cell death*. A double main chain/side rail scission on the same "rung" of the DNA ladder results in *irreparable* damage or *cell death*. Faulty repair of main chain breakage can result in "cross-linking."

Damage to the nitrogenous bases, that is, damage to the base itself or to the rungs connecting the main chains, can result in alteration of base sequences causing a *molecular lesion/point mutation*. Any subsequent divisions result in daughter cells with incorrect genetic information.

The majority (approximately 90%) of cell damage is repairable. However, subsequent or multiple "hits" to the same cell are more likely to leave permanent damage.

Cellular and Relative Tissue Radiosensitivity

These types of molecular damage can occur to any of the somatic cells or to genetic cells. For example, high levels of radiation exposure to the bone marrow (where blood cells are produced) can cause a decrease in the number of circulating blood cells.

Tissue radiosensitivity is closely related to the cell (life and division) cycle. Cells divide for the purposes of reproduction, repair, and growth, and the cell cycle is an orderly arrangement of events. The cell cycle can be divided into two parts: interphase and *mitosis*. Interphase is further divided into three steps: gap 1 (G_1), synthesis (S), and gap 2 (G_2). Important, radiologically, is the fact that cells are *particularly radiosensitive* during late G_2 and mitosis (M). DNA replication occurs during the S phase, which is the *least radiosensitive* stage of the cell cycle (Fig. 7–9).

Lymphocytes, a type of white blood cell that plays an important role in the immune system, are particularly radiosensitive. If lymphocytes suffer radiation damage, the body loses its ability to fight infection and becomes more susceptible to disease.

Epithelial tissue, which lines the respiratory system and intestines, is also a highly radiosensitive tissue. In contrast, *muscle* and *nervous* tissues are comparatively insensitive to radiation. Because nerve cells in the adult do not undergo mitosis, they comprise the most *radioresistant* somatic tissue. However, nervous tissue *in the fetus* (particularly the second to eighth week) is highly mitotic and, hence, highly *radiosensitive*.

The *genetic cells* of the gonads are considered especially radiosensitive tissues. Exposure to ionizing radiation can cause temporary infertility, permanent sterility, or mutations in succeeding generations. In particular, the reproductive cells of the fetus and young

Types of DNA Damage

- Main chain, double-side rail break
- Main chain, single-side rail break
- Main chain breakage, cross-linking
- Base damage, point mutations

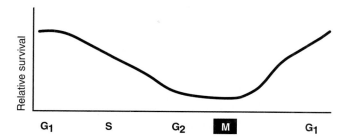

Figure 7–9. Cell radiosensitivity during cell cycle. Cells in late G_2 and in mitosis are most radiosensitive.

children are exceptionally radiosensitive. Other factors that determine tissue response, and can modify radiation injury, include the following:

1. *Fractionation and protraction:* Small doses delivered over a long period of time produce a lesser effect. (The greatest effect of irradiation will be observed if a *large quantity* of radiation is delivered in a *short time* to the *whole body*.)

2. *Oxygen:* The greater the oxygen content of tissues, the greater their radiosensitivity. Dissolved oxygen in tissues increases stability and toxicity of free radicals. The oxygen enhancement ratio can be determined by dividing the dose required to cause an effect *without* oxygen *by* the dose required to cause that effect *with* oxygen.

3. *Temperature:* Tissues are more radiosensitive at higher temperatures; chromosome aberrations are more likely to occur at lower temperatures because repair processes are inhibited.

4. *Age:* Fetal tissue is most radiosensitive. As the individual ages, tissue sensitivity decreases. Radiosensitivity increases again in old age, but only slightly.

Remember, as the LET of the ionizing radiation increases, the radiation's ability to produce biologic damage also increases. This is described quantitatively as RBE; LET, and RBE are directly related.

It is well established that sufficient quantities of ionizing radiation can cause a number of serious *somatic* and/or *genetic* effects. What is not clear, however, are the long-term effects of low-level (diagnostic and occupational) x-radiation.

Health care professionals involved in prescribing and delivering radiologic examinations have an obligation to keep nonproductive radiation exposure to all individuals as low as possible. Possible abusive overuse of radiologic (and other diagnostic) examinations is currently being scrutinized by many health care facilities as part of a continuous quality improvement program. Some formerly routine examinations are now considered excessive and unnecessary, for example, routine chest x-ray on admission to the hospital, are no longer performed unless the patient is admitted to the pulmonary medicine or surgical service; preemployment chest and/or lumbar spine examinations are frequently considered to have little benefit.

In states having no *licensure* requirements for radiographers, physicians, and hospitals often assume the responsibility of hiring only credentialed radiographers. Participation in *quality assurance* ensures that imaging equipment is functioning optimally and that image quality is up to expected standards.

Radiographers must consider patient dose when selecting exposure factors. One component of a radiographer's professionalism, as stated in the principles of the *ARRT Code of Ethics*, is to consistently employ every means possible to decrease radiation exposure to the population.

Radiographers must follow the *ALARA* principle (keeping exposure As Low As Reasonably Achievable) as they carry out their tasks. The radiologic facility must undergo appropriate radiation surveys. Staff must be properly oriented and regular inservice reviews of radiation safety must take place. Proper radiation monitoring and review of monthly radiation reports is essential.

Summary

- The Law of Bergonié and Tribondeau states that the most radiosensitive cells are young, undifferentiated, and highly mitotic cells.
- LET is another means of expressing radiation quality and determining the radiation-weighting factor.
- W_r and W_t are needed because identical doses of different kinds of radiation to different tissues will cause different biologic effects.
- EqD = absorbed dose $\times W_r$.
- $EfD = W_r \times W_t \times$ absorbed dose (D).
- Diagnostic x-radiation is low-energy, low-LET radiation.
- Ionizing radiation effect on cells is named according to the interaction site, namely, direct effect and indirect effect.
- The most radiosensitive cell is the lymphocyte.
- As radiation professionals, we are obligated to keep radiation exposure to our patients and ourselves ALARA.

GENETIC EFFECTS

Pregnancy

There are a number of situations that require the radiographer's special attention. Irradiation during *pregnancy*, especially in early pregnancy, must be avoided. The fetus is particularly radiosensitive during the first trimester, during much of which time pregnancy may not even be suspected. *Especially high-risk examinations* include pelvis, hip, femur, lumbar spine, cystograms and urograms, upper gastrointestinal (GI) series, and barium enema examinations.

During the first trimester, specifically the second to tenth week of pregnancy (i.e., during major organogenesis), if the radiation dose is sufficient, fetal anomalies can be produced. *Skeletal and/or organ anomalies* can appear if irradiation occurs in the early part of this time period, and *neurologic anomalies* can be formed in the latter part; *mental retardation,* childhood *malignant diseases*, such as cancers or leukemia, and retarded growth/development can also result from irradiation during the first trimester.

Fetal irradiation during the second and third trimesters is not likely to produce anomalies, but rather, with sufficient dose, some type of childhood malignant disease. Fetal irradiation during the first 2 weeks of gestation can result in *embryonic resorption or spontaneous abortion.*

It must be emphasized, however, that the likelihood of producing fetal anomalies at doses below 5–15 rad (0.05–0.15 Gy) is exceedingly small and that most general diagnostic examinations are likely to deliver fetal doses of less than 1–2 rad.

Females

Elective Scheduling/10-Day Rule. In consideration of the potential risk, female patients of childbearing age should be questioned regarding their last menstrual period (LMP) and the possibility of their being pregnant. Figure 7–10 is an example algorithm for questioning female

> **Ways to Reduce Risk to Recently Fertilized Ovum**
>
> - Elective scheduling/10-day rule
> - Patient questionnaire
> - Posting

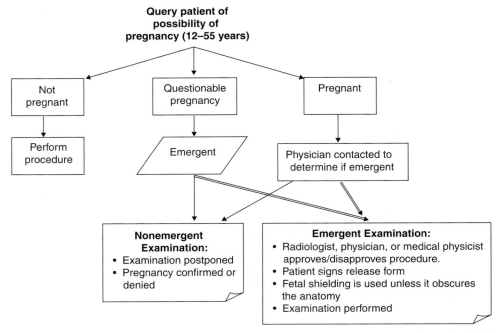

Figure 7–10. Algorithm for questioning female patients having reproductive potential. (Courtesy of Tom Piccoli, DABR.)

patients having reproductive potential. Facilities offering radiologic services should make inquiries of their female patients regarding LMP and advise them of the risk associated with radiation exposure during pregnancy. The *10-day rule* identifies the first 10 days following onset of the menses as the safest time to schedule elective procedures of the abdomen/pelvis.

Patient Questionnaire. In addition to supporting the ALARA concept, many institutions also use a patient questionnaire as a guide for scheduling elective abdominal x-ray examinations on women of reproductive age. The patient completes a form that requests information concerning her LMP and the possibility of her being pregnant.

Posting. In place of either or both of the above—or in addition to them—posters can be obtained, or signs can be made, that caution the patient to tell the radiologic technologist if she suspects that she might be pregnant. Most facilities will post these signs in waiting rooms, dressing rooms, and radiographic rooms.

Concern is occasionally expressed regarding dose received during diagnostic *mammography*. Yet the risk associated with the x-ray dose received is minimal compared with the benefits of early detection of breast cancer. The use of dedicated mammography equipment with digital or screen–film technique performed by credentialed radiographers delivers a very low skin and glandular dose.

Males

Because of the location of the gonads and *shielding* restrictions thus imposed in the female patient, the female gonads (ovaries) receive more radiation exposure than the male gonads (testes) undergoing similar examinations. The ovaries lie within the abdominal cavity and frequently cannot be effectively shielded during abdominal, pelvic, and lumbar spine radiography. Therefore, they can receive far more organ dose than the shielded testes (which are located outside the abdominal cavity) during diagnostic examinations of the abdominal region (e.g., lumbar spine, upper and lower GI, intravenous, or retrograde pyelography).

It is important to note that the ovarian stem cells, the oogonia, reproduce only during fetal life. During childbearing years, there are only 400–500 mature ova accessible for fertilization, that is, one ovum per menstrual cycle for each of the fertile years. The male germ cells, spermatogonia, are being produced continuously and longevity of fertility is quite different than in the female.

Children

The female oogonia of fetal life and early childhood and male spermatogonia are especially radiosensitive because of their immature stage of development. Consequently, particular care should be taken to adequately shield the reproductive organs of pediatric patients. All too often a radiographer will conscientiously shield adult patients of reproductive age, but fail to consider children whose reproductive lives are ahead of them and whose reproductive cells are particularly radiosensitive.

Very sizable doses of radiation to children are also thought to be associated with increased incidence of leukemia and other radiation-induced malignancies. Examples of high-risk examinations might include pelvic and abdominal radiography and examinations requiring periodic follow-ups, such as scoliosis series. It is advisable to shield the hematopoietic bones of children to reduce radiation dose to blood-forming cells.

Genetically Significant Dose

Each member of the world's population bears a particular genetic dose of radiation. Its sources include environmental exposure, radiation received for medical and dental purposes, and occupational exposure. The quantity of exposure to each individual depends on that individual's geographic location (environmental radiation and elevation of terrain), overall general health, the accessibility of health care, and the occupational worker's adherence to radiation protection guidelines. Generally speaking, the genetic dose to an *individual* is very small. Some individuals may receive no genetic dose in a given year, some individuals are past their reproductive years, and some individuals will not or cannot bear children. Even if some individuals receive larger quantities of radiation exposure, its impact is "diluted" by the total number of population. This concept is referred to as *genetically significant dose*, defined as the average annual gonadal dose to the population of childbearing age and estimated to be 20 mrem.

It is appropriate to mention *repeat radiographs* at this time. Poor images resulting from technical error (e.g., incorrect positioning, improper selection of technical factors), or equipment malfunction must be repeated, thereby subjecting the patient to twice the necessary exposure dose. An exceedingly important feature with significant impact on patient dose is appropriate *collimation*. An important part of radiation protection, then, is care and attention to detail to avoid technical errors requiring repeat images. Another component is a quality assurance program (through an ongoing preventive maintenance program and appropriate inservice education) that assures proper equipment function and compliance with established standards.

SOMATIC EFFECTS

Somatic effects of radiation are those that affect the irradiated body itself. Somatic effects are described as being *early* or *late*, depending on the length of time between irradiation and manifestation of effects.

Early somatic effects are manifested within minutes, hours, days, or weeks of irradiation, and occur only following a very large dose of ionizing radiation. It must be emphasized that doses received from diagnostic radiologic procedures are not sufficient to produce these early effects. An exceedingly *high dose of radiation delivered to the whole body in a short period of time* is required to produce *early* somatic effects.

Carcinogenesis

Late somatic effects are those that can occur years after initial exposure and are caused by low, chronic exposures. Occupationally exposed personnel are concerned with the late effects of radiation exposure. Some somatic effects like *carcinogenesis* have been mentioned earlier: the *bone malignancies* developed by the radium watch-dial painters as a result of radiation exposure to bone marrow, the *thyroid* cancers of the individuals irradiated as children for thymus enlargement, the leukemia eventually developed by patients whose pain from ankylosing spondylitis was relieved by irradiation, and the *skin cancers* developed by early radiology pioneers working so closely with the "unknown ray." These malignancies are examples of somatic effects of radiation.

Cataractogenesis

Another example of somatic effects of radiation is *cataract* formation to the lenses of eyes of those individuals accidentally exposed to sufficient quantities of radiation (e.g., early cyclotron experimenters).

Lifespan Shortening

The lives of many of the early radiation workers were several years shorter than the lives of the general population. Statistics revealed that radiologists, for example, had a shorter lifespan than physicians of other specialties. *Lifespan shortening*, then, *was* another somatic effect of radiation. Certainly, these effects should *never be experienced today.* So much has been learned about the biologic effects of radiation since its discovery and a part of what we have learned has, sadly, been as a result of the experiences of the radiology pioneers.

Reproductive Risks

The human reproductive organs are particularly radiosensitive. *Fertility* and *heredity* are greatly affected by the *germ cells* produced within the testes (*spermatogonia*) and ovaries (*oogonia*). Excessive radiation exposure to the gonads can cause *temporary or permanent sterility*, and/or *genetic mutations*.

Embryologic/Fetal Effects

Embryologic/fetal effects are those experienced by the body of the developing embryo or fetus. Spontaneous abortion, skeletal or neurologic anomalies (mental retardation and microcephaly), and leukemia are examples of embryologic or fetal somatic effects.

Acute Radiation Syndrome (ARS)

After a large dose (at least 2 Gy or 200 rad) of radiation to the *skin*, a mild *erythema* will result in 1 or 2 days. With a large enough dose, in approximately 2 weeks, a moist *desquamation* can occur followed by a dry desquamation. It takes approximately 5 Gy or 500 rad to produce skin erythema (*skin erythema dose; SED*) in 50% of a population so exposed. This is termed the SED_{50}. Another skin response is *epilation*, that is, hair loss as a result of damage to hair follicles and associated structures.

Most blood cells in circulation are manufactured by the bone marrow. The most radiosensitive of these cells are the *lymphocytes*—cells involved in immune response. They are the first to demonstrate depletion after a large enough exposure (0.25 Gy or 25 rad threshold), although all cells will decrease in number following a large dose of ionizing radiation.

Acute Radiation Syndrome (ARS), sometimes referred to as radiation sickness, is an acute condition caused by a large external penetrating exposure of ionizing radiation (at least 50–100 rad/0.5–1.0 Gy), all at one time or in a very short period of time, and to all or most of the body.

There are three types of ARS. *Hematopoetic*, or bone marrow, syndrome can cause nausea, vomiting, diarrhea, decreased blood count, infection, and hemorrhage. *Gastrointestinal* (GI) syndrome generally occurs at doses between 1000–10,000 rad (10–100 Gy). GI syndrome causes severe damage to the (stem) cells lining the GI resulting in nausea, vomiting, diarrhea, blood changes, and hemorrhage; death usually occurs within 2 weeks. *Central nervous system* (CNS) or *cardiovascular* (CV) syndrome usually occurs at doses greater than 5000 rad (50 Gy). The normally radioresilient central nervous and/or cardiovascular systems are affected very quickly. There is collapse of the circulatory system, as increased pressure in the cranial vault, vasculitis, meningitis, ataxia, and shock. Death occurs in 3 days. Certainly, these syndromes are most likely to occur as a result of a nuclear accident or attack, atomic bomb fallout—and never should be a concern in diagnostic radiology. Acute radiation syndrome has four stages:

- Prodromal stage: Symptoms are nausea, vomiting, and diarrhea that occur 1 hour to 2 days following exposure.

Acute Radiation Syndromes

- Hematopoietic
- Gastrointestinal
- Central Nervous System

Stages of Acute Radiation Syndrome

- Prodromal
- Latent
- Manifest illness
- Recovery or death

- Latent stage: Symptoms disappear; the exposed individual seems generally healthy for up to a few weeks. The length of the latent stage depends upon the amount of exposure received (inversely related).
- Manifest Illness stage: Symptoms depend on the specific syndrome and last up to several months, depending on severity.
- Recovery or death: Individuals who do not recover will die within weeks or months of exposure; recovery process can take from several weeks up to 2 years. Those who recover must be concerned about long-term effects.

Summary

- Delivery of ionizing radiation during early pregnancy is particularly hazardous.
- Possible responses to irradiation in utero include spontaneous abortion, congenital anomalies, mental retardation, microcephaly, and leukemia or other childhood malignancies.
- Elective booking, patient questionnaire, and posting are suggested ways to avoid irradiation of a new embryo/fetus.
- Gonadal shielding is easier in the male patient because the reproductive organs are located externally.
- All children should be shielded whenever possible.
- Genetic effects refer to damage to reproductive cells, affecting the reproductive capacity of the individual, or creating mutations that will be passed on to future generations.
- The genetic dose of radiation borne by each member of the reproductive population is called the genetically significant dose.
- Somatic effects include those manifesting themselves in the exposed individual and can be described as early or late effects.
- Early somatic effects can occur only after a very large single exposure of radiation to the whole body (ARS).
- Late somatic effects include carcinogenesis, cataractogenesis, embryologic effect, lifespan shortening, reproductive risks, and systemic effects.
- Occupationally exposed personnel are concerned with the late effects of radiation exposure.

COMPREHENSION CHECK

Congratulations! You have completed this chapter. If you are able to answer the following group of very comprehensive questions, you should feel confident that you have really mastered this section. You are then ready to go on to "Registry-type" questions that follow. For greatest success, do not go to the multiple-choice questions without first completing the short-answer questions below.

1. List various kinds of electromagnetic radiation (p. 225).

2. Identify the way in which all electromagnetic radiations are similar and in what respects they differ (p. 225).

3. Define the terms *wavelength* and *frequency* (p. 225).

4. Explain how wavelength and energy, and how frequency and energy, are related (p. 225).

5. Describe what is meant by the term *ionizing* radiation and how it differs from other electromagnetic radiations (p. 226).

6. Give examples of natural and artificial/man-made background radiations and identify the percentage each contributes to the population's annual radiation dose (p. 226).

7. What are the two ways in which x-ray photons are produced at the tungsten anode? Describe each. Which occurs more often (p. 227)?

8. Describe the photoelectric effect and Compton scatter. The following should be included in your description (p. 228, 229).

   A. Energy required for production of each

   B. Electron shell involved

   C. Any electron shell vacancy or occupancy changes

   D. Type of absorber (atomic number) most likely involved

   E. Retention or loss of energy of incoming photon

   F. Interaction associated with a recoil electron

   G. Effect on image contrast

   H. Impact on patient dose

9. Describe the purpose of dose–response (dose–effect) curves (p. 230).

10. Describe the difference between linear and non-linear dose–response curves (p. 230).

11. Describe the difference between threshold and nonthreshold dose–response curves (p. 231).

12. Differentiate between stochastic and nonstochastic effects (p. 231, 232).

13. Name the type of dose–response curve that identifies *no* safe dose (p. 231).

14. Explain why occupationally exposed individuals are mainly concerned with the late, or long-term, effects of radiation exposure (p. 231, 232).

15. List possible long-term effects of radiation exposure (p. 231, 232).

16. List the three types of cells described by Bergonié and Tribondeau in 1906 as being the most radiosensitive (p. 233).

17. Discuss deterministic versus stochastic risks; give examples of each (p. 232).

18. What is described as the rate at which radiation deposits energy in tissue (p. 234)?

19. Why is a W_r assigned to different types of radiation; a W_t assigned to different tissue types (p. 233)?

20. How can effective dose (*EfD*) be determined (p. 233)?

21. How are LET and RBE related (p. 234)?

22. With respect to the molecular effects of radiation, describe the difference between the direct and indirect effects; identify the one that occurs more frequently in the diagnostic range (p. 234, 235).

23. What type(s) of DNA damage is/are repairable; which can result in cell death; mutation (p. 234, 235)?

24. Identify each of the following as either radiosensitive or radioresistant: muscle, nerve (fetal and adult), and epithelial tissue; lymphocytes; and reproductive cells (p. 233, 235).

25. How does each of the following affect the response of tissue to irradiation: tissue age, oxygen content, fractionation/protraction of radiation delivery (p. 236)?

26. Identify the meaning of the acronym ALARA and how it relates to the radiographer (p. 236).

27. What is the most radiosensitive portion of the human gestational period? List four possible results of excessive radiation exposure during this period (p. 237).

28. What can result from excessive radiation exposure during the second and third trimesters of pregnancy (p. 237)?

29. How much radiation exposure is necessary to produce fetal anomalies? Approximately how much fetal radiation do most diagnostic examinations deliver (p. 237)?

30. List three methods the radiology department can use to avoid irradiating a newly fertilized ovum (p. 237, 238).

31. Explain the value of determining the LMP for female patients of childbearing age (p. 237, 238).

32. Describe the effectiveness of gonadal shielding in the male versus female patient; discuss the importance of shielding children (p. 238, 239).

33. Describe the concept of genetically significant dose (p. 239, 240).

34. Why are we concerned with genetic dose? When do genetic effects manifest themselves (p. 239, 240)?

35. Distinguish between early and late somatic effects; when does each occur with respect to initial exposure? Can you give historic examples of each (p. 240).

36. What kind of radiation exposure would be required to cause early somatic effects? Give examples of early somatic effects (p. 240, 241).

37. What kind of radiation exposure is characteristic of late somatic effects? Give examples of late somatic effects (p. 240, 241).

CHAPTER REVIEW QUESTIONS

1. The type of dose–response curve used to predict stochastic effects is the
   - (A) Nonlinear nonthreshold
   - (B) Nonlinear threshold
   - (C) Linear nonthreshold
   - (D) Linear threshold

2. A dose of 0.25 Gy or 25 rad to the fetus during the third or fourth week of pregnancy is more likely to cause which of the following:
   - (A) Spontaneous abortion
   - (B) Skeletal anomalies
   - (C) Neurologic anomalies
   - (D) Organogenesis

3. Linear energy transfer (LET) is
   1. A method of expressing radiation quality
   2. A measure of the rate at which radiation energy is transferred to soft tissue
   3. Absorption of polyenergetic radiation
   - (A) 1 only
   - (B) 1 and 2 only
   - (C) 1 and 3 only
   - (D) 1, 2, and 3

4. What is the effect on relative biologic effectiveness (RBE) as linear energy transfer (LET) decreases?
   - (A) As LET decreases, RBE increases
   - (B) As LET decreases, RBE decreases
   - (C) As LET decreases, RBE stabilizes
   - (D) LET has no effect on RBE

5. The effects of radiation to biologic material are dependent on several factors. If a quantity of radiation is delivered to a body over a long period of time, the effect
   - (A) will be greater than if it were delivered all at one time
   - (B) will be less than if it were delivered all at one time
   - (C) has no relation to how it is delivered in time
   - (D) is solely dependent on the radiation quality

6. Which of the following account(s) for x-ray beam heterogeneity?
   1. Incident electrons interacting with several layers of tungsten target atoms
   2. Electrons moving to fill different shell vacancies
   3. Its nuclear origin
   - (A) 1 only
   - (B) 1 and 2 only
   - (C) 1 and 3 only
   - (D) 1, 2, and 3

7. What is used to account for the relative radiosensitivity of various tissues and organs:
   1. Tissue weighting factors (W_t)
   2. Radiation weighting factors (W_r)
   3. Absorbed dose
   - (A) 1 only
   - (B) 1 and 2 only
   - (C) 2 and 3 only
   - (D) 1, 2, and 3

8. How are wavelength and energy related?
   - (A) Directly
   - (B) Inversely
   - (C) Chemically
   - (D) Empirically

9. The useful x-ray beam can be accurately described as having what sort of nature?
   - (A) Homogeneous
   - (B) Heterogeneous
   - (C) Homologous
   - (D) Focused

10. Long-term effects of radiation exposure include
    1. Formation of cataracts
    2. Cancer
    3. Genetic effects
    - (A) 1 only
    - (B) 1 and 2 only
    - (C) 2 and 3 only
    - (D) 1, 2, and 3

Answers and Explanations

1. (C) The linear nonthreshold curve is used to illustrate responses such as leukemia, cancer, and genetic effects. These are also referred to as stochastic effects. Stochastic effects occur randomly and are "all-or-nothing" type effects; that is, they do not occur with degrees of severity. Remember that *in a nonthreshold curve there is no safe dose*, that is, no dose below which there will definitely be no biologic response. Theoretically, even one x-ray photon can cause a biologic response. The linear nonthreshold curve is the curve of choice to predict effects of low level (e.g., medical and occupational) exposure to ionizing radiation.

2. (B) During the first trimester, specifically the second to eighth week of pregnancy (during major organogenesis), if the radiation dose is at least 0.2 Gy or 20 rad, fetal anomalies can be produced. *Skeletal anomalies* usually appear if irradiation occurs in the early part of this time period, and *neurologic anomalies* are formed in the latter part; mental retardation and childhood malignant diseases, such as cancers or leukemia, can also result from irradiation during the first trimester. Fetal irradiation during the second and third trimesters is not likely to produce anomalies, but rather, with sufficient dose, some type of childhood malignant disease. Fetal irradiation during the first 2 weeks of gestation can result in *spontaneous abortion.*

It must be emphasized, however, that the likelihood of producing fetal anomalies at doses less than 5–15 rad (0.05–0.15 Gy) is exceedingly small and that most general diagnostic examinations are likely to deliver fetal doses of less than 1–2 rad.

3. (B) When biologic material is irradiated, there are a number of modifying factors that determine what kind and how much response will occur in the biologic material. One of these factors is LET, which expresses the rate at which particulate or photon energy is transferred to the absorber. Because different kinds of radiation have different degrees of penetration in different materials, it is also a useful way of expressing the quality of the radiation.

4. (B) LET expresses the rate at which photon or particulate energy is transferred to (absorbed by) biologic material (through ionization processes) and is dependent on radiation type and tissue absorption characteristics. RBE describes the degree of response or amount of biologic change we can expect of the irradiated material, and is *directly related to LET*. As the amount of transferred energy (LET) *increases* (from interactions occurring between radiation and biologic material), the amount of biologic effect or damage (RBE) will also *increase*; as the amount of LET *decreases,* the RBE will also *decrease.*

5. (B) The effects of a quantity of radiation delivered to a body is dependent on a few factors, including the amount of radiation received, the size of the irradiated area, and how the radiation is delivered in time. If the radiation is delivered in portions over a period of time, it is said to be fractionated and has a less harmful effect than if the radiation was delivered all at once. Cells have an opportunity to repair and some recovery occurs between doses.

6. (B) The x-ray photons produced at the tungsten target comprise a heterogeneous beam, that is, a spectrum of photon energies. This is accounted for by the fact that the incident electrons have different energies. Also, the incident electrons travel through several layers of tungsten target material, lose energy with each interaction, and therefore produce increasingly weaker x-ray photons. During characteristic x-ray production, vacancies may be filled in the K, L, or M shells, differing with each other in binding energies, and therefore, a variety of energy photons are emitted.

7. (A) The *tissue weighting factor* (W_t) represents the relative tissue radiosensitivity of irradiated material (e.g., muscle vs. intestinal epithelium vs. bone, etc.). The radiation weighting factor (W_r) is a number assigned to different types of ionizing radiations to better determine their effect on tissue (e.g., x-ray vs. alpha particles). The W_r of different ionizing radiations is dependent on the LET of that particular radiation. The following formula is used to determine *effective dose (EfD)*.

Effective dose (*EfD*) = Radiation weighting factor (W_r)
$\times$ Tissue weighting factor (W_t)
$\times$ Absorbed dose (D)

8. (B) Frequency and wavelength are closely associated with the relative energy of electromagnetic radiations. *More energetic radiations have shorter* *wavelengths and higher frequency*; thus, they are inversely related. The relationship between frequency, wavelength, and energy is illustrated in the electromagnetic spectrum (Fig. 7–1). Some radiations are energetic enough to rearrange atoms in materials through which they pass, and can therefore be hazardous to living tissue.

9. **(B)** Electrons may undergo any one of a few types of interactions as they encounter the target. The emitted photons can therefore have a variety of energies and thus are termed heterogeneous or polyenergetic. It is only at extremely high energies that photon energy becomes more homogeneous; only gamma radiation can be accurately termed homogeneous or monoenergetic.

10. **(D)** Occupationally exposed individuals are concerned principally with *late* (i.e., *long-term* or *delayed*) effects of radiation, such as *genetic effects*, *leukemia*, *cancers*, and *cataractogenesis*, which can occur many years following initial exposure to low levels of ionizing radiation. These long-term, or delayed, effects are represented by the linear, non-threshold, dose–response curve, with the exception of cataractogenesis, which is represented by the linear, threshold, dose–response curve. An acute dose of approximately 200 rad would be required to cause radiogenic cataracts. A far greater occupational (i.e., fractionated) dose of approximately 1,000 rad would be required to induce cataracts.

Patient Protection | 8

Medical imaging has demonstrated itself to be an invaluable diagnostic tool and its use has grown dramatically in recent years. However, the benefits of imaging technology must be carefully balanced with the risks associated with ionizing radiation exposure. We must remember that the risks are *invisible, long term,* and *cumulative. Ionizing radiation dose is directly and linearly related to risk.*

Statistics indicate that the number of radiologic imaging examinations performed annually is steadily increasing. Many individuals receiving ionizing radiation doses, multiplied by extensive testing (approximately 60 million computed tomographies performed annually in the United States) involves a significant population risk. The ascribed cancer risk will rise correspondingly—at least 5% of cancers could result from diagnostic radiation.

The risk model of Biological Effects of Ionizing Radiation (BEIR) Committee VII for exposure to low-level radiation predicts that approximately 1 in 100 people are likely to develop solid cancer or leukemia from an exposure of 100 mSv above background dose.

All radiologic imaging professionals have the ethical responsibility to keep radiation exposure to patients (and themselves) to an absolute minimum. One exceedingly important consideration in reducing patient exposure is *good patient communication.* Explaining the examination and answering the patient's questions will better ensure understanding and cooperation and reduce the chance for retakes. *Quality Assurance programs* are in place to ensure that retakes will not be required as a result of equipment malfunction. Employees receive orientation on new equipment to ensure that it is used to best advantage and to reduce retakes as a result of unfamiliarity with equipment operation.

The concern about the risk of possible long-term effects of x-ray exposure obliges us to practice the *ALARA* (As Low As Reasonably Achievable) principle. This chapter reviews means of achieving this goal.

Effective Dose per Exam

- *Conventional and Fluoroscopy:*
Chest	0.1 mSv
C spine	0.2 mSv
L spine	1.5 mSv
Pelvis	3.0 mSv
UGI	6.0 mSv
BE	8.0 mSv

- *Interventional:*
ERCP	4.0 mSv
Vertebroplasty	16 mSv

- *CT:*
Head	2 mSv
Chest	7 mSv
Abd/pelvis	10 mSv
Heart angio	20 mSv

(from NCRP #160, 2009)

Beam Restriction

- Reduces patient dose
- Reduces production of scattered radiation
- Improves image quality

Beam Restrictor Types

- Aperture diaphragm
- Cone/cylinder
- Collimator

BEAM RESTRICTION

Purpose

Beam restriction, that is, limitation of irradiated field size, is probably the single most important factor in keeping patient dose to a minimum. The primary beam must be confined to the area of interest, so that only tissues of diagnostic interest should be irradiated.

Another benefit of beam restriction is that, because a smaller quantity of tissue is irradiated, less scattered radiation will be produced. Remember, scattered radiation does not carry useful information; it degrades the radiographic image by adding a layer of fog that impairs detail visibility.

There are three basic types of *beam restrictors*: aperture diaphragms, cones, and collimators.

Types

Aperture Diaphragms. The *aperture diaphragm* is the most elementary of the three types and is occasionally used in dedicated chest units, dental x-ray units, and trauma imaging equipment. It is simply a flat piece of lead (Pb) having a central opening with a size and shape that determines the size and shape of the x-ray beam. Regardless of the type, the aperture diaphragm should demonstrate adequate beam restriction by providing an unexposed border around the edge of the x-ray image.

Cones and Cylinders. *Cones* are circular, lead-lined devices that slide into place on the collimator housing. They may be the straight *cylinder* type, with proximal and distal diameters that are identical, or the infrequently used *flare type*, with a distal diameter that is greater than its proximal diameter. Cylinder cones are frequently able to extend, like a telescope, by means of a simple thumbscrew adjustment (Fig. 8–1). Although their use is limited, cylinder cones are most efficient because they provide beam restriction *closer to* the anatomic part being imaged.

A disadvantage of both the aperture and cone is their fixed opening size, which will provide only one field size at a given distance. To change the size of the irradiated field, the radiographer must change to a different size aperture or cone. In addition, the cylinder cone can be used only for relatively small field sizes, such as the paranasal sinuses, L5–S1, or other small areas of interest.

Collimators. The *collimator* is, overall, the most efficient beam-restricting device. The collimator box is attached to the tube head, and its upper aperture, the first set of shutters, is placed as close as possible to the x-ray tube port window (Fig. 8–2). This is done to control the amount of image degrading "off-focus" (or "stem") radiation leaving the x-ray tube (i.e., radiation produced when electrons strike surfaces other than the focal track). The next set/stage of *lead shutters* ("blades" or "leaves") actually consists of two pairs of adjustable shutters—one pair for field length and another pair for field width. It is these shutters that are used to regulate the length and width of the irradiated field.

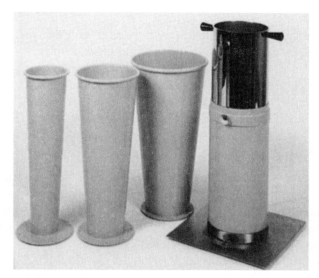

Figure 8–1. Cylinder cones (especially the extendible type) are generally considered more efficient than aperture diaphragms because they restrict the size and shape of the x-ray beam for a greater distance. The closer the distal end of the beam restrictor is to the area of interest, the greater its efficiency. (Courtesy of Burkhart Roentgen, Inc.)

Light-Localization Apparatus

Another important part of the collimator assembly is the *light-localization apparatus.* It consists of a small light bulb (to illuminate the field) and a 45-degree angle mirror to deflect the light. For the light field and x-ray field to correspond accurately, *the x-ray tube focal spot and the light*

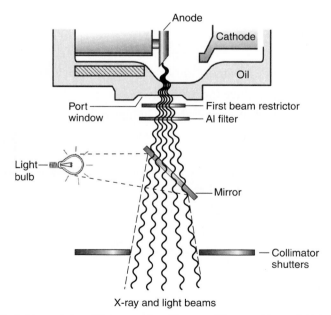

Figure 8–2. X-ray tube, filters, and collimator. The position of the collimator shutters can be seen. Note the position of the first beam restrictor, located at the x-ray tube port window. The oil coolant surrounding the x-ray tube contributes to inherent filtration. Added filtration includes the aluminum filter, the mirror, and collimator.

bulb must be exactly the same distance from the center of the mirror (Fig. 8–2). If the light and x-ray fields are not congruent, the image receptor can be misaligned enough to require repeat examination.

Collimator accuracy should be regularly checked as part of the quality assurance program. National Council on Radiation Protection and Measurements (NCRP) guidelines state that collimators must be accurate to within 2% of the source-to-image-receptor distance (SID).

Accuracy

Cylinder cones are sometimes attached to the tube housing and used in conjunction with collimators. It is important to collimate to the approximate cone diameter size; wide-open collimator shutters can lead to excessive scattered radiation production and can degrade the resulting radiographic image.

As a backup to the illuminated light field, should the light bulb burn out, there is a calibrated scale on the front of the collimator that indicates the x-ray field size at various SIDs.

An important safety feature of collimators (radiographic and fluoroscopic) is *positive beam limitation (PBL)*. Sensors located in the Bucky tray or other IR holder signal the collimator to open or close according to the Image Receptor (IR) size being used in the Bucky tray. A properly calibrated PBL system will provide a small unexposed border on all sides of the finished image and is required by NCRP guidelines to be accurate to within 3% of the SID for a single side, and within 4% of the SID total for all sides (e.g., if PBL inaccurate by 2.75% in one direction, it is acceptable as long as inaccurate less than 1.25% in other directions). The NCRP guideline for *manual* collimation is to be within 2% of the SID. The FDA regulation requiring PBL for all x-ray equipment was removed in 1994, therefore many new x-ray units no longer have the PBL feature.

Summary

- Beam restriction is the most important way to reduce patient dose.
- Beam restrictors reduce the production of scattered radiation.
- Beam restriction improves visibility of image details.
- Types of beam restrictors include aperture diaphragms, cones and cylinders, and collimators.
- A properly calibrated PBL device will provide an unexposed border on all sides of the finished radiograph.
- For the light and x-ray field to correspond accurately, the focal spot and light bulb must be exactly the same distance from the mirror.

EXPOSURE FACTORS

mAs and kV

Selection of exposure factors has a significant impact on patient dose. Remember that the unit milliampere-seconds (mAs) is used to control the *quantity* of ionizing radiation delivered to the patient, and *kV*

Factor	Function
mAs	controls quantity—no effect on quality
kV	controls quality, affects quantity

(kilovoltage) determines the *penetrability* of the x-ray beam. As kilo-voltage is increased, more high-energy photons are produced and the overall average energy of the beam is increased. An increase in mAs increases the *number* of photons produced at the target, but mAs is unrelated to photon energy.

Generally speaking then, in an effort to keep radiation dose to a minimum, it makes sense to use the lowest mAs and the highest kV that will produce the desired radiographic results. An added benefit is that at high-kV and low-mAs values, the heat delivered to the x-ray tube is lower and tube life is extended.

Generator Type

Three-phase or high-frequency generators predominate in stationary radiologic equipment today. They produce a nearly constant potential waveform, thereby offering the advantage of somewhat *reduced patient dose*. If voltage never drops to zero, more high-energy photons are produced—that have less likelihood of being absorbed by the patient. High-frequency generators are often smaller, more efficient, and less costly than the older high-voltage generators.

FILTRATION

X-ray photons emanating from the target/focal spot comprise a *polyenergetic* primary beam. There are many low-energy (or "soft") x rays that, if not removed, would contribute significantly to patient *skin dose*. These low-energy photons are diagnostically useless; they are too weak to penetrate the patient and expose the image receptor; they simply penetrate a small thickness of tissue before being absorbed. Filters, usually made of aluminum, are used in radiography to reduce patient dose by removing these low-energy photons (i.e., *decreased* beam *intensity*), and resulting in an x-ray beam of *higher average energy*. *Total filtration* is composed of *inherent filtration* plus *added filtration*.

Inherent Filtration

Inherent filtration is that in which a filtration is "built-in" and it is composed of materials that are a permanent part of the x-ray tube and its tube housing. Once x rays are produced at/within the tungsten target, many low-energy photons are absorbed by the anode surface itself. Other low-energy photons are removed by the *window* of the *glass envelope* (~0.5 mm Al equivalent) of the x-ray tube. Still other low-energy photons will be removed by the thin layer of oil coolant/insulation surrounding the x-ray tube. The glass envelope window in *mammographic* x-ray tubes is often made of *beryllium*, that is, a substance having a low-atomic number ($Z\# = 4$) and that has an inherent filtration of approximately 0.1 mm Al equivalent.

Inherent filtration tends to increase as the x-ray tube ages. With use, tungsten evaporates and is deposited on the inner surface of the glass envelope, effectively acting as additional filtration and decreasing x-ray output.

Filtration Summary

<50 kV = 0.5 mm Al equivalent
50–70 kV = 1.5 mm Al equivalent
>70 kV = 2.5 mm Al equivalent

Added Filtration

Added filtration refers to the *thin sheets of aluminum* that are added (Fig. 8–2) to make the necessary total thickness of aluminum equivalent filtration. For equipment operated above 70 kV, the total filtration requirement is 2.5 mm Al equivalent. Included in added filtration are the *collimator* and its *mirror* (~1.0 mm Al equivalent).

The effect of total aluminum filtration is to remove the low-energy photons, thereby *decreasing patient skin dose*, and resulting in an x-ray beam having *higher average energy* and greater penetrability.

NCRP Guidelines

NCRP guidelines state that equipment operating above 70 kV must have a minimum *total* (inherent plus added) filtration of *2.5 mm Al equivalent.* Equipment operating between 50 and 70 kV must have at least 1.5 mm Al equivalent filtration. X-ray tubes operating below 50 kV must have at least 0.5 mm Al equivalent filtration. Mammography equipment with a molybdenum target will have 0.025–0.03-mm molybdenum filtration. For magnification studies, a fractional tungsten target tube, having at least 0.5 mm Al equivalent total filtration, may be used.

Summary

- Low mAs and high kV factors help keep patient dose to a minimum.
- Proper calibration of equipment is essential for predictable results.
- Proper selection of technical factors and an effective quality assurance (QA) system help reduce radiation exposure.
- Filtration removes low-energy x-rays from primary beam, thereby
  - reducing patient skin dose and
  - increasing the average energy of the beam.
- Filtration is usually expressed in mm of Al equivalent.
- Inherent + added filtration = total filtration.
- Inherent filtration includes the glass envelope, oil coolant/insulation.
- Added filtration consists of thin layers of Al, and includes the collimator and its mirror.
- Equipment operated above 70 kV must have at least 2.5 mm Al equivalent.
- Inherent filtration increases with tube age, thereby decreasing tube output.

SHIELDING

Rationale for Use

Protective shielding is used to reduce unnecessary radiation exposure to especially radiosensitive organs (i.e., gonads, blood-forming organs) and should be provided to patients whenever possible during radiographic and fluoroscopic examinations (Fig. 8–3).

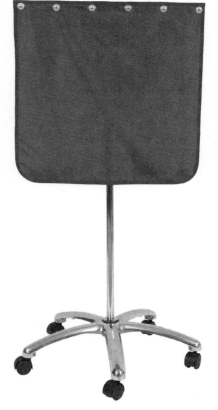

Figure 8–3. Portable lead shielding is useful for patient protection during diagnostic procedures. It can be moved easily and features adjustable height. (Courtesy of Shielding International.)

There are three indications for the effective use of gonadal shields. If the gonads lie in or within 5 cm of a well-collimated field, shielding should be used. A patient with reasonable reproductive potential should be shielded; a generally accepted procedure is to include all women under the ages of 55 years and men under the age of 65 years. Gonadal shielding should be used if diagnostic objectives permit, that is, as long as the shield does not obscure important diagnostic information. Protective shields must be carefully placed; superimposition on diagnostically important anatomic structures can cause retakes and exposure to unnecessary radiation. Accurate positioning and beam restriction must always accompany gonadal shielding. When positioning body parts such as the extremities or the breast, the radiographer must be certain that the unshielded gonads do not intercept any of the primary/useful x-ray beam.

Gonadal shielding is far more effective in the male patient because the reproductive organs lie outside the body. Male patients are therefore more easily shielded, and shielding is much less likely to interfere with the diagnostic objectives of the examination. Female reproductive organs are located within the abdominal cavity, where shielding becomes a much less feasible option.

The use of protective shielding during *mobile radiography* should not be neglected.

Gonadal Shielding Should Be Used if
• the gonads lie in, or within 5 cm of, the collimated field;
• the patient has reasonable reproductive potential;
• diagnostic objectives permit.

Types and Placement of Shields

There are three types of gonadal shields available: flat, contact shields; shadow shields; and contour (shaped) contact shields.

Flat, Contact. The simplest types are flat, *contact shields*, such as pieces of lead-impregnated vinyl that are placed over the patient's gonads. Because they are difficult to secure in place, flat contact shields are useful primarily for anteroposterior (AP) or posteroanterior (PA) recumbent projections. Some flat contact shields now are equipped with straps for easy adjustment and a comfortable fit; without this feature flat contact shields cannot be secured adequately for oblique, lateral decubitus, erect, or fluoroscopic procedures.

Shadow. *Shadow shields* attach to the x-ray tube head. They consist of a piece of leaded material attached to an arm extending from the tube head (Fig. 8–4). The leaded material casts a shadow within the illuminated field that corresponds to the shielded area. Although shadow shields are initially more expensive, they are likely to be a one-time expense. Shadow shields can be used for more projections than flat contact shields and may also be used without contaminating a sterile field. They cannot be used for fluoroscopic procedures.

Contour (Shaped) Contact Shields. *Contour* (shaped) *contact shields* are very effective gonadal shields. They are shaped to enclose the male reproductive organs and held in place by disposable briefs (Fig. 8–5). They are effective for a variety of projections, including oblique, erect, and fluoroscopic procedures.

Breast Shields. *Breast shields* should be used for female patients during scoliosis series. Scoliosis series are typically performed at ages when developing breast tissue is particularly radiosensitive. Breast shields are

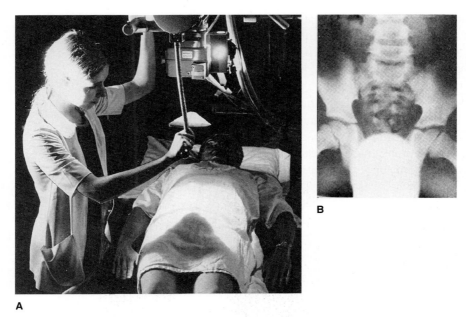

A

B

Figure 8–4. (**A**) A shadow shield is attached to the collimator housing. It has a movable arm that allows a shield of the desired size and shape to be placed in the radiation field over the gonadal area. It is manually operated and swings away when not in use. (Courtesy of Nuclear Associates.) (**B**) Correct placement of shadow shield. (Courtesy of C.B. Radiology Design, Jamestown, New York.)

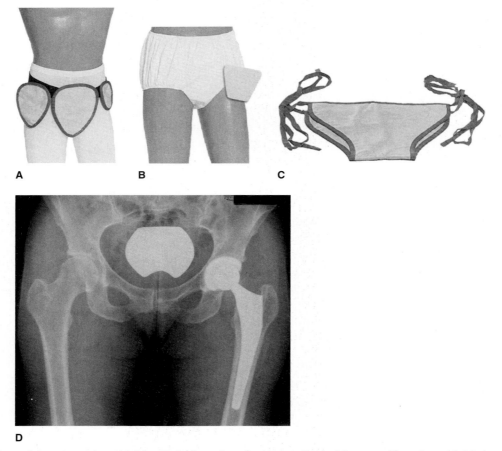

A

B

C

D

Figure 8–5. (**A**) Gonadal and ovarian shield with belt system features attachable gonad/ovarian shields in assorted sizes. (**B**) Male gonadal shield Insert, made of flexible vinyl coated lead, fits securely into front pouch of disposable brief. (**C**) Infant/child/adult diaper shields are available and provide front and back gonad region protection. (Courtesy of Shielding International.) (**D**) Excellent shielding of an AP female pelvis for hips. (Courtesy of Department of Radiology & Imaging, Hospital for Special Surgery, New York, NY.)

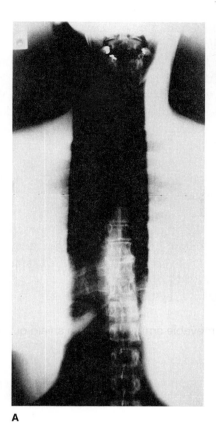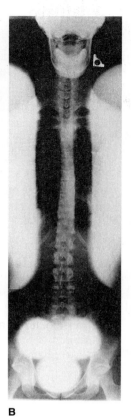

A   **B**

Figure 8–6. Spinal column studies are often required for evaluation of adolescent scoliosis, thus presenting a twofold problem: radiation exposure to youthful gonadal and breast tissues and significantly differing tissue densities and thicknesses. Both problems can be resolved with the use of a compensating filter (for uniform density) that incorporates lead shielding for the breasts and gonads. **(A)** Performed without the filter/shield. **(B)** Performed with the filter/shield. Note the improved visualization of the entire vertebral column and appropriate protection of the breasts and gonads. (Courtesy of Nuclear Associates.)

available incorporated in vertebral column compensating filters (Fig. 8–6), and as leaded vinyl vests ("spinal stoles"; Fig. 8–7) that can be used in upright or recumbent projections. In addition, when performed *PA*, radiation dose to the breast can be reduced to *0.1%* of that received in the AP projection; magnification considerations are minimal.

Some companies have environmentally friendly recycle/renew programs. They will recycle frontal or full protection aprons into smaller/half aprons, thyroid shields, gonad shields, and so on, for up to half the price of a new shield. Some companies will safely dispose of old lead aprons for a small fee.

In addition, there are some new types of "lead" shields that are completely lead-free, very light-weight, provide 0.5 mm lead equivalency, and are environmentally friendly.

Patient Position

Because the primary x-ray beam has a *polyenergetic* (heterogeneous) nature, the entrance dose or skin dose is significantly greater than the exit dose. This principle may be employed in radiation protection by placing particularly radiosensitive organs away from the entrance of primary beam.

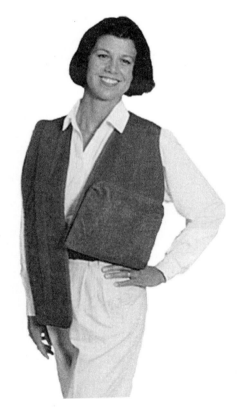

Figure 8–7. Breast shields are available as leaded vinyl vests, "spinal stoles," which can be used in upright or recumbent positions. (Courtesy of Shielding International.)

To place the gonads further from the primary beam and reduce gonadal dose, abdominal radiography should be performed in the PA projection whenever possible. Dose to the lens is significantly decreased when skull radiographs are performed in the PA projection.

The same principle applies when performing scoliosis series on young children in an effort to reduce gonadal dose and to decrease dose to breast tissue in young girls. Dose to breast tissue during scoliosis survey can also be reduced with the use of breast shields (see Figs. 8–6 and 8–7). The PA projection does not generally cause a significant adverse effect on recorded detail and is advocated to decrease dose to the reproductive organs and other radiosensitive areas.

Lead aprons can also be placed over chest/abdomen during radiography of various body parts to protect radiosensitive organs from unnecessary exposure to scattered radiation. Half aprons, or portable mobile shielding, can be used to protect the gonads from scattered radiation in chest radiography. Lead aprons/shielding can be placed *under* the patient during fluoroscopic procedures if they do not interfere with the objectives of the examination.

Summary

- Especially radiosensitive organs include the gonads, and blood-forming organs.
- Gonadal shielding should be used
  - if the gonads lie in or within 5 cm of *collimated* beam,
  - if the patient has reproductive potential, and
  - if diagnostic objectives permit.
- Three types of gonadal shields are
  - flat contact,
  - shadow, and
  - contour contact.
- Male gonads are more easily and effectively shielded.
- Breast shields should be used as needed.
- To reduce exposure to reproductive organs and/or breasts, it is helpful to perform abdominal radiography and scoliosis series in the PA projection whenever possible.

REDUCING PATIENT EXPOSURE

Patient Communication

Gaining the patient's confidence and trust through effective communication is an essential part of the radiographic examination. Some patients will require a greater use of the radiographer's communication skills—patients who are seriously ill or injured; traumatized patients; patients who have impaired vision, hearing, or speech; pediatric patients; non–English-speaking patients; the elderly and infirm; the physically or mentally impaired; alcohol and drug abusers—the radiographer must adapt his or her communication skills to meet the needs of many types of individuals and their condition/affliction. It is imperative that the radiographer take adequate time to thoroughly explain the procedure or examination to the patient.

The radiographer requires the cooperation of the patient throughout the course of the examination. A thorough explanation will alleviate the patient's anxieties and permit fuller cooperation. Better understanding and cooperation will yield a good radiographic image and reduce the likelihood of repeat exposures. *Repeat exposures contribute to a significant increase in unnecessary patient exposure.*

Positioning of Patient

Another means of reducing patient exposure is by careful and accurate positioning. As already mentioned, retake exposures/examinations contribute to a significant increase in unnecessary patient exposure, as well as increased facility expense.

Exact positioning and centering is particularly critical when using automatic exposure control (AEC). The anatomic part of interest must be positioned (centered) accurately with respect to the AEC's sensors; otherwise, the resulting image can be over- or underexposed.

Automatic Exposure Control

An *AEC* is used to automatically regulate the amount of ionizing radiation delivered to the patient and image recorder, thereby serving to produce consistent and comparable radiographic results time after time. When AEC is installed in the x-ray circuit, it is calibrated to produce radiographic densities as required by the radiologist. AECs have sensors that signal to terminate the exposure once a predetermined, known-correct exposure has been reached. When using film/screen systems, it is essential to use the correct speed screen and film combination with the AEC—the screen and film combination that it has been programmed for. The AEC cannot compensate for a speed system that it does not "know" about. For example, if the system has been programmed for a 400 system and 200 speed intensifying screens are used, the image will exhibit half the expected density.

Whether using traditional or computerized/digital imaging equipment, *exact positioning and centering* is particularly critical when using equipment with AECs. The anatomic part of interest must be positioned (centered) accurately with respect to the AEC's sensors; otherwise, the resulting image can demonstrate insufficient or excessive densities.

There are two types of AECs: *ionization chambers* and *phototimers*.

Ionization Chamber. A parallel plate *ionization chamber* consists of a radiolucent chamber just beneath the tabletop above the IR and grid (Fig. 8–8). As x-ray photons emerge from the patient, they enter the chamber and ionize the air within. When a predetermined quantity of ionization has occurred (as determined by the selected exposure factors), the exposure automatically terminates.

Phototimer. In the *phototimer*, a small fluorescent screen is positioned beneath the IR (Fig. 8–8). When remnant radiation emerging from the patient exits the IR, the fluorescent screen emits light. The fluorescent light charges a photomultiplier tube and, once a predetermined charge has been reached, the exposure is terminated.

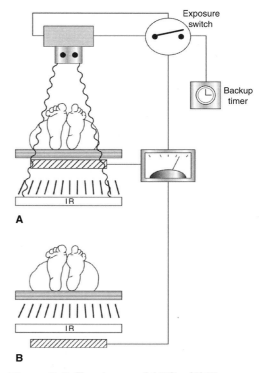

Figure 8–8. Two types of AECs. **(A)** The ionization chamber is positioned between the tabletop and IR. **(B)** The phototimer is located below the IR. Note that a backup timer, which serves to terminate the exposure in the event of AEC failure, is used in conjunction with both AECs.

Backup Timer. In either case, the manual timer should be used as *backup timer*. This ensures that, in case of AEC malfunction, the exposure will terminate and *avoid patient overexposure and tube overload.*

Minimum Response Time. Another important feature of the AEC to be familiar with is its *minimum response/reaction time*. This is the length of the *shortest exposure possible* with a particular AEC. If less than the minimum response time is required for a particular exposure, the radiograph will exhibit excessive density. Decreasing the mA (preferable) or decreasing the kV will result in requiring an increase in exposure time—bringing the minimum response time within the established range of the AEC.

Summary

- Effective communication can increase patient cooperation and decrease repeats.
- Repeat exposures result in an increase in patient dose.
- When used properly, AECs ensure consistency of radiographic density.
- There are two types of AECs: ionization chamber type and phototimer type.
- The ionization chamber type is located between the patient and IR.
- The phototimer type is located beneath the IR.
- Every AEC has a minimum response time.
- AECs require accurate positioning and centering to produce predictable results.
- The manual timer must be used as backup timer to avoid patient overexposure and tube overload.

IMAGE RECEPTORS

When a film/screen system is used, higher speed (faster) systems require a smaller dose of radiation to produce a diagnostic radiograph. As one component of the effort to reduce population dose, rare earth phosphors are used almost exclusively in general film/screen radiography. Rare earth phosphors are at least four times faster than the earlier calcium tungstate phosphors, and the recorded detail they provide is entirely satisfactory. In general, the fastest film/screen combination consistent with diagnostic requirements should be used.

An advantage of *digital fluoroscopy* (DF) and digital static imaging is reduced patient dose. The lower DF dose is because DF x-ray beams are *pulsed*, rather than continuous. The static DF images are also lower dose because the TV camera tube or the CCD (charge-coupled device) has greater sensitivity than the spot film emulsion.

GRIDS AND AIR-GAP TECHNIQUE

Grids, both stationary and moving, function to *remove a large percentage of scattered* (primarily Compton) radiation from the remnant beam before it reaches the image receptor, thereby *improving radiographic contrast*.

Because scattered radiation often makes a significant contribution to the overall radiographic density, the addition of a grid (or increase in the grid ratio) must be accompanied by an appropriate *increase in exposure factors* (usually mAs) to maintain adequate density. The improvement in image quality is usually more significant than the *increased exposure to the patient* (Fig. 8–9).

However, the use of high-ratio grids at low kV levels is discouraged because of the unnecessary patient exposure required. Higher ratio grids are more effective in reducing the amount of scattered radiation reaching the IR; however, their use requires more mAs (more patient dose, more heat buildup) and decreases positioning latitude (of the x-ray tube). Lower ratio grids (5:1, 6:1) are often used in mobile imaging because they often more (grid) positioning latitude.

An 8:1 grid is satisfactory for radiography up to 90 kV. A 16:1 grid ratio is frequently recommended for exams using more than 100 kV. General radiographic fixed equipment generally has a 10:1 or 12:1 grid.

It is interesting to note that, to produce a given density, a moving grid generally requires more exposure than a stationary grid of the same ratio. Because, as the lead strips continually change position as they move back and forth, some of the perpendicular rays will unavoidably be "caught" by the lead strips moving into their path.

An *air-gap* technique can function similar to, or in place of, a low ratio grid. A distance is introduced between the patient/part and the image receptor. Scattered photons emerging from the patient will continue to diverge and never reach the image receptor.

A "natural" air gap exists in the *lateral* projection of the cervical spine and a 72-inch SID can be used *without* a grid (Fig. 8–10). *Transmitted* photons reach the IR, but *scattered* photons diverge and never reach the IR. Because no air gap is introduced in the *AP* projection of the cervical spine, it is usually radiographed at 40-inches SID *with* the use of a grid.

The Object-to-Image Receptor-Distance (OID) required in *magnification radiography* is an air gap and therefore grids are rarely needed when this special imaging technique is performed.

Air-gap technique may also be used in place of a grid in chest radiography. However, to maintain optimum recorded detail and avoid excessive magnification, the SID must be increased considerably (usually a 6-inch OID and a 7-feet SID), compensated for by an appropriate increase in mAs. Air-gap technique is limited to imaging of fairly thin parts, as more thick and dense tissues would require excessive and impractical radiation exposures.

In addition, equipment must be properly calibrated to produce consistently predictable results; specifically, the equipment must have *linearity* and *reproducibility*. When adjacent mA stations are tested, for example 100 and 200 mA, and the exposure time is kept constant, the 200-mA station should produce twice exposure rate of the 100-mA station—this is *linearity*. *Reproducibility* refers to consistency in exposure output during repeated exposures at a particular setting.

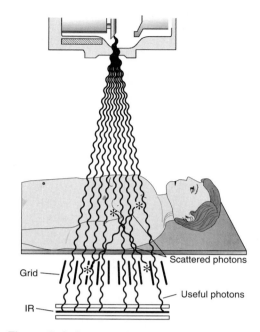

Figure 8–9. Scattered radiation generated within the patient can cause serious degradation of image quality. The improvement in image quality afforded by the use of grids more than makes up for the required increase in patient exposure.

FLUOROSCOPY

Fluoroscopy is potentially a higher patient dose procedure. The principal reason for this is that the source of x-ray photons is so much closer

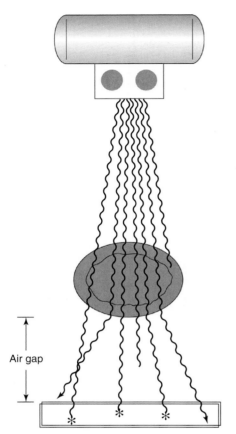

Figure 8–10. When an air gap is used, much of the scattered radiation generated within the patient never reaches the image receptor. An air gap may occasionally be used in place of a grid.

Ways to Decrease Patient Fluoroscopic Dose

- Decrease length of fluoroscopic exposure
- Employ use of last image hold
- Keep patient as close to the Image Intensifier (I.I.) as possible
- Use Automatic Brightness Control (ABC) setting with highest kV/lowest mA combination
- Minimize use of "boost" and "magnification" modes
- Collimation; use smallest Field of View (FOV)
- Use lowest practical pulse rate
- Change tube angle or patient position to spread dose over larger area

to the patient than in overhead radiography. On September 30, 1994, the FDA issued the following advisory: "The FDA has received reports of occasional but at times severe radiation-induced burns to patients resulting from prolonged fluoroscopically-guided, invasive procedures." This is probably due to the increasing number and duration of fluoroscopically guided medical procedures.

There are NCRP recommendations that provide guidelines for minimum source-to-skin distance (SSD), maximum tube output, collimation, timer and exposure switch specifications, etc. Many of these important guidelines are listed in the following section.

An advantage of *digital* fluoroscopy is reduced patient dose. The principal reason for lower patient dose in DF is that DF x-ray beams are *pulsed*, rather than continuous. In addition, the TV camera tube or CCD has greater sensitivity than does film emulsion.

Remember that the entrance dose or skin dose is significantly greater than the exit dose; this holds true in fluoroscopy as well as radiography. This principle may be employed in radiation protection by placing particularly radiosensitive organs away from the primary beam. Moreover, lead aprons or half aprons can be placed *under* particularly radiosensitive areas (when using under table fluoroscopy), as long as those areas are not of clinical significance.

High-kilovoltage exposure factors are preferred to reduce patient dose in fluoroscopy as well as radiography. The length of the fluoroscopic examination must be monitored by a 5-minute cumulative timer.

NCRP RECOMMENDATIONS FOR PATIENT PROTECTION

Note: Many of the means of patient protection serve to protect the operator as well.

- Equipment operating above 70 kV must have a minimum total (inherent plus added) *filtration* of 2.5 mm Al equivalent.
- *Reproducibility:* for a given group of exposure factors, output intensity must be consistent from one exposure to the next; any variation in output intensity must not exceed 5%.
- *Linearity:* output intensity must be constant when adjacent mA stations are used, with exposure times adjusted to maintain the same mAs; any variation in output intensity must not exceed 10%.
- X-ray tube *housing* must keep leakage radiation to less than 100 mR/hr when measured 1 m from the tube.
- A device (*centering light*) must be provided to align the center of the x-ray beam with the center of the image receptor.
- *Beam limiting devices* must be provided; the *collimated* x-ray field must correspond with the visible light field within 2% of the SID in manual collimation and within 4% in PBL.
- The x-ray timer must be accurate. Single-phase equipment can be tested with a simple *spinning-top* test tool. Three-phase equipment is tested with a *synchronous spinning top* or an oscilloscope.
- *SSD* must not be fewer than 12 inches for all radiographic procedures other than dental radiography.

- The SSD must be at least 15 inches in stationary (fixed) fluoroscopic equipment, and at least 12 inches for mobile fluoroscopic equipment.
- The tabletop intensity of the *fluoroscopic* beam must be fewer than 10 R/min.
- A *cumulative timing device* must be available to signal the fluoroscopist (audibly, visibly, or both) when a maximum of 5 minute of fluoroscopy time has elapsed.
- The *SID indicator* must be accurate to within 2% of the indicated SID.
- When more than one x-ray tube can be energized from a single control panel, there must be an obvious indicator on the control panel and on or near each tube housing that indicates which tube is being operated.
- The location of the *focal spot* must be indicated on the outside of the tube housing.
- Film–screen combinations should be the *fastest possible*, consistent with the diagnostic objectives of the examination.
- Radiographic *intensifying screens* should be cleaned and checked regularly, at least every 6 months.
- X-ray *film* must be stored in an adequately protected place.
- Radiographic equipment should undergo regular QA testing.
- The radiographer must be able to see and communicate with the patient at all times.
- The exposure switches must be the "*dead-man*" type.

Summary

- In film/screen imaging, the fastest screen–film combination consistent with diagnostic requirements should be used.
- When used correctly, digital imaging can significantly reduce patient dose.
- Grids improve the radiographic image by reducing the amount of scattered radiation fog, but necessitate an increase in exposure.
- An air gap can have the same effect as a low-ratio grid in decreasing the amount of scattered radiation reaching the image receptor; however, SID must be increased to decrease magnification and preserve recorded detail.
- Fluoroscopy generally delivers a higher patient dose because of decreased SSD.
- There are several important NCRP recommendations governing patient protection with which the radiographer should be familiar.

COMPREHENSION CHECK

Congratulations! You have completed your review of this chapter. If you are able to answer the following group of very comprehensive questions, you should feel confident that you have really mastered this section. You are then ready to go on to "Registry-type" questions that follow.

For greatest success, do not go to the multiple-choice questions without first completing the short-answer questions below.

1. What are some methods of achieving the ALARA goal (p. 249, 250)?

2. What is the most important factor in minimizing patient exposure? Give an example of how it affects patient dose (p. 252, 253).

3. List the three types of beam restrictors; describe the particular use(s) and efficiency of each (p. 250).

4. What effect does beam restriction have on the production of scattered radiation (p. 250)?

5. What degree of accuracy must beam restrictors maintain (both manual and PBL) (p. 252)?

6. How is "off focus" radiation minimized (p. 250)?

7. Describe the relationship between the focal spot and collimator light bulb with respect to IR alignment (p. 251, 252).

8. Explain the importance of an AEC's backup timer (p. 259, 260).

9. What is meant by the minimum response time of an AEC (p. 260)?

10. Why is positioning and centering so critical when using AECs (p. 259)?

11. What combination of exposure factors should be used, in general, to keep patient dose to a minimum (p. 252, 253)?

12. How does filtration affect patient dose (p. 254)?

13. Describe the two types of filtration that comprise total filtration (p. 253, 254)

14. What are the NCRP filtration requirements (p. 254)?

15. How and why does inherent filtration change as the x-ray tube ages; how does it affect tube output (p. 253)?

16. List the three criteria for determining when gonadal shielding should be used (p. 255).

17. Describe the three types of gonadal shielding and indicate the effectiveness of each (p. 255).

18. When might a breast or lens shield be used (p. 255-257).

19. Explain the value of performing scoliosis series, abdominal, and skull radiography in the PA projection (p. 255-258).

20. How do film–screen combinations impact patient dose (p. 259, 260)?

21. The NCRP makes several recommendations that can impact patient dose. Briefly describe the recommendations for each of the following (p. 262, 263).

    A. Patient visibility during examination

    B. QA testing

    C. Speed and care of intensifying screens

    D. External indication of focal spot

    E. Energizing multiple x-ray tubes from one control panel

    F. Minimum SSD in fluoroscopy units

    G. X-ray timer testing and accuracy

    H. Beam limitation accuracy (manual and PBL) required

    I. Beam alignment

    J. Leakage radiation

    K. Quantity of filtration

    L. Linearity and reproducibility

CHAPTER REVIEW QUESTIONS

1. Which of the following is (are) a feature(s) of x-ray equipment, designed especially to eliminate unnecessary radiation to the patient?
   1. Filtration
   2. Minimum SSD of 12 inches
   3. Collimator accuracy
   (A) 1 only
   (B) 1 and 2 only
   (C) 1 and 3 only
   (D) 1, 2, and 3

2. The quality assurance term used to describe consistency in exposure at adjacent mA stations is:
   (A) Automatic exposure control
   (B) Positive beam limitation
   (C) Linearity
   (D) Reproducibility

3. How does filtration affect the primary beam?
   (A) Filtration increases the average energy of the primary beam
   (B) Filtration decreases the average energy of the primary beam
   (C) Filtration results in an increased patient dose
   (D) Filtration increases the intensity of the primary beam

4. Patient dose is affected by:
   1. Inherent filtration
   2. Added filtration
   3. Source–image distance
   (A) 1 only
   (B) 1 and 2 only
   (C) 1 and 3 only
   (D) 1, 2, and 3

5. Which of the following groups of exposure factors will deliver the *greatest* amount of exposure to the patient?
   (A) 20 mAs, 100 kV
   (B) 40 mAs, 90 kV
   (C) 80 mAs, 80 kV
   (D) 160 mAs, 70 kV

6. The principal function of x-ray beam filtration is to:
   (A) Reduce operator dose
   (B) Reduce patient skin dose
   (C) Reduce image noise
   (D) Reduce scattered radiation

7. Patient dose can be *decreased* by using:
   1. High-speed film and screen combination
   2. High-ratio grids
   3. Air-gap technique
   (A) 1 only
   (B) 1 and 2 only
   (C) 1 and 3 only
   (D) 1, 2, and 3

8. Which of the following are included in the types of gonadal shielding?
   1. Flat contact
   2. Shaped (contour) contact
   3. Shadow
   (A) 1 only
   (B) 1 and 2 only
   (C) 2 and 3 only
   (D) 1, 2, and 3

9. The advantages of beam restriction include:
   1. Production of less scattered radiation
   2. Irradiation of less biologic material
   3. Patient shielding will not be required
   (A) 1 only
   (B) 1 and 2 only
   (C) 2 and 3 only
   (D) 1, 2, and 3

10. A backup timer for the automatic exposure control device serves to:
    1. Protect the patient from overexposure
    2. Protect the x-ray tube from excessive heat
    3. Eventually increase inherent filtration
    (A) 1 only
    (B) 1 and 2 only
    (C) 1 and 3 only
    (D) 1, 2, and 3

Answers and Explanations

1. (D) According to NCRP regulations, radiographic, and fluoroscopic equipment must have a total Al *filtration* of at least 2.5 mm Al equivalent whenever the equipment is operated at 70 kV or greater, to reduce excessive exposure to low-energy radiation. *Collimator* and beam alignment must be accurate to within 2% for manual, 4% for PBL. The *SSD* must not be less than 12 *inches* for all procedures other than dental radiography. Distance is the single best protection from radiation. Excessively short SIDs/SSDs cause a significant increase in patient skin dose.

2. (C) Equipment must be properly calibrated to produce consistently predictable results; specifically, the equipment must have *linearity* and *reproducibility*. When adjacent mA stations are tested, for example 100 and 200 mA, and the exposure time is kept constant, the 200-mA station should produce twice exposure rate of the 100-mA station—this is *linearity*. *Reproducibility* refers to consistency in exposure output during repeated exposures at a particular setting.

3. (A) X-rays produced at the target comprise a heterogeneous primary beam. Filtration serves to eliminate the softer, less-penetrating photons leaving an x-ray beam of higher average energy. Filtration is important in patient protection because unfiltered, low-energy photons not energetic enough to reach the image receptor are absorbed by the body and contribute to total patient dose.

4. (D) *Inherent* filtration is composed of materials that are a permanent part of the tube housing; that is, the glass envelope of the x-ray tube and the oil coolant. *Added* filtration, usually thin sheets of aluminum, is present to make a total of 2.5 mm Al equivalent for equipment operated above 70 kV. Filtration is used to decrease patient dose by removing the weak x rays having no value but contributing to skin dose. According to the inverse square law of radiation, exposure dose increases as *distance* from the source decreases, and vice versa.

5. (D) mAs regulates the quantity of radiation delivered to the patient. kV regulates the quality (penetration) of the ionizing radiation delivered to the patient. The higher the mAs, the greater the patient dose. Higher energy (more penetrating) radiation—which is more likely to *exit* the patient—accompanied by a lower mAs is the safest combination for the patient.

6. (B) It is our ethical responsibility to minimize radiation dose to our patients. X rays produced at the target comprise a heterogeneous primary beam. There are many "soft" (low-energy) photons that, if not removed, would contribute to only greater patient dose. They are too weak to penetrate the patient and expose the image receptor; they just penetrate a small thickness of tissue and are absorbed. Filters, usually made of aluminum, are used in *radiography to reduce patient dose by removing this low-energy radiation*, resulting in an x-ray beam of higher average energy. Total filtration is composed of inherent filtration plus added filtration.

7. (A) The *higher the speed* of the film and screen system, the *smaller the dose* of radiation required to produce a diagnostic radiograph. As one component of the effort to reduce population dose, rare earth phosphors are used almost exclusively today in general radiography, as they are at least four times faster than calcium tungstate phosphors.

Grids, both stationary and moving, function to remove a large percentage of scattered (primarily Compton) radiation from the remnant beam before it reaches the image receptor, thereby improving radiographic contrast. Because scattered radiation often makes a significant contribution to the overall radiographic density, the addition of a *grid* (or an increase in the grid ratio) must be accompanied by an appropriate *increase in exposure factors* (usually mAs) to maintain adequate density. The improvement in image quality is usually more significant than the increased exposure to the patient (Figs. 8–9 and 8–10).

Air-gap technique functions similar to, or in place of, a grid. A distance is introduced between the patient and the image receptor. However, to maintain optimum recorded detail and avoid excessive magnification, the SID must be increased considerably, followed by a *significant increase in mAs*.

8. (D) Gonadal shielding should be used whenever appropriate and possible during radiographic and fluoroscopic examinations. *Flat contact* shields (flat sheets of flexible leaded vinyl) are useful for recumbent studies, but when the examination necessitates that oblique, lateral, or erect projections be obtained, they become less efficient. *Shaped contact (contour)* shields are best because they enclose the male reproductive organs, remaining in oblique, lateral, and erect positions—but they can be used only for male patients. *Shadow* shields that attach to the tube head are particularly useful for surgical sterile fields.

9. (B) With greater beam restriction (i.e., smaller field size), less biologic material is irradiated, thereby reducing the possibility of harmful effects. If less tissue is irradiated, less scattered radiation is produced, resulting in improved image contrast. Protective shielding is used to reduce unnecessary radiation exposure to especially radiosensitive organs (i.e., gonads, lens, blood-forming organs) and should be provided to patients *whenever possible* during radiographic and fluoroscopic examinations. Beam restriction and shielding are essential components of patient protection.

10. (B) A parallel plate *ionization chamber* consists of a radiolucent chamber just beneath the tabletop (Fig. 8–8). As x-ray photons emerge from the patient, they enter the chamber and ionize the air within. When a predetermined quantity of ionization has occurred (as determined by the selected exposure factors), the exposure automatically terminates. In the *phototimer*, a small fluorescent screen is positioned beneath the IR (Fig. 8–8). When remnant radiation emerging from the patient exits the IR, the exposure is terminated. The *manual* timer should be used as *backup timer*, in case the AEC fails to terminate the exposure, *thus protecting the patient from overexposure and the x-ray tube from excessive heat load*. The backup timer is unrelated to filtration.

Personnel Protection | 9

GENERAL CONSIDERATIONS

Occupational Exposure

Radiographers must avoid unnecessary radiation exposure to themselves and strive to keep patient dose to an absolute minimum. The sources of radiation exposure to radiographers are the primary beam and secondary radiation (scattered and leakage). *Radiographers must never be exposed to the primary, or useful, x-ray beam.*

The patient is the principal source of scattered radiation; protection guidelines address secondary radiation exposure. The National Council on Radiation Protection and Measurements (NCRP) recommends *personal monitoring* for individuals who may receive 10% of the occupational dose-equivalent limit of 5 rem/y (50 mSv/y).

Time, *distance*, and *shielding* are the cardinal principles of radiation protection; dosimeter *monitoring* evaluates their effectiveness. Minimizing the length of a fluoroscopic procedure employs the principle of *time*. Increasing the distance between the x-ray source and the technologist, as in mobile radiography or in fluoroscopy, employs the principle of *distance*. Wearing a lead apron during fluoroscopy and providing the patient with gonadal shielding are examples of employing the principle of *shielding*. The principles of time, distance, and shielding apply to both patient exposure and occupational exposure.

ALARA Principle

The use of radiation-monitoring devices helps us evaluate the *effectiveness* of radiation protection practices. Anyone who might receive 0.1 of the annual dose (i.e., 0.5 rem) limit must be provided a dosimeter. Reports received, often monthly, from dosimeter laboratories are official legal documents. They are reviewed, and attempts should be made to reduce *any* exposure no matter how small. Radiographers must follow the *ALARA* (*As Low As Reasonably Achievable*) principle as they carry out their tasks. Radiologic facilities undergo regular radiation surveys. New radiologic staff participate in radiation safety orientation, and regular in-service education on radiation safety is conducted annually. Proper radiation monitoring and regular official review of radiation dosimeter reports are essential.

OCCUPATIONAL RADIATION SOURCES

Scattered Radiation

When primary x-ray photons intercept an object and undergo a change in direction, *scattered radiation* results.

The most significant occupational radiation hazard in diagnostic radiology is scattered radiation from the *patient*, particularly in *fluoroscopy*, where use of high kilovoltage results in energetic Compton scatter emerging from the patient. This poses a real occupational hazard to the radiologist and radiographer.

The intensity of scattered radiation 1 m from the patient is approximately 0.1% of the intensity of the primary beam. That is why, in terms of radiation protection, *the patient is considered the most important source* of scattered radiation exposure. Other scattering objects include the *x-ray table*, *Bucky-slot cover/closer*, and *control booth* wall.

Leakage Radiation

Leakage radiation is that which is emitted from the x-ray tube housing in directions *other* than that of the primary beam. NCRP guidelines state that any leakage radiation from lead-lined x-ray tubes must not exceed 100 mR/h when measured at a distance of 1 m from the x-ray tube.

NCRP Guidelines

NCRP guidelines regulate equipment design, among other things, in an effort to reduce exposure to personnel and patients. Among the guidelines that serve to reduce exposure to personnel are as follows:

- The control panel must somehow indicate when the x-ray tube is energized (i.e., "exposure-on" time) by means of an audible or visible signal/sign.
- The x-ray exposure switch must be a "deadman" switch and situated so that it cannot be operated outside the shielded area of the control booth.

Some patients, such as infants and children, are unable to maintain the required radiographic position. Mechanical immobilizing and restraining devices, carefully and intelligently used, serve to prevent motion on the resulting image. Additional help with immobilization, though infrequently required, can be a non pregnant relative or friend (older than age 18 years) or, as last recourse, another hospital employee. The services of radiology personnel must *never* be used to help immobilize patients for x-ray procedures.

NCRP guidelines regarding protection of the *patient* and/or *personnel* during *fluoroscopic* procedures include the following:

- During fluoroscopic procedures, the *image intensifier* serves as a protective barrier from the primary beam and must be the equivalent of 2.0-mm Pb.
- The exposure switch must be the "deadman" type.
- With undertable fluoroscopic tubes, a Bucky-slot cover having at least the equivalent of 0.25-mm Pb must be available to attenuate scattered radiation (which is about at gonadal level).

Rules for Selecting Someone to Assist the Patient in the Radiographic Department

- A male (older than 18 years) is preferred; however, a female who is older than 18 years and not pregnant may also assist.
- The individual must be provided with protective apparel.
- The individual must be as far as possible from the useful beam.
- The individual must not stand in the path of the useful beam.

- A cumulative timing device must be available to signal the fluoro-scopist (audibly, visibly, or both) when a maximum of 5 minutes of fluoroscopy time has elapsed.

- A leaded screen drape and tableside shield, having at least the equiv-alent of 0.25-mm Pb, to reduce scattered radiation to the operator must be available.

- The tabletop intensity of the fluoroscopic beam must be fewer than 10 R/min.

- Protective *lead aprons* must be *at least 0.25-mm Pb* equivalent and must be worn by the workers in the fluoroscopy department.

- Protective *lead gloves* must be at least 0.25-mm Pb equivalent. The un-shielded hand must not be placed in the unattenuated or useful beam.

- When fluoroscopy is performed with an undertable image intensifier (as in "remote" x-ray units), palpation must be performed mechanically.

Summary

- Time, distance, and shielding are the principal guidelines for reduc-ing radiographic exposure; monitoring evaluates their effectiveness.

- Radiology professionals must practice the ALARA principle, that is, keeping exposure to ionizing radiation *as low as reasonably achievable*.

- The principal scattering object is the patient; others include the x-ray table, Bucky-slot cover, and control booth walls.

- It is important to be familiar with pertinent guidelines established by NCRP reports: medical x-ray, electron beam and gamma-ray protec-tion for energies up to 50 MeV (Equipment Design, Performance and Use [1989; NCRP Report No. 102]; Radiation Protection for Medical and Allied Health Personnel [1989; NCRP Report No. 105]; Limita-tion of Exposure to Ionizing Radiation [1993; NCRP No. 116]); and Ionizing Radiation Exposure of the Population of the United States (2009; NCRP No. 160).

- Mechanical restraining devices should be used to immobilize the patient/part when necessary during radiographic examinations.

- Persons occupationally exposed to radiation must never assist (hold) patients during radiographic examinations.

- If someone is required to assist a patient during an examination, it is essential that radiation safety guidelines be adhered to.

- There are several NCRP guidelines regarding protection during fluoroscopic procedures with which the radiographer should be familiar.

FUNDAMENTAL METHODS OF PROTECTION

Cardinal Rules

The practice of effective radiation safety depends chiefly on common sense. That is, to safeguard yourself from something harmful, you gen-erally remove yourself from it as soon as possible, stay as far away from it as possible, and keep a barrier between it and yourself—hence, the cardinal principles of *time*, *distance*, and *shielding*.

Radiation Protection Rules

- Time
- Distance
- Shielding

Primary Barriers

- Protect from the useful beam

Secondary Barriers

- Protect from scattered and leakage radiation

Attenuation Characteristics of Lead Aprons

X-ray attenuation at:

Pb-equivalent thickness	75 kV	100 kV
0.25 mm	66%	51%
0.50 mm	88%	75%
1.0 mm	99%	94%

The greatest amount of occupational exposure is received in *fluoroscopic* procedures and *mobile* radiography. It is here that the radiographer must place special emphasis on the cardinal rules of radiation protection: time, distance, and shielding. Federal government controls also regulate manufacturing standards for the protection of both personnel and patients.

Inverse Square Law

Reducing the length of time exposed to ionizing radiation, as in reducing fluoroscopy time, results in a reduction of occupational exposure. Increasing the distance from the source of radiation results in a reduction of occupational exposure, as illustrated by the *inverse square law*. Placing a barrier, such as a lead wall or lead apron, between you and the source of radiation results in a reduction of occupational exposure. Review the following examples:

- *Time:* If 10 mrem is received in 30 minutes of fluoroscopic procedure, how much will be received if the fluoroscopic time is reduced to 15 minutes? (If the fluoroscopic exposure time is cut in half, from 30 to 15 minutes, the exposure dose received would be correspondingly one-half of the original, or 5 mrem.)
- *Distance:* If 40 mrem (0.4 mSv) is received at a distance of 40 inches from the x-ray source, what dose will be received at a distance of 80 inches from the source? (According to the inverse square law, if the distance from the radiation source is doubled, exposure dose will be one-fourth of the original quantity, or 10 mrem/0.1 mSv.)

To reduce exposure dose to health care professionals, patients, and the general population, we must minimize the *time* of exposure to the source of radiation, provide effective *shielding* from the radiation source, and most importantly, maximize the *distance* from the source of radiation.

PRIMARY AND SECONDARY BARRIERS

NCRP Guidelines

Primary radiation barriers protect against direct exposure from the primary (useful) x-ray beam and have much greater attenuation capability than *secondary barriers*, which protect only from leakage and scattered radiation.

Examples of primary barriers are the lead walls and doors of a radiographic room, that is, any surface that could be struck by the useful beam. Primary protective barriers of typical installations generally consist of walls with 1/16-inch (1.5-mm) lead thickness and 7-feet height.

Secondary radiation is defined as leakage and/or scattered radiation. The x-ray tube housing protects from leakage radiation, as stated previously. The patient is the source of most scattered radiation.

Secondary radiation barriers include the portion of the walls above 7 feet in height; this area requires only 1/32-inch lead. The control booth is also a secondary barrier, toward which the primary beam must never be directed (Fig. 9–1). The radiographer must be protected by the control booth shielding during exposures, and the exposure switch

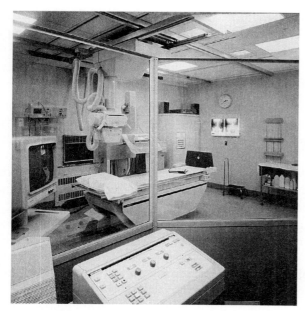

Figure 9–1. The control booth permits the operator to view the patient. The leaded booth and glass protect the operator from exposure to scattered radiation. The control booth is a secondary barrier toward which the primary beam must never be directed. (Courtesy of Nuclear Associates.)

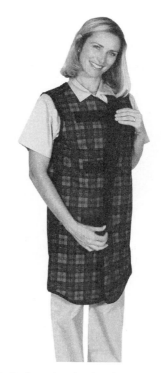

Figure 9–2. A protective lead apron must be worn during fluoroscopic procedures. Various types/styles of lead aprons are available. The figure shows a wraparound-type protective apron. (Courtesy of Shielding International.)

or cord must be positioned and attached so that the exposure can be made only *within* the control booth. Leaded glass, usually 1.5-mm Pb equivalent, should be available for patient observation.

Protective Apparel and Its Care

During fluoroscopic procedures requiring the radiographer's presence in the radiographic department, the radiographer must wear protective apparel, to include a lead apron (Fig. 9–2). Lead aprons are secondary radiation barriers and *must* contain *at least* 0.25 (¼)-mm Pb equivalent (according to 10 CFR Part 20), usually in the form of lead-impregnated vinyl. Many radiology departments routinely use lead aprons containing 0.5-mm Pb. (The NCRP recommends 0.5-mm Pb equivalent minimum.) These aprons are heavier, but they attenuate a higher percentage of scattered radiation (see Attenuation Characteristics table).

Other useful protective apparel includes sterile attenuating gloves (Fig. 9–3), thyroid shields, and leaded eyewear (Fig. 9–4). Lead aprons, lead gloves, and other apparel are secondary barriers; *they do not provide protection from the useful beam.*

Proper care of protective apparel is essential to ensure effectiveness. Lead aprons and gloves should be hung on appropriate racks, not dropped on the floor or folded. Careless handling can result in formation of cracks. Lead aprons and gloves should be imaged annually (either fluoroscopically or radiographically) to check for cracks.

Some companies have environment-friendly recycle/renew programs. They recycle frontal or full-protection aprons into smaller/half aprons, thyroid shields, gonadal shields, and so on, for up to half the price of a new shield. Some companies safely dispose of old lead aprons for a small fee.

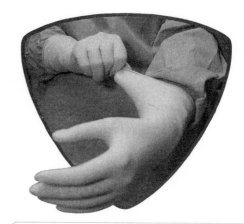

Protection Data:			
kV level	60 kV	80 kV	100 kV
% attenuation	59%	49%	42%

Figure 9–3. Attenuating sterile gloves are available for interventional procedures, diagnostic heart catheterization, coronary angioplasty, angiocardiography, pain management, orthopedics, and other fluoroscopic procedures. (Courtesy of Shielding International.)

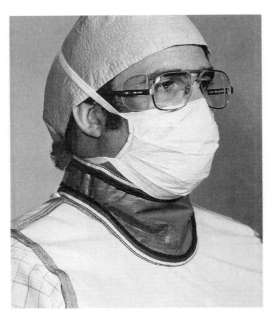

Figure 9–4. Other protective apparel available for fluoroscopic procedures include leaded eyewear. (Courtesy of Nuclear Associates.)

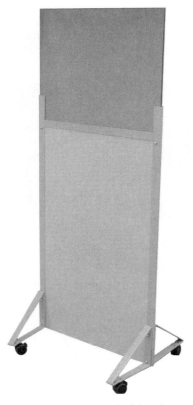

Figure 9–5. Movable leaded barriers provide full-body protection for individuals required to remain in the radiographic or fluoroscopic room. Mobile barriers provide protection from secondary radiation and are available in a variety of sizes and lead equivalents. (Courtesy of Shielding International.)

Additionally, there are some new types of "lead" shields that are completely *lead free*, lightweight, provide 0.5-mm lead equivalency, and are environment friendly.

Protective Accessories

Attenuating sterile gloves are also available for the interventional fluoroscopist. They are thin enough to permit good tactile sensitivity, yet effectively attenuate a good portion of x-ray exposure to the hands (see Fig. 9–3 and its table). The gloves are nonlatex and are lead- and powder free. They are useful for interventional procedures, diagnostic heart catheterization, coronary angioplasty, angiocardiography, pain management, orthopedics, and other fluoroscopic procedures.

Another device available for individuals required to remain in the fluoroscopy department is a mobile lead barrier (Fig. 9–5). These barriers feature optically clear and shatter-resistant lead acrylic windows and provide full-body protection from scattered radiation. They are usually available in a variety of lead equivalents.

Lead aprons can be placed under the patient's pillow during GI and BE examinations when the radiographer's assistance is required at the head end of the table during fluoroscopy.

SPECIAL CONSIDERATIONS

Pregnancy

Deserving special consideration in protection from occupational exposure is the *pregnant radiographer*. As soon as the radiographer knows she is pregnant, it is advisable that she declare her pregnancy in writing. At that time, her occupational radiation history will be reviewed. She must be provided with a second (fetal) monitor. Modifications can be made to the pregnant radiographer's work assignments (e.g., no fluoroscopic assignments), but this is unnecessary if routine radiation safety guidelines are followed.

A radiographer who wears his or her radiation monitor on the collar outside the lead apron usually receives fewer than 100 mrem (1 mSv)/y. If a *fetal monitor* were worn under the lead apron at waist level, it would receive 10% of that dose, or fewer than 10 mrem (0.1 mSv). Because the *gestational dose limit* to the fetus during the gestation period must not exceed *500 mrem (5 mSv)*, under typical conditions, when sufficient protection measures are taken, modification of work assignments is not usually necessary. If a fetal, or "baby," monitor is worn, it must be clearly identified and not confused with the radiographer's regular monitor.

However, radiation protection standards should be reviewed during pregnancy and monthly dosimeter reports closely monitored. Many facilities document the counseling received by the pregnant radiographer from the time she advises her supervisor of her pregnancy and makes the signed documents part of the employee's records.

Mobile Units

Each *mobile x-ray unit* should have a *lead apron* assigned to it. The radiographer should wear the apron while making the exposure at the furthest distance possible from the x-ray tube. The mobile unit's exposure cord must permit the radiographer to stand at least *6 feet* from the x-ray tube and patient. In *mobile fluoroscopic* units, there must be a source-to-patient skin distance of at least 12 inches.

Fluoroscopic Units and Procedures

All *fluoroscopic* equipment must provide at least 12 inches (30 cm), and preferably 15 inches (38 cm), between the x-ray source (focal spot) and the x-ray tabletop (patient), according to NCRP Report No. 102. The *tabletop intensity* of the fluoroscopic beam must not exceed *10 R/min*, or 2.1 R/min/mA. With undertable fluoroscopic tubes, a Bucky-slot cover having at least the equivalent of 0.25-mm Pb must be available to attenuate scattered radiation. Fluoroscopic milliamperes must not exceed 5, although image-intensified fluoroscopy usually operates between 1 and 3 mA.

Because the image intensifier functions as a primary barrier, it must have a lead equivalent of at least 2.0 mm. A cumulative timing device must be available to signal the fluoroscopist (audibly, visibly, or both) when a maximum of 5 minutes of fluoroscopy time has elapsed. Beam collimation must be apparent through visualization of unexposed borders on the TV monitor, and *total filtration* must be at least *2.5-mm Al* equivalent. Because occupational exposure to scattered radiation is of considerable importance in fluoroscopy, a *protective curtain/drape* of at least *0.25-mm Pb* equivalent must be placed between the patient and the fluoroscopist.

The effect of kV and mA adjustment on fluoroscopic images is similar to that on radiographic images. The automatic exposure control automatically varies the exposure required when viewing body tissues of widely differing tissue densities (e.g., between the abdomen and the chest). *As in radiography, high kV and low mA s (milliampere-seconds) values are preferred in an effort to reduce dose.*

Summary

- The cardinal principles of radiation protection are time, distance, and shielding.
- Primary barriers protect from the useful (primary) beam, for example the walls and doors of the radiographic department.
- Secondary barriers protect from sources of leakage and scattered radiation, for example x-ray tube housing and the patient.
- Secondary barriers (e.g., control panel wall and lead apron) do not afford protection from the primary beam.
- There are several NCRP guidelines with which the radiographer should be familiar regarding required thickness and uses of protective shielding (see p. 270, 271, 274).
- A pregnant radiographer should advise her supervisor of her condition as soon as possible.
- A pregnant radiographer wears a special second radiation monitor at waist level under her lead apron.
- Most occupational exposure is received in fluoroscopy and mobile radiography (especially C arm).

COMPREHENSION CHECK

Congratulations! You have completed your review of this chapter. If you are able to answer the following group of very comprehensive questions, you should feel confident that you have really mastered this section. You are then ready to go on to "Registry-type" questions that follow. For greatest success, do not go to the multiple-choice questions without first completing the short-answer questions below.

1. What are the three cardinal rules, or principal guidelines, for radiation protection (p. 269)?

2. When is personal radiation monitoring required (p. 269)?

3. What is the most significant scattering object in fluoroscopy? Why? List other scattering objects (p. 270).

4. What are the NCRP guidelines on leakage radiation, exposure switches, and exposure indicators (p. 270)?

5. What resources should be employed to assist and immobilize patients during radiographic examinations (p. 270)?

6. What rules apply if an individual is required in the radiographic department for assistance during a procedure (p. 270)?

7. Describe the NCRP guidelines that are in place for the patient and personnel protection during fluoroscopic procedures with respect to (p. 270, 271):

    A. Image intensifier lead equivalent

    B. Exposure switch

    C. Bucky-slot cover

    D. Cumulative timer

    E. Lead drape or curtain

    F. Tabletop intensity maximum

    G. Apron and glove lead equivalency

    H. Palpation with remote fluoroscopy units

8. Distinguish between, and give examples of, primary and secondary barriers (p. 272, 273).

9. What is the usual recommended thickness and recommended height of x-ray department walls (p. 272)?

10. What protects from leakage radiation (p. 272)?

11. Identify each of the following as primary or secondary barriers: x-ray room walls, control panel, lead aprons, and gloves (p. 272, 273).

12. How should lead aprons and gloves be cared for (p. 273, 274)?

13. Describe how a pregnant radiographer may use a second personal monitor (p. 274).

14. What is the gestational fetal dose limit (p. 274)?

15. What kinds of counseling and documentation are recommended for the pregnant radiographer (p. 274)?

16. What areas of an x-ray facility generally have the highest occupational exposure (p. 274, 275)?

17. What NCRP guidelines govern mobile radiography with respect to availability of lead aprons, exposure cord, and fluoroscope source-to-skin distance (SSD) (p. 274, 275)?

18. What NCRP guidelines govern fluoroscopy equipment with respect to SSD, tabletop intensity, maximum mA, image intensifier lead equivalent, and fluoroscopy exposure switch (p. 275)?

19. What NCRP guidelines govern fluoroscopy equipment with respect to collimation, total filtration, protective curtain, Bucky-slot cover, and cumulative timer (p. 275)?

CHAPTER REVIEW QUESTIONS

1. Each time an x-ray photon scatters, its intensity at 1 meter from the scattering object is what fraction of its original intensity?
   - (A) 1/10
   - (B) 1/100
   - (C) 1/500
   - (D) 1/1,000

2. If an individual received 45 mR while standing at 4 feet from a source of radiation for 2 minutes, which of the options listed below will *most* effectively reduce his or her radiation exposure?
   - (A) Standing 6 feet from the source for 2 minutes
   - (B) Standing 5 feet from the source for 1 minute
   - (C) Standing 4 feet from the source for 3 minutes
   - (D) Standing 3 feet from the source for 2 minutes

3. How much protection is provided from a 100-kV x-ray beam when using a 0.50-mm lead equivalent apron?
   - (A) 65%
   - (B) 75%
   - (C) 88%
   - (D) 99%

4. Radiation dose to personnel is reduced by the following exposure cord guidelines:
   1. Exposure cords on mobile equipment must allow the operator to be at least 6 feet from the x-ray tube
   2. Exposure cords on fixed equipment must allow the operator to be at least 6 feet from the x-ray tube
   3. Exposure cords on fixed and mobile equipment should be the coiled expandable type
   - (A) 1 only
   - (B) 1 and 2 only
   - (C) 2 and 3 only
   - (D) 1, 2, and 3

5. Which of the following groups of exposure factors will deliver the *least* exposure to the patient?
   - (A) 5 mAs, 90 kV
   - (B) 10 mAs, 80 kV
   - (C) 20 mAs, 68 kV
   - (D) 40 mAs, 66 kV

6. Some patients, such as infants and children, are unable to stay in the necessary radiographic position and require assistance. If mechanical restraining devices cannot be used, who of the following is *best* suited to hold these patients?
   - (A) Floor nurse
   - (B) Transporter
   - (C) Friend or relative
   - (D) Student-radiographer

7. Guidelines used to reduce personnel and/or patient dose in fluoroscopy include:
   1. Maximum tabletop intensity of 10 R/min
   2. Maximum SSD of 12 inches
   3. Minimum filtration of 2.5 mm Al equivalent
   - (A) 1 only
   - (B) 1 and 2 only
   - (C) 1 and 3 only
   - (D) 1, 2, and 3

8. Features of fluoroscopic equipment designed especially to eliminate unnecessary radiation to the patient and personnel include:
   1. Protective curtain
   2. Filtration
   3. Collimation
   - (A) 1 only
   - (B) 1 and 2 only
   - (C) 1 and 3 only
   - (D) 1, 2, and 3

9. Primary radiation barriers must be at least how high?
   - (A) 5 feet
   - (B) 6 feet
   - (C) 7 feet
   - (D) 8 feet

10. The protective control booth from which the radiographer makes the x-ray exposure is a:
   - (A) Primary barrier
   - (B) Secondary barrier
   - (C) Useful beam barrier
   - (D) Remnant radiation barrier

Answers and Explanations

1. (D) One of the radiation protection guidelines for the occupationally exposed is that the x-ray beam must scatter twice before reaching the operator. Each time the x-ray beam scatters, its intensity at 1 m from the scattering object is approximately 0.1% of the intensity of the primary beam, that is, *one-thousandth* of its original intensity. That is why, in terms of radiation protection, the patient is considered the most important source of scatter. Of course, the operator should be behind a shielded booth while making the exposure, but multiple scatterings further reduce danger of exposure from scattered radiation. Other scattering objects include the x-ray table, Bucky-slot cover, and control booth wall.

2. (B) A quick survey of the distractors reveals that options C and D will *increase* exposure dose; thus, they are eliminated as possible correct answers. Both A and B will serve to reduce radiation exposure, as distance is increased and exposure time is decreased in each case. It remains to be seen then which is the more effective. Using the inverse square law of radiation, it is found that the individual would receive *20 mR at 6 feet in 2 minutes* and would receive *14.4 mR at 5 feet in 1 minute:*

$$\frac{I_1}{I_2} = \frac{D_2^2}{D_1^2}$$

Substituting known values from distractor A:

$$\frac{45\,\text{mR}}{x} = \frac{6\,\text{feet}^2}{4\,\text{feet}^2}$$

$$\frac{45}{x} = \frac{36}{16}$$

$$36x = 720$$

$$x = 20\ mR\ at\ 6\ feet\ for\ 2\ minutes$$

$$\frac{I_1}{I_2} = \frac{D_2^2}{D_1^2}$$

Substituting known values from distractor B:

$$\frac{45\,\text{mR}}{x} = \frac{5\,\text{feet}^2}{4\,\text{feet}^2}$$

$$\frac{45}{x} = \frac{25}{16}$$

$$25x = 720$$

$$x = 28.8\ \text{mR at 5 feet for 2 minutes,}$$
$$\text{therefore, 14.4 mR in 1 minute}$$

Note the inverse relationship between the distance and the dose. As distance from the source of radiation increases, dose rate significantly decreases.

3. (B) Lead aprons are worn by occupationally exposed individuals using fluoroscopic procedures. Lead aprons are available with various lead equivalents; 0.25, 0.5, and 1.0 mm are the most common. The *1.0-mm* lead equivalent apron will provide close to 100% protection at most kV levels, but it is rarely used because it weighs anywhere from 12 to 24 lb. A *0.5-mm* apron will attenuate approximately 99% of a 50-kV beam, 88% of a 75-kV beam, and 75% of a 100-kV beam. A *0.25-mm* lead equivalent apron will attenuate approximately 97% of a 50-kV x-ray beam, 66% of a 75-kV beam, and 51% of a 100-kV beam.

4. (A) Radiographic and fluoroscopic equipment is designed to help decrease the exposure dose to the patient and operator. One of the design features is the exposure cord. Exposure cords on *fixed* equipment must be short enough to prevent the exposure from being made outside the control booth. Exposure cords on *mobile* equipment must be long enough to permit the operator to stand at least 6 feet from the x-ray tube.

5. (A) mAs regulates the *quantity* of radiation delivered to the patient. kV regulates the *quality* (penetration) of the radiation delivered to the patient. Therefore, higher energy (more penetrating) radiation—which is more likely to exit the patient—accompanied by lower mAs is the safest combination for the patient, delivering the *lowest* dose. Higher mAs at lower kV values *increases* patient dose.

6. (C) If mechanical restraint is impossible, a friend or relative accompanying the patient should be requested to hold the patient. If a friend or relative is not available, a nurse or transporter may be asked for help. Protective apparel, such as lead apron and gloves, should be provided to the person(s) holding the patient. *Radiology personnel must never assist in holding patients, and the individual assisting should never be in the path of the primary beam.*

7. (C) All *fluoroscopic* equipment (both stationary and mobile) must provide *at least* 12 inches (30 cm), and preferably 15 inches (38 cm), between the x-ray source (focal spot) and the x-ray tabletop, according to NCRP Report No. 102. The tabletop *intensity* of the fluoroscopic beam must not exceed *10 R/min*, or 2.1 R/min/mA. Required filtration must be at least the equivalent of 2.5-mm aluminum. Fluoroscopic mA must not exceed 5, although image-intensified fluoroscopy usually operates between 1 and 3 mA. The image intensifier functions as a primary barrier and has a lead equivalent of 2.0 mm.

8. (D) The *protective* curtain is usually made of leaded vinyl with at least 0.25-mm Pb equivalent. It must be positioned between the patient and the fluoroscopist, and it greatly reduces exposure of the fluoroscopist to energetic scatter from the patient. Just as overhead radiation barrier equipment, fluoroscopic total *filtration* must be at least 2.5-mm Al equivalent to reduce excessive exposure to low-energy radiation. *Collimator* or beam alignment must be accurate to within 2%.

9. (C) Radiation protection guidelines have established that *primary radiation barriers* must be at least 7 feet high. Primary radiation barriers are walls that the primary beam might be directed toward. They usually contain 1.5-mm lead, but this can vary depending on the *use factor* and other factors.

10. (B) *Primary barriers* are those that protect us from the primary or useful beam. They have much greater attenuation capability than secondary barriers that protect only from leakage and scattered radiation. The radiographic room walls are therefore considered primary barriers because the primary beam is often directed toward them, as in chest radiography. Most control booth barriers, however, are *secondary barriers* and the primary beam is never directed toward them. They are usually constructed of four thicknesses of gypsum board and/or 0.5 to 1 inch of plate glass. Remnant radiation penetrates the patient and forms the latent image on the image receptor.

Radiation Exposure and Monitoring | 10

UNITS OF MEASUREMENT

W.C. Röntgen's paper "On a New Kind of Rays" described the ionizing effect of x-rays on air, their penetrating effects on all forms of matter, and their effect on photographic emulsions. Röntgen's work was so thorough and complete that we know little more today than was originally presented in his paper. We still use these principles today to detect and quantify radiation exposure.

The (traditional/conventional) radiation units of measurement, the roentgen, rad, and rem, are of importance to the radiographer—the SI (Standard International) units of measure have gained in usage and must also be understood by the radiographer. The ARRT (American Registry of Radiologic Technologists) Content Specifications for the Examination in Radiography indicate that the certification examination generally uses the conventional units of measurement. However, it is stated that questions referenced to specific reports, such as the National Council on Radiation Protection and Measurements (NCRP) reports, will use SI units to be consistent with those reports.

Roentgen/Gy$_a$

The ARRT examination does not capitalize "roentgen" as a unit of measurement, and no "s" is used to indicate plural (i.e., 10 roentgen, *not* 10 Roentgens; the same is true for the terms rad and rem). When used to express *rate*, it is abbreviated to R/min or R/hr. The *roentgen* is a unit of measure of *ionization in air*, and can be referred to as the *unit of exposure*. Because x-rays ionize air, all the ions of *either* sign (positive *or* negative) formed in a particular quantity of air are counted and equated to a quantity of radiation expressed in the unit *roentgen*. The roentgen is valid only for *x* and *gamma radiations* at energies up to 3 MeV (million/mega electron volts). The roentgen is the traditional unit of measure for exposure to x- or gamma radiations.

The term *kerma* is used to express *kinetic energy released in matter*. X-rays expend kinetic energy as they ionize the air. Joule/kilogram is used to measure air kerma and $1 \text{ J/kg} = 1 \text{ Gy}_a$. The subscript *a* represents *air* as the absorber. The mGy$_a$ is the Standard International (SI) unit of measure of radiation intensity.

Roentgen

- Measures ionization in air (negative *or* positive ions counted)
- Measures x- or gamma radiation only
- Is valid up to 3 MeV

Traditional and SI Units

Roentgen	Air Kerma (Gy$_a$)
Rad	Gray (Gy$_t$)
Rem	Sievert (Sv)

TABLE 10–1. Quality Factor for Different Types of Radiation

Ionizing Radiation Type	Quality Factor
Gamma rays	1
X-ray photons	1
Alpha particles	20
Beta particles	1
Fast neutrons	20

Rad/Gray (Gy$_t$)

The *rad* is an acronym for *radiation absorbed dose*. As ionizing radiation passes through matter, a certain amount of its energy is deposited in that matter; note that we again are referring to energy released in matter, i.e.: *kerma*. The rad has been described as equivalent to *100 ergs* of energy deposited *per gram* of irradiated material. The SI unit is *Gray* (Gy$_t$) – the subscript *t* representing *tissue*. Absorbed dose and energy deposited is strongly related to chemical change and biologic damage. The amount of energy deposited and possible biologic damage are dependent on the following:

- Type of ionizing radiation
- Atomic number of the tissue
- Mass density of the tissue
- Energy of the radiation

Rem/Sievert

The *rem* is an acronym for *radiation equivalent man*. The rem uses the information collected for the rad, but also uses a quality factor (QF) to predict biologic effects from different types of radiation (Table 10–1). Thus, the equation rad × QF = rem. Radiations having a high QF have a higher linear energy transfer (LET) and greater potential to produce biologic damage. The rem is described as the unit of *dose equivalency* (DE) and used to express occupational exposure.

The rem SI unit of measurement is the Sv (Sievert), where 1 Sv = 100 rem.

Similar absorbed doses of *different kinds* of radiation can cause different biologic effects to *tissues of differing radiosensitivity*. A *radiation weighting factor* (W$_r$) is a number assigned to different types of ionizing radiations so that their effect(s) may be better determined (e.g., x-ray vs. alpha particles). The W$_r$ of different ionizing radiations is dependent on the LET of that particular radiation. A *tissue weighting factor* (W$_t$) represents the relative tissue radiosensitivity of the irradiated material (e.g., muscle vs. intestinal epithelium vs. bone, etc.). The weighting factor is like the *SI* equivalent of the *traditional* QF; for example, rad × QF = rem, whereas, Gy × W$_r$ = Sv.

Particulate Radiation

Particulate radiation (alpha, beta, etc.) is highly ionizing. As an *internal* source of radiation, it increases LET, and a significant biologic effect can result. As an *external* source of radiation, most is virtually innocuous. However, some beta particles (e.g., Mo-99 and Co-60 beta) are very energetic and can cause serious external damage.

As the *atomic number* of the irradiated tissue increases, a greater number of x-ray photons is absorbed by the tissue (i.e., the photoelectric interaction increases), and LET increases. As the *energy* of the ionizing radiation increases, it becomes more penetrating and LET decreases, thereby decreasing the likelihood of biologic effects.

Because the rad does not take into account the biologic effect of various types of radiation, it is not used to express occupational exposure.

MONITORING DEVICES

National Council on Radiation Protection and Measurements (NCRP) Guidelines for Use

Radiation monitoring is used to evaluate the effectiveness of the radiation safety policies and practices in place. The Code of Federal Regulations (CFR) states that monitoring be provided for occupationally exposed individuals in a controlled area who are likely to receive more than 1/10 *the dose-equivalent limit.*

Optically Stimulated Luminescence

Optically stimulated luminescence (OSL) dosimeters are gradually replacing the long-used film badges. The OSL contains a thin layer of *aluminum oxide* (Al_2O_3). Aluminum oxide absorbs and stores the energy associated with exposure to ionizing radiation. OSL dosimeters are available with various combination of filter packs (Fig. 10–1). Some

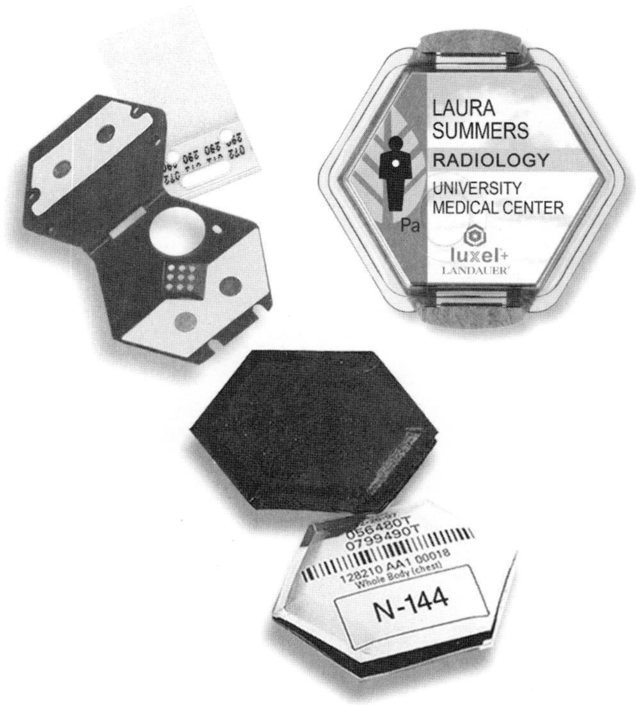

> **Personal Radiation Monitors**
>
> - Optically stimulated luminescence
> - Thermoluminescent dosimeter
> - Film badge
> - Pocket dosimeter

Figure 10–1. OSL dosimeters are available with various combinations of filters. Some contain a filter pack of tin, copper, and an open window. Others are available with aluminum, copper/aluminum, plastic, and an open window. Still others contain lead, copper/aluminum, plastic, and an open window. These various filters serve to identify the type and energy of radiation. (Courtesy of Landauer Inc, Glenwood, IL.)

contain a filter pack of tin, copper, and an open window. Others are available with aluminum, copper/aluminum, plastic, and an open window. Still others contain lead, copper/aluminum, plastic, and an open window. In any case, these various *filters* serve to identify the type and energy of *ionizing radiation* that interacted with the dosimeter; for example photons that penetrate the copper to interact with the dosimeter are more energetic than those that might have only enough energy to pass through the plastic filter.

When the OSL is returned to the laboratory for processing, the Al_2O_3 chips are stimulated with green light from either a laser or light-emitting diode source. The resulting blue light emitted from the Al_2O_3 is proportional to the amount of radiation exposure. The quantity of light emitted is equated to a radiation quantity expressed in mrem on the written report returned to the user. Both high- and low-energy photons and beta particles can be measured with this technique.

The OSL dosimeter allows for multiple readouts and can be used to reconfirm reported radiation doses. This is because only a fraction of the radiation exposure signal contained in the Al_2O_3 material is used up upon stimulation with the green light. Other advantages of the OSL dosimeter include the ability to measure radiation doses as low as 1 mrem (with a precision of ±1 mrem) and to be reanalyzed, if necessary. Their tamper-proof plastic package is unaffected by heat, moisture, and pressure. Although many facilities prefer monthly radiation reports, because OSL dosimeters are so accurate and stable, they can be used for longer periods and "read" quarterly.

Film Badge

The ionizing radiation monitor used for many years was the *film badge*. The film badge consists of special radiation dosimetry film packaged like dental film and enclosed in a special plastic holder. The plastic holder features an open window (through which the user's name appears) and various *filters* (which serve to identify the *type* and *energy of ionizing radiation* received by the user; Fig. 10–2).

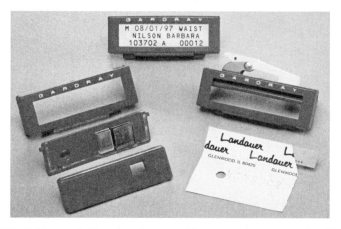

Figure 10–2. The radiation monitor used for many years was the *film badge,* consisting of special film packages such as dental film and enclosed in a special plastic holder. The plastic holder has an open window and various filters, which serve to identify the type and energy of radiation. (Courtesy of Landauer Inc, Glenwood, IL.)

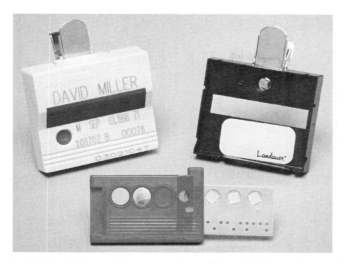

Figure 10–3. The TLD contains crystalline chips of LiF, which absorb and store the energy associated with exposure to ionizing radiation. (Courtesy of Landauer Inc, Glenwood, IL.)

Radiation that exposes the film behind an aluminum filter is more energetic than a radiation that passes through only the open window and less energetic than a radiation penetrating a copper filter. Film badges are used for 1 *month*, collected, and sent to a special laboratory for processing. The degree of exposure is carefully evaluated and equated to a dose usually expressed in *mrem*; the film badge can measure doses as low as 10 mrem.

Film badges had been the most widely used personal radiation monitors, but are being replaced by the OSL dosimeters.

Thermoluminescent Dosimeter

The thermoluminescent dosimeter (TLD) (Fig. 10–3) contains crystalline chips of *lithium fluoride* (LiF). LiF absorbs and stores the energy associated with exposure to ionizing radiation. When the TLD is returned to the laboratory for processing, the LiF chips are heated. This process causes a release of visible light from the chips in proportion to the amount of ionizing radiation absorbed. The quantity of light emitted is equated to a radiation quantity expressed in mrem on the written report returned to the user.

The TLD is more sensitive and precise than the film badge because it can measure doses as low as 5 mrem. The TLD is unaffected by heat or humidity and can be worn up to 3 months before processing. However, in the unlikely event that the user had unknowingly received excessive radiation exposure, the user should be made aware of it as soon as possible, and the event should be recent enough to be able to recall. This is often considered the single disadvantage of the TLD. The OSL, film badge, and TLD measure a variety of energies of x-, beta-, and gamma radiations.

Pocket Dosimeter

The use of a *pocket dosimeter* (Fig. 10–4) is indicated when working with high exposures or large quantities of radiation for a short period of time, so that an immediate reading is available to the user. The pocket

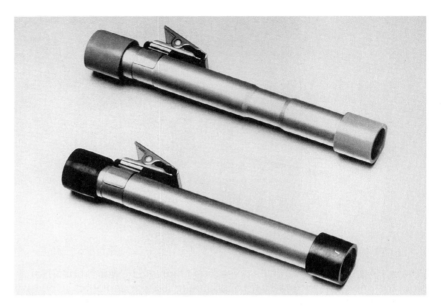

Figure 10–4. The pocket dosimeter contains a small ionization chamber that counts charges in proportion to the exposure received. (Courtesy of Nuclear Associates.)

dosimeter is sensitive and accurate, but has limited application in diagnostic radiography.

The pocket dosimeter, or *pocket isolation chamber*, resembles a penlight. Within the dosimeter is a thimble ionization chamber. In the presence of x- or gamma radiations, a particular quantity of air is ionized and causes the fiber indicator to register radiation quantity in milliroentgen (mR). The self-reading type may be "read" by holding the dosimeter up to the light and, looking through the eyepiece, observing the fiber indicator, which indicates a quantity of 0 to 200 mR. One disadvantage of the pocket dosimeter as a personal monitor is that it does not provide a permanent legal record of exposure.

Evaluation and Maintenance of Records

Personal monitors should be worn consistently in the same place and facing forward (i.e., with the open window and user's identification visible). If the badge is correctly worn at the collar outside the lead apron, it will approximate dose to the head and neck and will provide an overestimation of dose to the shielded organs.

The use of a second monitor is occasionally indicated. The *pregnant radiographer* may wear a second, waist-level, dosimeter *under* her lead apron to approximate fetal dose (Fig. 10–5). Some procedures require the hands to be near the useful beam (e.g., some fluoroscopic and vascular procedures). A finger, or ring, monitor provides information on exposure to the hands (Fig. 10–6).

The radiographer is occupationally exposed to *low-energy, low-LET* radiation. Monitoring devices are worn *only for occupational purposes* and never if the individual is exposed for medical or dental reasons. The radiographer should review his or her record monthly (or quarterly, if a quarterly system is used) as the report is received by the institution. The radiation safety officer (RSO) is responsible for reviewing all dosimeter

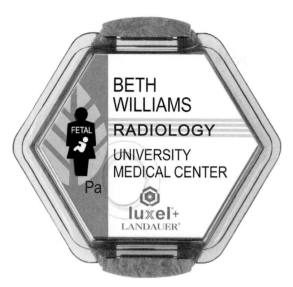

Figure 10–5. The *pregnant radiographer* should wear a second, waist-level, dosimeter under her lead apron that will measure the approximate fetal dose. (Courtesy of Landauer Inc, Glenwood, IL.)

reports and being certain that the staff is monitored, educated, and regularly updated.

An *official written report* is sent to the sponsoring institution (Fig. 10–7) to document doses received from the OSL, TLD, or film badge. A number of columns of specific data are reported. Exposure data that are

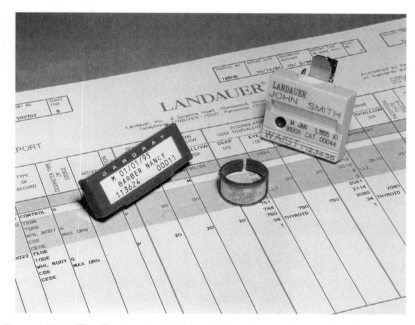

Figure 10–6. The film badge (*left*) contains filters to determine the type and energy of radiation received by the wearer. The TLD (*right*) contains thermoluminescent crystals that emit quantities of light proportional to their degree of exposure. The ring badge (*center*) is particularly useful for individuals whose hands are in close proximity to radioactive nuclides or the fluoroscopic x-ray field. A report similar to the one shown is returned monthly, documenting the radiation dose received by each of the personal monitors. (Courtesy of Landauer Inc, Glenwood, IL.)

LANDAUER®

Landauer, Inc. 2 Science Road   Glenwood, Illinois 60425-1586
Telephone: (708) 755-7000   Facsimile: (708) 755-7016
www.landauerinc.com

SAMPLE ORGANIZATION
RADIATION SAFETY OFFICER
2 SCIENCE ROAD
GLENWOOD, IL 60425

RADIATION DOSIMETRY REPORT

luxel®

ACCOUNT NO.	SERIES CODE	ANALYTICAL WORK ORDER	REPORT DATE	DOSIMETER RECEIVED	REPORT TIME IN WORK DAYS	PAGE NO.
103702	RAD	992150087	6/13/07	06/09/07	4	1

PARTICIPANT NUMBER	NAME (ID NUMBER / BIRTH DATE / SEX)	DOSIMETER	USE	RADIATION QUALITY	DOSE EQUIVALENT (MREM) FOR PERIODS SHOWN BELOW — DEEP DDE	EYE LDE	SHALLOW SDE	YEAR TO DATE DOSE EQUIVALENT (MREM) — DEEP DDE	EYE LDE	SHALLOW SDE	LIFETIME DOSE EQUIVALENT (MREM) — DEEP DDE	EYE LDE	SHALLOW SDE	RECORDS FOR YEAR	INCEPTION DATE (MM/YY)
FOR MONITORING PERIOD:					05/01/07 - 05/31/07			2007							
0000H	CONTROL	J	CNTRL		M	M	M							5	07/97
	CONTROL	P	CNTRL		M	M	M								07/97
	CONTROL	U	CNTRL				M								07/97
00189	ADAMS, HEATHER 336235619 08/31/1968 F	P	WHBODY		M	M	M	9	10	12	29	31	42	5	07/01
00191	ADDISON, JOHN 471563287 10/04/1968 M	J	WHBODY	PN	90	90	90	100	100	100	200	200	200	5	07/01
				P	60	60	60	70	70	70	170	170	170		
				NF	30	30	30	30	30	30	30	30	30		
00202	HARRIS, KATHY 587582144 06/09/1960 F	P	WHBODY		M	M	M	M	M	M	M	M	M	5	02/02
		U	RFINGR				M			30			30		02/02
00005	MEYER, STEVE 982778955 07/15/1964 M	P	COLLAR	PL	119	119	113							5	08/97
		P	WAIST	P	10	11	11								08/97
			ASSIGN		19	119	113	33	185	174	1387	2308	2320		
			NOTE		ASSIGNED DOSE BASED ON EDE 1 CALCULATION										
		U	RFINGR				140			690			2180		08/97
00203	STEVENS, LEE 335478977 08/25/1951 M	P	WHBODY		ABSENT			M	M	M	M	M	M	4	07/02
		U	RFINGR		ABSENT					M			M		07/02
00204	WALKER, JANE 416995421 03/21/1947 F	P	WHBODY		3	3	3	12	11	11	22	21	21	5	11/02
00188	WEBSTER, ROBERT 355381469 05/15/1972 M	P	WHBODY NOTE		40 CALCULATED	40	40	200	200	200	240	240	240	5	07/01

M: MINIMAL REPORTING SERVICE OF 1 MREM
ELECTRONIC MEDIA TO FOLLOW THIS REPORT

QUALITY CONTROL RELEASE: LMR

1 - PR   6774 - PT131 - N1

-21587

NVLAP
NVLAP LAB CODE 100518-0 **

Figure 10–7. An *official written report* documents doses received from the OSL, TLD, or film badge. Columns of specific data are reported, including the current period exposure, annual cumulative exposure, and separate readings for special dosimeters, such as fetal or extremity dosimeters. (Courtesy of Landauer Inc, Glenwood, IL.)

required to appear are the current period exposure, the annual cumulative exposure, and separate readings for special dosimeters, such as fetal or extremity dosimeters.

NCRP RECOMMENDATIONS

A part of the professional radiographer's responsibility lies in keeping occupational exposure to a minimum. The use of radiation-monitoring devices helps evaluate the effectiveness of radiation protection practices. The periodic reports received from OSL, film badge, or TLD laboratories are official legal documents that must be reviewed, and an attempt should be made to reduce *any* exposure no matter how small (i.e., the ALARA principle).

NCRP Report No. 116 and the CFR (10 CFR §20) require that occupationally exposed individuals 18 years of age and older do not receive exposures in excess of 5 rem (50 mSv)/y. A radiography student participating in clinical education before the age of 18 years must not receive an annual dose of more than 0.1 rem (100 mrem). Since the general population is not in the vicinity of man-made ionizing radiation on a daily basis, their annual dose limit is 1/10 that of ours, that is 0.5 rem (5 mSv)/y.

The lifetime cumulative exposure for the occupationally exposed individual is determined using the following formula: 1 rem × age in years. Thus, a 26-year-old radiographer's lifetime occupational exposure must not exceed 26 rem (260 mSv). The pregnant radiographer's *gestational* exposure to the fetus must not exceed 0.5 rem (500 mrem, 5 mSv); the *monthly* fetal dose must not exceed 0.05 rem (0.5 mSv).

These are the recommended maximum dose-equivalent limits. The *actual* mean annual exposure to occupationally exposed medical personnel is 100 to 140 mrem (1–1.4 mSv), well below the recommended limit. This seems to indicate that we are performing our tasks in a safe, conscientious, and ethical manner.

Summary

- The roentgen (R unit), or unit of exposure, is the unit used to describe the quantity of ionization in air.
- The rad describes absorbed dose.
- The rem is the unit of dose equivalency (DE), used to quantify biologic effectiveness.
- The OSL is the newest, most accurate personal dosimeter; it can be processed monthly or quarterly. It uses a thin layer of Al_2O_3 to store information.
- Film badges are convenient, low-cost radiation monitors that are processed monthly.
- TLDs use LiF crystals to store exposure information. They are more precise and more expensive than film badges and may be processed quarterly.
- Film badges and TLDs measure exposure to x-, beta-, and gamma radiations.
- Pocket dosimeters are thimble ionization chambers used to monitor larger quantities of radiation exposure, up to 200 mR.
- Radiographers must strive to keep their occupational dose ALARA.
- NCRP Report No. 116 and the CFR (10 CFR §20) establish limits for exposure to ionizing radiation with which radiographers should be familiar.

COMPREHENSION CHECK

Congratulations! You have completed your review of this chapter. If you are able to answer the following group of very comprehensive questions, you should feel confident that you have really mastered this section. You are then ready to go on to "Registry-type" questions that follow. For greatest success, do not go to the multiple-choice questions without first completing the short-answer questions below.

1. Discuss the R as a unit of measurement, including what it measures, the radiation(s) it measures, and up to what energy (p. 281).

2. What does the acronym rad mean? Define rad. Discuss/convert the rad to SI unit (p. 282).

3. Name the three factors influencing the amount of energy deposited (rad) in tissue (p. 282).

4. Relate particulate radiation to degree of ionization in tissue, LET, and possible biologic effects (p. 282, 283).

5. Discuss the function of quality factor and weighting factors (p. 282).

6. What does the acronym rem mean? Discuss/convert the rem to SI unit (p. 282).

7. Why can the rem be accurately used to describe occupational DE, whereas the rad cannot (p. 282)?

8. Describe the film badge. Include the following in your description (p. 284, 285).
   A. Construction
   B. Purpose of filters
   C. Length of time used
   D. Type(s) of radiation detected
   E. How it is "read" and in what unit
   F. Any advantages or disadvantages

9. Describe the TLD. Include the following in your description (p. 285).
   A. Construction
   B. Type of crystals used and their unique characteristics
   C. Length of time used
   D. Type(s) of radiation detected
   E. How it is "read" and in what unit
   F. Any advantages or disadvantages

10. Describe the pocket dosimeter. Include the following in your description (p. 285, 286).
   A. Construction
   B. Indications for use
   C. How it is "read," in what unit, and up to what maximum
   D. Any advantages or disadvantages

11. Describe the OSL to include (p. 283, 284):
   A. Component parts
   B. Type of crystal used, and how it reacts to radiation exposure
   C. Types and purpose of filters
   D. How the OSL is "read"
   E. Degree of accuracy
   F. How affected by environmental condition

12. What is the NCRP-recommended dose limit for occupational exposure in individuals younger than 18 years and older than 18 years (p. 288, 289)?

13. How is lifetime cumulative occupational exposure determined (p. 289)?

14. What is the NCRP-recommended dose limit for gestational fetal exposure (p. 289)?

CHAPTER REVIEW QUESTIONS

1. Which of the following is a measure of dose to biologic tissue?

   (A) Roentgen

   (B) Rad (Gy)

   (C) Rem (Sv)

   (D) RBE

2. What is the annual dose limit for a student radiographer who is younger than 18 years and beginning clinical assignments?

   (A) 0.1 rem (1 mSv)

   (B) 0.5 rem (5 mSv)

   (C) 5 rem (50 mSv)

   (D) 10 rem (100 mSv)

3. The purpose of filters in a film badge is:

   (A) To eliminate harmful rays

   (B) To measure radiation quality

   (C) To prevent exposure from alpha particles

   (D) To support the film contained within

4. The dose limits established for the OSL, TLD, film badge, and pocket dosimeter are valid for:

   (A) Alpha-, beta-, and x radiations

   (B) X- and gamma radiations only

   (C) Beta-, x-, and gamma radiations

   (D) All ionizing radiations

5. The operation of personal radiation monitoring devices can depend upon:

   1. Ionization

   2. Thermoluminescence

   3. Resonance

   (A) 1 only

   (B) 1 and 2 only

   (C) 2 and 3 only

   (D) 1, 2, and 3

6. What is the established monthly fetal dose-limit guideline for pregnant radiographers?

   (A) 0.05 rem (0.5 mSv)

   (B) 0.5 rem (5 mSv)

   (C) 5.0 rem (50 mSv)

   (D) 10.0 rem (100 mSv)

7. Which of the following crystals are used in an optically luminescent dosimetry system?

   (A) Silver bromide

   (B) Aluminum oxide

   (C) Lithium fluoride

   (D) Ferrous sulfate

8. Potential ionizing radiation damage to tissue is dependent upon the:

   1. Z number of the tissue

   2. Type of ionizing radiation

   3. Mass density of the tissue

   (A) 1 only

   (B) 1 and 2 only

   (C) 2 and 3 only

   (D) 1, 2, and 3

9. The unit of measurement used to express occupational exposure is the:

   (A) Roentgen

   (B) Rad (Gray)

   (C) Rem (Sievert)

   (D) Relative biologic effectiveness (RBE)

10. The NCRP recommends an annual effective occupational dose-equivalent limit of:

    (A) 25 mSv (2.5 rem)

    (B) 50 mSv (5 rem)

    (C) 100 mSv (10 rem)

    (D) 200 mSv (20 rem)

Answers and Explanations

1. (C) Roentgen is the unit of exposure; it measures the quantity of ionization in air. The rad is an acronym for radiation-absorbed dose; it measures the energy deposited in any material. The rem is an acronym for radiation equivalent man; it includes the RBE specific to the tissue irradiated, thereby being a valid unit of measurement of dose to biologic material.

2. (A) Because the established dose limit formula guideline is used for occupationally exposed persons 18 years of age and older, guidelines had to be established in the event a student entered training prior to age 18 years. The guideline states that the occupational dose limit for students younger than 18 years is 0.1 rem (100 mrem or 1 mSv) in any given year.

3. (B) Film badge filters (usually aluminum and copper) serve to help measure radiation quality (energy). Only the most energetic radiation will penetrate the copper; radiation of lower levels will penetrate the aluminum, and the lowest energy radiation will pass readily through the unfiltered area. Thus, radiation of different energy levels can be recorded, measured, and reported.

4. (C) The occupational dose limit is valid for x-, beta-, and gamma radiations. Because alpha radiation is so. Traditional personal monitors will not record alpha radiation because alpha particles are rapidly ionizing and capable of penetrating only a few centimeters of air. They are practically harmless as an external source of radiation but, potentially, the most harmful as an *internal* source. Pocket dosimeters measure x- and gamma radiations only; alpha and beta particles are not energetic enough to penetrate the device and enter the ionization chamber.

5. (B) Ionization is the fundamental principle of operation of both the film badge and the pocket dosimeter. In the film badge, the film's silver halide emulsion is ionized by x-ray photons. The pocket dosimeter contains an ionization chamber, and the number of ionizations taking place may be equated to exposure dose. Resonance refers to motion and has no application to personal radiation monitoring.

6. (A) The declared pregnant radiographer poses a special radiation protection consideration, for the safety of the unborn individual must be considered. It must be remembered that the developing fetus is particularly sensitive to radiation exposure. Therefore, established guidelines state that the occupational radiation exposure to the fetus must not exceed 0.5 rem (500 mrem or 5 mSv) during the entire gestation period; the *monthly* fetal dose must not exceed 0.05 rem (0.5 mSv).

7. (B) OSL dosimeters are personal radiation monitors that use aluminum oxide crystals. These crystals, once exposed to ionizing radiation and then stimulated with a laser, give off light proportional to the amount of radiation received. OSL dosimeters are very accurate personal monitors. TLDs use lithium fluoride as the sensitive crystal.

8. (D) Absorbed dose refers to the amount of energy deposited per unit mass and is strongly related to chemical change and biologic damage. The amount of energy deposited and, thus, the amount of possible biologic damage are dependent on the *type of ionizing radiation*, the *atomic (Z) number of the tissue*, the *mass density of the tissue*, and the *energy of the radiation*.

A radiation weighting factor (W_r) is a number assigned to different types of ionizing radiations so that their effect(s) may be better determined. The W_r of different ionizing radiations is dependent on the LET of that particular radiation. A tissue weighting factor (W_t) represents the relative tissue radiosensitivity of the irradiated material.

LET is another means of expressing radiation quality and determining the W_r. As the LET of radiation increases, the radiation's ability to produce biologic damage also increases. This is described quantitatively by RBE; LET and RBE are directly related.

Most sources of ionizing radiation have a mixture of high- and low-LET radiations. Low-LET radiations deposit less energy in cells/tissues along their path than high-LET radiations, and is considered less destructive as it traverses tissues.

9. (C) *Roentgen* is the unit of exposure; it measures the quantity of ionizations in air. The *rad* is an acronym for *r*adiation-*a*bsorbed *d*ose; it measures the energy deposited in any material. The *rem* is an acronym for *r*adiation *e*quivalent *m*an; it includes the RBE specific to the tissue irradiated, thereby being a valid unit of measurement of dose to biologic material.

10. (B) A 1984 review of radiation exposure data revealed that the average annual dose equivalent for monitored radiation workers was approximately 2.3 mSv (0.23 rem). The fact that this is approximately 1/10 the recommended limit indicates that the limit is adequate for radiation protection purposes. Consequently, the NCRP reiterates its 1971 recommended annual limit of 50 mSv (5 rem) (*NCRP Report No. 105, pp. 14–15*).

Technical Factors and Image Quality | 11

The last 10 years have seen the process of x-ray image production undergo the most amazing changes since the discovery of x-ray itself in 1895. The majority of x-ray images produced today are probably produced *electronically*—that is, Computerized Radiography (CR) or Digital Radiography (DR).

Although most radiographers and radiography students might be dealing with electronic imaging (CR, DR), it is still essential to comprehend and employ the fundamentals of image production—and to learn a bit about what might be referred to as *projection radiography* or *traditional radiography*, that is, screen-film (SF) imaging. Additionally, we can better appreciate today's tools and achievements if we understand the strides taken along the path that lead to today's technology.

If radiography students found "technique," that is, exposure factors to be confusing in the past, I can only believe that the subject is now even more complex and bewildering. We have a still-quite-new technology being operated by a generational mix of imaging professionals.

Seasoned radiographers that used SF imaging for years are now performing digital imaging. Students that work side-by-side with them have learned much digital imaging in the classroom but, in clinical, the students might still be putting "cassettes" into Bucky trays, reviewing their "films," and perhaps even getting "wet readings." Experienced radiographers that may have developed their own technique charts at one time are now using APR—Anatomically Programmed Radiography— that is, preprogrammed technical factors.

However, there is much that is *unchanged* in the x-ray imaging chain. And, more importantly, there is much that is still dependant upon the knowledge and skill of the radiographer—in order to obtain quality images, under ALARA conditions.

It is true that there are more variables than there are constants in x-ray imaging. How can one comprehend all the variables and control image quality when the equipment *seems* to make all the decisions? The most obvious variable, and the one in which the least modification is possible, is the *patient*. Body habitus, muscle tone, pathology, trauma, and age all require accurate assessment prior to the intelligent selection of technical

Image Quality:

- Density/Brightness ⎤ *Visibility*
- Contrast/Gray Scale ⎦ *Factors*
- Detail/Resolution ⎤ *Geometric*
- Distortion ⎦ *Factors*

Exposure Factors:

- mA
- time
- kV
- distance

Factors Affecting Recorded Detail/Resolution:

- OID (magnification distortion)
- SID (magnification distortion)
- Focal spot size (focal spot blur)
- Patient factors (structural shape/position)
- Intensifying screens (screen blur)
- Motion (obliterates detail)

Distortion:

- Size distortion (magnification)
- Shape distortion (elongation/foreshortening)

Factors Affecting Distortion:

- Size distortion/Magnification
    OID
    SID
- Shape distortion:
    Alignment of x-ray tube, anatomic part, and IR (elongation/foreshortening)

factors and/or preprogrammed exposure algorithms. The importance of careful and accurate patient evaluation cannot be overemphasized.

Even when using *APR, Automatic Exposure Control* (AEC) or *computerized* or *digital imaging* (CR/DR), the radiographer's accurate evaluation of the patient will result in more knowledgeable and efficient use of the technical equipment.

After the patient is evaluated, various aspects of the procedure and imaging accessories that affect image quality must be considered: SID, tube angle techniques, grid ratios, and filters, to name a few.

Fortunately, these items are fairly standard from one radiographic room to the next within a given department. When it comes to mobile radiography or being able to move from one facility to another, however, a good working knowledge of a variety of imaging accessories and their particular use is required.

What about circumstances that require deviation from the normal SID, or the introduction of an OID? What if the patient is unable to move from stretcher or wheel chair, is unable to maintain the required position or suspend their respiration, is in pain or semiconscious? How does collimation affect the radiographic image? How does scattered radiation affect a PSP differently than it affects film emulsion? Why does kilovoltage (kV) affect image density as well as regulate radiographic contrast—how does that compare to digital imaging? What is meant by the terms . . . *contrast resolution, spatial resolution, and APR?* . . . How do all these variables affect the image, and how can we use them to achieve optimal image quality? We are concerned with producing high quality x-ray images—so how is image quality defined? Of what does it consist?

Image quality consists of image *density* (*brightness* is the electronic/CR/DR term), *contrast* or *gray scale, recorded detail* (*spatial resolution* is the electronic/CR/DR term), and *distortion.* The *visibility,* factors are density/brightness and contrast/gray scale. The *geometric* factors are recorded detail/spatial resolution and distortion.

The *exposure/technical factors* we use to create the image are milliamperage (*mA*), exposure time (*s*), kilovoltage (*kV*), and *SID. Patient variables* that have significant impact on factor selection and the radiologic image are *tissue density,* tissue *thickness,* any *pathology,* and ability to cooperate.

This chapter will review the factors affecting Image Quality in both traditional *SF* imaging and *electronic* (CR/DR) imaging. Factors related to SF imaging will be related to any application in CR/DR and covered within the scope required by the radiography examination content specifications published by the ARRT.

GEOMETRIC FACTORS

Detail/Resolution and Distortion

All of the geometric factors—OID, SID, Focal Spot Size, Distortion, Structural position and shape, and Motion—(*except* intensifying screens) *apply to digital imaging as well as SF imaging.*

The term *recorded detail* refers to the *clarity,* or *resolution,* with which anatomic structures are represented in the x-ray image.

If the tiny image details (e.g., bony trabeculae, minute calcifications) of a variety of images made under different circumstances were compared, especially with the use of a magnifying glass, it would be noted that the image details appear with varying degrees of clarity. On some of the images, details would be clearly defined, while on other images the edges of tiny details would have varied degrees of unsharpness, that is, these would not be defined as sharply or with the same degree of resolution. This is the basic concept of recorded detail. The term used to describe the IR's impact on recorded detail in CR/DR is *spatial resolution*.

The term *distortion* refers to misrepresentation of the actual *size* (*magnification*) or *shape* (*foreshortening* or *elongation*) of the structures imaged, which may be partly or wholly caused by inherent object unsharpness.

The degree of resolution transferred to the image receptor (IR) is a function of the resolving power of each of the system components and is expressed in line pairs per millimeter (lp/mm) (Fig. 11–1). *One line pair refers to one line and the one space adjacent to it.* Resolution describes how closely fine details may be associated and still be recognized as separate details before seeming to blend into each other and appear "as one" (Fig. 11–2).

The term *visibility of detail* refers to *how well the recorded detail can be seen*; for example, excessive density, brightness, or scattered radiation fog impairs detail visibility because it obscures the details. Density and fog have no effect on how sharply an image detail is rendered; they do,

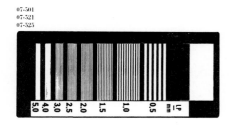

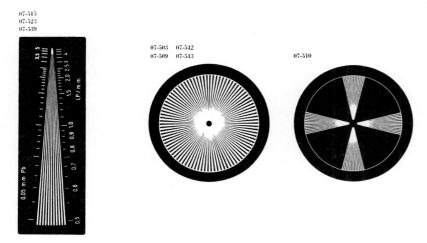

Figure 11–1. Resolution is measured with a *resolution test pattern* and expressed in lp/mm. Resolution test tools are pictured. The *star pattern* is generally used for focal spot size evaluation. (Courtesy of Nuclear Associates.)

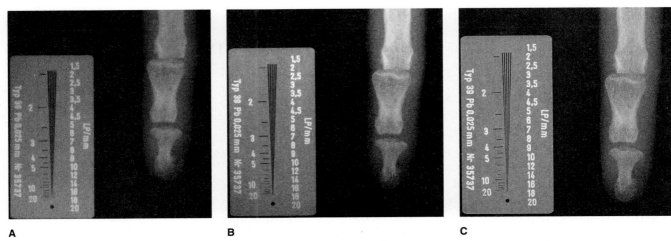

A   B   C

Figure 11–2. *Magnified views of the second phalanx and resolution test pattern.* **(A)** Significant blur or unsharpness of image details; resolution is approximately *6 lp/mm.* **(B)** Improved recorded detail; resolution of approximately 8 lp/mm. **(C)** Best recorded detail (least blur); resolution of approximately 12 *lp/mm.* (From the American College of Radiology Learning File. Courtesy of the American College of Radiology.)

however, determine how easily we are able to recognize those details. In *digital imaging,* the term frequently used to describe this quality is *contrast resolution.*

Each of the factors having an effect on recorded detail will be discussed in the following sections.

Summary

- OID, SID, Focal Spot Size, Motion—all *apply to digital imaging as well as SF imaging.*
- Recorded Detail refers to the sharpness of structural detail borders.
- Recorded detail can be measured using a resolution test pattern and expressed in lp/mm.
- The term used to describe the IR's impact on recorded detail in CR/DR is spatial resolution.
- Distortion relates to the size and/or shape of the *imaged* part compared with the actual size and shape of the *anatomic* object.
- The terms *magnification, elongation,* and *foreshortening* are used when describing distortion.
- Anything that affects density/brightness or contrast affects visibility of detail; in electronic/digital imaging, the term often used to describe this quality is *contrast resolution.*

Distance

If you place your hand between a flashlight and a wall, or any flat surface of a dimly lighted room, the shadow of your hand will vary in *size and clarity* as it changes position with respect to the flashlight and surface. As your hand moves farther from the surface, the shadow becomes larger and less distinct. As your hand is brought closer to the surface

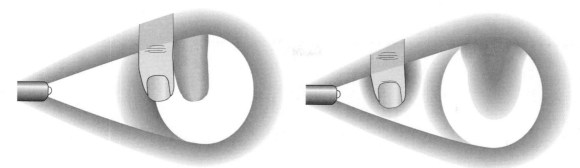

Figure 11–3. *Effect of OID on magnification and detail.* As the finger moves *away* from the surface (toward the light source), the shadow image becomes *magnified* and *blurry*.

(and farther from the flashlight), the shadow becomes more like the actual size of your hand and appears with more clarity (Fig. 11–3).

OID. The above experiment and Figure 11–3 illustrate the effect *OID* has on recorded detail. Because (like visible light) the x-ray beam diverges as it leaves its source, an increase in OID will increase *magnification.* X-ray photons strike all parts of the object, continue traveling in a divergent fashion, and "deposit" the (now magnified and unsharp) image on the IR (Fig. 11–4). *Geometrically recorded detail improves as OID decreases.*

OID has a much greater effect on magnification than SID. The significance of the effect can be realized when recalling that each inch of OID is remedied by seven inches increase in SID!

SID. A similar example can be used to show the effect of *SID* on image geometry and recorded detail. If your hand is placed at a given distance from the flat surface, any change in the *distance between the light source and surface* will affect the magnification and clarity of the shadow image. As the flashlight moves closer to your hand, the shadow will become larger and less distinct. As the flashlight is moved farther from the surface, the shadow approaches the actual size of your hand and becomes sharper and more distinct (Fig. 11–5). Similarly, as the distance between the x-ray source and IR increases, the x-ray image is less magnified and more distinct (Fig. 11–6). *Geometrically recorded detail improves as SID increases.*

Summary

- Recorded detail and magnification are *inversely* related, that is, recorded detail *increases* as magnification *decreases.*
- SID and OID regulate magnification and therefore influence the geometric properties, and hence recorded detail, of the radiographic image.
- SID is *inversely* related to magnification (↑ SID = ↓ magnification) and *directly* related to recorded detail (↑ SID = ↑ recorded detail).
- OID is *directly* related to magnification (↑ OID = ↑ magnification) and *inversely* related to recorded detail (↑ OID = ↓ recorded detail).
- Changes in OID impact detail more significantly than similar changes in SID.

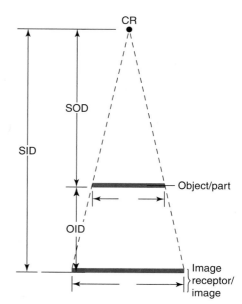

Figure 11–4. As distance from the object to the image receptor (OID) increases, the projected size of the image increases, that is, magnification increases.

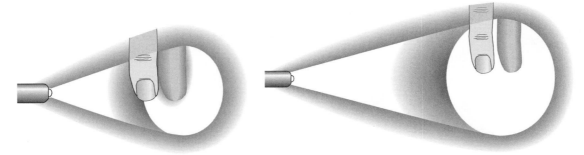

Figure 11–5. *Effect of SID on magnification and detail*. As the light source moves closer to the finger, the shadow image becomes magnified and blurry.

Patient Factors

A certain amount of object unsharpness is an inherent part of every radiographic image because *of the position and shape of anatomic structures within the body*.

Structure Position. Structures within the three-dimensional human body lie in different planes. For example, the frontal sinuses are more anterior than the sphenoids, the ureters are more anterior than the kidneys, the upper renal poles lie in a plane posterior to the lower renal

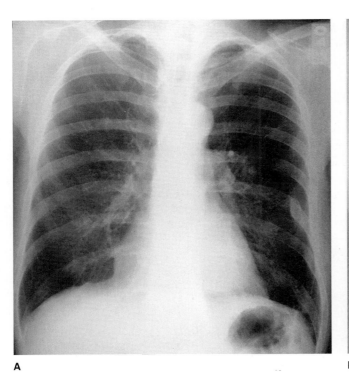

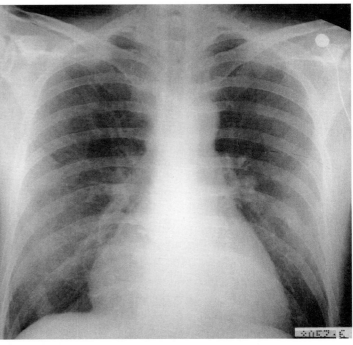

A

B

Figure 11–6. **(A)** *Posteroanterior* (PA) erect chest taken at a distance of 6 *feet* demonstrates an accurate representation of the heart shadow and various parenchymal and bony structures. **(B)** *Anteroposterior* (AP) erect at 50 *in*. of the same patient taken within 24 hours and with no change in patient condition. The *heart appears markedly larger* (15.5 cm on PA and 20 cm on AP) for two *reasons*: (1) the heart is farther from the image receptor in the AP projection and (2) the SID is decreased; thus, the heart is magnified. (From the American College of Radiology Learning File. Courtesy of the American College of Radiology.)

poles, the fundus of the stomach is more posterior than the body and pylorus, and the posterior portions of the sacroiliac joints are more medial than their anterior portions.

Structural Shape. Additionally, the three-dimensional shape of solid anatomic structures rarely coincides with the shape of the divergent beam. Consequently, some structures are imaged with more inherent distortion than others, and shapes of anatomic structures can be entirely misrepresented. Structures *farther* from the IR will be distorted (i.e., *magnified*) more than those *closer* to the IR.

For the *shape* of anatomic structures to be accurately recorded, the structures must be *parallel* to the x-ray tube and the IR and aligned with the central ray (CR). The shape of anatomic structures lying at an angle within the body or placed away from the CR will be misrepresented on the IR (Fig. 11–7). *There are two types of shape distortion.* If a linear structure is angled within the body, that is, not parallel with the long axis of the part/body and not parallel to the IR, that anatomic structure will appear *smaller*—it will be *foreshortened*. A good example of fore-shortening is demonstrated in the PA projection of the wrist. The curved carpal scaphoid appears smaller than its actual size because of foreshortening. On the other hand, *elongation* occurs when the x-ray tube is angled. This is often used to advantage in radiography. In the Towne method of the skull, the occipital bone is better visualized when the CR is angled 30 degree caudally because the facial bones are projected down away and removed from superimposition on the occipital bone. Similarly, the tortuous sigmoid colon can be "opened up" in the *anteroposterior* (AP) projection by employing a cephalad angle. Thus, distortion can be used to improve visualization of some structures.

Subject/Object Unsharpness Results When:

- Object shape does not coincide with the shape of x-ray beam
- Object plane is not parallel with x-ray tube and/or IR
- Anatomic object(s) of interest are not in the path of the CR
- Anatomic object(s) of interest are a distance from the IR

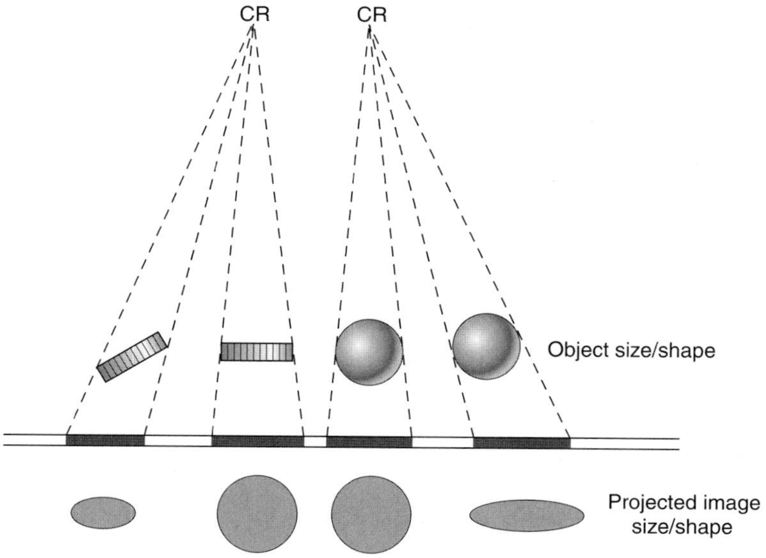

Figure 11–7. The shape of various structures can be radiographically mis-represented (i.e., *foreshortened or elongated*) as a result of their position in the body. That misrepresentation can be exaggerated when the part is away from the central axis of the x-ray beam.

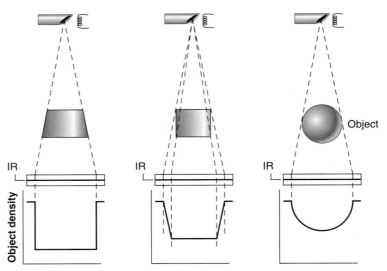

Figure 11–8. Blur or unsharpness results when the *shape* of a three-dimensional object does not coincide with that of the x-ray beam. Blur is accompanied by changes in image density/brightness as a result of differing thicknesses traversed by the x-ray beam.

Image details placed away from the path of the CR will be exposed by more divergent rays, resulting in *rotation distortion*. This is why the CR must be directed to the part of greatest interest. For example, if bilateral hands are requested, it might be better to image them individually; if imaged simultaneously, the CR will be directed to no anatomic part (between the two hands) and rotation distortion will occur.

Unless the edges of a three-dimensional *object* conform to the shape of the x-ray beam, blur or unsharpness will occur at the partially attenuating edge of the object. As Figure 11–8 illustrates, this will be accompanied by changes in radiographic/image density, according to the thickness of areas traversed by the x-ray beam.

Summary

- Some geometric unsharpness is intrinsic because of the shape and position of the structure of interest within the body.
- Structures that do not parallel the x-ray tube and IR and/or that lie outside the central axis of the x-ray beam will be foreshortened or elongated.
- Structures within the body lie at varying distances from the x-ray IR, producing varying degrees of magnification.

Focal Spot Size

Another factor influencing the geometry of the image, and having a significant impact on resolution, is focal spot size. If x-ray photons were emitted from a single point source, structures would be recorded

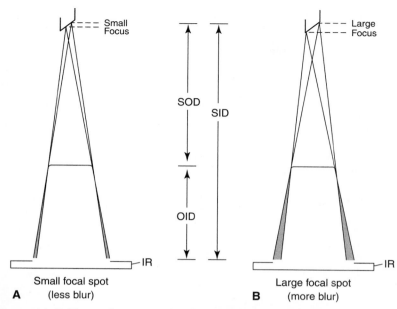

Figure 11–9. X-ray photons emitted from a small but measurable focal spot (**A**) will produce a small zone of blur or unsharpness around each image detail. X-ray photons emitted from a larger focal spot (**B**) will produce a larger degree of unsharpness/blur. The degree of blur is directly related to the *size of the focal spot.*

and resolved with great clarity. However, because x-ray photons emerge from a measurable focus, image details are represented with unsharp edges.

As shown in Figures 11–9 and 11–10, photons emerging from various points on a measurable focal spot are responsible for producing blurred, unsharp edges of anatomic details. The extent or size of the unsharp area is directly related to the focal spot size and OID and inversely related to the SID, that is, unsharpness increases as focal spot size and OID increase and as the SID decreases.

This border of unsharpness around image details is often referred to as *focal spot blur, geometric unsharpness,* or *edge gradient.* The *smaller* the focal spot size, the *better the recorded detail.*

A distinction is made between the *actual focal spot* (AFS) and the *effective (or projected) focal spot* (EFS). The AFS is the finite area on the tungsten target that is actually bombarded by electrons from the filament. The EFS is the foreshortened size of the focus as it is projected down toward the IR. This is called *line focusing* or the *line focus principle* (Fig. 11–11). We generally speak in terms of the effective, or projected, focal spot; manufacturers state EFS size.

The angle of the anode can have a significant effect on recorded detail. Differences in anode angle, all other factors remaining constant, will affect the size of the EFS, as illustrated in Figure 11–11C–E. The AFSs in Figure 11–11C and 11–11D are of the same size, but the anode angle in Figure 11–11D is half of that in Figure 11–11C. Note how much smaller the *effective* or *projected* focal spot is in Figure 11–11D.

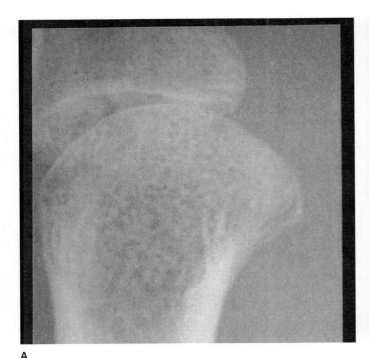
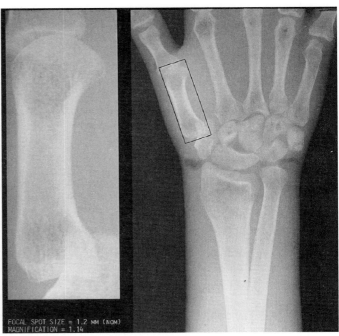

A   B

Figure 11–10. *Effect of focal spot on recorded detail.* Both images were produced using direct exposure technique to better show the effect of focal spot size on detail, independent of the influence of intensifying screens. **(A)** Magnified image of the first metacarpal, made with a 0.6-mm focal spot. Note the blur or unsharpness associated with bony trabeculae, especially noticeable on the magnified image. **(B)** Image made under identical conditions but using a 1.2-mm focal spot; more severe degradation of recorded detail is demonstrated as a result of blur from the use of a larger focal spot. *Note*: Magnification views must be made with a 0.3-mm *(fractional)* focal spot, or smaller, to preserve recorded detail/spatial resolution. (From the American College of Radiology Learning File. Courtesy of the American College of Radiology.)

Hence, when using a very small anode angle, a larger actual anode area can be bombarded (Fig. 11–11E) while maintaining a small EFS. Thus, a "fractional" (0.3 mm or smaller) EFS can be maintained, recorded detail is improved, and anode heat load tolerance is not compromised. This type of x-ray tube is useful in magnification and visualization of small blood vessels.

The size of the EFS, with its associated blur or unsharpness, actually *varies along the length of the IR*, being largest in size (and associated with most blur) at the cathode end of the IR and smallest at the anode end (Figs. 11–12 and 11–13).

If the use of a smaller focal spot size provides us with better recorded detail, why is the smallest available focal spot not always used? Simply because focal spot size is also associated with the buildup of *heat* within the x-ray tube. Large quantities of heat delivered to the x-ray tube, especially in a short period of time, can be very damaging to the tube and can shorten its life span.

If the focal spot is small, heat is confined to a tiny area; localized melting of the target material and anode *pitting* and/or cracking can occur more easily. The larger the focal spot, the greater the surface area available for heat dispersion (via conduction, convection, and radiation). The perfect combination would, of course, be a large actual focus that could withstand heat and still provide a small effective focus for

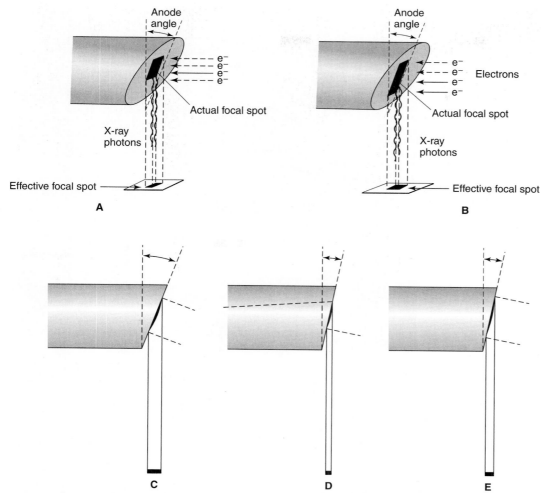

Figure 11–11. (A) and **(B)** Demonstrate how the effective focal spot will differ from the actual focal spot as a result of the *line focus principle*. **(C)** and **(D)** Demonstrate how the *angle*/bevel of the actual focal spot will affect the effective focal spot. **(E)** Demonstrates how a small anode angle combined with a large actual focal spot can result in a small effective focal spot. *The size of the effective focal spot, with its associated blur, actually varies along the length of the image receptor*, being largest at the cathode end of the image receptor and smallest at the anode end (see Figs. 11–12 and 11–13).

optimum-recorded detail. This can be achieved by using an x-ray tube with a small anode *angle* of approximately 7 to 10 degrees. As previously mentioned, the smaller angle enables a larger "face" to be presented to the electron stream, that is, a larger surface area over which to disperse heat (Fig. 11–11). The slight anode angle causes significant foreshortening of the AFS, creating a very small *EFS*.

A difficulty associated with the use of a small anode angle, however, is maintaining a large (14 × 17) field size. The small anode angle produces a pronounced *anode heel effect* (Fig. 11–14). Using a small anode angle, a typical radiographic distance of 40 in. SID, and a 14 × 17-in. IR, there will be approximately 2 in. of unexposed area at the anode end of the image. This can be remedied with an increase in SID, which must be accompanied by an appropriate increase in exposure factors.

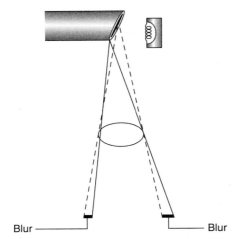

Figure 11–12. Because of the angle of the anode, unsharpness or blur is greatest at the cathode end of the image receptor.

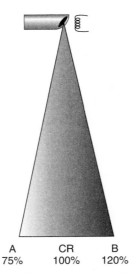

Figure 11–14. *The anode heel effect.* As x-ray photons are produced at the anode focus, a portion of the divergent beam nearest the anode end (**A**) is absorbed by the anode's "heel." This represents a decrease in x-ray beam intensity at the anode side of the x-ray beam. The smaller/steeper the anode angle/bevel, the more pronounced the heel effect.

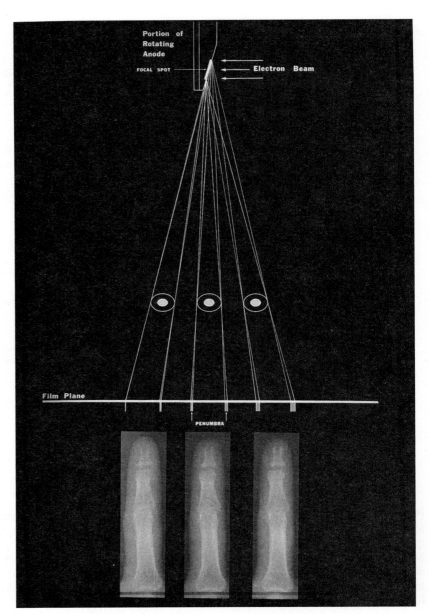

Figure 11–13. *Variation of effective focal spot size along the longitudinal tube axis.* Three images of the third phalanx are shown: one taken at the anode end of the x-ray beam, one at the central portion of the beam, and one at the cathode end. The images clearly illustrate gradual loss of recorded detail toward the cathode end of the x-ray beam. (From the American College of Radiology Learning File. Courtesy of the American College of Radiology.)

Summary

- Focal spot size affects detail by influencing the degree of blur or unsharpness: ↑ focal spot size = ↑ blur = ↓ detail.

- Unsharpness/blur is *directly* related to focal spot size and OID, and *inversely* related to SID.

- The use of a small focal spot improves recorded detail but generates more heat at the anode.

- The effective or projected focal spot size is always smaller than the AFS according to the line focus principle.
- EFS size varies along the longitudinal axis of the IR, being largest at the cathode end and smallest at the anode end of the x-ray beam.
- Smaller anode angles can permit larger AFS sizes while maintaining small EFS sizes—at the expense of accentuating the *anode heel effect*.
- Use of a small anode angle can limit IR coverage at traditional and short SIDs.
- The anode heel effect is most pronounced using large IRs, short SIDs, and small anode angles.

PHOTOGRAPHIC FACTORS

Motion

Motion is probably the greatest challenge to good image detail. Image blur or unsharpness, as a result of motion, can cause severe degradation of recorded detail (Fig. 11–15A). The best method of minimizing *voluntary motion* is through good *communication* and suspended respiration. A patient who understands what to expect and what is expected of him or her is better prepared and more likely to cooperate than a patient whose concerns have been inadequately addressed.

Involuntary motion, such as peristaltic activity, muscle spasms, and heart action, cannot be controlled by the patient. The best way to minimize involuntary motion is by using the shortest possible *exposure time*.

Detail Factors:

- OID
- SID
- SOD
- Focal Spot Size
- Motion
- Distortion
- Structural position and shape *all apply to digital imaging as well as SF imaging.*

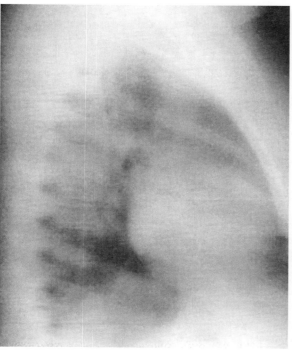

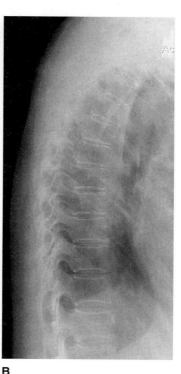

A   B

Figure 11–15. **(A)** Loss of recorded detail as a result of part motion. **(B)** Intentional motion, as a result of respiration during a long exposure, is used to blur ribs and pulmonary vascular markings thereby promoting better visualization of thoracic vertebrae. (Courtesy of Stamford Hospital, Department of Radiology.)

To Minimize Voluntary Motion:

• Good communication
• Suspended respiration

To Minimize Involuntary Motion:

• Short exposure time
• Part support and stabilization
• Special immobilization devices

Motion is often a problem in mobile radiography with machines of limited output (thereby prohibiting the use of short exposure times).

Special positioning devices (such as pediatric immobilizers), positioning sponges, and carefully placed sandbags are frequently used to assist the patient in maintaining the required position.

Equipment motion can cause an effect similar to that caused by patient motion. Bucky/grid motion can cause motion of the part during tabletop examinations; x-ray equipment sometimes has a switch to turn off the bucky/grid when doing tabletop work. Bumping an improperly balanced x-ray tube housing just before making the exposure can result in motion blur or unsharpness if the exposure is made while the x-ray tube is still vibrating.

Motion blur is probably the greatest enemy of recorded detail and is most obvious when the motion is close to the IR (i.e., part motion is more damaging to recorded detail than tube motion) (Fig. 11–16).

Deliberate motion is occasionally used to blur out unwanted structures so that the area of interest can be seen to better advantage. The "breathing techniques" of lateral thoracic spine (see Fig. 11–15B) and transthoracic shoulder are typical examples. Another is the infrequently performed procedure of (conventional) *tomography*, in which a preselected structure plane will be clearly delineated while structures above and below that plane are blurred (see Fig. 11–17).

Summary

• Motion is the greatest adversary of recorded detail.
• Voluntary patient motion can be minimized through good communication.
• Involuntary patient motion is best minimized by using the shortest possible exposure time.
• Various radiographic accessories are available to help minimize both voluntary and involuntary patient motion.
• Equipment motion can also result in loss of recorded detail in the form of image blur.
• Special techniques that introduce motion are sometimes employed to see some structures particularly well.

Intensifying Screens

In the very early days of radiography, before *intensifying screens* were available, images were produced by exposure of photographic emulsion to x-rays alone. Tremendously lengthy exposures were required for even the smallest parts; the very famous image of Mrs. Röntgen's hand was probably a 20+ minute exposure! These exposures took their toll on the fragile, scarcely understood equipment and, of course, on the unsuspecting victims of excessive radiation exposure. Intensifying screens are a component of SF imaging only—*they are not a component of digital imaging.*

In 1896, Thomas Edison developed the *calcium tungstate* intensifying screen that served to reduce the required to reduce the required exposure to a fraction of the original exposure. Calcium tungstate screens gained wide acceptance during World War I and were used almost exclusively until the advent of *rare earth phosphors* in the early 1970s.

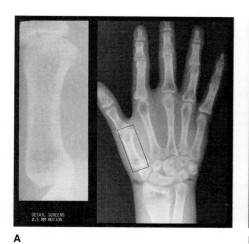
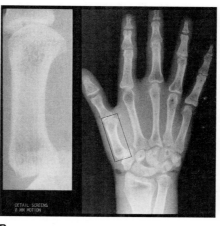
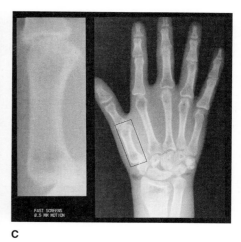

A **B** **C**

Figure 11–16. (A) Image made using 100 speed system; 0.5 mm of motion was introduced. Motion blur is noticeable, particularly in the magnified view of the first metacarpal. Compare the recorded detail of image A with that of image B. (B) Also made using 100 speed but having no motion. (C) Made with 400 speed and 0.5-mm motion. Note how much more obvious detail loss becomes with a faster imaging system. (From the American College of Radiology Learning File. Courtesy of the American Collegeof Radiology.)

The active ingredient in intensifying screens is the fluorescent *phosphor* that functions to change x-ray photon energy to fluorescent light energy. More than *98% of the exposure received by the film emulsion is from fluorescent light* emitted by intensifying screen phosphors. For every x-ray photon absorbed by the phosphor, many light photons are emitted. They *intensify* the action of x-rays and permit the use of much smaller exposures.

In the production of intensifying screens, phosphors are powdered and mixed with a transparent binding substance. A somewhat reflective plastic base material is used as a support upon which the phosphor mixture is spread—this is called the *phosphor layer* or *active layer* (Fig. 11–18).

Rare Earth Phosphors

Gadolinium

Lanthanum

Yttrium

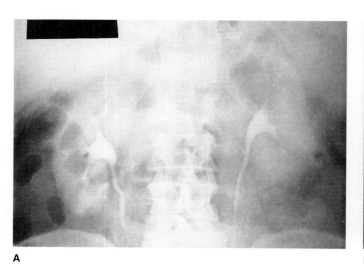
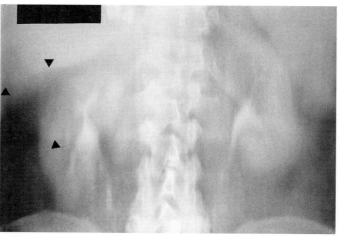

A **B**

Figure 11–17. (A) Plain IVU image with no visible abnormalities. (B) An 8-cm tomographic section of the same patient clearly depicting a 7-cm renal cyst overlying the R midrenal cortex. (From the American College of Radiology Learning File. Courtesy of the American College of Radiology.)

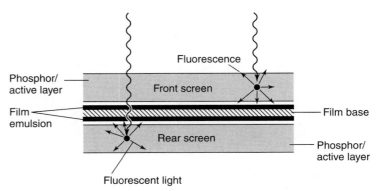

Figure 11–18. *A cross section of screens and film.* The illustration shows how duplitized x-ray film is sandwiched between two intensifying screens. Phosphors of the adjacent intensifying screens absorb x-ray energy and convert it to fluorescent light, which then exposes the neighboring film emulsion as shown in Figure 11–19.

Different phosphors have different x-ray absorbing and fluorescent light-emitting properties. A particular phosphor's ability to absorb x-ray energy and convert it to fluorescent light energy is referred to as its *conversion efficiency* (CE). Phosphors having greater sensitivity (i.e., speed) have greater CE.

Factors that contribute to the speed of intensifying screens include the type of phosphor, phosphor size, active/phosphor layer thickness, and reflective backing.

Phosphors. Phosphors with a *high atomic number* react to x-ray photons more efficiently and possess greater speed. This is referred to as *detective quantum efficiency* (DQE). The more fluorescent light each phosphor emits, the greater its Conversion Efficiency (CE) and speed.

Fluorescence should terminate at the same time as the x-ray source; continued fluorescence is termed *lag* and contributes to an overexposed image. The color light emitted must match the sensitivity of the film emulsion used. This is known as *spectral matching.* Blue-emitting screens must be matched with blue sensitive film; green-emitting screens must be matched with green sensitive film.

Phosphorescence refers to the luminescence from fluoroscopic screen phosphors (cesium iodide; zinc cadmium sulfide). Their unique characteristic is brief lingering luminescence *after* the termination of x-ray (*afterglow*)—permitting continued viewing of the part without additional exposure.

Rare earth phosphors possess a high DQE and CE. The rare earth phosphors used in radiography are oxysulfides and oxybromides of *lanthanum, gadolinium,* and *yttrium.* The phosphors used in fluoroscopy are *cesium iodide* and *zinc cadmium sulfide.*

Speed Charcteristics. Screen speed is directly related to phosphor size, phosphor layer thickness, and degree of reflective backing. As each of these increases, there is a greater number of light photons directed toward the film emulsion. Some manufacturers incorporate a *dye* in the

---

Intensifying Screen Speed Increases As:

- Phosphor size increases
- Active/phosphor layer thickness increases
- Phosphor sensitivity increases
- Screen reflectance increases but, *as screen speed increases,*
- Recorded Detail Decreases

Recorded Detail/Spatial Resolution Increases As:

- Focal spot size decreases
- SID increases
- OID (magnification) decreases
- Motion decreases
- (Shape) distortion decreases
- Screen speed decreases

phosphor layer that functions to reduce light *diffusion*, thus improving resolution.

Loss of recorded detail may be a result of intensifying screen blur or unsharpness. Fluorescent light emerging from the phosphors diffuses and spreads over a larger area (Fig. 11–19). It is this diffusion of fluorescent light that causes indistinct, blurry anatomic details. The degree of diffusion, and hence, the degree of blurriness, is primarily dependent on the factors that regulate intensifying screen speed (Fig. 11–20).

Another way intensifying screens have a significant impact on recorded detail is through *screen/film contact*. Imperfect contact results in blurriness that severely degrades recorded detail (Fig. 11–21A). Causes of poor contact include damaged cassette frames and foreign bodies in the cassette. Areas of poor contact allow light to diffuse over a larger area, thus exaggerating screen blur. Proper care of intensifying screens includes periodic evaluation of screen contact by using a specially designed *wire mesh* (Fig. 11–21B).

A related problem associated with fast screens is *quantum mottle*. As screen speed and/or kV are increased, mAs may be reduced to such a small amount that image *graininess*, or quantum mottle, becomes a problem (Figs. 11–22 and 11–23). This graininess becomes apparent and increases as the system speed increases.

Summary

- As intensifying screen speed increases, patient dose decreases and x-ray tube life increases.
- Intensifying screen phosphors absorb x-ray photons (DQE) and emit a quantity of fluorescent light (CE); the greater the DQE and CE, the faster the speed screen.
- Fluorescent light is responsible for more than 98% of film emulsion exposure.
- The color light emitted by the phosphors must be correctly matched with the film emulsion sensitivity (spectral matching).
- Higher speed screens produce poorer recorded detail, as a result of greater fluorescent light diffusion.
- Intensifying screen speed is influenced by the type and size of phosphor used, the thickness of the active/phosphor layer, and the degree of base reflectance.
- Quantum mottle is more likely to occur when using fast screens with low mAs and high kV factors.
- Phosphors that continue to fluoresce after the x-ray source has terminated are said to possess "lag" or "afterglow."
- Phosphorescence is associated with fluoroscopic screens.
- Perfect SF contact is required for good detail; screens are tested for SF contact with a specially designed wire mesh.
- Intensifying screens are unrelated to digital imaging.

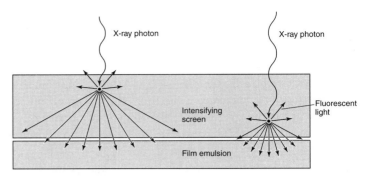

Figure 11–19. Screen thickness and diffusion of fluorescent light versus recorded detail. As intensifying screen thickness increases, the film is exposed by diffused light from distant phosphors. The phosphors of thinner intensifying screens fluoresce closer to the film; therefore, light is diffused to a lesser degree and recorded detail is maintained.

VISIBILITY FACTORS

Factors affecting density and contrast in SF imaging have little to no effect on similar characteristics seen in digital x-ray images. Though its use is rapidly declining, there are still some SF systems in use and our certification exam specifications still require some knowledge of this system.

In order to understand the fundamentals of these imaging factors and characteristics, SF imaging with its terminology will be reviewed first. Digital imaging review will follow.

Density: SF Imaging

Radiographic, or image density is defined as the overall amount of blackening on a radiographic image or a particular portion of the image.

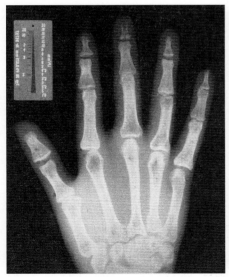
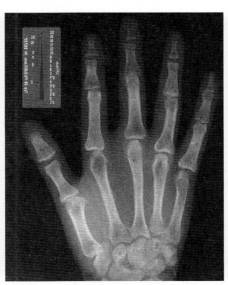
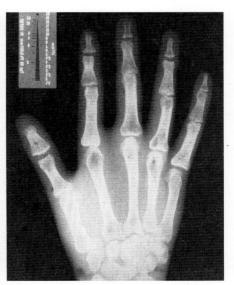

A   B   C

Figure 11–20. Imaging system speed versus required exposure and resolution. Image *A* was made without intensifying screens but required 128 mAs exposure. Image *B* was made using 100 speed screens and 10 mAs exposure. Image *C* was made with 400 speed screens and 1.33 mAs exposure. Note the progressive loss of recorded detail accompanying the increase in system speed. (From the American College of Radiology Learning File. Courtesy of the American College of Radiology.)

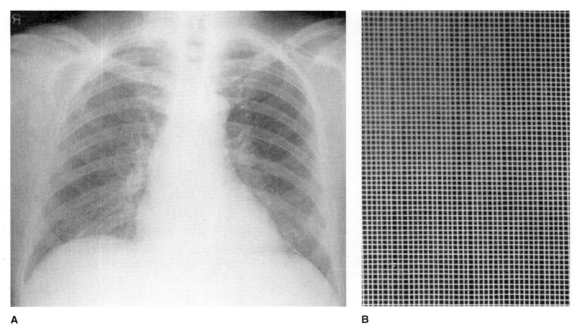

A   **B**

Figure 11–21. *Demonstration of poor SF contact.* (A) Blur as a consequence of poor SF contact in the apical region of the chest. (B) Wire mesh test of a different cassette illustrates blur caused by poor film-to-screen contact in the central region of the cassette. (From the American College of Radiology Learning File. Courtesy of the American College of Radiology.)

It provides the correct degree of background blackening for the anatomic image.

Excessive density can obscure image details; insufficient density can mask or simulate pathology. Radiographic density is a *quantitative* factor, that is, it describes an *amount* of image blackening determined by the *number* of x-ray photons used to create the image. Thus, radiographic density is regulated by the *exposure rate* or *number* of x-ray photons reaching the IR.

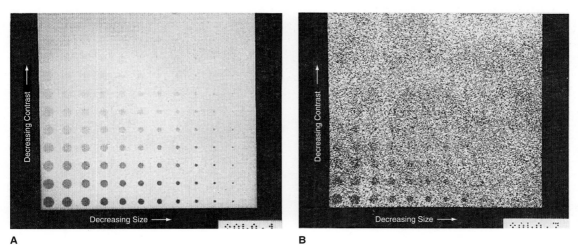

A   **B**

Figure 11–22. (A) and (B) The contrast–detail quality assurance device imaged illustrates the effect of x-ray exposure and resulting quantum mottle. Image *B* was made using a much lower mAs value (fewer x-ray photons) than image *A*; note the striking graininess in *B*. (From the American College of Radiology Learning File. Courtesy of the American College of Radiology.)

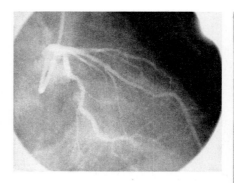
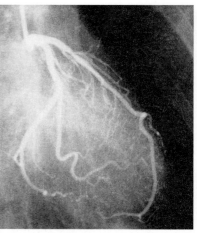

Figure 11–23. Quantum mottle/graininess can make visibility of small vessels difficult. (From the American College of Radiology Learning File. Courtesy of the American College of Radiology.)

In SF imaging, *optical/image density* is generally thought of as being optimal, excessive, or insufficient, when in fact it can be precisely measured and quantified. Optical density can be described as the relationship between the amount of light *incident* upon the film image (i.e., from the illuminator) compared with the amount of light *transmitted* through the film image. This relationship is expressed in the following equation:

$$OD = \log_{10} \frac{I_0 (\text{incident light})}{I_t (\text{transmitted light})}$$

The diagnostically useful range of optical image density is 0.25 to 2.5 (Figs. 11–24 and 11–25).

mAs and Density. Milliampere-seconds (*mAs*) is the *product* of milliamperes (mA) and exposure time (seconds). Technical factors are usually expressed

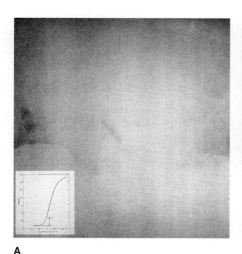
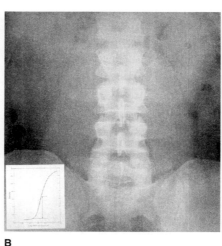
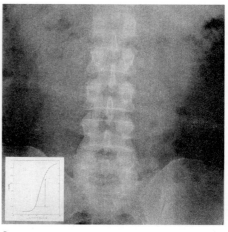

A   B   C

Figure 11–24. **(A–C)** *The diagnostically useful range of optical densities is approximately* 0.25 to 2.5. Note the range of densities visualized on each of these radiographs. **(A)**: density range 0.2 to 0.7 (*too light*); **(B)**: density range 0.5 to 2.3 (*appropriate*); **(C)**: density range 1.2 to 2.9 (*too dark*). (From the American College of Radiology Learning File. Courtesy of the American College of Radiology.)

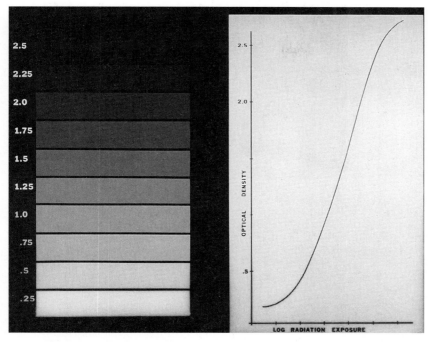

Figure 11–25. A sensitometric curve, like the one above, is used to illustrate the relationship between the x-ray exposure given the *film emulsion* and the resulting density. The study of film emulsion response to exposure is called *sensitometry*. (From the American College of Radiology Learning File. Courtesy of the American College of Radiology.)

in terms of mAs because there are a number of possible combinations of mA and time that will produce the desired mAs.

For example, if 10 mAs is required to produce a given image density, each of the following combinations should produce identical results: 100 mA and 100 msec, 200 mA and 50 msec, 300 mA and 33 msec, 400 mA and 25 msec, and so on. Any combination of mA and time that will produce a given mAs (i.e., a particular *quantity* of x-ray photons) will produce identical image density. This is known as the *reciprocity law.*

Density is a quantitative factor describing the *amount* of image blackening; mAs is a quantitative factor regulating the *number* of x-ray photons produced (i.e., x-ray beam *intensity, exposure rate, quantity*). mAs is the single most important technical factor associated with image density and is the factor of choice for regulating image density.

mAs is directly proportional to image density. If the mAs is doubled, twice the exposure rate and twice the image density results. If the mAs is cut in half, the exposure rate and image density are reduced by half (Fig. 11–26).

An underexposed or overexposed film image requires an mAs increase or decrease of at least 30%. For example, a particular image was produced using 25 mAs and 78 kV and exhibited *somewhat insufficient density*. What factors would be required to produce an image having the desired image density? (25 mAs + 30% = 32.5 mAs).

If the image were *significantly* lacking in density, it would have been appropriate to double the mAs.

Reciprocity Law:

Any combination of mA and exposure time that will produce a particular mAs, will produce identical image density.

Quantitative Terms:

Density

Describes the *amount* of blackening on an x-ray image or a part of the image

mAs

Directly proportional to the *intensity/exposure rate/number* of x-ray photons produced

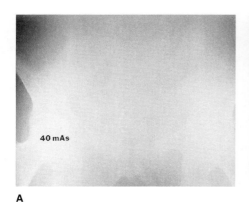
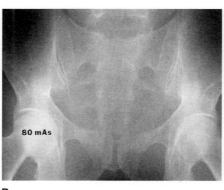
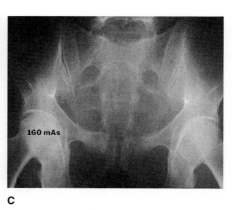

A   B   C

Figure 11–26. *Image density is directly proportional to mAs.* (A) Image made using 40 mAs. (B) Image made of the same subject using 80 mAs, all other factors remaining constant; doubling the mAs has produced twice the image density. (C) Image made using 160 mAs, resulting in another doubling of image density. (From the American College of Radiology Learning File. Courtesy of the American College of Radiology.)

Summary

- mAs is the product of mA and exposure time in seconds.
- Any combination of mA and time that will produce a given mAs will produce identical radiographic density according to the *reciprocity law*.
- Radiographic image density and mAs are quantitative factors and are directly related.
- Doubling the mAs will double the radiographic density; halving the mAs will reduce the density to half.
- At least a 30% change must be made in mAs for there to be a perceptible change in radiographic density.

SID and Density. As a child, you may have been told to "read your book next to the lamp, where you will have more light." Perhaps your youthful eyes could see just fine where you were, but in fact your advisor was correct in saying that more light was available closer to its source (the lamp).

As distance from a light source increases, the light diverges and covers a larger area; the quantity of light available per unit area becomes less and less as distance increases. The intensity (quantity) of light decreases according to the *inverse square law*, that is, the intensity of light at a particular distance from its source is inversely proportional to the square of the distance (Fig. 11–27). For example, if you decreased the distance between your book and the lamp from 6 to 3 feet, you would have four times as much light available.

Similarly, SID has a significant impact on x-ray beam intensity and, hence, radiographic density. *As the distance between the x-ray tube and IR increases, exposure rate (and therefore radiographic density/brightness) decreases according to the inverse square law.*

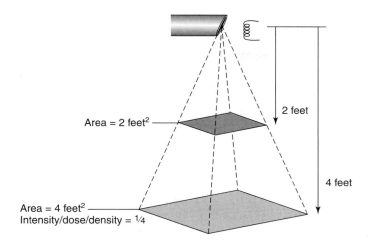

Figure 11–27. *The inverse square law.* Because x-ray beam coverage (area) increases with the square of the distance, the number of x-ray photons per unit area decreases by the same amount.

Notice that according to the *inverse square law*, the exposure rate is *inversely* proportional to the square of the distance, whereas using the *density maintenance formula* to determine new mAs because of diminished exposure rate, mAs is *directly* proportional to the distance squared.

The two equations that will be used are:

$$\frac{I_1}{I_2} = \frac{D_2^2}{D_1^2} \qquad \text{Inverse square}$$

$$\frac{mAs_1}{mAs_2} = \frac{D_1^2}{D_2^2} \qquad \text{Density maintenance formula}$$

In the inverse square law equation, I represents intensity (a quantitative term referring to exposure rate; expressed as R/time or mR/time) and D represents distance (SID). The original intensity is represented by I_1, the original distance squared is represented by D_1^2, and the new distance squared is represented by D_2^2. I_2 represents the new intensity (i.e., the new exposure rate). Note that the relationship is an *inversely proportional* one. Also note that the *opposite* is true in the density maintenance formula, that is, the relationship is *directly* proportional.

An x-ray image made using 12 mAs and 82 kV at 52-in. SID resulted in an exposure rate of 40 mR/min. Another image of the same part will be made at 44-in. SID. What is the exposure rate at the new distance?

Using the inverse square law and substituting known factors,

$$\frac{40}{x} = \frac{1,936}{2,704} \frac{\left(44^2\right)}{\left(52^2\right)}$$

$$1,936x = 108,160$$

$$x = 55.86 \text{ mR / min at } 44'' \text{ SID}$$

> **Use the Inverse Square Law to Determine the New Exposure Rate at a New Distance**
>
> $$\frac{I_1}{I_2} = \frac{D_2^2}{D_1^2}$$

Use the Density Maintenance Formula to Determine the New mAs at a New Distance

$$\frac{mAs_1}{mAs_2} = \frac{D^2}{D_2^2}$$

This illustrates the relationship between distance and x-ray intensity. As the *distance* is *decreased*, the *intensity* of the x-ray beam *increases* (according to the inverse square law). The *resulting increase in radiographic density* will require an adjustment of technical factors, specifically mAs (according to the density maintenance formula), to reproduce the original density.

In the same example (above), what new mAs value will be required at the new distance (44 in.) to maintain the original density?

Using the distance maintenance formula and substituting known factors,

$$\frac{mAs_1}{mAs_2} = \frac{D_1^2}{D_2^2}$$

$$\frac{12}{x} = \frac{2,704}{1,936} \frac{(52^2)}{(44^2)}$$

$$2,704x = 23,232$$

$$x = 8.59 \text{ mAs at } 44'' \text{ SID}$$

At 44-in. SID, 8.59 mAs will be required to produce the same radiographic/image density that was produced at 52-in. SID using 12 mAs.

Summary

- Relatively small changes in SID can have a significant effect on image density.
- As the SID increases, exposure rate and image density decrease.
- With changes in SID, the inverse square law is used to calculate the *new exposure rate*.
- With changes in SID, the density maintenance formula is used to calculate the *new mAs*.

X-ray Photons Can:

- *Penetrate* through the part
- *Scatter* within the part
- Be *absorbed* by the part

kV and Density. As kV is increased, *more* electrons are driven to the anode with greater speed and energy. More high-energy electrons will result in production of *more high-energy x-rays*. Thus, kV affects both quality (energy) and quantity of the x-ray beam. However, although kV and radiographic density are directly *related*, they are not directly proportional, that is, twice the radiographic density does not result from doubling the kV. The effect of kV on quantity is not proportional because an increase in kV produces an increase in photons of *all energies*.

With respect to the effect of kV on image density, the *15% rule* can be used. If it is desired to double the film density, yet impossible to adjust the mAs, a similar effect can be achieved by *increasing the kV by 15%*. Conversely, the density may be reduced to half by decreasing the kV by 15% (Fig. 11–28).

An x-ray image was made using the following technical factors: 400 mA, 25 msec, and 84 kV. It is necessary to produce another image with twice the radiographic density. The maximum mA available is

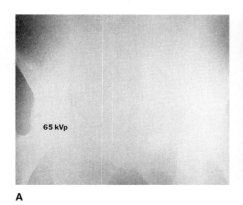
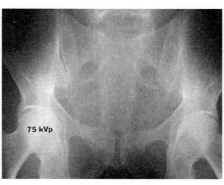
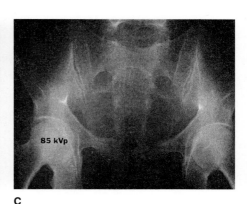

A   B   C

Figure 11–28. *Illustration of the 15% rule.* Image B was made using 15% more kV than image A and demonstrates twice the density of image A. Image C was made using 15% more kV than image B and demonstrates twice the density of image B. (From the American College of Radiology Learning File. Courtesy of the American College of Radiology.)

400 and the exposure time cannot be increased because of involuntary motion. What alternate kV can be employed to produce a radiograph with the desired image density?

If twice the original density is needed, the kV may be increased 15% to produce the desired effect. Fifteen percent of 84 is 12.6. Therefore, using the same mAs and increasing the kV to 97 should produce an image with twice the original density. *Note:* Changing the kV will change the scale of contrast.

Summary

- Increased kV produces *more* high-energy x-ray photons, that is, exposure rate increases.

- An increase in kV will result in an increase in image density; a decrease in kV will result in a decrease in density.

- When mAs manipulation is not possible, density can be doubled or halved by using the 15% rule.

Intensifying Screens and Density. Intensifying screens amplify the effect of x-rays on film emulsion by means of fluorescence. For every one x-ray photon interacting with screen phosphors, many light photons are emitted. This effect becomes more pronounced as screen speed increases.

Therefore, with any given group of exposure factors, as screen speed increases, image density increases.

Screen speed and image density are directly proportional. An increase in intensifying screen speed from 200 to 400 doubles the image density and enables the radiographer to reduce the mAs to half, thus reducing patient dose (Fig. 11–29) and tube wear (heat units) considerably.

Intensifying screens are a component of SF imaging only—*they are not a component of digital imaging.*

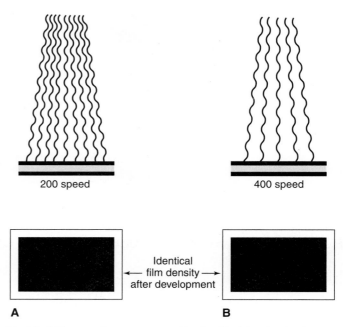

Figure 11–29. 200 speed screens used in *A* with 20 mAs. In *B*, an increase in screen speed to 400 permits an exposure reduction to 10 mAs with the same resulting film density.

Summary

- Intensifying screens amplify the action of x-rays through their property of fluorescence.
- All other factors remaining constant, an increase in screen speed will result in an increase in image density.
- Screen speed and image density are directly proportional; screen speed and patient dose are inversely proportional.
- Screen speed and image resolution/sharpness are inversely related.
- Intensifying screens are a component of SF imaging only—*they are not a component of digital imaging.*

Grids and Density

Use of Grids. As x-ray photons travel through a part, they either pass all the way through to the IR or undergo interaction(s) that result in the photon's either being absorbed by the part or being deviated in direction. Photons that change direction (*scattered radiation*) undermine and degrade the image.

Part III discussed the origin of most scattered radiation: that is, Compton scatter interactions. With respect to radiographic image quality, Compton interaction is responsible for the scattered radiation that reaches the IR. *Scattered radiation* adds unwanted *degrading* densities to the x-ray image.

The single most important way to reduce the production of scattered radiation is to restrict the size of the x-ray field. Although *collimation*, optimum *kV*, and *compression* can be used (Fig. 11–30), a significant amount of scattered radiation is still generated within the part being imaged and can have a severely deleterious effect on image quality, as illustrated in the pelvis images shown in Figure 11–31.

A *grid* is a device interposed between the part and IR that functions to absorb a large percentage of scattered radiation before it reaches the IR. It is constructed of alternating strips of lead foil and radiolucent filler material. X-ray photons traveling in the same direction as the primary beam pass between the lead strips. X-ray photons, having undergone interactions within the body and deviated in various directions, are absorbed by the lead strips; this is referred to as "cleanup" of scattered radiation (Fig. 11–32).

The use of grids is recommended for body parts measuring 10 cm and greater. The major exception to this rule is the chest, which can frequently be examined without a grid because its contents (mostly air) do not generate significant quantities of scattered radiation. Even so, many institutions perform most chest examinations using a grid and high-kV factors.

When imaging large body parts without the use of a grid, scattered radiation contributes to more than 50% of the total IR exposure. If a grid is introduced, there will be significantly *fewer* photons reaching the IR, hence a very significant decrease in radiographic *density*. To maintain adequate density then, the addition of a grid must be accompanied by an appropriately substantial increase in *mAs*. Before beginning a discussion of the impact of grids on technical factors, a more complete study of them is in order.

Types of Grids. A grid may be *stationary* or *moving*. Stationary grids are the simplest type and consist of alternating *vertical* lead strips (i.e., a *parallel* grid) and radiolucent interspace filler material. A grid cassette is an example of a stationary grid. Another example is the "slip-on," or

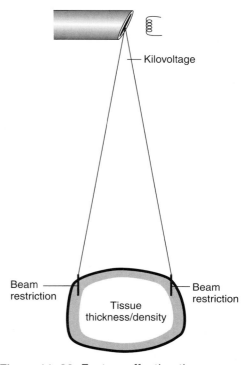

Figure 11–30. *Factors affecting the production of scattered radiation:* kV level, beam restriction, and thickness and density of tissues.

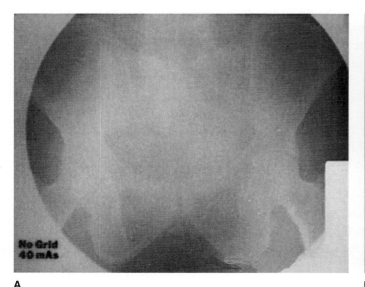

A

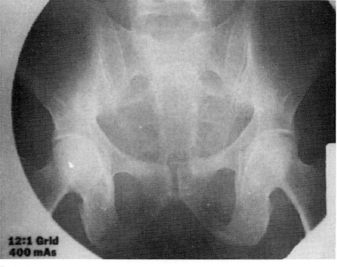

B

Figure 11–31. **(A)** Image made at 40 mAs without a grid. Because of the thickness and nature of the part imaged, a significant amount of scattered radiation was generated and exposed the (undiagnostic) film. **(B)** Image made using a 12:1 grid. Although an exposure increase to 400 mAs was required, a large percentage of the scattered radiation generated was removed before it reached the image receptor. (From the American College of Radiology Learning File. Courtesy of the American College of Radiology.)

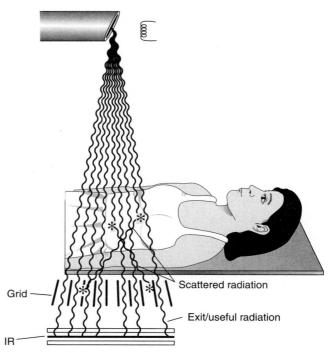

Figure 11–32. Scattered radiation generated in the object is removed with the use of a grid.

Origin of Scattered Radiation and Methods for Controlling Its Production

- The larger the x-ray field size, the more SR produced. *Solution:* collimate!

- The higher the kV, the greater the production of SR (a result of the higher incidence of Compton scatter interactions). *Solution:* use optimum kV.

- The thicker and more dense the body tissues, the greater the amount of SR produced. *Solution:* when possible, part compression or use of prone position to decrease effect of fatty abdominal tissue.

Grids can be:

- Parallel or focused
- Stationary or moving

"wafer," grid that may be placed over a regular cassette. *Stationary grids* are useful in mobile radiography and horizontal beam (cross-table lateral) radiography; they are usually low ratio. A potential disadvantage of stationary grids is visibility of grid lines.

A *moving grid* is in motion during the exposure, and grid lines are effectively blurred out of the radiographic image. The lead strips and interspace material of a moving grid are slightly *angled* so that, at a given distance from the focal spot, the angle of the lead strips will conform with the divergence of the x-ray beam. A grid with lead strips angled thus is called a *focused grid*; if an imaginary line is extended up from each lead strip, the point of intersection is called the *convergence line*, and the distance from the convergence line to the surface of the grid is the *focusing distance* (Fig. 11–33). That focusing distance is the ideal SID, although grids usually specify a *focal range* in which they can be safely used.

Another type of grid is the *crossed grid*; it has a second series of lead strips aligned perpendicular to the first. Crossed grids may be parallel or focused and are extremely efficient in absorbing scattered radiation; however, their use prohibits any x-ray tube angulation and requires that the x-ray tube be exactly centered to the center of the grid. Any misalignment or tube angulation can result in severe *grid cutoff* (absorption of the useful beam). Crossed grids are not frequently used in general radiography.

Grid Errors. Care must be taken to avoid errors common to the use of focused grids, including angulation errors, off-level errors, off-focus errors, off-center errors, and upside-down grid placement.

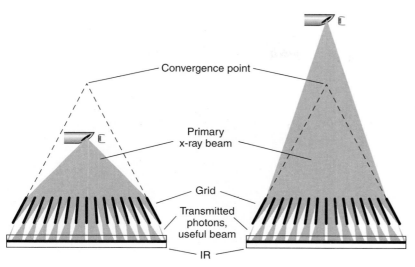

Figure 11–33. Grid cutoff will be apparent if the SID is above or below the specified focal range limits and will be characterized by density loss at the periphery of the image. This is described as an *off-focus error* or *focus–grid distance decentering.*

- *Angulation errors:* The x-ray tube may be safely angled in the direction of the lead strips; angulation "against" the lead strips causes *grid cutoff,* that is, absorption of the useful beam with resulting loss of density across the image.

- *Off-level errors:* If the planes of the x-ray tube and grid surface are not parallel, *grid cutoff* will occur. This can happen if the x-ray tube is angled "against" the lead strips or if the grid cassette is tilted under the patient during mobile radiography. To avoid cutoff, the grid surface must be perpendicular to the central ray and, if CR angulation is required, that the tube angle is parallel with the direction of the lead strips.

- *Off-focus errors:* If the SID is below the lower limits, or above the upper limits, of the specified focal range—*grid cutoff* will occur. This type of error is also referred to as *focus–grid distance decentering.* Off focus errors are usually characterized by loss of density at the *periphery* of the image.

- *Off-center errors:* If the x-ray beam is not centered to the grid (i.e., if it is shifted laterally), *grid cutoff* will occur. This type of error is referred to as lateral decentering and characterized by a *uniform density loss* across the radiographic image (Fig. 11–34).

If the x-ray beam is both off-center *and* off-focus *below* the focusing distance, the portion of the image below the focus will show *increased* density; if the x-ray beam is off-center *and* off-focus *above* the focusing distance, the image below the focus will show *decreased* density.

- *Upside-down grid:* A focused grid placed upside down has its lead strips angled exactly opposite the path/direction of the x-ray beam. So, except for the central area where the lead strips and x-ray beam are vertical, *grid cutoff* will be severe (Fig. 11–35).

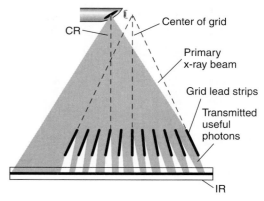

Figure 11–34. *A uniform density loss* across the radiographic image will occur if the x-ray beam is off-center laterally.

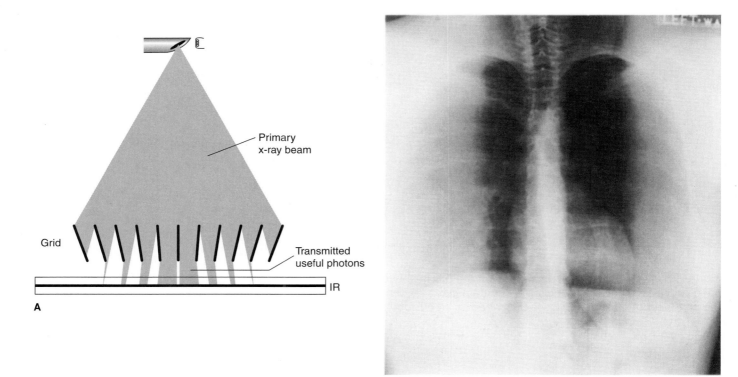

Figure 11–35. **(A,B)** An *upside-down focused grid* presents its lead strips in the opposite direction to that of the x-ray beam. This results in severe grid cutoff everywhere except in the central portion of the radiographic image.

Figure 11–36. Cross section of a grid. *Grid ratio* is defined as the height of the lead strips (*H*) to width of the interspace material (*W*). Grid ratio = *H/W*.

Grid Characteristics. Two of a grid's *physical characteristics* that determine its degree of efficiency in the removal of scattered radiation are grid ratio and number of lead strips per inch.

• *Grid ratio:* Grid ratio is defined as the height of the lead strips compared with the distance between them (Fig. 11–36):

$$\text{Grid ratio} = \frac{\text{Height of Pb strip}}{\text{Width of interspace material}}.$$

For example, a grid having lead strips 1.5-mm tall separated by interspace material 0.15-mm wide has a grid ratio of 10:1.

As the lead strips are made taller, or the distance between them decreases, scattered radiation is more likely to be trapped before reaching the IR. A 12:1 ratio grid will absorb more scattered radiation than an 8:1 ratio grid.

• *Number of lead strips per inch:* The number of lead strips per inch is also referred to as *grid frequency*. The advantage of many lead strips per inch is that there is less *visibility* of the lead strips. As the number of lead foil strips per inch increases, the lead foil strips must become *thinner*, and therefore *less visible*. There is, of course, a disadvantage here. If the lead strips get thinner, more energetic scattered radiation can pass through them and reach the IR. So, to maintain the efficiency of a grid having many lead strips per inch, its grid *ratio* is often increased as well, that is, the lead strips are made taller to increase the likelihood of their trapping scattered radiation before it reaches the IR.

The radiolucent interspace material is most frequently made of plastic or fiber, particularly in pediatric imaging and mammography; some grids use aluminum as the interspace material. Aluminum is sturdier; it gives the image a smoother appearance free of objectionable *grid lines* and can perhaps have an additional filtering effect on scattered radiation. However, a greater increase in patient dose is required with aluminum interspaced grids.

Other ways of expressing and measuring grid efficiency include the following:

- *Grid factor*—the *grid factor* (G) of a particular grid is the ratio of the total amount of radiation (primary and scattered) incident upon the surface of the grid compared with the amount of radiation transmitted through the grid:

$$G = \frac{\text{Incident total}}{\text{Transmitted total}}$$

The grid factor is the grid conversion factor, that is, that amount by which the mAs must be changed to compensate for the radiation absorbed by the grid (Fig. 11–37). This is discussed in further detail later in this section.

- *Contrast improvement factor*—the ratio of radiographic contrast obtained with a grid compared with the contrast obtained without a grid is referred to as the contrast improvement factor (CIF). Grids have a major impact on contrast resolution:

$$CIF = \frac{\text{Contrast with grid}}{\text{Contrast without grid}}.$$

- *Selectivity*—the ratio between the quantity of *useful photons transmitted* through the grid and the quantity of *scattered photons transmitted* is referred to as the selectivity (S) of the grid:

$$S = \frac{\text{Useful photon transmission}}{\text{Scattered photon transmission}}.$$

An undesirable but unavoidable characteristic of grids is that they do absorb some useful photons as well as scattered photons. The higher the grid ratio, the more pronounced this will be. The higher the useful to scattered photon transmission ratio, the more desirable the grid.

- *Lead content*—this is perhaps least familiar to the radiographer because it applies little to the practical use of the grid. While the definitions of *grid ratio* and *grid frequency* do not take into account the thickness of the lead strip, the term *lead content* does express this. Lead content is measured in g/cm^2 and expresses the amount of lead contained within a particular grid.

How must exposure factors be adjusted to maintain appropriate density when changing from nongrid to grid? How can exposure factors be changed to preserve the density level when changing from one ratio grid to another?

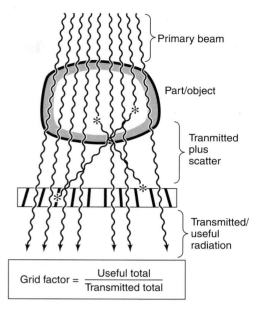

Figure 11–37. The grid factor (G) is the *grid conversion factor* and expresses the x-ray quantity/exposure at the grid surface compared to the quantity of x-ray transmitted through the grid.

Grid Conversion Factors for Various Ratio Grids

Grid ratio	Conversion factor
No grid	1
5:1	2
6:1	3
8:1	4
10 or 12:1	5
16:1	6

In actual practice, the grid conversion factor varies slightly according to kV range used. The ARRT recognizes that different textbooks cite slightly different grid conversion factors and has stated that the distractors in calculation problems will not be so close as to cause conflict with the keyed correct answer. The conversion factors listed in the accompanying table are probably the most commonly used factors and can be used to calculate grid conversions in exposure factor problems.

Example:

A particular examination was performed tabletop/nongrid at 40-in. SID using 7 mAs and 90 kV. To reduce the amount of image-degrading scattered radiation, another image will be made using a 12:1 ratio grid. What new mAs factor will be required to maintain the original level of radiographic/image density?

The grid conversion formula is:

$$\frac{mAs_1}{mAs_2} = \frac{Grid\ factor_1}{Grid\ factor_2}.$$

Substituting known quantities

$$\frac{7}{x} = \frac{1}{5}$$

$$x = 35\ mAs\ required\ with\ 12:1\ grid.$$

Example:

A lumbar spine was imaged laterally at 40-in. SID using 40 mAs and 95 kV and an 8:1 ratio grid. To improve scattered radiation cleanup, another image will be made using a 12:1 grid. What new mAs factor will be required to maintain the original level of radiographic/ image density?

Using the grid conversion formula shown above and substituting known quantities,

$$\frac{40}{x} = \frac{4}{5}$$

$$4x = 200$$

$$x = 50\ mAs\ required\ with\ 12:1\ grid.$$

In general, an 8:1 grid is satisfactory for radiography up to 90 kV. A 16:1 grid ratio is frequently advocated for radiography greater than 100 kV. General radiographic fixed equipment usually has a 10:1 or 12:1 grid.

The use of high-ratio grids at low-kV levels is discouraged because of the unnecessary patient exposure required. Higher-ratio grids are more effective in reducing the amount of scattered radiation reaching the IR; however, their use requires more mAs and decreases positioning latitude (of the x-ray tube). Lower-ratio grids (5:1, 6:1) are often used in mobile imaging because they offer more (grid) positioning latitude.

Remember, to avoid detrimental changes in radiographic density, mAs adjustments are essential when changing grid ratios.

A word of caution regarding the use of an *inverted (SF) cassette* in place of a grid: the results are unpredictable and this practice is discouraged. Appropriate selection and careful use of a grid provides a far more predictable outcome and a diagnostically superior radiographic image. An inverted computed radiography (CR) image plate produces characteristic artifacts on the processed image.

An *air gap* introduced between the object and IR can have an effect similar to that of a grid. As energetic scattered radiation emerges from the body, it continues to travel in its divergent fashion and, much of the time, will bypass the IR (Fig. 11–38). A 6-in. air gap produces an effect similar to an 8:1 grid, while a 10-in. air gap is equivalent to a 16:1 grid. It is necessary to increase the SID to reduce the magnification caused by the air gap/OID.

Summary

- Scattered radiation is a result of x-ray photon interaction with tissue via Compton scattering processes.

- Scattered radiation adds quality-degrading densities to the radiographic image (increased density and lower contrast).

- The production of scattered radiation increases with increases in field size, kV, thickness, and volume of tissue.

- The single most important way to decrease the production of scattered radiation is to limit the field size, that is, collimate.

- The amount of scattered radiation reaching the IR is decreased through the combined use of collimators and grids.

- Grids are made of alternating strips of lead and radiolucent material; they are placed between the patient and IR to absorb scattered radiation exiting from the part.

- Grids may be stationary or moving, parallel, or focused.

- Focused grids require that
  - the correct surface be facing the x-ray tube (i.e., not upside down)
  - tube angulation parallels the lead strips, that the long axis of the x-ray tube and grid surface are parallel, that the SID should be within the stated focusing distance/range
  - the x-ray beam should not be off-center (laterally) with the center of the grid.

- If focused grid requirements are not met, the resulting image will demonstrate a loss of density as a consequence of grid cutoff (i.e., absorption of the useful beam).

- The most common way of expressing grid efficiency is by grid ratio and number of lead strips per inch.

- Because grids remove many x-ray photons that would have contributed to image density, the addition of a grid requires a significant increase in mAs.

- When implementing a grid or changing grid ratio, a grid-conversion factor must be used to determine required mAs change to avoid undesirable changes in radiographic/image density.

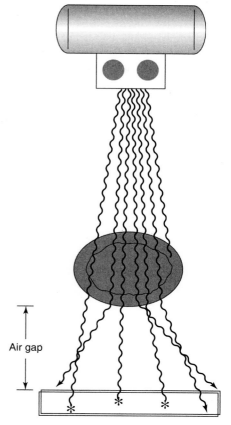

Figure 11–38. Air-gap technique. As scattered radiation emerges from the part, it continues to travel in its divergent fashion, bypassing the image receptor.

Filtration:

- Reduces patient skin dose
- Minimum 2.5-mm Al equivalent
- Inherent × added = total filtration
- Increases overall average energy of x-ray beam

Compensating Filtration:

- Used for anatomic parts having very different thickness/absorption properties
- Used to "balance" tissue densities; improves visualization of all tissues

Filtration and Density. As discussed in Chapter 8, the primary beam generally has a total filtration of 2.5-mm Al equivalent for patient protection purposes. In general-purpose radiographic tubes, the glass envelope usually accounts for approximately 0.5-mm Al equivalent, and the collimator provides approximately 1.0-mm Al equivalent. These are considered *inherent filtration.* The manufacturer adds another 1.0-mm Al (*added filtration*) to meet the minimum requirements of 2.5-mm Al equivalent total filtration for radiographic tubes operated above 70 kV.

This type of filter serves to remove the diagnostically useless x-ray photons that contribute only to patient (skin) dose. Because this radiation is "soft" (low energy) and would not reach the IR anyway, the x-ray tube total filtration *has no effect on image density.* Filtration increases the *overall average energy* of the x-ray beam.

Compensating filters can be used to provide more uniform radiographic density when imaging structures having widely different *attenuation coefficients* (x-ray absorbing properties) because of thickness or tissue composition. Usually made of aluminum or clear plastic, they slide into tracks in the collimator housing similar to a cylinder cone or attach magnetically to the undersurface of the collimator housing.

If a SF x-ray image of a foot demonstrates well-exposed tarsals, the toes will frequently be overexposed (Fig. 11–39A). If the exposure is adjusted to improve the image of the toes, the tarsals will then be underexposed. Because the foot varies so greatly in thickness and tissue density along its long axis, it is difficult to achieve uniform image density. A simple *wedge*-shaped compensating filter can remedy the situation (Figs. 11–39E, 11–40B, and 11–40C). The filter is attached to the collimator housing so that the thin portion is over the tarsals and the thick portion over the toes. Exposure factors appropriate for tarsals are used, and the thick portion of the filter removes enough of the primary beam to prevent overexposure of the toes. Thus, a foot image having uniform density throughout is achieved (Figs. 11–39A and 11–39B). A wedge filter is also useful for femur examinations and decubitus abdomen images (Figs. 11–39C and 11–39D).

Another type of compensating filter is the *trough* filter (Fig. 11–40A), so named because its central portion is thin and the portions extending laterally are thicker, thus forming a central trough. A trough filter can be used in chest radiography to permit visualization of the more dense mediastinal structures without overexposing the more radiolucent lungs and pulmonary vascular markings.

Another simple, yet effective, application of compensating filtration is the use of a saline or similar solution bag. The saline bag is placed over the thinner body part and serves to filter out excessive exposure. This technique is effectively employed in the AP projection of the thoracic spine; however, its use should be noted as it can cause a slight image artifact.

Balancing uneven tissue densities is less problematic in digital imaging. Probably the single greatest advantage of digital imaging is its contrast resolution.

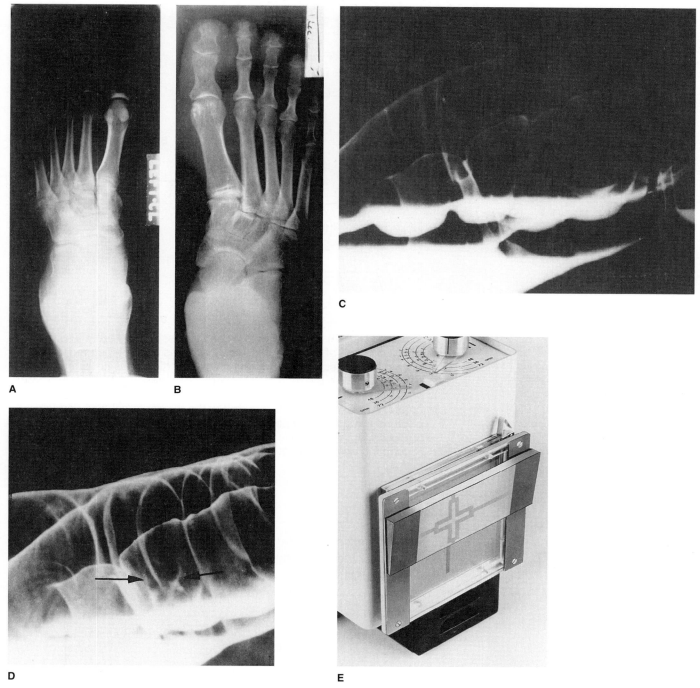

Figure 11–39. (A) Typical foot imaged without the use of a *compensating filter*; although the tarsals and metatarsals are well demonstrated, the phalanges are significantly overexposed. (B) Image made using a compensating filter whose thicker portion was placed over the phalanges to balance radiographic densities. (C) Lateral decubitus image of an air- and barium-filled colon. Abdominal tissues often shift to the dependent side in the decubitus position, making the "down" side thicker than the "up" side. Excessive density of the air-filled structures can obliterate pathology. (D) Use of a wedge-shaped compensating filter can equalize tissue density differences, thus providing more uniform radiographic/image density and improved visualization of any pathology (a polypoid lesion is demonstrated). (E) Compensating (wedge) filter magnetically attached to the x-ray collimator housing. (Courtesy of Nuclear Associates.)

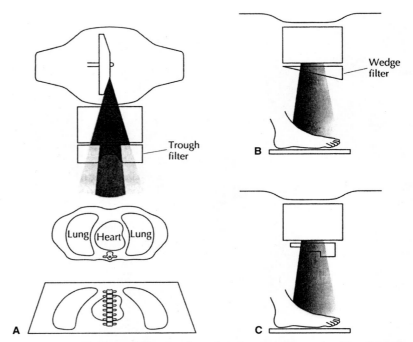

Figure 11–40. (A) *Trough filter* in place for chest radiography. The thicker lateral portions of the trough reduce the intensity of the beam directed toward the lungs, while the thinner central portion does not attenuate the beam directed to the more dense mediastinal structures. (B,C) Two types of *wedge filters* used to "graduate" the x-ray beam intensity, with a greater number of photons directed to the thicker tarsal area and fewer photons toward the thinner areas of metatarsals and phalanges. (Reproduced, with permission, from Shephard CT. *Radiographic Image Production and Manipulation.* New York: McGraw-Hill, 2003.)

Summary

- When anatomic parts vary greatly in thickness or tissue composition, compensating filters may be used to "even out" radiographic densities.
- Protective x-ray tube filtration of 2.5-mm Al has no effect on radiographic/image density.
- Compensating filters slide into place by means of tracks on the collimator housing.
- Compensating filters are available in various shapes: their thicker portions absorb more of the x-ray beam and are therefore placed over thinner body parts, while their thinner portions (absorbing fewer x-rays) are placed over thicker body parts.

Patient Factors and Density. Normal tissue variants and pathologic processes that alter tissue thickness and composition can have a significant effect on image density. The radiographer must be aware of these variants and processes to make an appropriate and accurate selection of technical factors.

In 1916, R. Walter Mills presented an article at the American Roentgen Ray Society meeting in Chicago (published in *American Journal of Roentgenology*, April 1917) describing "The Relation of Bodily Habitus to Visceral Form, Position, Tonus and Motility." In his article, he coined the terms *hypersthenic*, *sthenic*, *hyposthenic*, and *asthenic* (defined in Chapter 5) to describe the various body types. He noted that most physicians came into the field prejudiced by their early anatomic teachings and had fixed conceptions, "which the revelations of the roentgen ray ruthlessly outraged."

Radiographers still use these terms today to describe *body habitus* and its normal variants. Knowledge of each of the body types and its associated tissue characteristics, position and tonus of associated organs, and so on helps us to position more accurately and to select appropriate technical factors.

For example, the same body part, such as the stomach, in two different individuals will require very different central ray points of entry if one individual is hypersthenic and the other asthenic. A particular body part, such as the shoulder, might measure the same on two different individuals, yet it may not be appropriate to select identical exposure factors for each if one is a muscular sthenic build and the other a hyposthenic type with little muscle tone.

Other factors that influence image density, and consequently the selection of technical factors, are age, gender, and pathology. Various abnormal pathologic conditions, disease processes, and trauma can affect tissue density and, hence, density. Normal variants of muscle development result from different lifestyles, occupations, and age and will affect image density.

Some pathologic conditions are referred to as *destructive*, such as osteoporosis and conditions involving necrosis or atrophy. These conditions can cause an undesirable increase in image density unless they are recognized and appropriate changes are made in exposure factors. Other conditions such as ascites, rheumatoid arthritis, and Paget disease are *additive*, and an increase in exposure factors is required to maintain adequate density/brightness.

Examples of *Additive* Pathologic Conditions

- Ascites
- Rheumatoid arthritis
- Paget disease
- Pneumonia
- Atelectasis
- Congestive heart failure
- Edematous tissue

Examples of *Destructive* Pathologic Conditions

- Osteoporosis
- Osteomalacia
- Pneumoperitoneum
- Emphysema
- Degenerative arthritis
- Atrophic and necrotic conditions

Summary

- Variations in tissue density will be noted as image density variations in the x-ray image.
- Normal tissue density differences exist as a result of body habitus, age, gender, and level of activity.
- Abnormal density differences can be observed as a result of trauma or pathologic conditions.
- The radiographer must be knowledgeable about conditions affecting normal and abnormal changes in tissue density to make appropriate selection of technical factors.

Generator Type and Density. *Three-phase* x-ray generation is much more efficient than *single phase* because the voltage never drops to zero.

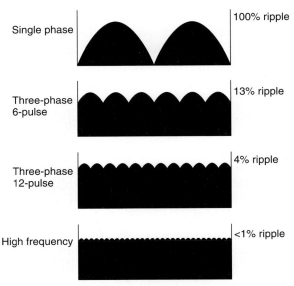

Figure 11–41. *Single-phase (1ø) and three-phase (3ø) waveforms.* Compared with the one useful impulse available per 1/60th second with alternating current, single-phase rectified current has two useful impulses, 3ø 6p rectified has 6 useful impulses, and 3ø 12p has 12.

Three-phase equipment has a small-voltage ripple and thus produces more high-energy x-ray photons (Fig. 11–41). Therefore, if two x-ray images were made of the same part and using the same factors, one made with a single-phase machine and one with a three-phase machine, the three-phase image would show considerably more image density. Consequently, to reproduce similar image densities when using different generators, exposure factor adjustment is necessary.

If 92 kV and 60 mAs were used for a particular abdominal exposure using single-phase equipment, what mAs would be required to produce a similar image using three-phase, six-pulse equipment?

The correction table in the box in this section indicates that only two-thirds of the original single-phase mAs would be required to produce similar image density with three-phase equipment.

Thus,

$2/3 \times 60 = 40$ mAs with 3ø 6p equipment (note that kV remains the same).

It should be noted that approximately the same quantity of radiation is delivered to *the IR* from each x-ray machine (1ø and 3ø) to produce similar images. The entrance skin exposures (ESE), however, differ significantly (Fig. 11–42). This is because the single-phase machine produces many more low-energy photons, contributing to patient skin dose but not to image density.

When technical factors are modified for single-phase or three-phase changes, it is usually the mAs that is adjusted; however, kV adjustment is also workable. Changing from single-phase to three-phase requires a 12% decrease in kV; conversely, changing from three-phase to single-phase requires a 12% increase in kV.

Correction Factors

Single phase	Three phase
x mAs	2/3x for 3φ (6p)
x mAs	1/2x for 3φ (12p)
x kV	x − 12% for 3φ

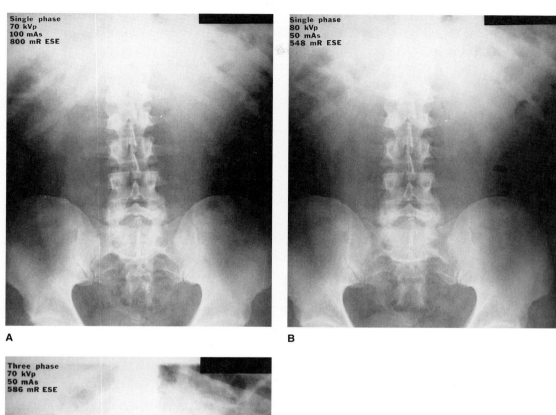

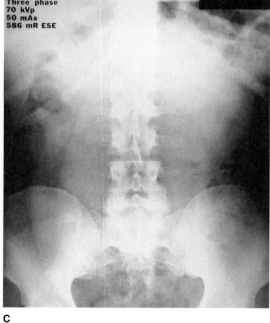

Figure 11–42. Images *A* and *C* are good examples of 1ø to 3ø conversion and the difference in entrance skin exposure (ESE). Images *A* and *B* demonstrate the radiation protection factor is increasing from 70 kV at 100 mAs to 80 kV at 50 mAs; note the big difference in ESE. (From the American College of Radiology Learning File. Courtesy of the American College of Radiology.)

Conventional 60-Hz full-wave rectified power is converted to a higher frequency of 500 to 25,000 Hz in the most recent generator design—the *high-frequency generator*. The high-frequency generator is small in size, in addition to producing an almost constant potential waveform. High-frequency generators first appeared in mobile x-ray units and were then adopted by mammography and CT equipment.

Today, more and more radiographic equipment uses high-frequency generators. Their compact size makes them popular, and the fact that they produce nearly constant potential voltage helps to improve image quality and decrease patient dose (fewer low-energy photons to contribute to skin dose).

Correction for generator type is unnecessary in digital imaging.

Summary

- Three-phase (3ø) equipment produces nearly peak potential voltage, whereas single-phase (1ø) voltage drops periodically to zero between voltage peaks.
- mAs is usually adjusted to compensate for differences between 1ø and 3ø waveform equipment.
- When changing from 1ø to 3ø 6p, two-thirds less mAs is required; from 1ø to 3ø 12p, one-half the original mAs is required (the reverse is true when changing from 3ø to 1ø).

Beam Restriction and Density. A change in image density will occur with changes in the size of the irradiated field, all other factors remaining constant. *Beam restriction* (i.e., reducing the volume of tissue irradiated) reduces the production of scattered radiation and, consequently, decreases image density. The reverse is also true: as field size increases, image density increases as a result of increased production of scattered radiation fog. *Therefore, as changes are made in the size of the irradiated field, an accompanying change in mAs is required to maintain the same image density.*

Anode Heel Effect and Density. The anode heel effect was discussed earlier with respect to focal spot size and recorded detail. Figures 11–43 and 11–44 illustrate how a portion of the divergent x-ray beam is absorbed by the anode, resulting in diminished image density at the anode end of the image.

When using general x-ray tubes at standard distances, the heel effect is noticeable only when imaging parts of uneven thickness, such as the femur and thoracic spine. In these cases, the heel effect may be used to advantage by placing the thicker body portion under the cathode end of the x-ray beam, thus having the effect of "balancing/evening out" tissue densities.

Film Processing and Density. Radiographic film emulsion is very sensitive to even small changes in chemical processing. A decrease in developer temperature of 2°F to 3°F will produce a dramatic decrease in optical density (Fig. 11–45) and, conversely, even a small rise in developer temperature results in a noticeable density increase

---

The Anode Heel Effect Is Emphasized Under the Following Conditions

- At short SIDs
- With large size image receptors
- With small anode angle x-ray tubes

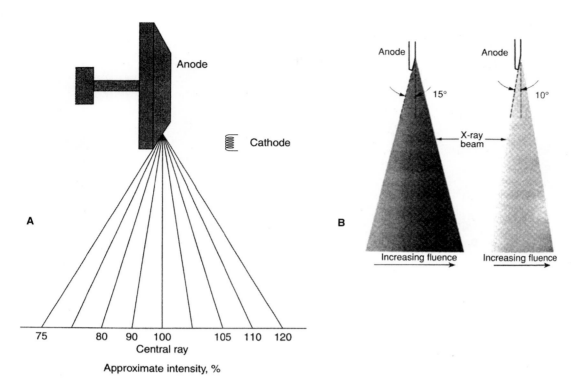

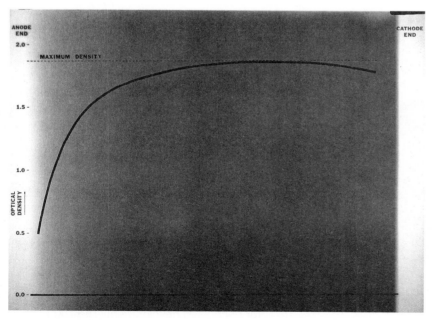

Figure 11–43. (**A**) and (**B**) *The anode heel effect*. As x-ray photons are produced within the anode, a portion of the divergent beam is absorbed by the anode's "heel." This represents a decrease in x-ray beam intensity at the anode end of the x-ray beam. (Reproduced, with permission, from Shephard CT. *Radiographic Image Production and Manipulation*. New York: McGraw-Hill, 2003.)

Figure 11–44. *Radiographic illustration of the anode heel effect*. Note the gradual increase in radiographic density toward the cathode end of the beam. (From the American College of Radiology Learning File. Courtesy of the American College of Radiology.)

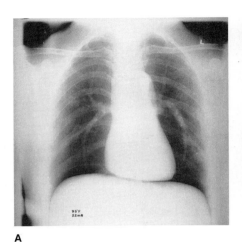
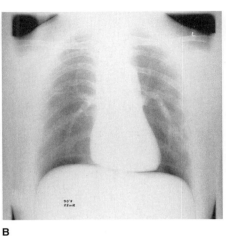
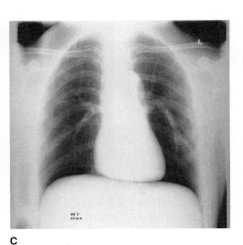

A   B   C

Figure 11–45. *Developer temperature* vs. *image density* and *patient exposure.* (A) Radiograph of chest phantom made using 22 mR and processed at recommended temp. of 95°F. (B) The same conditions except that the developer temp. was 5_ lower, at 90°F; note the significant change in radiographic density. (C) Radiograph using the same 90°F developer, but with exposure compensated to provide the required density; note the increase in exposure dose to 35 mR. (From the American College of Radiology Learning File. Courtesy of the American College of Radiology.)

(Fig. 11–46). Figure 11–47 illustrates the impact of developer temperature on the sensitometric curve.

Optical density is also directly related to the length of development and replenishment rate, that is, density increases as development time increases or as replenishment rate increases.

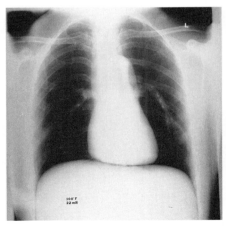

Figure 11–46. This radiograph was exposed under the same conditions as the radiograph in Figure 11–45A but was processed at a developer temperature 5° above normal (at 100°F), producing a dark radiograph. (From the American College of Radiology Learning File. Courtesy of the American College of Radiology.)

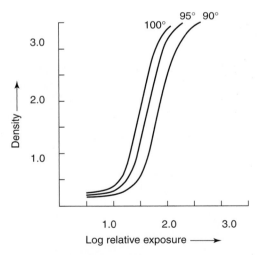

Figure 11–47. The sensitometric curve illustrates the effect of the *developer temperature* changes seen in Figures 11–45 and 11–46. The position of the 90°F curve is to the right of the optimal temperature (95°F) curve; to achieve the same density, the exposure must be increased to compensate for decreased development. The 100°F curve is to the left, therefore less exposure is required to compensate for decreased development. (From the American College of Radiology Learning File. Courtesy of the American College of Radiology.)

Summary

- Changing the size of the irradiated field affects image density as a result of increased or decreased scattered radiation production.
- The anode heel effect is characterized by greater x-ray intensity (i.e., quantity) at the cathode end of the beam. The anode heel effect is most pronounced at short SIDs, with large IRs, and with x-ray tubes having small anode angles.
- The anode heel effect can be used to compensate for a difference in tissue density/thickness (e.g., femur, thoracic spine).
- Optical density increases as developer temperature increases and as the replenishment rate and/or length of development increase.

Contrast: SF imaging

Factors affecting density and contrast in SF imaging have little to no effect on similar characteristics seen in digital x-ray images. Though its use is rapidly declining, there are still some SF systems in use and our certification exam specifications still require some knowledge of this system.

In order to understand the fundamentals of these imaging factors and characteristics, SF imaging with its terminology is reviewed first. Digital imaging review will follow.

Radiographic contrast exists whenever two or more differing densities are present in a radiographic image. These density differences exhibit a particular gray scale. The function of contrast is *to make details visible*. When there are just a few densities, with noticeable difference between the densities, radiographic *contrast* is said to be *high* or *short scale*. When there are many shades of densities (grays) with only slight difference between them, radiographic *contrast is low* or *long scale*.

Radiographic (SF) contrast is the *sum of subject contrast and film contrast*.

Subject contrast is a result of *differential absorption* by tissues of varying densities and thicknesses. X-ray photons undergo attenuation by various body tissues to differing degrees—with *less* exit radiation from thicker/more dense structures (i.e., structures having higher *attenuation coefficients*), and *more* exit radiation from thinner/less dense structures. Subject contrast, then, is the primary cause of the various density *differences* visible on the x-ray image. It is exhibited as a *scale of grays* having varying tones representative of differential tissue absorption.

SF subject contrast is regulated by the quality (energy, wavelength, penetrability) of x-ray photons.

Film contrast describes the response of the film emulsion to the variety of x-ray photons emerging from the irradiated part. Film contrast is affected by the manufacturing process, processing conditions, and fluorescent properties of the intensifying screens; film contrast characteristics are illustrated by the sensitometric (*D* log *E*) curve.

- The function of contrast is to make details visible.

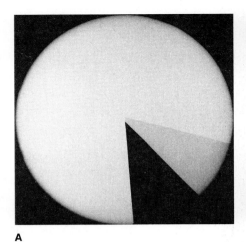
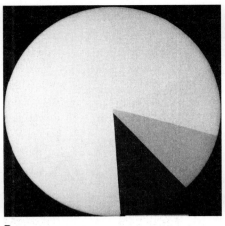
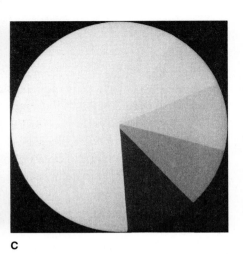

A   B   C

Figure 11–48. *Contrast functions to make details visible*. Images were made of a circular phantom having a variety of wedge-shaped thicknesses; a circular "lesion" of greater density is embedded in each wedge. Note that the level of contrast between adjacent areas is strongly related to the degree of visibility of the "lesions." **(A)** Illustrates the highest contrast; only two wedges (thicknesses) are visualized and only one "lesion" is barely visible. **(B)** The contrast scale is a little longer; a third wedge begins to be seen and two "lesions" are visualized. **(C)** Five wedges are visualized (hopefully the printing process can demonstrate them) and at least three "lesions" can be seen clearly. From the American College of Radiology Learning File. Courtesy of the American College of Radiology.)

Contrast Terminology

High *contrast is*	Low *contrast is*
• short-scale contrast	• long-scale contrast

It displays:	It displays:
• few, very different, image/tissue densities	• many similar image/tissue densities

It is a *product of*	It is a *product of*
• lower kV	• higher kV
• few, dissimilar tissue densities	• many similar tissue densities
• more, "tighter" collimation	• larger field sizes

An x-ray image exhibiting a range of different shades of gray, with *little difference* among the various shades, possesses *long-scale* (low) *contrast*. An image that exhibits only a few gray shades possesses *short scale* (high) *contrast*.

The function of the contrast scale is to make image details visible.

Most anatomic structures have an infinite number of details representing a variety of tissue densities and having different x-ray absorption properties. If the anatomic part is represented radiographically by only a few shades of gray, many anatomic details are not being visualized at all. If, however, the image displays a wide range of gray tones, more anatomic details will be represented and visualized (Fig. 11–48). Therefore, long-scale contrast *usually* provides more information (but short-scale, i.e., high, contrast may be required for certain examinations or body parts) (see Fig. 11–49).

A number of factors affect the production of image contrast and each is discussed individually.

Summary

• The function of contrast is to make details visible.
• Radiographic contrast refers to the degree of difference between image densities.
• SF radiographic contrast is the sum of subject contrast and film contrast.
• Subject contrast is the result of differential absorption of x-rays by body tissues having different attenuation coefficients (various thicknesses and densities).
• Subject contrast is regulated by selection of x-ray beam quality (kV).

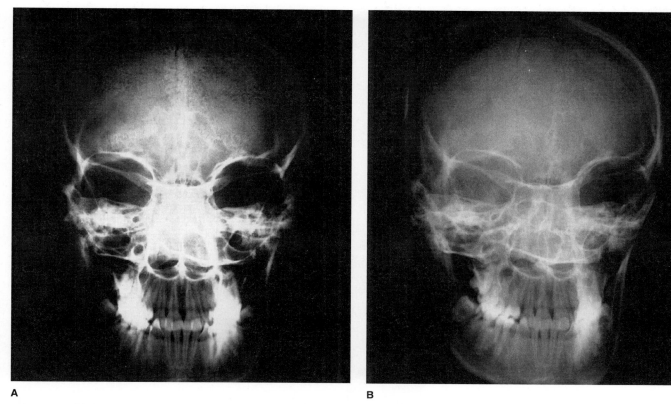

A   B

Figure 11–49. (A) Example of *high*, or *short-scale, contrast*. **(B)** Example of *low, or long-scale, contrast*. Rotation of the part is also seen. (From the American College of Radiology Learning File. Courtesy of the American College of Radiology.)

- Film contrast is the result of manufacturing, processing, and intensifying screens.
- Radiographic images having many different shades of gray, varying slightly from one another, are said to possess long-scale (or low) contrast.
- Radiographic images possessing few density differences, markedly different from each other, are said to possess short-scale (or high) contrast.
- Digital imaging significantly improves dynamic range and contrast resolution.

kV and Contrast. Kilovoltage governs x-ray *penetrability* and is the primary exposure factor regulating radiographic contrast in SF imaging. In general, as kV increases, so does the scale of contrast (Fig. 11–50).

As a general rule, parts having *low subject contrast* are likely to produce long-scale contrast. If high kV technical factors are used to image these parts, unacceptably low radiographic contrast will result because of scattered radiation fog.

Scattered radiation fog impairs the visibility of low-contrast object details, degrading the diagnostic quality of the image. When imaging structures having *low subject contrast*, use of *lower kV* frequently helps emphasize what little contrast exists in the subject tissues.

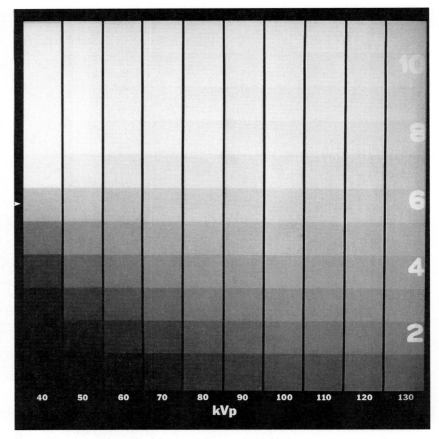

Figure 11–50. *Aluminum step wedge test.* As kV increases, a greater number of steps (and the subtle differences between them) are discernible. (From the American College of Radiology Learning File. Courtesy of the American College of Radiology.)

Because kV determines the penetrating ability of the x-ray photons, *low kV* can be used to *emphasize differences* between tissue densities, for example, in mammography, foreign-body localization, and iodine-containing renal collecting systems (Fig. 11–51).

Anatomic parts having *high subject contrast* will produce short-scale radiographic contrast, and if low kV is used to image these parts, unacceptably high radiographic contrast will result (Fig. 11–52). Visibility of structures within the very light and very dark areas is greatly diminished. When imaging structures having *high subject contrast*, the use of *higher kV* will promote more uniform penetration of the part; thus, it "evens out" big differences in tissue densities and brings about visualization of small image details (as in high-kV chest radiography).

Kilovoltage also affects the degree of *exposure latitude.* Exposure latitude is the leeway, or margin of error, one has with a given group of exposure factors. At higher kilovoltages, a difference of a few kV will make little, if any, difference radiographically. At low kilovoltages, however, an error of just a few kV can make a very noticeable difference in the radiographic image. There is, therefore, a larger "margin for error" in kV selection at higher kV ranges.

Short-Scale Contrast results as:

- Subject contrast increases
- kV decreases
- Scattered radiation decreases
- Grid ratio increases
- Film latitude decreases

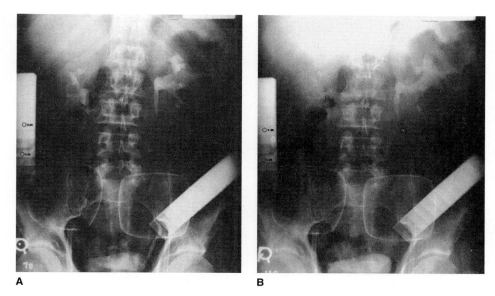

A   **B**

Figure 11–51. In anatomic regions having *low subject* contrast, such as the abdominal viscera, artificial contrast agents are often introduced to enhance subject contrast. **(A)** IVU made using 70 kV. **(B)** IVU using 110 kV. The use of excessive kV with iodinated media and the resulting production of more scattered radiation has almost obliterated the contrast-filled collecting systems in image **B.** (From the American College of Radiology Learning File. Courtesy of the American College of Radiology.)

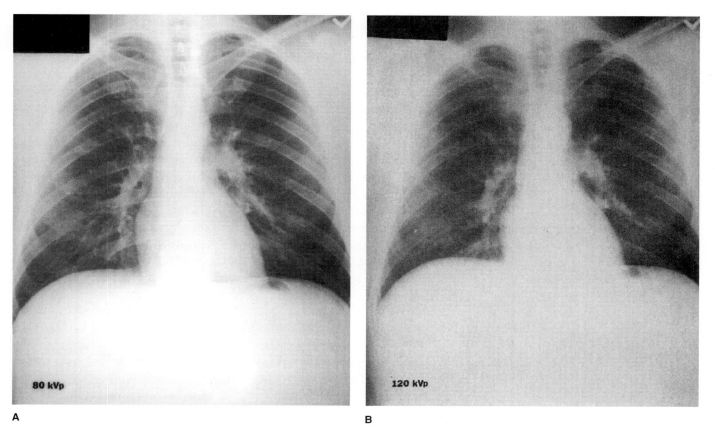

80 kVp

120 kVp

A   **B**

Figure 11–52. Posteroanterior (PA) chest images made using 80 kV **(A)** and 120 kV **(B)**. Image A PA chest image made using 80 kV demonstrates shorter scale contrast, and pulmonary vascular markings are not well visualized. **(B)** Chest image made using 120 kV demonstrates longer scale contrast, and visualization of pulmonary vascular markings *through* the bony rib details, and requires a smaller patient dose. (From the American College of Radiology Learning File. Courtesy of the American College of Radiology.)

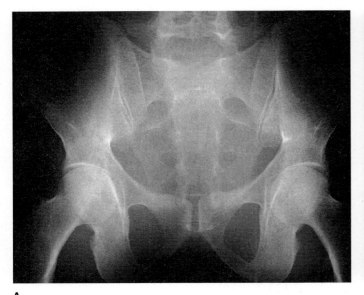

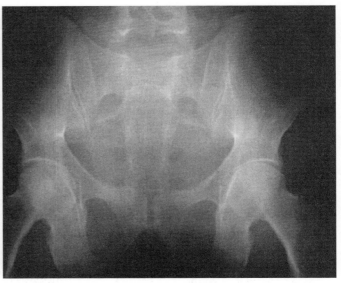

A

B

Figure 11–53. *Kilovoltage is directly related to the production of scattered radiation.* (A) Image made using 80 kV and 75 mAs. (B) Image made using 100 kV and 18 mAs, all other factors remaining the same. As kV is increased, the percentage of scattered radiation relative to primary radiation increases. Use of optimum kV for each anatomic part is helpful in keeping scatter to a minimum. (From the American College of Radiology Learning File. Courtesy of the American College of Radiology.)

Factors that Determine Production of SR:

- Field size/beam restriction
- Kilovoltage
- Thickness/volume and density of tissues

Scattered Radiation and Contrast. High kV may be desirable in terms of patient dose, x-ray tube life, and making more anatomic details visible, but use of too high kV results in production of excessive amounts of scattered radiation and fog, resulting in *diminished* visibility of image details (Fig. 11–53).

Much of the scattered radiation produced is highly energetic and exits the patient along with the useful image-forming radiation. However, scattered radiation carries no useful information but adds *noise* in the form of fog, thereby impairing visibility of detail.

Because scattered radiation can have such a devastating effect on image contrast, it is essential that radiographers are knowledgeable about methods of controlling its production. The three factors that have a significant effect on the *production of scattered radiation* are beam restriction, kV, and thickness (volume) and density of tissues.

Perhaps the most important way to limit the production of scattered radiation and improve contrast is by *limiting the size of the irradiated field*, that is, through *beam restriction* (Fig. 11–54).

As the size of the x-ray field is reduced, there is less area and tissue volume for scattered radiation to be generated. As the volume and/or density of the irradiated tissues increase(s), so does quantity of scattered radiation produced (Fig. 11–55). Thicker and more dense anatomic structures will generate more scattered radiation. *Compression* of certain parts can occasionally be used to minimize the effect of scatter, but "tighter" *collimation* can *always* be used effectively.

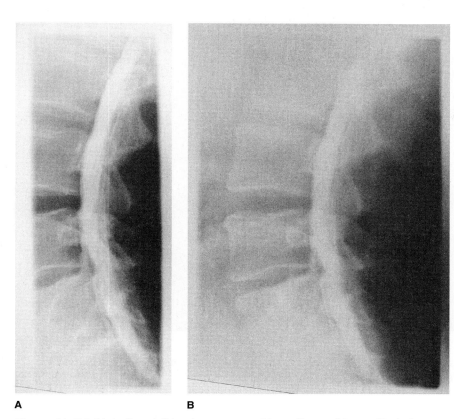

A   **B**

Figure 11–54. Note the striking improvement in radiographic quality in image A as beam restriction is increased in this lateral lumbar myelogram. Although a 50% increase in exposure was required to maintain appropriate density in image A (to compensate for less scattered radiation reaching the image receptor), radiation protection is maintained because the volume of irradiated tissue is decreased. (From the American College of Radiology Learning File. Courtesy of the American College of Radiology.)

Introduction of an OID (*air gap*) can have a noticeable effect on image contrast. An air gap introduced between the object and IR has an effect similar to that of a grid. A 6-in. air gap is equivalent to the effectiveness of an 8:1 grid; a 10-in. air gap is equivalent to the effectiveness of a 16:1 grid. As energetic scattered radiation emerges from the body, it continues to travel in its divergent fashion and, much of the time, will bypass the IR (see Fig. 11–38).

Patient Factors and Contrast. Various tissue types and pathologic processes can alter tissue thickness and composition and thereby have a significant effect on radiographic contrast. Anatomic structures having high atomic number and pathologic conditions that increase tissue density tend to produce a higher contrast.

The greater the radiographer's awareness of the tissue nature and/or pathology under investigation, the more intelligently and accurately exposure factors can be selected.

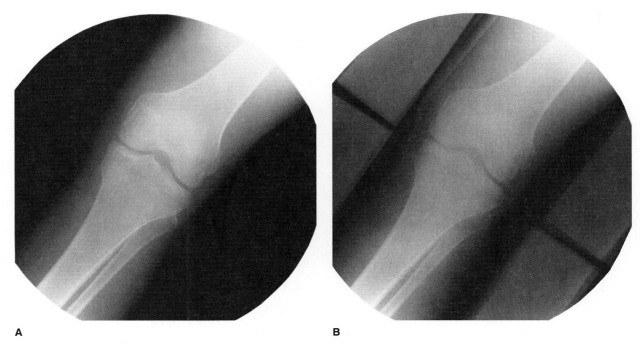

A   B

Figure 11–55. *The volume of irradiated tissue is directly related to the quantity of scattered radiation generated*. (**A**) Anteroposterior (AP) of knee. (**B**) AP with paraffin absorbers *around* the knee. The loss of contrast exhibited in *B* is caused by increased *volume* of irradiated material within the beam, resulting in increased scattered radiation fog. Note that the part need not be *thicker* to generate significant scatter, just that the total *irradiated volume* be greater. (From the American College of Radiology Learning File. Courtesy of the American College of Radiology.)

Summary

- kV selection determines the energy of x-ray photons and therefore degree of penetration of various tissues, thereby determining the contrast characteristics of the image.

- Images of structures having low subject contrast often benefit from the use of lower kV, while structures having high subject contrast can be represented with a longer range of grays by using higher kV.

- The use of high kV reduces patient dose and reduces the production of x-ray tube heat but increases the production of scattered radiation fog.

- Scattered radiation carries no useful information but, rather, adds noise that impairs visibility of image details. Production of scattered radiation can be minimized by using optimum kV techniques and by restricting the size of the x-ray beam as much as possible.

- As the thickness and density of tissues increase, so does the production of scattered radiation; tissue thickness can sometimes be minimized with compression.

- As normal tissues undergo pathologic change, their penetrability frequently also changes in ways characteristic of the disease process (i.e., additive vs. destructive disease processes).

Grids and Contrast. An image produced using a grid differs considerably from an image produced without a grid (see Fig. 11–31). Since thicker, denser parts can generate significant amounts of scattered radiation, a grid should be used whenever a part measures 11 cm or greater in thickness. A possible exception to this rule is the chest, although much chest radiography performed today employs high kV and grids.

Although collimation, optimum kV, and compression may be used, a large amount of scattered radiation can still be generated within the part being imaged and can have a severely deleterious effect on image contrast. Without the use of a grid, scattered radiation can contribute 50% to 90% of the total image exposure. The function of a grid, then, is to remove scattered radiation exiting the patient *before* it reaches the IR, thereby improving contrast (Fig. 11–56).

As discussed earlier in this chapter, two of a grid's physical characteristics that determine its degree of efficiency in the removal of scattered radiation are *grid ratio* (the height of the lead strips compared with the distance between them—see Fig. 11–36) and number of *lead strips per inch*. Other familiar ways of expressing and measuring grid efficiency include the *grid factor* (grid conversion factor), *CIF*, and *selectivity*. Higher-ratio grids are more effective in reducing the amount of scattered radiation reaching the IR; however, their use requires more mAs and decreases grid positioning latitude.

The *grid factor* (G) is the ratio of the total amount of radiation (useful and scattered) incident upon the surface of the grid to the amount of radiation transmitted through the grid (see Fig. 11–37):

$$G = \frac{\text{Total incident}}{\text{Total transmitted}}$$

The *CIF* is the ratio of radiographic contrast obtained with a grid to that obtained without a grid:

$$CIF = \frac{\text{Contrast with grid}}{\text{Contrast without grid}}$$

Selectivity (S) is the ratio between the quantity of primary photons transmitted through the grid and the quantity of scattered photons transmitted:

$$S = \frac{\text{Useful photon transmission}}{\text{Scattered photon transmission}}.$$

As previously discussed, the introduction of an *air gap* can have an effect similar to that obtained through the addition of a grid.

Filtration and Contrast. The primary beam usually has a total (protective) filtration of 2.5-mm Al equivalent. Inherent filtration includes 0.5-mm Al from the glass envelope and 1.0-mm Al from the collimator. The manufacturer adds another 1.0-mm Al to meet the minimum

As Grid Ratio Increases:

- Scattered radiation cleanup increases and contrast improves
- Contrast scale decreases (i.e., higher contrast results)
- Exposure factors (usually mAs) must increase
- Patient dose increases
- Positioning latitude decreases

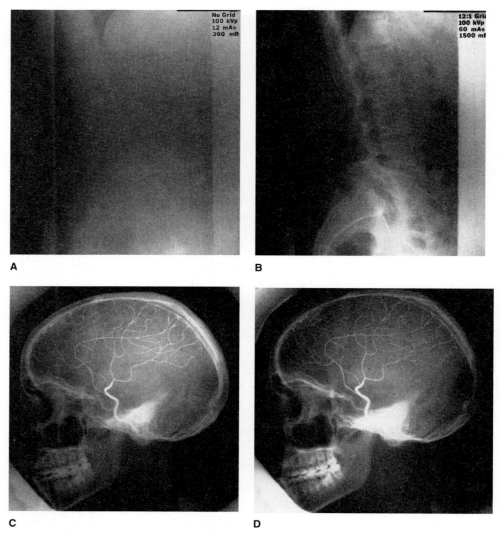

Figure 11–56. *Effect of grids on image contrast* and quality. (A) Made using 100 kV, 12 mAs, no grid; scattered radiation fog obliterates anatomic details almost completely. (B) Made with 100 kV, 60 mAs, and a 12:1 grid, all other factors constant; scattered radiation is "cleaned up" and image details are more readily perceptible. (C) Made without a grid using 70 kV and 4 mAs. (D) Made with 12:1 grid, 70 kV and 20 mAs. Note the improved contrast and detail visibility. (From the American College of Radiology Learning File. Courtesy of the American College of Radiology.)

requirements of 2.5-mm Al equivalent total filtration for radiographic tubes operated above 70 kV.

Filtration serves to increase the overall average energy of the beam; it "hardens" the x-ray beam. The 2.5-mm Al equivalent functions to remove the diagnostically useless x-ray photons that contribute to patient dose. Since these photons do not have sufficient energy to reach the IR, the usual required filtration in the x-ray tube *has no effect on image contrast* (Fig. 11–57).

The addition or removal of *compensating* filters (as discussed in Section II, F) will impact the radiographic contrast unless exposure factors are adjusted to compensate for the change (see Figs. 11–39 and 11–40).

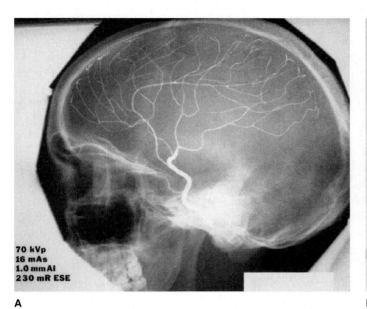

70 kVp
16 mAs
1.0 mm Al
230 mR ESE

A

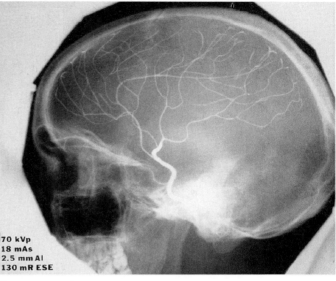

70 kVp
18 mAs
2.5 mm Al
130 mR ESE

B

Figure 11–57. **(A)** and **(B)** *The effect of filtration on image contrast*. The contrast displayed in *A* and *B* is very similar. An increase in filtration, however, results in a lower ESE (entrance skin exposure) and greater tube load (mAs). As filtration is increased above 2.5 mm Al, minimal dose reduction occurs and tube loading is significantly increased. (From the American College of Radiology Learning File. Courtesy of the American College of Radiology.)

Summary

- X-rays scattering within a part and having enough energy to exit the body and reach the IR produce scattered radiation fog (noise), thus degrading contrast.

- Grids function to absorb scattered radiation before it reaches the IR.

- Scattered radiation cleanup increases as grid ratio increases.

- The higher the grid ratio, the higher (shorter scale) the resulting contrast.

- X-ray tube filtration ordinarily has no effect on image contrast; it functions primarily for patient protection.

- Compensating filters added or removed from the x-ray beam will affect contrast unless exposure adjustment is made.

AUTOMATIC EXPOSURE CONTROL

AEC is used to automatically regulate the amount of ionizing radiation delivered to the anatomic part and IR, thereby serving to produce consistent and comparable radiographic results time after time. When AEC is installed in the x-ray circuit, it is calibrated to terminate the exposure once a predetermined (known correct) exposure has been made.

When using SF systems, it is essential to use the SF combination for which the AEC has been programmed. For example, if the system has been programmed for a 400 system, and a 200-speed cassette is used, the image will exhibit half the expected density.

Two Types of AECs:

- Phototimer
- Ionization chamber

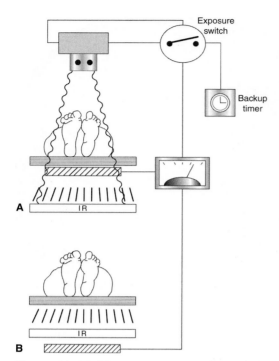

Figure 11–58. The two types of *automatic exposure devices* are the *ionization chamber* (located just below the tabletop) **(A)** and the *phototimer* (located below the IR) **(B)**. Note the *backup timer* that functions to terminate the exposure, should the AEC fail to operate properly.

Whether using traditional or digital imaging equipment, *exact positioning and centering* is particularly critical when using AEC. The anatomic part of interest must be positioned (centered) accurately with respect to the AEC's sensors; otherwise, the result can be over- or underexposure.

Types

In one type of AEC, there is a (radiolucent) parallel plate *ionization chamber* just beneath the tabletop, *above* the IR (Fig. 11–58). The part to be examined is centered to the sensor and imaged. As x-ray photons emerge from the patient, they enter the chamber and ionize the air within. When a predetermined quantity of ionization has occurred, indicating that correct exposure has been reached, the exposure automatically terminates.

The other type of AEC is the (radiopaque) *phototimer* type in which a small fluorescent screen is positioned *beneath* the IR. When the exit radiation emerging from the part interacts with and exits the IR, the fluorescent screen emits light and charges a photomultiplier tube (PMT). Once a predetermined charge has been reached, the exposure is automatically terminated.

In either case, the *manual* timer should always be used as a *backup timer*. In case of AEC malfunction, the backup timer would terminate the exposure, thus *avoiding patient overexposure and tube overload*.

Another important feature of the AEC is its *minimum response/reaction time*. This is the length of the *shortest exposure possible* with a particular AEC (10–30 msec). If less than the minimum response time is required for a particular exposure, the resulting image will exhibit overexposure. The only way to remedy this is to decrease the mA or decrease the kV. Each maneuver will result in increased exposure time to within the response time capabilities of the AEC. If the contrast scale is to be maintained, the mA adjustment is preferable.

Positioning Accuracy

To achieve the expected radiographic density (*in SF imaging*), the appropriate detector(s)/sensor(s) must be selected and the part of interest must be correctly positioned directly above the appropriate detector(s)/sensor(s).

If a structure having less tissue density than the part of interest is positioned above the detector, or if the detector is incompletely covered, the detector will terminate the exposure sooner and the area of interest will be *underexposed*. Similarly, if the incorrect sensor for the anatomic part is selected, a density error will result.

On the other hand, if the sensor is positioned under a structure having greater tissue density than the part of interest (e.g., if the center detector is used for a PA chest image), the exposure will be greater than required and an *overexposed* image will result.

Consequently, although the exposure is "automatic," knowledge of anatomy, accurate positioning skills and correct equipment use are essential to producing proper image density.

Pathology

The presence of pathology often modifies tissue composition. Changes that occur are generally spoken of as *additive* or *degenerative*. Additive pathology is that which increases tissue density, requiring an increase in exposure factors (e.g., ascites). Degenerative pathology involves deterioration of the part (e.g., osteoporosis) and requires a decrease in exposure factors.

Because the function of an automatic exposure device is to "recognize" differences in tissue density and thickness, it will compensate for most pathologic changes by adjusting the mAs. In the event further compensation is necessary, most AECs have a *master density control* (on the control panel) that allows the radiographer to modify its output.

Using the master density control, normal exposure and density can usually be varied in increments of 25%, plus or minus—usually displayed on the control panel as +1 and −1. It must be noted that if an image is overexposed because an exposure shorter than the *minimum reaction time* (shortest possible exposure) is required, a reduction in master density control will not resolve the situation. Rather, a lower-mA station should be selected so that an exposure time within the machine's capability can be used.

Summary

- The function of AECs is to produce consistent and comparable radiographic images.
- There are two types of AECs: ionization chamber and phototimer.
- Ionization chambers are located between the x-ray table and cassette; phototimers are located beneath the IR.
- Backup timers are used in conjunction with AECs and function to terminate the exposure in case of AEC malfunction.
- Minimum reaction time is the shortest exposure time possible with a particular AEC.
- The successful use of AECs requires accurate patient positioning and proper detector/sensor selection.
- Pathologic conditions may be either additive or degenerative; correct use of the AEC will compensate for pathologic conditions.
- AECs have a master density control, usually adjustable in increments of 25%.

TECHNIQUE CHARTS

Fixed vs Variable kV Technique

In a *variable kV technique* chart, the mAs is fixed and the kV is increased as part thickness increases. For each centimeter increase in thickness, the kV is increased by 2. Accurate measurement with calipers is required. The variable kV technique chart is not frequently used today because it is associated with increased scattered radiation production and inconsistent contrast and density.

Examples of Additive Pathologic Conditions

- Ascites
- Rheumatoid arthritis
- Paget disease
- Pneumonia
- Atelectasis
- Congestive heart failure
- Edematous tissue

Examples of Destructive Pathologic Conditions

- Osteoporosis
- Osteomalacia
- Pneumoperitoneum
- Emphysema
- Degenerative arthritis
- Atrophic and necrotic conditions

Fixed kV Technique Chart

	Fixed kV*	Grid
Extremities	55	No grid
Skull	75	Grid
Abdomen	75	Grid
Lateral lumbar	90	Grid
Barium studies	120	Grid
Chest examinations	120	Grid

*For 3ø equipment factors, single ø will require approximately 12% higher kV.

A *fixed kV technique* chart specifies a particular kV for each body part or type of examination. A kV is selected that will provide adequate penetration and the appropriate scale of contrast. mAs is used to compensate for variation of patient size and condition.

Accurate *measurement of the part* to be imaged is essential with the *variable* kV technique chart because the kV increases by 2 for every 1-cm increase in part thickness. *Fixed* kV charts may specify a specific kV for the "small," "medium," or "large" patient, which corresponds to measurements within a particular range (e.g., 10–12 cm = small, 13–15 cm = medium, and 16–18 cm = large). Accurate measurement may be essential for the correct application of each method. Structures imaged using AECs do not require measurement because the AEC automatically adjusts the exposure for tissue variations.

AECs and Technique Charts

Fixed kV techniques are generally used with AECs. An optimum kV for each body part (femur, abdomen, hip, chest, etc.) is selected and the exposure is automatically terminated once the predetermined correct exposure (mAs) has been reached.

The AEC automatically adjusts the exposure required for body parts that have *different thicknesses and tissue densities*. Proper functioning of the AEC depends on *accurate positioning* by the radiographer. The *correct photocell*(s) must be selected, and the anatomic part of interest must completely *cover the photocell* to achieve the desired image quality. If *collimation* is inadequate and a field size larger than the part is used, excessive scattered radiation from the body or tabletop can cause the AEC to terminate the exposure prematurely, resulting in an underexposed radiograph.

Backup time always should be selected on the manual timer to prevent patient overexposure and to protect the x-ray tube from excessive heat production should the AEC malfunction. Selection of the optimal kilovoltage for the part being radiographed is essential—no practical amount of milliampere- seconds can make up for inadequate penetration (kilovoltage). Excessive kilovoltage can cause the AEC to terminate the exposure prematurely.

A *technique chart*, therefore, is strongly recommended for use with AEC; it should indicate the optimal *kilovoltage* for the part, the *photocells* that should be selected, and the *backup time* that should be set.

Other Considerations

Body position plays an important role in obtaining the expected radiographic results. For example, a well-exposed image of a normal adult abdomen measuring 24 cm in the recumbent AP position cannot be duplicated using the same factors if the patient is turned prone or positioned decubitus or erect.

A *plain* image of a particular abdomen requires different exposure factors from the same abdomen having a *barium*-filled stomach.

Different exposures will be required for extremities with and without *casts*.

Body parts undergoing additive or destructive *pathologic changes* can require substantial exposure changes to maintain the required density and contrast.

Limitations of SF Systems:

- Narrow exposure latitude
- Chemical processing
- Increased cost
- Storage space requirements
- No image enhancement capability
- No electronic transmission capability

AECs will compensate for thickness and tissue density differences (including those caused by position and respiration), pathologic changes, and beam restriction. However, it should be emphasized that the radiographer's skill and accuracy in *positioning* and *photocell selection* play an important role in the proper function of AECs.

A particular chest properly exposed on *inspiration* using a 14 × 17 in. IR cannot be duplicated, without a change in factors, when the exposure is made on *expiration* or the field size is *collimated* to an 8 × 10 in. anatomic area.

This concept, and many others, changes when considering *electronic/digital imaging* technology—begun in the following section.

Limitations of SF Imaging

The limitations of SF radiography include narrow exposure latitude, chemical processing requirements, increased cost for film and labor, storage space requirements, incapable of image enhancement or electronic transmission.

The chief advantages of SF imaging are high spatial resolution and uniformity in image appearance. Another possible advantage is availability of many highly skilled professionals experienced in using SF imaging.

SF images can be converted to a digital form using a *film digitizer*. The output digitized image characteristics are essentially those of the SF. There are two major types of digitizers; one using laser scanning and the other using an array of CCD sensors. The laser system generally results in better density and contrast duplication than the CCD, but the CCD type provides better duplicated resolution and better overall operational dependability. In general, film digitizers add noise to the digital image and limit its grayscale range. Poor original film image quality cannot be compensated for with digitization and windowing.

> **Advantages of SF Systems:**
>
> - High spatial resolution
> - Image consistency

ELECTRONIC/DIGITAL IMAGING

Electronic imaging consists of computed radiography (CR) and digital radiography (DR). As electronic/digital imaging technology continues to develop, descriptive terms also evolve. The most current terms are described and used here.

Electronic Imaging (CR/DR) imaging is the *same* as SF (or *projection*) imaging with respect to the production of x-rays, x-ray interaction and production of scatter, x-ray beam geometry, and factors affecting detail and distortion.

Electronic imaging *differs* from SF imaging in its method of acquisition; in a one (*direct conversion*) or two (*indirect conversion*) step process, remnant x-ray photons are converted into an electric charge image. Computer hardware and software are required in both CR and DR; analog-to-digital conversion is required in CR.

In *SF technology* the film functions as the vehicle of detection, display, and storage. In *digital imaging*, each of these functions is carried out by a separate component of the digital system.

In *SF imaging* the density and contrast are determined by exposure factor selection.

In *digital imaging* brightness and contrast are determined by computer software.

Emergence and Growth of Digital Imaging

Diagnostic radiography is undergoing probably its most significant changes since the discovery of x-rays. Sonography and nuclear medicine had made the change to electronic; CT and MRI are intrinsically electronic; thus, radiography is the last imaging modality to make the transition to electronic/digital. Incentive for the transition was initially low because SF systems are reliable and produce excellent image quality. Additionally, radiography's high spatial resolution and field of view (FOV) demand that electronic images carry a large amount of digital data. To illustrate: a typical PA chest image carries between 4 to 32 MB of digital data, while a single CT image holds approximately 0.5 MB. Therefore, radiographic images require lots of digital storage space, a high bandwidth in PACS, and require costly high-resolution monitors for (diagnostic) display.

Nevertheless, although some imaging offices and hospital imaging departments might still utilize traditional SF imaging, it is clear that digital/filmless imaging will soon replace what some still think of as "traditional" imaging methods. The language of electronic radiography includes, but is far from limited to, terms such as *computed radiography* (CR), *digital* (both *direct*, and *indirect*) *radiography* (DR), PSPs, *storage phosphor screens* (SPSs), *charge-coupled devices* (CCDs), thin-film transistors (TFTs), and *picture archiving and communication systems* (PACSs).

Resolution in Digital Imaging

In radiography, *recorded detail* and *detail visibility* are the two major terms that have been used to describe image quality. They can be updated, particularly with respect to digital imaging to *spatial resolution* and *contrast resolution*, respectively. A mathematical expression of spatial resolution is modulation transfer function (MTF). One of the outstanding features of electronic imaging is its ability to provide excellent contrast resolution, which can often be more important than spatial resolution.

Spatial resolution is the term used to describe the IR's impact on recorded detail in CR/DR, and is usually expressed in terms of line pairs/mm. The spatial resolution of electronic imaging cannot compare with that of SF imaging. SF resolution is much better, but CR/DR's ability to perceive small differences in tissue densities (i.e., better contrast resolution) is often more valuable, particularly when viewing soft tissues. For example, SF imaging provides a spatial resolution of about 10 lp/mm, while CR/DR ranges between 2.5 and 5 lp/mm! However, because of the wide dynamic range (i.e., the IR's ability to respond to the exposure) of CR/DR, the number of subtle densities able to be recorded is far greater, resulting in far better contrast resolution.

Digital Radiographic Images Require:

- large amount of digital storage space
- high bandwidth in PACS
- high resolution display monitors

- One outstanding quality of digital imaging is its exceptional *contrast resolution*

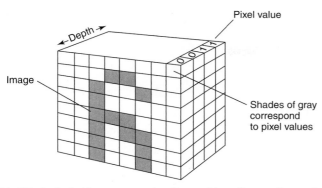

Figure 11–59. A digital image may be likened to a three-dimensional object made up of many small cubes, each containing a binary digit or bit. The image is seen on one surface of the block, whose depth is the number of bits required to describe each pixel's gray level.

Pixel Matrix. A digital image is formed by a *matrix of pixels* (*picture* elements, measured in the "XY" direction) in rows and columns. A matrix that has 512 pixels in each row and column is a 512 × 512 matrix (a typical CT image), as seen in Figures 11–59 and 11–60. The third dimension, "Z" direction, in the matrix of pixels is the *depth* that is referred to as the *voxel* (volume element) (Fig. 11–60).

Pixel depth is directly related to shades of gray—called *dynamic range*—and is measured in *bits*. The greater the number of bits, the more shades of gray. For example, a 1-bit (2^1) pixel will demonstrate 2 shades of gray, whereas a 6-bit (2^6) pixel can display 64 shades and a 7-bit (2^7) pixel 128 shades. However, pixel depth is unrelated to resolution.

Bit depth in *CT* is approximately 2^{12} with a dynamic range of almost 5,000 gray shades, approximately 2^{14} in *CR/DR* with a dynamic range of more than 16,000 gray shades, and approximately 2^{16} in digital *mammography* with a dynamic range of more than 65,500 gray shades.

The *matrix* is the number of pixels in the XY direction. *As matrix size increases, for a fixed FOV, pixel size is smaller and better image resolution results* (Fig. 11–61). An electronic/digital image is formed by a *matrix* of pixels in *rows* and *columns*. A matrix having 512 pixels in each row and column is a 512 × 512 matrix (a typical CT image).

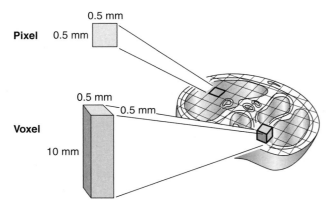

Figure 11–60. The third dimension in the matrix of pixels is the depth, which together with the pixel is referred to as the voxel (volume element).

Pixel:

- Two dimensional
- *Pic*ture *el*ement
- Measured in XY direction
- Pixel pitch = distance between pixels (impacts spatial resolution)

Voxel:

- The third dimension, depth
- *Vol*ume *el*ement
- Measured in Z direction

Matrix:

- Number of pixels in XY direction

Field of View (FOV)

- How much of the part/patient is included in the matrix

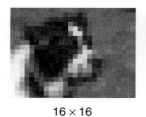 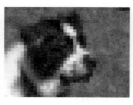 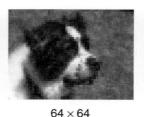 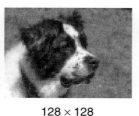 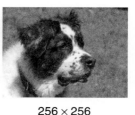

| 16 × 16 | 32 × 32 | 64 × 64 | 128 × 128 | 256 × 256 |

Figure 11–61. The matrix is the number of pixels in the XY direction. The larger the matrix size, the better the image resolution.

The term *field of view* (FOV) is used to describe how much of the patient (e.g., 150 mm diameter) is included in the matrix. The matrix and the FOV can be changed independently without one affecting the other, but changes in either will change pixel size.

As *matrix size is increased* (e.g., from 512 × 512 to 1,024 × 1,024) there are more and smaller pixels in the matrix and, therefore, *improved resolution*. Fewer and larger pixels result in poor resolution, a "pixelly" (or "mosaicked") image, that is, one in which you can actually see the individual pixel boxes (Fig. 11–61).

If FOV is increased, pixel size increases. Pixel size is inversely related to resolution; as pixel size increases, resolution decreases.

As in SF radiography, spatial resolution is measured in line pairs per millimeter (lp/mm). Another factor impacting CR resolution is *pixel pitch*, that is the distance between adjacent pixels, as determined by the scanning/*sampling frequency*. Pixels/mm, or pixel density, is used to express sampling frequency. Spatial resolution is improved with a smaller pixel pitch and greater pixels/mm (sampling frequency).

SNR. In describing *signal-to-noise ratio* (SNR), "signal" refers to the photons that have penetrated the part without interaction (i.e., unattenuated), and "noise" refers to Compton scatter and any other form of image-degrading fog.

SNR is used to describe contrast resolution; the higher the SNR, the better the contrast resolution. Generally speaking, SNR increases as mAs increases, but so does patient dose.

Compared with SF imaging, *patient dose* should be less in CR and DR (especially DR). Images should not be repeated because of brightness or contrast imperfections. Average *exposure index* guidelines should be established and maintained.

DQE. The DQE (Detective Quantum Efficiency i.e., ability of receptor material to perceive and interact with x-ray photons) of the PSP storage plate can be regarded as an x-ray absorption coefficient and is highly dependent on photon energy (kV) as well as the composition and thickness of the PSP layer.

The PSP receptor screens in CR/DR receptors use cesium iodide, barium fluorohalide, and amorphous selenium. The DQE of these receptors is higher than that of the intensifying screens used in SF imaging; thus, another reason CR/DR imaging should require less patient dose than SF imaging.

While x-ray photons are still required to produce the images, CR and DR utilize computer technology to convert the analog image to a digital image: to "read" (process) that image, to *display and manipulate* that image, and *to store* that image (see Fig. 11–62).

Pixel Size Affected By:

- Change in matrix size
- Change in FOV

CR Spatial Resolution Improves with:

- Smaller pixel pitch
- Greater pixels/mm
- Greater sampling frequency

Functions of Digital Imaging System:

- Sensor function
- Display function
- Storage function

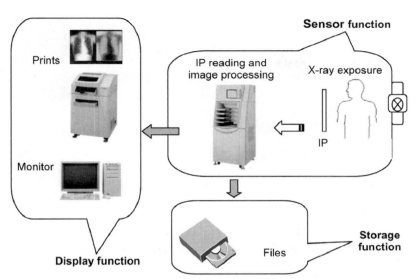

Figure 11–62. An electronic/digital imaging system is composed of various devices having separate functions: (1) the *sensor* function, x-ray exposure of a photostimulable phosphor (PSP) image plate that then goes to the scanner/reader for image processing; (2) the *display* function, image is viewed on a monitor and/or hard copy prints are made; and (3) the *storage* function, records are kept of all images for later retrieval. (Courtesy of FUJIFILM Medical Systems USA, Inc.)

ANATOMICALLY PROGRAMMED RADIOGRAPHY (APR)

The appearance of a CR or DR control panel differs greatly from its earlier predecessors. Using APR, the radiographer no longer selects specific exposure factors but, rather, uses console graphics or a touch screen to *select the anatomic part and its relative size* (S, M, L) to be imaged. The unit's microprocessor chooses the appropriate mAs and kV for that particular part and size—from the "internal technique chart" predetermined and stored upon installation.

APR is used in conjunction with AEC and is therefore still highly dependent upon the skillfulness of its user. Accurate positioning, photocell selection, and control of scattered radiation is essential to the production of quality images. See the AEC section(s) for review of these important factors.

COMPUTED RADIOGRAPHY

The Image Plate

Traditional x-ray *cassettes* contain a pair of intensifying screens with film sandwiched between the two screens. In computed radiography (CR), the cassette-like device is termed an image plate (IP). IPs have no intensifying screens or film within (Fig. 11–63), hence the term *filmless radiography*. The IPs have a *protective* function (for the flexible PSP storage plate within) and can be conveniently placed in the bucky tray or under the anatomic part.

The IPs need not be light-tight because the PSP storage plate inside is *not sensitive* to brief exposures to white light. One corner of the IP's rear panel has a *memory chip* for patient information; the IP also has a thin *lead foil backing* (similar to intensifying screen cassettes) to absorb any backscatter.

Abbreviations

IP	Image Plate
PSP	Photostimulable phosphor
PSL	Photostimulable luminescence
SPS	Storage phosphor screen
CR	Computed Radiography
SNR	Signal-to-Noise Ratio
MTF	Modulation Transfer Function
PMT	Photomultiplier tube
PD	Photodiode
ADC	Analog-to-Digital Converter
APR	Anatomically Programmed Radiography
DQE	Detective Quantum Efficiency
CCD	Charge Coupled Device
TFT	Thin-Film Transistor
HIS	Hospital Information System
RIS	Radiology Information System
PACS	Picture Archiving and Communication System
DICOM	Digital Imaging and Communications in Medicine
EDR	Exposure Data Recognition
DEL	Detector Element
SF	Screen/film

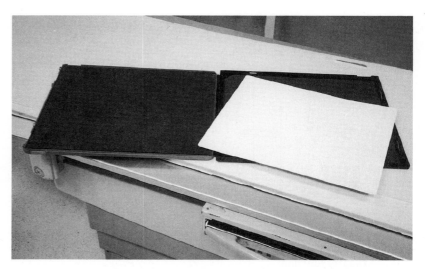

Figure 11–63. The IP holds a photostimulable storage phosphor (PSP – the image receptor) between its front and rear panels. (Reproduced, with permission, from Shephard CT. *Radiographic Image Production and Manipulation*. New York: McGraw-Hill, 2003.)

The Photostimulable Phosphor (PSP)

Inside the IP is the all-important *PSP*, also called SPS, which is the actual IR.

The PSP storage plate within the IP has a layer of europium-activated barium fluorohalide ($BaFX:Eu^{2}+$; X = halogen) mixed with a binder substance. This layer serves as the *IR* when exposed in the traditional manner; it looks very much like an x-ray cassette intensifying screen.

The barium fluorohalide is usually *granular* or *turbid* phosphors. Other examples of turbid phosphors are gadolinium oxysulfide and rubidium chloride. *"Needle"*-shaped or *columnar* phosphors (usually cesium iodide) have the advantage of *better x-ray absorption* and *less light diffusion* (Fig. 11–64).

Just under the barium fluorohalide layer is a *reflective layer* that helps direct emitted light up toward the CR reader. Below the reflective layer is the *base*, behind that is an *antistatic layer*, and then the *lead foil* to absorb backscatter. Over the top of the barium fluorohalide is a *protective layer*.

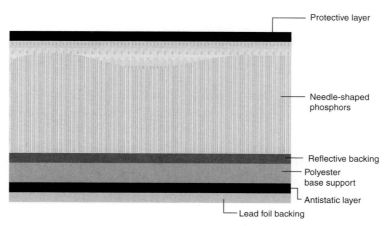

Figure 11–64. Barium fluorohalide is either granular or "needle shaped." The "needlelike" phosphors have the advantage of *better x-ray absorption and less light diffusion.*

Some PSP storage plates are manufactured specifically for better resolution (e.g., for mammography). Some higher-resolution PSP storage plates "read" the information from *both* sides of the PSP storage plates.

X-ray Absorption by PSP

When the barium fluorohalide absorbs x-ray energy, *electrons are released and they divide into two groups*. One electron group initiates *immediate luminescence* (primary excitation) during the excited state of Eu^{2+}. The other electron group *becomes trapped* within the phosphor's halogen ions, forming a "color center" (also called "F center"). These are the phosphors that ultimately form the radiographic image because, when exposed to a *monochromatic* laser light source, these phosphors emit *polychromatic* light (secondary excitation), termed *photostimulated luminescence* (PSL).

The PSP layer can *store* its latent image for several hours; however, after approximately 8 hours, noticeable image *fading* will occur. The europium activator is important for the *storage* characteristic of the PSPs; it also has a function similar to the sensitization specks within film emulsion—without europium the image will not become manifest.

Reading the PSP

After exposure, the IP is placed into the CR *scanner/reader* (Fig. 11–65), where the PSP screen is automatically removed. The latent image on the PSP is changed to a *manifest image* as it is moved at a *constant* speed and scanned by a narrow monochromatic *high-intensity helium–neon laser* or a *solid-state* laser to obtain the pixel data.

The longer wavelength light from the newer *solid-state lasers* has the advantage of being unlikely to interfere with the light being emitted by the PSPs (Fig. 11–66). This appropriate (red, 430–550 nm) wavelength is absorbed by the "color center" and the electrons trapped there, causing PSL to occur during the excited state of Eu^{2+}(secondary excitation).

The phosphors are activated by a *monochromatic* laser light; however, PSL is a *different* color (bluish-purple, blue–green, etc.). These two lights (PSL and laser) must not interfere with each other. To improve the image SNR, the PSL (carrying the x-ray image) must be a different

> ### PSP Storage Plate Layers
>
> - Protective coat
> - $BaFX:Eu^{2+}$ phosphors in binder material
> - Reflective backing
> - Polyester base support material
> - Antistatic layer
> - Lead foil backing

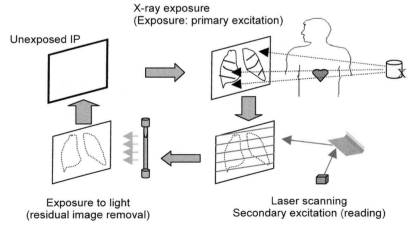

Figure 11–65. The *recording, reading,* and *erasure* cycle of an IP and its PSP. The PSP, within the IP, is exposed to x-ray photons, scanned/read, and then erased for reuse. (Courtesy of FUJIFILM Medical Systems USA, Inc.)

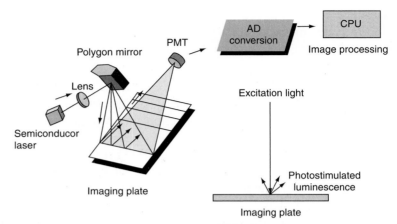

Figure 11–66. The latent image on the PSP screen is changed to a manifest image as it is moved at a constant speed and scanned by a narrow high-intensity helium–neon laser or a solid-state laser to obtain the pixel data. (Courtesy of FUJIFILM Medical Systems USA, Inc.)

wavelength/color than, and physically separate from, the laser excitation light. An *optical filter* is used that permits *transmission* of the PSL but *attenuates* the laser light; this filter is mounted in front of a PMT.

The PMT or photodiode (PD) is used to detect the PSL and convert it to electrical signals (see Fig. 11–66). The electrical energy is sent to an *analog-to-digital converter (ADC)* where it becomes the *digital* image that is displayed, after a short delay, on a high-resolution monitor and/or printed out by a laser printer (hard copy). The digitized images can also be manipulated in *postprocessing*, electronically *transmitted*, and stored/ *archived*. Postprocessing manipulation can include *edge enhancement*; this technique can be used to improve the visibility of structures such as chest tubes by accentuating their edges.

An artifact associated with digital imaging and grids is "aliasing" (see Fig. 13–31B). If the direction of the lead strips and the grid lines per inch (i.e., grid frequency) matches the scan frequency of the scanner/ reader, this artifact can occur. Aliasing appears as superimposed images slightly out of alignment, an image "wrapping" effect. This most commonly occurs in mobile radiography with stationary grids and can be a problem with DR flat panel detectors.

Once the PSP reading process is completed, any remaining data stored on the PSP are erased by exposing it to high-intensity light (called "erasure"); the PSP storage plate is then ready for reuse (see Fig. 11–65).

As previously mentioned, image *"fading"* will occur if there is a delay in reading the PSP. This is because after a time, trapped photoelectrons are released from the "color center" and are therefore unable to participate in PSL. PSL intensity *decreases* in the interval between x-ray exposure and the image-reading process. If the exposed PSL is not delivered to the reader/processor for 8 hours, PSL decreases by approximately 25%. Fading also increases as environmental temperature increases.

PSP Sensitivity

PSP storage plates are very sensitive (more than film emulsion) not only to x-rays but ultraviolet, gamma, and particulate radiation. Environmental conditions are therefore an important consideration in the storage of PSP/storage screens and their IPs.

Steps in Reading the PSP Storage Plate:

- IP into scanner/reader
- PSP automatically removed
- PSP moved at constant speed, scanned by a monochromatic laser to obtain pixel data
- PSL occurs during scanning
- Scanning laser and PSL must be different wavelengths and must not interact
- For better SNR, an optical filter attenuates the laser, while transmitting the PSL
- PMT/PD detects the PSL and convert it to electrical signals
- Electrical signals sent to ADC and is displayed on monitor
- PSP erased by exposing it to high-intensity light; ready for reuse

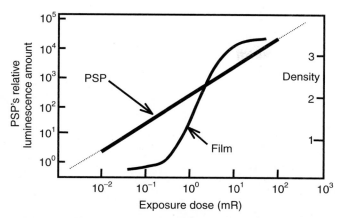

Figure 11–67. It compares the sensitometric curve of a typical film emulsion with that of PSP storage plates. The *wide dynamic range* (scale of contrast) of the PSP storage plate enables the correct detection of slight differences in x-ray absorption characteristics among various tissue densities. (Courtesy of FUJIFILM Medical Systems USA, Inc.)

Building materials such as concrete, marble, and so on, constantly emit natural radiation; bedrock in some geographic areas contributes significantly to background radiation. If PSP storage plates are stored for extended periods of time, the possibility of artifacts must be considered. These artifacts typically appear as randomly placed small black spots. *If an IP and its PSP storage plate has been stored, unused, for an extended period of time (i.e., for 48 hours), the PSP storage plate should be erased prior to use.*

The mechanical consistency and accuracy of the laser optics and transport systems of the CR scanner/reader is extremely important for image quality—inconsistent scanning motion can result in a wavy, or otherwise distorted, image. This is sometimes referred to as *"laser jitter"* and should be evaluated monthly as part of the CR QA monitoring.

Dynamic Range and Exposure Latitude

In CR, there is a *linear* relationship between the exposure given the PSP storage plate and its resulting luminescence (Fig. 11–67) as it is scanned by the laser. One of the biggest advantages of CR is the *dynamic range* it offers.

Earlier in this chapter, we studied the sensitometric curve of typical film emulsion and saw that there is a certain "range of correct exposure," limited by the toe and shoulder of the curve, which determines the emulsion's *latitude* characteristics.

The term *latitude* is used in SF imaging; the term *dynamic range* is used in CR. CR's wide dynamic range permits visualization of anatomic details having only slightly different absorption differentials and also permits the use of exposure data recognition (EDR), which automatically adjusts image density and contrast to meet diagnostic requirements.

This affords much greater *dynamic range* and *exposure latitude*; technical inaccuracies can be effectively eliminated. Overexposure of up to 500% and underexposure of up to 80% are reported as recoverable, thus eliminating most retakes (Fig. 11–68). *This surely affords increased efficiency; however, this does not mean that images can be exposed arbitrarily.*

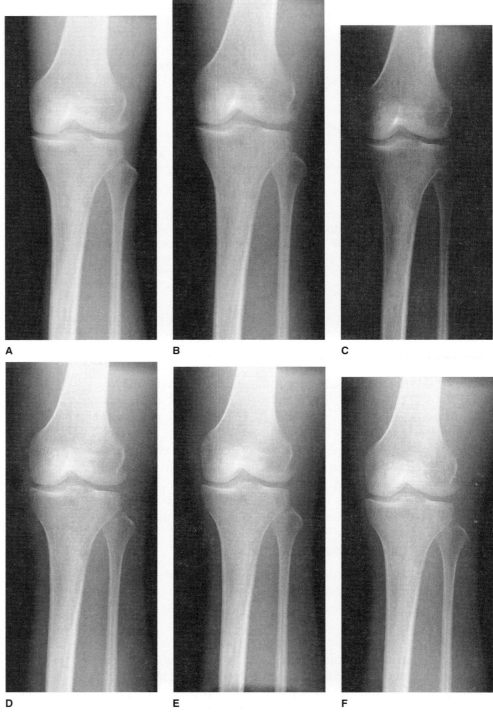

Figure 11–68. CR affords much *an almost infinite dynamic range/gray scale*; technical inaccuracies can be effectively eliminated, but *exposure* dose must still be considered. In the images seen above, *A*, *B*, and *C* were made with conventional SF using at 65 kV and at 3.2, 6.3, and 12.5 mAs, respectively. Density changes are easily identified. Images *D*, *E*, and *F* were made with CR again using 3.2, 6.3, and 12.5 mAs, respectively. The images are identical—demonstrating how *technical inaccuracies can be effectively eliminated* with CR. Although the radiographic/image densities are identical, the *exposure dose* is not! An approximation of the *exposure* dose can be determined from the *exposure indicator*: an"S" (sensitivity) number, "EI" (exposure index), or other "relative exposure index," depending on the manufacturer use.

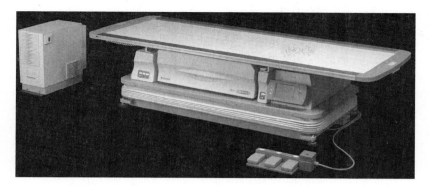

Figure 11–69. Direct-capture (cassette-less) digital radiographic unit. (Courtesy of FUJIFILM Medical Systems USA, Inc.)

The radiographer must keep dose reduction in mind. The *same* exposure factors as SF systems, *or less*, are generally recommended for CR.

Whereas CR uses IPs, DR does not. CR's use of IPs offers the advantage of continued use of existing equipment, and CR is convenient for mobile radiographic applications, for tabletop/nongrid work, and for crosstable/horizontal beam work.

INDIRECT AND DIRECT DR

CR/DR Differences

While CR utilizes traditional x-ray tables and cassette-like devices (IPs) to enclose and protect the flexible PSP, *DR* requires the use of somewhat different equipment. DR does not use cassettes/IPs or a traditional x-ray table; it is a *direct-capture*, or *indirect-capture*, system of x-ray imaging (Fig. 11–69). DR eliminates IPs and their handling, DR affords the advantage of immediate display of the image (compared with CR's slightly delayed image display), and DR exposures can be lower because of the detector's higher DQE (i.e., ability to perceive and interact with x-ray photons). DR, like CR, also offers the advantage of image preview and postprocessing.

While CR uses IPs that require an *identification process*, DR uses no such device. In DR, patient identification and demographics are selected from the RIS or HIS list.

Indirect-Capture DR

One type of *indirect*-capture flat-panel detector uses *cesium iodide* or *gadolinium oxysulfide* as the *scintillator*—which captures x-ray photons and emits light. That light is then transferred via a photodetector-coupling agent—a CCD or TFT.

CCD Method

Each CCD chip within the CCD array flat-panel detector has many pixel electronics on its photosensitive silicon surface. As CsI or GdOS *scintillation* falls upon each pixel, electrons are liberated and built up within the pixel—the greater the light intensity, the greater the number of electrons liberated. The image is still analog at this point. As the electronic charge within each pixel is read out, an electronic signal is produced and transmitted to the ADC for digitization. This method provides spatial resolution of up to 5 lp/mm.

Terminology Comparison

SF imaging	CR/DR imaging
Latitude	Dynamic range
Contrast	Contrast resolution
Density	Brightness
Recorded detail/sharpness	SNR
Resolution	Spatial frequency

CR Resolution Increases As

- PSP phosphor size decreases
- Laser beam size decreases
- Monitor matrix size increases

CR/DR Feature Comparisons:

CR:
- Traditional X-ray Equipment
- Uses IPs/Cassettes
- Delayed Image Display
- Image Preview/Post-processing

DR:
- Needs New Equipment
- Uses No IPs/Cassettes
- Immediate Image Display
- Image Preview/Post-processing
- Higher DQE/Lower Patient Dose

TFT Method

A TFT is composed of glass with amorphous (i.e., in fluid form rather than crystalline) selenium on both sides. CsI or GdOS scintillation light must be able to pass through the detector material to reach the ADC. As silicon is opaque, glass is the most commonly used (though delicate) interface because it is highly transparent and compatible with the system. Since glass is not a semiconductor like silicon, a thin film of amorphous selenium (a-Se) is deposited on its top and bottom—the transistors are made using this thin layer; hence, the name "*thin-film transistor.*" The electrical signal is transmitted to the ADC.

In both indirect-capture flat-panel detector methods, *scintillation* light is captured, read by a *photodetector* (CCD or TFT), changed to an electronic signal, and transmitted to the ADC for digitization.

Direct-Capture DR

In *direct*-capture flat-panel detector systems, x-ray energy is converted to an electrical signal in a single layer of material such as the semiconductor a-Se. Electric charges are applied to both surfaces of the a-Se, electron-hole pairs are created, and charges are read by TFT arrays located on the surfaces. The electrical signal is transferred directly to the ADC. The number of TFTs is equal to the number of image pixels.

Thus, the direct-capture system *eliminates the scintillator step* required in indirect DR. Since selenium has a relatively low Z number (compared with gadolinium [Z = 64] or cesium [Z = 55]), a-Se detectors are made thicker to improve detection, thus compensating for the low x-ray absorption of selenium. There is no diffusion of electrons (as there is light diffusion in intensifying screens), so spatial resolution is not affected in this manner.

The spatial resolution of direct digital systems is fixed and is related to the *detector element* (DEL) size of the TFT. The smaller the TFT DEL size, the better the spatial resolution. DEL size of 100 microns provides a spatial resolution of about 5 lp/mm (available only in some digital mammography systems). DEL size of 200 microns provides a spatial resolution of about 2.5 lp/mm (general radiography)—lower than that achieved with 400 speed intensifying screen system. A 100 speed intensifying screen system offers a spatial resolution of about 10 lp/mm—significantly greater than, and currently unachievable in, digital imaging.

Spatial resolution in digital imaging is fixed, but it is very important that radiographers are alert to the opportunities they have to utilize and control the remaining recorded detail factors (motion and geometric factors).

EXPOSURE INDICATION

CR offers *wide dynamic range* and *automatic optimization of the radiologic image.* When AEC is not used, CR can compensate for approximately 80% underexposure and 500% overexposure—this is termed *exposure data recognition* (EDR). This can be an important advantage particularly in trauma and mobile radiography. The radiographer must still be vigilant in patient dose considerations—overexposure, though correctable via EDR, results in *increased patient dose*; underexposure results in decreased image quality because of increased image *noise*.

CR systems provide some type of *exposure indicator*, its name varies according to manufacturer: an *S* (sensitivity) number, *EI* (exposure index), *REX* (reached exposure index), or other identifying exposure index depending on the manufacturer used. The manufacturer usually provides a chart identifying the acceptable *range* the exposure indicator numbers should be within for various examination types. While in one manufacturer's system a high S number is related to *under* exposure, a high *EI* number in another manufacturer's system is related to *over* exposure—it is essential for radiographers to be knowledgeable about the various types of equipment they use.

TECHNICAL FACTORS: DIGITAL IMAGING

In SF imaging, image quality components are density, contrast, detail, and distortion. Digital imaging quality still includes detail (*spatial resolution*) and *distortion*; however, *brightness* and *contrast* are determined by computer software. *Noise* and *Exposure Indication* are also very important image quality considerations in digital imaging.

The *number of x-ray photons* produced is still determined by mAs, but computer/digital processing algorithms will correct inaccurate selection of mAs.

X-ray *penetration* is still determined by kV but has much less an effect on image contrast because of the wide dynamic range afforded by digital imaging.

Additionally, *APR* enables the radiographer to select the *part* to be imaged (rather than specific exposure factors), and the most appropriate exposure factors are automatically selected.

GEOMETRIC FACTORS: DIGITAL IMAGING

The majority of SF geometric factors—OID, SID, Focal Spot Size, size and shape Distortion, Structural position and shape, and Motion *apply to digital imaging as well*. Although we might think of digital imaging as very automated, the radiographer has control of most of these Detail and Distortion factors and must be capable of using them to produce the best image with the smallest patient exposure dose.

Resolution

In addition to focal spot size, OID, SID, motion, structure position and shape, and tube angle, there are additional factors unique to digital imaging that affect resolution.

Matrix Size

The larger the matrix size, with the FOV unchanged, the better the resolution—because pixel size decreases.

FOV

As the FOV decreases, with matrix size remaining the same, the better the resolution—because pixel size decreases. Larger matrices are appropriate for large body parts, for example, the chest, to better visualize small anatomic details.

VISIBILITY FACTORS: DIGITAL IMAGING

Factors affecting density and contrast in SF imaging have little to no effect on similar characteristics seen in digital x-ray images.

Software processing algorithms control digital image *brightness*. The number of x-ray photons produced, as determined by the programmed algorithm, is probably the most important aspect of the digital imaging process.

The total number of x-ray photons exiting the part is divided among all the pixels—and each pixel must have enough x-ray photons to provide a *gray scale* range.

If there are insufficient x-ray photons for each pixel, noise (graininess) increases, that is, as SNR decreases, noise increases. Digital imaging EDR offers wide latitude and automatic optimization of the radiologic image. EDR, using the selected processing algorithm and its LUT, enables compensation for approximately 80% underexposure and 500% overexposure. While automatic/computerized optimization of the radiologic image is a wonderful tool, radiographers must be even more aware of their role in keeping patient dose to a minimum.

INFORMATION SYSTEMS AND NETWORK INTERFACES

Hospital information system (HIS) is a computer system that serves to track patient information: admission and discharge, diagnostic and treatment services, pharmaceutical and equipment information, billing information, and employee information. Functions of a *radiology information system* (RIS) include procedure ordering and scheduling, patient database maintenance, reporting and transcription, and billing. RIS can be a separate system, part of HIS, or part of PACS. Neither HIS nor RIS stores images, that is, the function of PACS.

An organization of computers *networked* together and capable of *storing* (archiving) and *transmitting* (communication) medical images is called a *PACS*. The PACS functions to obtain the images (*image acquisition*), to present the images for analysis (*image display and interpretation*), to store the images conveniently for future viewing (*image archival and retrieval*), and to provide a means of image transmission (*image communication*). This network can be limited to a single hospital or it can include distant sites. A PACS network is usually coupled with the *RIS* containing patient information regarding scheduling and imaging information and the *HIS* containing all other patient demographics. Patient confidentiality and unauthorized access, especially when networked with the Internet for image transmission, are serious concerns. Encryption software is used to prevent unlawful access to restricted information.

The recognized standard for format, services, and communication protocol affecting the transfer, storage, and display of diagnostic images in PACS and teleradiology systems has been established as *digital imaging and communications in medicine* (DICOM). Equipment from various vendors that conforms to the DICOM standard can be used together effectively to build PACS and teleradiology systems.

PACS Features

- Image acquisition
- Image display and interpretation
- Image archival and retrieval
- Image communication

Summary

- The fixed kV type chart uses an optimal kV for each anatomic part; its advantage is consistency of image contrast.

- The variable kV type chart increases/decreases the kV by 2 for each 1-cm increase/decrease in body thickness; thus, accurate part measurement is necessary.

- AECs will compensate for tissue thickness and density differences; they require accurate positioning and correct photocell selection.

- Electronic radiography includes CR, indirect DR, and direct DR.

- MTF is used to describe spatial resolution; SNR is used to describe contrast resolution.

- CR/DR's ability to provide better contrast resolution than SF is more valuable than the somewhat less spatial resolution it provides.

- As matrix size increases, for a fixed FOV, pixel size is smaller and better spatial resolution results.

- As FOV increases, for a fixed matrix size, the size of each pixel increases and spatial resolution decreases.

- CR and indirect DR convert x-rays to light and then to an electric signal; x-ray image on the monitor is somewhat delayed.

- Direct DR uses no cassette, no scintillation/fluorescent screen—x-rays interact with a-Se creating a charge that is interpreted by the TFT; x-ray image on the monitor is immediate.

- The electric signal from CR/DR is sent to the ADC, and from there to the computer monitor.

- The spatial resolution of direct digital systems is fixed and is related to the detector element DEL size of the TFT.

- In CR, PSP ($BaFX:Eu^{2+}$) screens emit retained x-ray energy as visible light when stimulated by a laser beam.

- CR image "fading" can occur if there is a delay in reading/ processing the PSP/SPS.

- If an IP and its PSP storage plate have been stored, unused, for an extended period of time, the PSP storage plate should be *erased* prior to use.

- CR offers wide latitude and automatic optimization of the radiologic image; CR/DR can compensate for approximately 80% underexposure and 500% overexposure.

- PACS is a system of computers networked together and capable of *storing* and *transmitting* medical images.

COMPREHENSION CHECK

1. What are some variables that contribute to difficulty in selection of exposure factors? What equipment features can help? What precautions must one observe when using these features (p. 297, 298)?

2. Define recorded detail; list other terms that can be used to refer to recorded detail (p. 298, 299).

3. To what does the term *resolution* refer; how is it measured and expressed (p. 298, 299)?

4. What does one "line pair" consist of (p. 299)?

5. Differentiate between *detail* and *distortion* (p. 298, 299).

6. How are the terms *magnification*, *elongation*, and *foreshortening* related to *distortion* (p. 299)?

7. Discuss the difference between detail and visibility of detail/contrast resolution (p. 298, 299).

8. What are the geometric factors affecting recorded detail (p. 298)?

9. What is the relationship among OID, recorded detail, and magnification; among SID, recorded detail, and magnification (p. 298, 299, 301)?

10. What are the two types of shape distortion? How can shape distortion be avoided (p. 299, 303)?

11. How is object unsharpness, with respect to its three-dimensional shape and OID, an inherent part of every radiographic image (p. 302, 303)?

12. Distinguish between actual and effective/projected/apparent focal spot size; what is the line focus principle (p. 304, 305)?

13. How is actual focal spot size related to recorded detail? How does the size of the projected focus vary along the length of the image receptor (p. 305)?

14. How are focal spot size and anode angle related to x-ray tube heat-loading capacity (p. 305-307)?

15. Discuss the difference between voluntary and involuntary motion, and describe the most effective means of avoiding each (p. 309, 310).

16. Why is motion intentionally introduced in some radiographic examinations? Give some examples (p. 310).

17. What is the relationship between the fluorescent light from intensifying screens and the total exposure received by the film emulsion (p. 310, 311)?

18. Discuss how phosphor type and size, active or phosphor layer thickness, and reflective backing affect the speed on intensifying screens (p. 311, 312).

19. What is lag or afterglow; how can it affect the radiographic image (p. 312)?

20. What are the three most commonly used rare earth phosphors (p. 312)?

21. What is the importance of spectral matching (p. 312)?

22. How is intensifying screen speed related to recorded detail? With what type of intensifying screens is quantum mottle usually associated (p. 313)?

23. What is the importance of screen and film contact? How is its accuracy tested (p. 313)?

24. Define radiographic density; describe optical density (OD); what is the term used in digital imaging to describe density (p. 314-316)?

25. Describe how radiographic density and mAs are related to the intensity and exposure rate of the x-ray beam (p. 315-317).

26. What is the reciprocity law, and how is it related to radiographic density? Give examples (p. 317).

27. What change in mAs is required to make a perceptible change in radiographic density (p. 317)?

28. How is SID related to x-ray beam intensity and technical factors (specifically mAs)? What law expresses this relationship (p. 318, 319)?

29. How is kV related to x-ray beam intensity and radiographic density (p. 320-322)?

30. What is the 15% rule? Give examples (p. 320).

31. What is the relationship among radiographic density, mAs, and intensifying screen speed? Give examples (p. 321, 322).

32. What three factors determine the quantity of scattered radiation produced? How can each be modified to limit the production of scattered radiation (p. 322, 323)?

33. How do grids affect the amount of scattered radiation reaching the image receptor? How do they impact radiographic density (p. 322, 323)?

34. What is a stationary grid? Give some examples of its use. What are its disadvantages (p. 323, 324)?

35. What is a moving grid? How does its construction generally differ from the stationary grid? What is its advantage over a stationary grid (p. 324)?

36. Define convergence line, focusing distance, focal range, crossed grid (p. 324).

37. Define grid cutoff, lateral decentering, focus–grid distance decentering (p. 324, 325).

38. Describe grid ratio, number of lead strips per inch, lead content; describe their relationship to *cleanup* and radiographic density (p. 326, 327, 328).

39. Of what material(s) is grid interspace material usually made? How is each related to efficiency, patient dose, sturdiness (p. 326, 327)?

40. Describe contrast improvement factor and selectivity (p. 327).

41. Describe how the grid-conversion factor can be used to determine the required mAs adjustment (p. 327, 328).

42. How can an air gap influence radiographic density (p. 329)?

43. What is inherent filtration? Of what does it consist (p. 330)?

44. What is added filtration? Of what does it consist (p. 330)?

45. What is the primary purpose of total filtration? What effect does it have on radiographic density (p. 330)?

46. Describe why and how compensating filters are used, how they affect radiographic density; give examples of common usage (p. 330, 331).

47. Describe how body position, condition, and pathology affect radiographic density (p. 332, 333).

48. Differentiate between and give examples of destructive and additive pathologic conditions (p. 332, 333).

49. How are different types of x-ray generators related to changes in radiographic density? How is mAs (or kV) changed when changing from single-phase equipment to 3ø 6P or 3ø 12P equipment? Which technical factor is preferable to change (p. 333-335)?

50. How can beam restriction affect radiographic density (p. 336)?

51. How can the anode heel effect impact radiographic density? Under what conditions is the heel effect most noticeable (p. 336, 337)?

52. How can automatic processing affect radiographic density (p. 336, 337)?

53. What is the function of radiographic contrast? What are its two components? What is *contrast resolution* (p. 339)?

54. Describe the difference between long-scale and short-scale contrast. What is the single most important technical factor regulating radiographic contrast (p. 339-341)?

55. What is subject contrast and how is it related to beam quality (p. 339, 340)?

56. Describe the impact of scattered radiation on radiographic contrast/contrast resolution; what is the most important way to limit the production of scattered radiation (p. 344)?

57. What kinds of pathologic conditions impact radiographic contrast (p. 345)?

58. How does the use of grids affect radiographic contrast/contrast resolution (p. 347)?

59. Describe the two types of AECs. Include in your description (p. 349, 350):

    (A) The location of each, relative to the tabletop and cassette

    (B) Operation of each and how exposure is terminated

60. Explain the importance of the backup timer used in AEC (p. 350).

61. Explain the importance of proper AEC photocell selection; describe typical errors in photocell selection and the subsequent radiographic results (p. 350, 352).

62. Explain how to correct a radiographic image overexposed as a result of the equipment minimum reaction time limitations (p. 350).

63. Why are fixed kV technique charts preferred over variable kV technique charts (p. 351, 352)?

64. Discuss why exposures made using an AEC do not require measurement of the part being examined, and why positioning accuracy is essential to proper function of the AEC (p. 350).

65. What are the types of electronic imaging? How do they differ from one another? What traditional x-ray image quality terms correlate to the terms *spatial resolution* and *contrast resolution* (p. 353)?

66. What is meant by FOV? How is it related to matrix size, pixel size, and spatial resolution (p. 354, 355, 356)?

67. What is the difference between turbid and columnar phosphors? How is it related to resolution (p. 358)?

68. Describe the difference between a SF x-ray cassette and the IP used in CR (p. 357).

69. Describe/list differences between CR and DR. (p. 363)

70. What is DQE? How does it differ from CR and DR? How does any difference potentially affect patient dose (p. 356, 357)?

71. How does the dynamic range of CR differ from the sensitometric curve of traditional SF radiography (p. 361)?

72. How does the PSP record the x-ray image (p. 358, 359)?

73. How is the exposed PSP "read" (p. 359-360)?

74. What kind of laser is used to stimulate the PSP? Of what importance is its motion (p. 359)?

75. What is the purpose of the optical filter (p. 360)?

76. What is the value of postprocessing (p. 360)?

77. What are some advantages of CR over traditional SF radiography (p. 361)?

78. What is image *fading*? How can it be avoided (p. 360)?

79. Why should PSPs be erased prior to use if they have been unused for an extended period (p. 361)?

80. Cite differences between indirect and direct DR (p. 363-364).

81. What are the two indirect digital methods; describe how each works (p. 363-364)?

82. What step of indirect DR is eliminated in direct DR (p. 364)?

83. What is a detector element? How is DEL size related to spatial resolution (p. 364)?

84. Discuss automatic optimization of the x-ray image offered by electronic imaging. How much over/underexposure can be corrected? In what way can the radiographer be made aware of over/underexposure (p. 364, 365)?

85. What is PACS? Identify its functions and component parts (p. 366).

CHAPTER REVIEW QUESTIONS

Congratulations! You have completed this chapter. You may go on to the "Registry-type" multiple-choice questions that follow.

1. Which of the following has (have) an effect on recorded detail?

    1. Focal spot size
    2. Shape of anatomic structure
    3. Object–image distance

    (A) 1 only
    (B) 1 and 2 only
    (C) 1 and 3 only
    (D) 1, 2, and 3

2. A wire mesh is used to test:

    (A) Focal spot size
    (B) For screen lag
    (C) SF contact
    (D) Screen speed

3. Misalignment of the tube–part–IR relationship results in:

    1. Shape distortion
    2. Magnification
    3. Focal spot blur

    (A) 1 only
    (B) 1 and 2 only
    (C) 1 and 3 only
    (D) 1, 2, and 3

4. The geometry of the radiologic image is affected by:

    1. OID
    2. SID
    3. Tube angle

    (A) 1 only
    (B) 1 and 2 only
    (C) 2 and 3 only
    (D) 1, 2, and 3

5. Although the stated focal spot size is measured directly under the AFS, EFS size actually varies along the width of the x-ray beam. At which portion of the x-ray beam is the EFS the smallest?

    (A) At its outer edge
    (B) Along the path of the central ray
    (C) At the cathode end
    (D) At the anode end

6. Which of the following will result in the best recorded detail?

    (A) 1.5-mm focal spot
    (B) 1.0-mm focal spot
    (C) 0.6-mm focal spot
    (D) 0.3-mm focal spot

7. All of the following are related to recorded detail, except:

    (A) Motion
    (B) Screen speed
    (C) Object–image distance
    (D) Grid ratio

8. Foreshortening may be caused by:

    1. The radiographic object being placed at an angle to the IR
    2. Insufficient distance between the focus and the IR
    3. Very little distance between the object and the IR

    (A) 1 only
    (B) 2 only
    (C) 1 and 2 only
    (D) 1, 2, and 3

9. When an intensifying screen continues to glow after the x-ray exposure has ended, the screen is said to possess:

    (A) Fluorescence
    (B) Incandescence
    (C) Luminescence
    (D) Lag

10. Which of the following has (have) an effect on distortion?
    1. Source–image distance
    2. Angulation of the x-ray tube
    3. Angulation of the part
    (A) 1 only
    (B) 1 and 2 only
    (C) 2 and 3 only
    (D) 1, 2, and 3

11. The ratio of a grid can be increased by:
    1. Increasing the width of the lead strips
    2. Increasing the height of the lead strips
    3. Decreasing the distance between the lead strips
    (A) 1 only
    (B) 1 and 2 only
    (C) 2 and 3 only
    (D) 1, 2, and 3

12. Of the following groups of (SF) exposure factors which will produce the greatest radiographic density?
    (A) 200 mA, 50 msec, 36-in. SID
    (B) 400 mA, 0.05 second, 72-in. SID
    (C) 400 mA, 0.10 second, 72-in. SID
    (D) 200 mA, 100 msec, 36-in. SID

13. How is SID related to exposure rate and image density?
    (A) As SID increases, exposure rate increases and image density increases
    (B) As SID increases, exposure rate increases and image density decreases
    (C) As SID increases, exposure rate decreases and image density increases
    (D) As SID increases, exposure rate decreases and image density decreases

14. If the radiographer is unable to adjust the mAs, yet needs to reduce the image density of a particular image by one-half, which of the following would best accomplish this?
    (A) Decrease the kV by 50%
    (B) Decrease the kV by 15%
    (C) Decrease the SID by 25%
    (D) Decrease the grid ratio

15. Exposure factors of 85 kV and 10 mAs are used for a particular nongrid exposure. What should be the new mAs if an 8:1 grid is added?
    (A) 20 mAs
    (B) 30 mAs
    (C) 40 mAs
    (D) 50 mAs

16. An x-ray image demonstrating poor contrast resolution can be attributable to insufficient:
    1. Beam restriction
    2. kV
    3. mAs
    (A) 1 only
    (B) 1 and 2 only
    (C) 2 and 3 only
    (D) 1, 2, and 3

17. The term used to describe image density in *digital* imaging is:
    (A) Blackening
    (B) Gray scale
    (C) Brightness
    (D) Resolution

18. An exposure was made using 200 mA, 50-msec exposure, and 75 kV. Each of the following changes will effectively double radiographic density, except:
    (A) Change to 0.1-second exposure
    (B) Change to 86 kV
    (C) Change to 20 mAs
    (D) Change to 100 mA

19. An exposure was made at 40-in. SID using 300 mA, 0.12-second exposure, and 70 kV with a 200 SF combination and an 8:1 grid. It is desired to repeat the image and, to produce improved detail, use 48-in. SID and 100 SF combination. Using 0.25-second exposure, and with all other factors remaining constant, what mA will be required to maintain the original radiographic density?
    (A) 100
    (B) 200
    (C) 300
    (D) 400

20. Radiographic density is directly related to x-ray:
    1. Beam intensity
    2. Exposure rate
    3. Photon quantity
    (A) 1 only
    (B) 1 and 2 only
    (C) 2 and 3 only
    (D) 1, 2, and 3

21. The effects of scattered radiation on the x-ray image include the following:
    1. It produces fog
    2. It decreases contrast resolution
    3. It increases grid cutoff
    (A) 1 only
    (B) 2 only
    (C) 1 and 2 only
    (D) 1, 2, and 3

22. In comparison to 90 kV, in SF imaging, 60 kV will:
    1. Permit greater exposure latitude
    2. Produce shorter scale contrast
    3. Produce less Compton scatter
    (A) 1 only
    (B) 1 and 2 only
    (C) 2 and 3 only
    (D) 1, 2, and 3

23. An increase in the kV applied to the x-ray tube increases the:
    1. X-ray wavelength
    2. Exposure rate
    3. Patient absorption
    (A) 1 only
    (B) 2 only
    (C) 1 and 3 only
    (D) 1, 2, and 3

24. All of the following are related to radiographic contrast *except*:
    (A) Photon energy
    (B) Grid ratio
    (C) Object–image distance
    (D) Focal spot size

25. Which of the following groups of exposure factors will produce the longest scale of contrast in SF imaging?
    (A) 200 mA, 1/20 second, 70 kV, 12:1 grid
    (B) 500 mA, 0.02 second, 80 kV, 16:1 grid
    (C) 300 mA, 30 msec, 90 kV, 8:1 grid
    (D) 600 mA, 15 msec, 70 kV, 8:1 grid

26. Which of the following anatomic parts exhibits the highest subject contrast?
    (A) Elbow
    (B) Kidney
    (C) Esophagus
    (D) Lumbar spine

27. An x-ray image that exhibits many shades of gray from white to black may be described as having:
    (A) Long-scale contrast
    (B) Short-scale contrast
    (C) More density
    (D) Good recorded detail

28. The advantages of high-kV chest radiography in SF imaging include:
    1. Greater exposure latitude
    2. Longer scale contrast
    3. Reduced patient dose
    (A) 1 only
    (B) 1 and 2 only
    (C) 1 and 3 only
    (D) 1, 2, and 3

29. Which of the following exposure factors is used to regulate radiographic contrast in SF imaging?
    (A) mA
    (B) Exposure time
    (C) mAs
    (D) kV

30. Which of the following contribute(s) to the radiographic contrast present on the finished image?
    1. Tissue density
    2. Pathology
    3. Beam restriction
    (A) 1 and 2 only
    (B) 1 and 3 only
    (C) 2 and 3 only
    (D) 1, 2, and 3

31. The use of optimum kV for small, medium, and large body parts is the premise of:
    (A) Fixed kV, variable mAs technique chart
    (B) Variable kV, fixed mAs technique chart
    (C) Fixed mAs, variable body part technique
    (D) Fixed mAs, variable SID technique

32. The function(s) of automatic beam limitation devices include:
    1. Increasing contrast resolution
    2. Absorption of scattered radiation
    3. Changing the quality of the x-ray beam
    (A) 1 only
    (B) 2 only
    (C) 1 and 2 only
    (D) 1, 2, and 3

33. What transforms the violet light emitted by the PSP into the image seen on the CRT?
    (A) The photostimulable phosphor
    (B) The scanner/reader
    (C) The ADC
    (D) The helium–neon laser

34. The sensitometric curve is used to illustrate the relationship between the:
    (A) SID and the resulting radiographic/image density
    (B) Exposure reaching the phosphors and the resulting fluorescence
    (C) Exposure given to the film and the resulting radiographic/image density
    (D) kV used and the resulting radiographic/image density

35. What component of an IP records the CR image?
    (A) The photostimulable phosphor
    (B) The scanner/reader
    (C) The film emulsion
    (D) The helium–neon laser

36. Image fading in CR can occur if:
    1. Unexposed PSPs are unused for extended periods
    2. Exposed PSPs are not processed soon after exposure
    3. Exposed PSPs are exposed to high temperatures
    (A) 1 only
    (B) 1 and 2 only
    (C) 2 and 3 only
    (D) 1, 2, and 3

37. If a part measuring 15 cm was imaged using 12 mAs and 72 kV, a similar part measuring 17 cm could be correctly exposed in SF imaging using:
    (A) 6 mAs 72 kV
    (B) 24 mAs 72 kV
    (C) 12 mAs 76 kV
    (D) 12 mAs 68 kV

38. Which of the following can be used to determine the sensitivity of a particular film emulsion?
    (A) Sensitometric curve
    (B) Dose–response curve
    (C) Reciprocity law
    (D) Inverse square law

39. The x-ray detection system that does not have a scintillation component is:
    (A) Indirect DR using CCD
    (B) Indirect DR using TFT
    (C) Direct DR
    (D) CR

40. Which of the following pathologic conditions would require an increase in exposure factors?
    (A) Pneumoperitoneum
    (B) Obstructed bowel
    (C) Renal colic
    (D) Ascites

Answers and Explanations

1. (D) Focal spot size affects recorded detail because of its effect on *blur*: the larger the focal spot size, the greater the blur produced. Recorded detail is significantly affected by distance changes because of their effect on magnification. As SID increases, magnification decreases and recorded detail increases. As OID increases, magnification increases and recorded detail decreases. Some structures are imaged with more inherent distortion than others, and shapes of anatomic structures can be entirely misrepresented. Structures *farther* from the IR will be distorted (i.e., magnified) more than those *closer* to the IR.

2. (C) Intensifying screens can have a considerable impact on recorded detail through *SF contact*. Areas of imperfect SF contact result in blurriness that severely degrades recorded detail (Fig. 11–21A). Causes of poor SF contact include warped screens, damaged cassette frames, and foreign bodies in the cassette. Larger cassettes are more susceptible to poor screen contact. Proper care of intensifying screens includes *periodic evaluation of screen contact using a specially designed wire mesh* (Fig. 11–21B). Focal spot testing uses a slit camera or star pattern.

3. (A) Shape distortion (foreshortening, elongation) is caused by improper alignment of the tube, part, and IR. Size distortion, or magnification, is caused by too great an object–image distance or too short a source–image distance. Focal spot size is associated with focal spot blur/unsharpness.

4. (D) OID and SID determine the degree of magnification (size distortion). The OID should be as short as possible and the SID should be as long as practical. The anatomic part should be accurately positioned as closely parallel to the IR as possible. If a linear structure is angled within the body and not parallel to the IR, that anatomic structure will appear *smaller*—it will be *foreshortened*. On the other hand, *elongation* occurs when the x-ray tube is angled. This can be used to advantage in radiography to improve visualization of some superimposed anatomic structures.

5. (D) X-ray tube anodes are constructed according to the *line focus principle*, that is, the focal spot is angled (usually 12–17 degrees) to the vertical. As the AFS is projected downward, it is foreshortened; thus, the EFS is always smaller than the AFS. As it is projected toward the cathode end of the x-ray beam, it

becomes larger and approaches its actual size. As it is projected toward the anode end, it gets smaller because of the anode "heel" effect.

6. (D) One factor influencing geometric sharpness is penumbra, or blur. The production of blur is inversely proportional to recorded detail. As focal spot size increases, blur increases, and recorded detail decreases.

7. (D) Motion is said to be the greatest enemy of recorded detail because it completely obliterates image sharpness. Screen speed can reduce recorded detail according to the degree of light diffusion from the phosphors. Object–image distance causes magnification and blurriness of recorded detail. Grid ratio is related to scattered radiation cleanup; it is unrelated to detail.

8. (A) Size distortion (magnification) is inversely proportional to SID and directly proportional to OID. Decreasing the SID and/or increasing the OID will increase size distortion. Aligning the tube, anatomic part, and IR so as to be parallel *reduces* shape distortion. *Angulation* of the long axis of the part with respect to the IR results in foreshortening of the object. *Tube* angulation causes elongation of the part.

9. (D) When intensifying screen phosphors absorb x-ray photons, the x-ray photon energy is converted to visible light energy. The light emitted by the phosphors is termed luminescence. There are two types of luminescence: fluorescence and phosphorescence. Fluorescence is luminescent light that ceases to be emitted *as soon* as the x-ray photon stimulation ceases. Phosphorescence, on the other hand, is when the phosphors continue to glow *after* x-ray photon stimulation ceases; another term for this is lag.

10. (D) Distortion can be described as being either size or shape. Size distortion is magnification, caused by either insufficient SID or excessive OID. Shape distortion results from misalignment of the x-ray tube, part, and IR. Tube angulation can cause elongation of the part. Angulation of the part with respect to the IR will foreshorten the image. Focal spot size is unrelated to distortion but strongly related to production of penumbral unsharpness.

11. (C) A grid consists of alternate strips of lead and interspace material. The lead strips are used to trap scattered radiation before it reaches the IR, thus decreasing the effect of scattered radiation fog on the image. *Grid ratio* is defined as the height of the lead strip to the distance between the strips (or width of the interspace material). Grid ratio increases as the lead strips are made taller, or the distance between them decreases—and scattered radiation is more likely to be trapped before reaching the IR. The thickness of the lead strips contributes to *lead content*. Lead content is measured in g/cm^2 and expresses the amount of lead contained within a particular grid.

12. **(D)** Using the formula mA $\times$ second = mAs, determine each mAs. The greatest radiographic density will be produced by the combination of greatest mAs and shortest SID. Groups A and C should produce identical radiographic density, according to the inverse square law, because group C is twice the distance and four times the mAs of group A. Group B has twice the distance of group A, but only twice the mAs; it has, therefore, less density than groups A and C. Group D has the same distance as group A, and twice the mAs, making it the group of technical factors that will produce the greatest radiographic density.

13. **(D)** According to the inverse square law of radiation, the intensity or exposure rate of radiation from its source is inversely proportional to the square of the distance. Thus, as distance from the source of radiation increases, exposure rate decreases. Because exposure rate and radiographic density are directly proportional, if the exposure rate of a beam directed to an IR is decreased, the resultant image density would be decreased proportionally.

14. **(B)** Image/optical density is proportional to mAs. However, other methods may be used to adjust image density. When correct adjustment of mAs is not possible, a decrease in kV by 15% will effectively halve the radiographic density. SID adjustment is not recommended for making density changes as image magnification and patient dose are affected as well. Decreasing the grid ratio will increase image density.

15. **(C)** To change nongrid to grid exposure, or to adjust exposure when changing from one grid ratio to another, recall the factor for each grid ratio:

no grid = 1 $\times$ original mAs

5:1 grid = 2 $\times$ original mAs

6:1 grid = 3 $\times$ original mAs

8:1 grid = 4 $\times$ original mAs

12:1 grid = 5 $\times$ original mAs

16:1 grid = 6 $\times$ original mAs

Therefore, to change from nongrid to 8:1 grid, multiply the original mAs by a factor of 4. A new mAs of 40 is required.

16. **(A)** An image that *lacks* sufficient *contrast/has poor contrast resolution* is one that is *too gray*—where similar tissue densities can be distinguished with difficulty or not at all. Insufficient beam restriction (i.e., not enough collimation) can certainly result in production of excess scattered radiation and therefore produce an image that is too gray/lacking sufficient contrast resolution. Insufficient kV would produce an image with *too much* (too high) contrast. The mAs factor has no *effect* on contrast scale.

17. **(C)** Radiographic, optical, or image density is defined as the overall amount of blackening on a radiographic *film* image or a particular portion of the film image. It provides the correct degree of background blackening for the anatomic image. In *digital* imaging, density is referred to as *brightness*. Excessive density can obscure image details; insufficient density can mask pathology. Radiographic density is a *quantitative* factor, that is, it describes an *amount* of image blackening determined by the *number* of x-ray photons used to create the image. Thus, radiographic density is regulated by the *exposure rate* or *number* of photons reaching the film emulsion or IR. Gray scale refers to image contrast. The degree of *resolution* transferred to the IR is a function of the resolving power of each of the system components and is expressed in *line pairs per millimeter* (lp/mm).

18. **(D)** Image density is directly proportional to mAs. If exposure time is doubled from 0.05 (1/20) second to 0.1 (1/10) second, image density will double. If the mAs is doubled from 10 to 20 mAs, image density will double. If the kV is increased by 15%, from 75 to 86 kV, image density will double according to the 15% rule. Changing to 100 mA will halve the mAs, effectively halving the image density.

19. **(D)** A review of the problem reveals that *three changes* are being made: an increase in SID, a change from 200 speed system to 100 speed system, and an increase in exposure time (to be considered last). Because the original mAs was 36, reducing the speed of the system to half (from 200 to 100) will require a doubling of the mAs, to 72, to maintain density. Now

we must deal with the distance change. Using the density maintenance formula (remember, 72 is now the *old* mAs), we find that the required new mAs at 48 in. is 103. Because the problem states that we are now using 0.25-second exposure, it is left to determine what mA, used with 0.25 second, will provide 103 mAs.

$$0.25x = 103$$
$$x = 412 \text{ mA}$$

20. (D) Density is a *quantitative* factor because it describes the *amount* of image blackening. mAs is also a quantitative factor because it regulates x-ray beam *intensity*, *exposure rate*, *quantity*, or *number* of x-ray photons produced. mAs is the single most important technical factor associated with image density and is the factor of choice for *regulating* image density.

mAs is directly proportional to the intensity (exposure rate, number, quantity) of x-ray photons produced and the resulting radiographic density. For example, if the mAs is doubled, twice the exposure rate and twice the density occurs. If the mAs is reduced to half, the exposure rate and resulting density are reduced to half (see Fig. 11–26).

21. (C) Scattered radiation is produced as x-ray photons travel through matter, interact with atoms and are scattered (change direction). If these scattered rays are energetic enough to exit the body, they will strike the IR from all different angles. They therefore do not carry useful information—merely producing a *gray fog* over the image, adding unwanted and undiagnostic densities, producing *less contrast resolution*. Grid cutoff increases contrast and is caused by improper relationship between the x-ray tube and grid.

22. (C) The lower the kV range, the less energetic/penetrating the x-ray photons. If fewer photons penetrate to reach the IR, fewer grays/densities appear and shorter scale contrast results. At lower-kV levels, less Compton scatter events occur—also accounting for fewer grays from scattered radiation. The lower the kV, the *less* the exposure latitude (margin of error in exposure).

23. (B) As the kV is increased, a *greater number* of electrons is driven across to the anode with *greater force*. Therefore, as energy conversion takes place

at the anode, *more high-energy* (short wavelength) photons are produced. However, because they are higher-energy photons, there will be less patient absorption.

24. (D) As photon energy increases, more penetration and greater production of scattered radiation occurs, producing a longer scale of contrast. As grid ratio increases, more scattered radiation is absorbed, producing a higher contrast. As OID increases, the distance between the part and IR acts as a grid and consequently less scattered radiation reaches the IR, producing a higher contrast. Focal spot size is related only to recorded detail.

25. (C) Of the given factors, kV and grid ratio will have a significant effect on radiographic contrast–contrast resolution. The mAs values are almost identical. Because an increased kV and low-ratio grid combination would allow the greatest amount of scattered radiation to reach the IR, thereby producing more gray tones, C is the best answer. D also uses a low-ratio grid, but the kV is too low to produce as much gray as C.

26. (A) The greatest subject contrast is found in body parts made of a few widely differing tissue densities. The elbow has but bone, some muscle, and soft tissues constituting high subject contrast. The abdomen, containing the kidneys, stomach, small and large intestines, and other viscera, is a heavy body part composed of many similar tissue densities and, thus, normally has very low subject contrast.

27. (A) Radiographic contrast is described as the difference between the densities present on an x-ray image. An image possessing many shades of gray between black and white is said to exhibit long-scale, or low, contrast. An image possessing only a few widely different shades of gray between black and white is said to exhibit short-scale, or high, contrast.

28. (D) The chest is composed of widely differing tissue densities (bone and air). In an effort to "even out" these tissue densities and better visualize pulmonary vascular markings, high kV is generally used. This produces more uniform penetration and results in a longer scale of contrast with visualization of the pulmonary vascular markings as well as bone (which is better penetrated) and air densities. The increased kV also affords the advantage of greater exposure latitude (an error of a few kV will make little, if any, difference). The fact that the kV is increased means that the mAs is accordingly reduced and, thus, patient dose is reduced as well.

29. (D) kV regulates the energy, and therefore penetration, of the photons produced at the target (anode). The greater the photon energy, the less the total absorption by dense tissues and the more that tissue densities will be "evened out," that is, showing a longer scale of grays. Time and mA are the quantitative exposure factors controlling radiographic density.

30. (D) The radiographic subject, that is, the patient, is composed of many different tissue types of varying densities, resulting in varying degrees of photon attenuation and absorption. This *differential absorption* contributes to the various shades of gray (i.e., scale of radiographic contrast) on the finished image. Normal tissue density may be significantly altered in the presence of pathology. For example, destructive bone disease can cause a dramatic decrease in tissue density. Abnormal accumulation of fluid (as in ascites) will cause a significant increase in tissue density. Muscle atrophy, or highly developed muscles, will similarly decrease or increase tissue density. Perhaps the most important way to improve contrast resolution and limit the production of scattered radiation is by limiting the size of the irradiated field through *beam restriction*. As the size of the field is reduced, there is less tissue volume irradiated; therefore, less scattered radiation will be produced.

31. (A) The optimum kV (or fixed kV) technique separates patients into small, medium, and large categories and assigns an optimum (or best) kV for that particular body part. Patient thickness (measurement in centimeters) determines mAs. This method of establishing exposure factors results in less variation in the scale of contrast than the variable kV method of technique selection.

32. (A) Beam restrictors function to limit size of the irradiated field. In doing so, they limit the volume of tissue irradiated (thereby decreasing the percentage of scattered radiation generated in the part) and help reduce patient dose. Because less scattered radiation is produced, less fog affects the x-ray image, thus improving contrast resolution. Beam restrictors do not affect the quality (energy) of the x-ray beam, that is, the function of kV and filtration. Beam restrictors do not absorb scattered radiation, that is, a function of grids.

33. (C) The exposed IR is placed into the CR reader, where the PSP screen is automatically removed. The latent image appears as the PSP is scanned by a narrow high-intensity *helium–neon laser*, *or solid-state laser*, to obtain the pixel data. As the PSP is scanned in the CR reader, it releases a violet light—a process referred to as *PSL*.

The luminescent light is converted to electrical energy representing the *analog* image. The electrical energy is sent to *an ADC* where it is digitized and becomes the *digital* image that is eventually displayed (after a short delay) on a high-resolution monitor and/or printed out by a laser printer. The digitized images can also be manipulated in post-processing, electronically transmitted, and stored/archived.

34. (C) The sensitometric (or H&D) curve is used to illustrate the relationship between the exposure given to the film and the resulting density. The relationship between the SID distance and resulting density is expressed in the inverse square law of radiation. The effect of kV on contrast can be illustrated using a penetrometer (aluminum step-wedge).

35. (A) Inside the IP is the PSP image storage plate. This PSP/SPS with its layer of europium-activated barium fluorohalide serves as the *IR* as it is exposed in the traditional manner and receives the latent image. The PSP can *store* the latent image for several hours; after approximately 8 hours, noticeable image fading will occur. Once the CR cassette is placed into the CR reader, the PSP screen is automatically removed. The latent image on the PSP is changed to a manifest image as it is scanned by a narrow high-intensity *helium–neon, or solid-state*, (monochromatic) *laser* to obtain the pixel data. As the PSP is scanned in the reader, it releases a (polychromatic) violet light—a process referred to as *photo-*(or light-) *stimulated luminescence.*

36. (C) Image "*fading*" will occur if there is a delay in reading the PSP/SPS. This is because after a time, trapped photoelectrons are released from the "color center" and are therefore unable to participate in PSL. PSL intensity *decreases* in the interval between

x-ray exposure and image reading/processing. If the exposed PSL is not delivered to the reader/processor for 8 hours, PSL decreases by approximately 25%. Fading also increases as environmental temperature increases. Since PSPs are very sensitive to exposure/fogging, when unexposed PSPs/SPSs are unused for extended periods, they should be erased before use.

37. **(C)** Using the variable kV method, a particular mAs is assigned to each body part. As part thickness increases, the kV (penetration) is also increased. The body part being imaged must be carefully measured and *for each centimeter increase in thickness, 2 kV is added* to the exposure.

38. **(A)** The sensitometric curve is used to show the relationship between the exposure given the film and the resulting film density. It can therefore be used to evaluate a particular film emulsion's response (speed, sensitivity) by determining how long it takes to record a particular density. A dose–response curve is used in radiation protection and illustrates the quantity of dose required to produce a particular effect. The reciprocity law states that a particular mAs, regardless of the combination of mA and time, should produce the same degree of blackening. The inverse square law illustrates the relationship between distance and radiation intensity.

39. **(C)** In both *indirect*-capture flat-panel detector methods, scintillation light is captured, read by a photodetector (CCD or TFT), changed to an electronic signal, and transmitted to the ADC for digitization. In *direct*-capture flat-panel detector systems, x-ray energy is converted to an electrical signal in a single layer of material such as the semiconductor a-Se. Electric charges are applied to both surfaces of the a-Se, electron-hole pairs are created, and charges are read by TFT arrays located on the surfaces. The electrical signal is transferred to the ADC. The number of TFTs is equal to the number of image pixels. Thus, the direct-capture system eliminates the scintillator step required in indirect DR.

40. **(D)** Because pneumoperitoneum is an abnormal accumulation of air or gas in the peritoneal cavity, it would require a decrease in exposure factors. Obstructed bowel usually involves distended, gas-filled bowel loops, again, requiring a decrease in exposure factors. With ascites, there is an abnormal accumulation of fluid in the abdominal cavity, necessitating an increase in exposure factors. Renal colic is the pain associated with the passage of renal calculi; usually no change from the normal exposure factors is required.

Image Processing and Quality Assurance | 12

SCREEN/FILM (SF) PROCESSING

Storage Conditions

The conditions under which x-ray film is stored can have considerable impact on the final x-ray image. The most common result of improper film storage is *fog*, which can have a severely degrading effect on image quality.

Boxes of unexposed film should be stored at a temperature no greater than 70°F. Excessive heat can accelerate the deterioration process and cause film fog. Atmospheric humidity should be kept between 40% and 60%. Excessively low humidity is conducive to the production of static electricity discharge (Fig. 12–1). High humidity levels encourage the production of fog. An *unopened* (i.e., hermetically sealed) bag of film protects the film from humidity, but not from excessive temperatures.

Boxes of film must also be stored away from chemical fumes that can fog film emulsion. Film can be fogged by ionizing radiation if stored too close to x-ray rooms or radionuclides.

Each box of x-ray film is identified with an expiration date before which the film must be used to avoid age fog. When replenishing film supply, film boxes should be rotated so that the oldest film is used first.

Film boxes should be stored in the upright position. If they are stacked upon one another, the sensitive emulsion (especially in the central portion) can be affected by pressure from the boxes above. Pressure marks (i.e., areas of fog) are produced and result in loss of contrast in that area of the x-ray image. Larger size film boxes (i.e., 14 × 17 in.) are particularly susceptible to this problem.

The *film bin* is a lighttight storage area where opened boxes of film are available for reloading empty cassettes. If a single door separates the darkroom from exterior white light, it is wise to have an automatic interlock system in place that prevents opening of the darkroom door while the film bin is open.

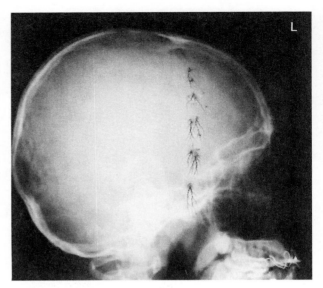

Figure 12–1. Plus-density artifact resulting from static electric discharge. (Courtesy of Stamford Hospital, Department of Radiology.)

Safelight Illumination

Adequate and safe darkroom lighting is an essential part of ensuring quality x-ray images. A source of white light is required for routine maintenance and cleaning. *Safelight* illumination must be appropriate for the type of film used, bright enough to provide adequate illumination, but must not expose the sensitive emulsions. Exposed film emulsion (i.e., having a latent image) is approximately eight times more sensitive than unexposed emulsion.

A frequently used *safelight* is the Kodak Wratten Series 6B, a brownish *safelight filter*, with a 7.5- to 15-W frosted lightbulb placed 4 feet above the work surface; it is used with a blue sensitive film. Another available safelight, somewhat brighter, is the Kodak GBX all-purpose filter, which provides a more reddish illumination. *Neither type can be safely used with laser film.*

Routine darkroom maintenance includes regular cleaning of all surfaces and walls and checks for white-light leaks. When checking for light leaks, all darkroom lights must be turned off, adequate time given for eyes to adjust to the darkness, and then a careful visual inspection made for white-light leaks.

Summary

- Boxes of unexposed film should be stored in a cool and dry environment, under 70°F, and between 40% and 60% humidity.
- Excessive temperatures cause film fog.
- Excessively low humidity encourages buildup of static electricity.
- Film should be stored away from radiation and chemicals.
- The film box expiration date should be noted and oldest film used first.

- Film boxes should be stored upright to avoid production of pressure marks.
- Kodak Wratten Series 6B and GBX darkroom filters are the most commonly used.
- Safelights should be placed 4 feet from the work surface with 7.5- to 15-W lightbulbs.

SCREEN/FILM CASSETTES

Routine Care

Routine documented care of all imaging system components is part of an efficient *quality assurance* program.

Cassettes require care and maintenance inside and outside. They should be stored *upright*, according to size and speed. Cassettes should be *inspected visually* for damage and cleanliness. The inside of cassettes should be *cleaned regularly* to keep them lint- and dust free; screens should be cleaned with special antistatic cleaner appropriate for the type of screen used.

Screens must also be *tested periodically* for screen-to-film contact with a *wire-mesh test*. The cassette to be tested is placed on the x-ray table and the wire-mesh device on *top* of the cassette, and an exposure is made at 5 mA s and 40 kV. The processed film should be viewed at a distance of at least 6 feet. Any *blurry* areas are indicative of poor contact between screens and film, and represent diminished image detail. The areas of poor contact also exhibit an increase in density and loss of contrast.

Screen/Film Artifacts

Radiographically speaking, an *artifact* is a fault, aberration, or any unnatural feature in an x-ray image. It can be the result of improper handling, automatic processing, or use of defective radiographic accessories. Artifacts are classified as *handling*, *processing*, and *exposure*.

Cassettes, screens, and film must be handled carefully to avoid leaving fingerprints or producing other film artifacts. Hands should be kept clean and dry, free from residue-leaving creams. Film should be handled carefully by the corners when loading and unloading cassettes. The technologist should not *slide* film into or out of the cassette, as the friction can cause static electricity buildup. Cassettes should be numbered or otherwise identified so that the artifact causing problems can be located and removed (Fig. 12–2).

Summary

- Cassettes should be stored upright according to size and speed.
- Cassettes should be tested periodically for adequate screen-to-film contact.
- Intensifying screens must be cleaned periodically with antistatic screen cleaner.

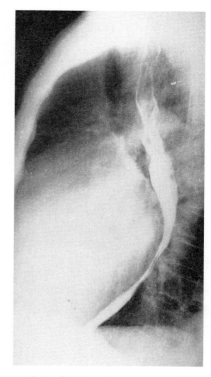

Figure 12–2. Dust or lint on intensifying screens. Small particles of dust, or other foreign objects, on intensifying screens keep the fluorescent light from reaching the film emulsion; hence, a clear (unexposed) area corresponds to each foreign particle. (From the American College of Radiology Learning File. Courtesy of the American College of Radiology.)

Types of Artifacts

- Handling (e.g., crinkle marks and static electrical discharge)
- Processing (e.g., chemical fog and guide shoe marks)
- Exposure (e.g., clothing and jewelry)

- Inadequate cleaning can result in white pinhole-type film artifacts (from dust/lint particles).
- Rough, improper handling or storage of cassettes can lead to damage, resulting in poor screen-to-film contact.
- Films must be handled carefully and properly to avoid artifacts such as static electricity, scratches, fog, or crescent/crinkle marks.

IMAGE IDENTIFICATION

Essential Information

X-ray images are often subpoenaed as court evidence in cases of medical litigation. In order to be considered as legitimate legal evidence, each x-ray image must contain certain essential and specific patient information. Essential information that must be included on each image is the identity of the patient, identity of the facility where the x-ray study was performed, date on which the study was performed, and a right- or left-side marker.

Other useful information that may be included, but that is not considered essential, is additional demographic characteristics of patients, such as their date of birth, the identity of the referring physician, the time of day when the study was performed, and the identity/initials of the radiographer performing the examination.

The identification of the radiographer performing the exam is recognized as an important medicolegal requirement, though not currently required that it be identified on each x-ray image.

Additionally, when multiple images are taken of a patient on the same day, it is important that the *time* the images were taken be included on the image. This permits the physician to chronologically follow the patient's progress.

Types of Systems

There are a number of *image identification* systems. Screen/film cassettes are purchased with a *lead blocker* to shield the underlying corner of film from x-ray exposure. This unexposed corner is then exposed with the essential patient information. Other types of image identification devices allow recording of patient information with the PSP storage plate inside the specially designed IP. In CR image plates a corner of the rear panel usually has a *memory chip* for patient information. DR imaging permits recording of patient demographic electronically.

Summary

- Medicolegal implications require that every image includes the patient's name or identification number, left- or right-side marker, examination date, and name of institution.
- When multiple images are taken of a patient the same day, the time of day should be indicated on each image.
- Some image identification systems can be used only in a darkroom.
- Other film/CR identification systems use special cassettes and are used in daylight conditions.

Information Required on Each X-ray Image

- Patient name/identification number
- Side marker, right or left
- Examination date
- Institution's name

Optional Information on Each X-ray Image

- Patient age or date of birth
- Attending physician
- Time of day
- Radiographer identification

FILM PROCESSING

Film emulsion consists of silver bromide (halide) grains/crystals suspended in gelatin. *Sensitization specks* are added to increase the sensitivity of the silver salts. *Positive silver ions* form the inner portion of the emulsion, whereas the *negative bromine ions* form the outer layer. At the time of exposure, the outer, negative, bromine ions are energized and their valence electrons ejected and absorbed by the (now negatively charged) sensitivity speck. The inner, positive, silver ions migrate to the negative charges and become metallic silver. Thus, the *latent* (exposed but invisible) *image* is formed. This is referred to as the *Gurney–Mott theory* of latent image formation. The chemical development process transforms the latent image to a *manifest* (visible) black metallic silver *image*.

Automatic film processing is carried out by a machine that *transports* the x-ray film through the necessary chemical solutions for a specific length of time in each solution, at the same time providing *agitation*, *temperature regulation*, and *chemical replenishment*. Within the processor are the *developer*, *fixer*, and wash tanks, followed by the dryer.

Rapid processing is accomplished by the use of increased solution temperatures, which requires that a *hardener* be added to the developer to control excessive emulsion swelling.

Each of the processor systems accomplishes specific functions; a basic understanding of these systems is required so that the processor can be used correctly and efficiently. A properly maintained and monitored processor ensures consistent radiographs that retain their quality images over a long period of time (good *archival quality*).

Chemistry Overview

The *developer* functions to convert the latent (invisible) image into the manifest (visible) silver image by *reducing the exposed silver bromide grains to black metallic silver*. Important factors affecting the development process are *time* (length of development), *temperature* (of the developer solution), and solution *activity* (strength and concentration).

The developer solution is alkaline in nature for optimal function of the *reducing agents*. Its *activator/accelerator* provides the necessary alkalinity and swells the gelatin emulsion, enabling the reducing agents to penetrate the emulsion and reach the exposed silver bromide grains.

One *reducing agent* builds up blacks in areas of greater film emulsion exposure and another produces gray tones in areas of less film emulsion exposure. With respect to sensitometry, the reducing agent that regulates the black areas controls the *shoulder (Dmax)* of the characteristic curve, whereas agent affecting the grays controls the toe (*Dmin*) area.

Developer solution is especially sensitive to oxygen, which weakens the solution and makes it less effective. A *preservative* is added to the developer to prevent its rapid oxidation. A *solvent* (water) for the concentrated chemicals is used to dilute the concentrate to the proper strength.

Rapid processing (90 sec) is achieved through the use of high temperatures that accelerate the development process. However, high temperatures can cause excessive emulsion swelling, resulting in roller transportation problems. A hardener is added to the developer to control emulsion swelling.

A *restrainer*, or antifog agent, is added to the developer to restrict its activity to only the exposed silver grains. Without the restrainer, the developing agents would attack the *unexposed* grains, creating *chemical fog*.

The function of the *fixer* (*hypo*) is to clear the film of the unexposed, undeveloped silver bromide grains. The fixer is an *acidic* solution, neutralizing any residual developer carried over and providing the required acid medium. The fixer contains a *hardener* whose function is to *shrink* and *reharden* the softened gelatin emulsion, protecting it from abrasion and promoting *archival quality*. Fixer preservative is the same as that found in the developer.

The *wash* rids the film of residual chemicals. Any remaining chemicals in the emulsion (e.g., as a result of defective wash cycle) will cause discoloration of the film with age. Since x-ray film records are kept for a number of years, it is important that they have sufficient *archival quality*.

Cold-water processors are, in general, less efficient in removing chemicals than warm-water processors. Agitation during the wash process help rid the emulsion of chemical residue.

Film Processing Steps

- *Developer: Reduces* exposed silver bromide to black metallic silver
- *Fixer: Clears* the film of the unexposed silver bromide and *rehardens* the emulsion
- *Wash: Removes* processing chemicals and *permits* archival quality
- *Dryer: Removes* water from film, and *shrinks* and *dries* the emulsion

---

Summary

- Developer solution reduces the exposed silver bromide grains to black metallic silver.
- The development process is greatly affected by development time and solution temperature and activity.
- The developer's preservative helps prevent the developer solution from oxidation.
- A hardener is added to the developer solution to control swelling.
- An antifog agent/restrainer is added to the developer to keep the reducing agents from attacking the unexposed silver bromide grains.
- The fixer is an acidic solution.
- The fixing, or clearing, agent removes unexposed silver grains from the emulsion, preventing further exposure.
- The fixer has a hardener to shrink and reharden the softened gelatin emulsion to protect it from abrasion.
- Adequate washing of residual chemicals from the film emulsion is essential for good archival quality.

Processor Overview

Transport System: The *transport system* functions to convey the film through the different processor sections by means of a series of rollers (Fig. 12–3). This is accomplished at a *prescribed speed*, which determines the length of time the film spends in each solution. The roller system also provides agitation of the solution at the film surface. The entire conveyance system consists of the *feed tray, crossover rollers, deep racks, turnaround assemblies,* and *receiving bin.*

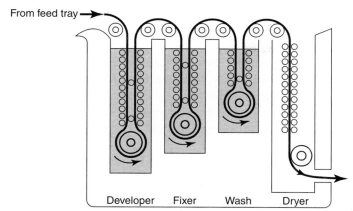

From feed tray →

Developer   Fixer   Wash   Dryer

Figure 12–3. Major components of an automatic processor. A series of rollers conveys the film through each processor section.

Film is aligned against one side of the feed tray as it is introduced into the processor. A sensor initiates solution replenishment as the film enters, and replenishment continues as the length of the film passes the sensor. Films should be fed into the processor along their *short* edge; feeding the film in "the long way" leads to *overreplenishment* and *increased image density*.

Crossover racks are out of solution and bridge the gaps between developer and fixer, fixer and wash, and wash and dry sections of the processor. Crossover rollers must be cleaned and kept free of crystallized solutions that can cause film artifacts as the soft emulsion passes by. The last set of rollers in each solution section has a *squeegee* action on film emulsion, thus removing excess solution before the film enters the next tank.

Turnaround assemblies are located at the bottom of the deep racks and serve to change the film direction as it changes from downward to upward motion. *Guide shoes*, or deflector plates, are also located where the film must change direction. They occasionally scratch the film, leaving characteristic *guide-shoe marks*, when they require adjustment.

When returning rollers to the processor after cleaning, care must be taken to seat them securely in their proper position. Transport problems (processor jam-up) result if racks are misaligned.

Replenishment System: As films travel from one processor section to another, chemical solution is carried away by the swollen film emulsion. The *replenishment* system keeps solution tanks full. Transport problems can arise from inadequate replenishment and low levels of solution. As film travels from one solution to the next, it carries residual chemicals over into the next section. Therefore, the activity of each solution is depleted through continual use. Diminished solution activity can have the same effects as low solution levels. The replenishment system assures that proper solution concentration is maintained.

Temperature Regulation: Developer solution is most dependent upon accurate temperature regulation; in a 90-second processor, developer temperature is usually maintained at 92°F to 95°F. The correct developer temperature must be constantly maintained. Even a minor fluctuation (i.e., 0.5°F) in developer temperature can cause a visible change in radiographic density and contrast.

Developer temperature is thermostatically controlled and developer solution is circulated through a heat exchanger under the fixer tank. Thus, the fixer temperature is regulated (in cold-water processors) by heat conducted from the developer solution. In older processors having stainless-steel tanks, fixer temperature is regulated by heat convection from the neighboring developer solution.

Recirculation System: As replenishment chemicals are added to the developer solution, the *recirculation system* provides agitation necessary for uniform solution concentration. As temperature adjustments are made, the recirculation system agitates the developer solution to promote temperature uniformity. *Agitation* provided by the system also functions to keep fresh solution in contact with the film emulsion. The recirculation system also functions to filter debris, such as gelatin particles, from the solutions.

Wash and Dry Systems: Thorough removal of chemical solutions from the film emulsion is required for good *archival film quality* and is provided by the wash section of the automatic processor. Agitation of the water makes the process more efficient. Any residual chemicals eventually result in film stain. *Residual fixer* eventually stains the film a yellowish brown that ultimately obscures the image and diminishes the archival quality. Films can be tested to determine their degree of fixer retention.

The dryer section functions to remove water from the film by blowing warm, dry air over the film surface. Dryer temperature is usually 120°F to 130°F, sufficient to shrink and dry the emulsion without being excessive. Excessive heat and overdrying can cause film damage. If films emerging from a properly heated dryer are damp, the problem may be excessive emulsion swelling and water retention as a result of inadequate developer or fixer replenisher (hardener).

Silver Recovery

X-ray film is expensive and can represent a large part of a radiology department annual budget. Approximately half of the film's silver remains in the emulsion after exposure and processing. The other half (unexposed silver) is *removed* from the film during the fixing process, and most of it is *recoverable* through *silver recovery* methods. A drain is connected to the fixer tank, and the fixer is allowed to flow directly into a *silver recovery unit* or to a large centrally located receptacle.

Silver recovery is desirable for *financial* and *ecologic* reasons. Fixer silver is toxic to the public water supply, and environmental legislation makes persons responsible for its direct passage into sewer lines, or other means of improper disposal, subject to severe fines and penalties.

There are two common types of silver recovery methods. Used fixer enters a *metallic displacement* (or metallic replacement) cartridge and metallic silver is precipitated onto the steel wool within. This method of silver recovery is most useful for low-volume locations.

Film Processor Systems

- Transport system
- Replenishment system
- Temperature regulation system
- Recirculation system
- Washer system
- Dryer system

Methods of Silver Recovery

- Electrolytic
- Metallic displacement

Electrolytic silver recovery units pass an electric current through the fixer solution, causing silver to be plated onto the cathode cylinder of the unit. The silver is periodically removed by scraping it from the stainless steel cathode. Electrolytic cells are best used in locations having medium-to-high volume.

Processor Maintenance

Accurate and consistent automatic processing contributes to radiographic consistency. Testing and monitoring procedures serve to indicate potential problems before they arise. Developer, fixer, and wash temperature should be checked twice a day. *Preventive maintenance* is frequently provided for by a commercial cleaning and parts-replacement service.

If solution levels in processor and replenisher tanks are frequently low, a bigger problem may exist and should be brought to the attention of the processor service company. Preprocessed and/or discarded processed films should *not* be used to clean rollers because they may contain residual fixer that can contaminate the developer solution.

The more effective the processor quality control program, the less troubleshooting will be required. Nevertheless, it is important that the radiographer be able to recognize and resolve some common processor problems.

Troubleshooting: Common Problems and Their Causes

Transport problems (film jam-ups)
- Inadequately maintained (dirty) rollers
- Too-rapid film feeding and overlapping
- Misaligned crossover or other racks
- Inadequate developer replenisher (hardener)

Excessive density (processor related)
- Elevated developer temperature
- Insufficient dilution of developer

Inadequate density (processor related)
- Too low developer temperature
- Excessive dilution of developer

Damp films
- Too low dryer temperature
- Faulty dryer blower
- Inadequate fixing
- Inadequate developer replenisher (hardener)

Fog (darkroom and/or film related)
- Unsafe safelight
- Contaminated developer
- Outdated film
- Improper film storage conditions
- Darkroom light leak

Summary

- The *transport system* conveys the film through the processor sections by means of a series of rollers.
- The last set of rollers in each solution section has a *squeegee* action on film emulsion, removing excess solution before the film enters the next tank.
- *Turnaround assemblies* are located at the bottom of the deep racks. *Guide shoes* are also located where the film must change direction.
- The *replenishment* system keeps solution tanks full and ensures that proper solution concentration is maintained.
- Developer temperature is *thermostatically controlled* and circulated through a *heat exchanger* under the fixer tank; developer temperature is usually 92°F to 95°F.
- The *recirculation system* provides agitation necessary for uniform solution concentration and keeps fresh solution in contact with the emulsion.
- Thorough removal of chemical solutions from the film emulsion is required for good *archival film quality* and is provided by the *wash* section of the automatic processor.
- Dryer temperature is usually 120°F to 130°F, which is sufficient to shrink and dry the emulsion without being excessive.
- Unexposed silver is removed from the film during the fixing process and most of it is recoverable through *silver recovery* methods; silver recovery is desirable for financial and ecologic reasons.

PROCESSING OF CR IMAGES

While an intensifying screen cassette contains light sensitive film as the image receptor, the image plate (IP) used in computed radiography (CR) houses a photostimulable storage phosphor (PSP) as the image receptor. For this reason, in its early days, CR was referred to as filmless radiography.

The digital processing of CR images is completely different from the chemical processing of film images. Digital imaging is covered in *Chapter 11* and in *Part V: Equipment Operation and Quality Control*.

Analog film images can be scanned and digitized by a film digitizer device.

IPs and PSPs

The IPs have a protective function (for the flexible PSP within), are used in the Bucky tray or under the anatomic part, and come in a variety of sizes (Fig. 12–4A). The IPs need not be light-tight because the PSP inside is not light sensitive. One corner of the IP's rear panel has a memory chip for patient information; the IP also has a thin lead foil backing to absorb any backscatter.

The PSP is composed of europium-doped barium fluorohalide (mixed with a binder) coated on a storage plate. Upon exposure, the x-ray photons interact with the (BaF:Eu2) crystals. As a result of this interaction, a small amount of visible light is emitted, but most of the

PSP: Three Stages

- X-ray exposure
- Scanning/reading
- Erasure

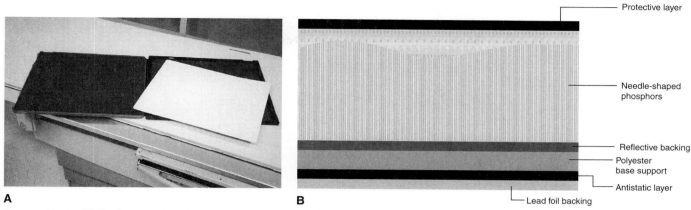

Figure 12–4. **(A)** An image plate (IP) holds the PSP between its front and rear panels. (Reproduced, with permission, from Shephard CT. *Radiographic Image Production and Manipulation.* New York: McGraw-Hill, 2003.) **(B)** Barium fluorohalide is either granular or "needle shaped." The "needlelike" phosphors have the advantage of *better x-ray absorption and less light diffusion.*

x-ray energy is stored (hence the term storage plate). This stored energy represents the latent image.

When the barium fluorohalide absorbs x-ray energy, electrons are released and they divide into two groups. One electron group initiates *immediate luminescence* (primary excitation) during the excited state of Eu^{2+}. The other electron group becomes trapped within the phosphor's halogen ions, forming a "color center." (also called "F center"). These are the phosphors that ultimately form the radiographic image because, when exposed to a *monochromatic* laser light source, these phosphors emit *polychromatic* light (secondary excitation), termed *photostimulated luminescence* (PSL).

The PSP layer can *store* its latent image for several hours; however, after approximately 8 hours, noticeable image *fading* will occur. The europium activator is important for the *storage* characteristic of the PSPs; it also has a function similar to the sensitization specks within film emulsion—without europium the image will not become visible.

The BaF is usually in the form of *granular* or *turbid* phosphors. Other examples of turbid phosphors are gadolinium oxysulfide and rubidium chloride. "*Needle*"-shaped (Fig. 12–4B) or *columnar* phosphors (usually cesium iodide) have the advantage of *better x-ray absorption* and *less light diffusion.*

Just under the barium fluorohalide layer is a *reflective layer* that helps direct emitted light toward the CR reader. Below the reflective layer is the base, behind that is an *antistatic layer*, and then the *lead foil* to absorb backscatter. Over the top of the barium fluorohalide is a *protective layer*.

Some PSP storage plates are manufactured specifically for better resolution (e.g., for mammography). Some higher-resolution PSPs "read" the information from both sides of the PSP storage plates.

After exposure, the IP is placed into the CR scanner/reader (See Fig. 12–5), where the PSP is automatically removed. A narrow (red) monochromatic high-intensity helium–neon laser or a solid-state laser beam scans back and forth across the PSP while it is simultaneously being pulled under the laser to progressively read the entire PSP. The movement of the PSP under the laser can be referred to as subscan motion.

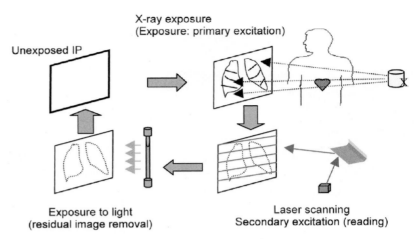

Figure 12–5. The recording, reading, and erasure cycles. The PSP, within the IP, is exposed to x-ray photons, scanned/read, and then erased for reuse. (Courtesy of FUJIFILM Medical Systems USA, Inc.)

The phosphors are activated by the monochromatic red laser light ($\approx$400 nm); however, PSL is a different color (bluish purple, blue–green, $\approx$550 nm). These two lights (PSL and laser) must not interfere with each other. To improve the image SNR, the PSL (carrying the x-ray image) must be a different wavelength/color than, and physically separate from, the laser excitation light. An optical filter is used that permits transmission of the PSL but attenuates the laser light; this filter is mounted in front of a photomultiplier tube (PMT). The optical filter is generally a blue glass filter placed between the light guide and PMT to filter out red laser light.

The PSL signal represents varying tissue densities and the latent image. The PMT or photodiode (PD) detects the PSL and converts it to electrical signals (see Fig. 12–6), which is then transferred to an analog-to-digital converter (ADC)—converting the analog electrical signal to digital data. This digital data is then transferred to a digital-to-analog converter (DAC) to be converted to a perceptible analog image on the display monitor. The monitor image can be electronically transmitted, windowed, manipulated, postprocessed, and stored efficiently (archived). Postprocessing functions can include edge enhancement; this technique can be used to improve the visibility of structures such as chest tubes by accentuating their edges.

After the scanning/reading process has been completed, any remaining information on the PSP is erased by exposing the PSP screen to high intensity laser light; the IP and its PSP storage plate is then ready for reuse.

An artifact associated with digital imaging and grids is "*aliasing*" (sometimes called "Moiré effect"). If the direction of the lead strips and the grid lines per inch (i.e., grid frequency) matches the scan frequency of the scanner/reader, this artifact can occur (Fig. 12–7). Aliasing appears as superimposed images slightly out of alignment, an image "wrapping" effect. This most commonly occurs in mobile radiography with stationary grids and can be a problem with DR flat panel detectors.

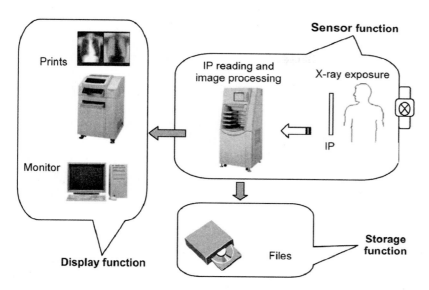

Figure 12–6. The latent image on the PSP is changed to a visible image as it is moved at a constant speed and scanned by a narrow high-intensity helium–neon laser or a solid-state laser to obtain the pixel data. (Courtesy of FUJIFILM Medical Systems USA, Inc.)

Once the PSP storage plate reading process is completed, any remaining data stored on the PSP are erased by exposing it to high intensity light (called "erasure"); the PSP storage plate is then ready for reuse. Thus, the PSP undergoes three cycles: (i) x-ray exposure, (ii) reading, and (iii) erasure (Fig. 12–5).

Image *"fading"* occurs if there is a delay in reading the PSP. After a time, trapped photoelectrons are released from the "color center" and are therefore unable to participate in PSL. PSL intensity *decreases* in the interval between x-ray exposure and the image-reading process. If the exposed PSL is not delivered to the reader/processor for 8 hours, PSL

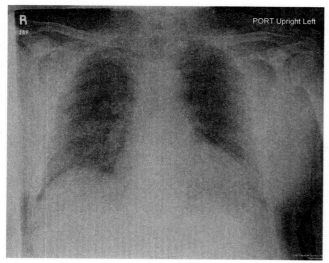

Figure 12–7. If the direction of the lead strips and the grid lines per inch/grid frequency matches the scan frequency of the scanner/reader, the "aliasing" artifact can occur.

decreases by approximately 25%. Fading also increases as environmental temperature increases.

PSP storage plates are very sensitive (more than film emulsion) not only to x-rays but ultraviolet, gamma, and particulate radiation. Environmental conditions are therefore an important consideration in their storage. Building materials such as concrete, marble, and others constantly emit natural radiation; bedrock in some geographic areas contributes significantly to background radiation. If PSPs are stored for extended periods of time, the possibility of artifacts must be considered. These artifacts typically appear as randomly placed small black spots. *If an IP and its PSP storage plate has been stored, unused, for 48 hours or more), the PSP storage plate should be erased prior to use.*

The mechanical consistency and accuracy of the laser optics and transport systems of the CR scanner/reader is extremely important for image quality—inconsistent scanning motion can result in a wavy, or otherwise distorted, image. This is sometimes referred to as *"laser jitter"* and should be evaluated monthly as part of the CR QA monitoring.

Histograms and Lookup Tables

In digital imaging there are numerous *brightness values* that represent various *tissue densities* (i.e., x-ray attenuation properties), for example bone, muscle, fat, blood-filled organs, air/gas, metal, contrast media, and pathologic processes. In CR, the CR scanner/reader recognizes all these values and constructs a representative gray-scale *histogram* of them, corresponding to the anatomic characteristics of the imaged part. Thus, all PA chest histograms are similar, all lateral chest histograms are similar, all pelvis histograms are similar, and so on.

A histogram is a *graphic representation* of pixel value distribution (Figs. 12–8B and C). The histogram is an analysis and graphic representation of all the densities from the PSP screen, demonstrating the quantity of exposure, the number of pixels, and their value. Histograms are unique to each body part imaged. Over time, if required diagnostic image characteristics change, the default histogram can be updated to reflect the latest required characteristics.

The radiographer selects a *processing algorithm* by selecting the anatomic part and particular projection on the computer/control panel – this is referred to as *Anatomically Programmed Radiography* (APR). After a part is exposed/imaged, its PSP is read/scanned and its own histogram is developed and analyzed. The resulting analysis, and histogram of the *actual* imaged part, is compared to the *programmed* representative histogram for that part.

The CR unit then matches that information with a particular *lookup table* (LUT)—a "characteristic curve" that best matches the anatomic part being imaged, to provide the appropriate gray-scale rendition. The observer is able to review the image and, if desired, change its appearance (through "windowing"); doing so changes the LUT. Hence, *histogram analysis* and use of the appropriate *LUT* together function to produce predictable image quality in CR.

It is important to note that *histogram appearance* and *patient dose* can be affected by the radiographer's knowledge and skill using digital

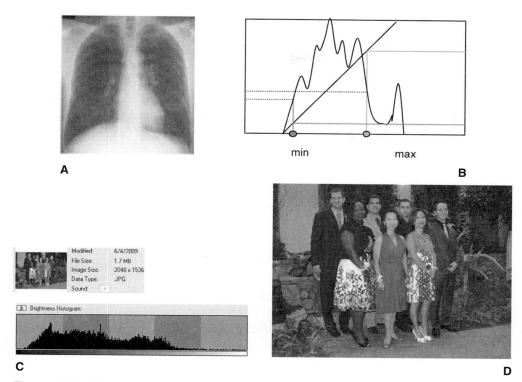

Figure 12–8. PA chest (**A**) and its histogram (**B**); a graphic representation illustrating the distribution of pixel values. (Courtesy of FUJIFILM Medical Systems USA, Inc.) Many of today's digital cameras can also display the histogram distribution (**C**) of pixel values, for example, for typical graduation photos (**D**). [Courtesy of Christina Cheong, RT(R)(M).]

imaging, in addition to their degree of accuracy in *positioning* and *centering*. Beam restriction is exceedingly important to avoid *histogram analysis errors*. Lack of adequate collimation can result in signals outside the anatomic area being included in the exposure data recognition/histogram analysis. This can result in a variety of histogram analysis errors including excessively light, dark, or noisy images.

As seen in Figure 12–9, because of poor collimation, the average exposure level and exposure latitude has changed; these changes are reflected in the images' informational numbers ("S number," "exposure index," etc.). Other factors affecting histogram appearance, and therefore these exposure indicator factors, include selection of the *correct processing algorithm* (e.g., chest vs. femur vs. cervical spine), changes in *scatter, source-to-image-receptor distance* (SID), *object-to-image-receptor distance* (OID), and *collimation*—in short, anything that affects scatter and/or dose. One other factor is *delay in processing* from time of exposure. Delay in processing can result in *fading* of the image. Normal examination times and short delays between projections are generally not a problem.

The image seen on the monitor, then, is the "default" image—one that has been obtained using parameters that have been prescribed consistent with department preferences.

Exposure Field Recognition

The CR reader can identify and separately analyze region(s) of interest (ROI) when more than one exposure is made to a single PSP. This

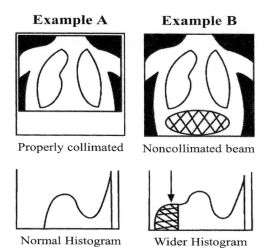

Figure 12–9. Average exposure level and exposure latitude in B has changed as a result of poor collimation. This will be reflected in the image informational numbers (e.g.,: "S number," "exposure index," etc.). Other factors affecting histogram appearance include selection of processing algorithm, any changes in SR, SID, OID, in addition to beam restriction. (Courtesy of FUJIFILM Medical Systems USA, Inc.)

is most typical in extremity imaging and the process is termed *exposure field recognition, partition pattern recognition, or segmentation.* For the best results, the collimated borders should be sharp and well defined. This ensures that unnecessary information outside the collimated edges, such as scatter, will be eliminated from the histogram analysis.

The scanner/reader distinguishes the number and orientation of images by identifying their collimated borders and analyzing only that exposure within the borders. If the entire PSP screen was analyzed, the histogram would be skewed and the resulting image far from optimum.

Other common conditions that can cause failure of exposure field recognition are poor or overlapping collimation (Fig. 12–10), scattered radiation (especially from adjacent field), and metallic bodies such as prostheses.

Postprocessing/Image Manipulation

Through *postprocessing* the radiographer can *manipulate,* that is change and enhance, the image displayed on the monitor.

One way to alter image contrast and/or brightness is through *windowing.* The term *windowing* refers to some change made to *window width* and/or window level, that is, a change in the LUT. Changes in window *width* affect change in the number of *gray shades.* Change in window *level* affects change in the image *brightness* (Fig. 12–11).

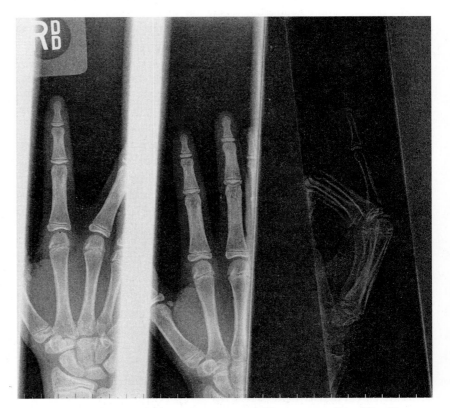

Figure 12–10. The "partition pattern recognition process" in CR will determine if the image is divided, and if so, how it is divided. In the CR image above, one image was not recognized. (Reproduced, with permission, from Shephard CT. *Radiographic Image Production and Manipulation.* New York: McGraw-Hill, 2003.)

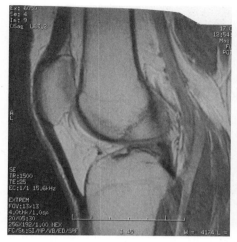

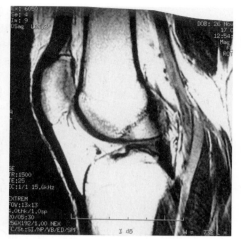

B

C

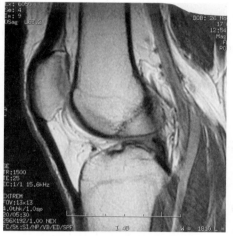

A

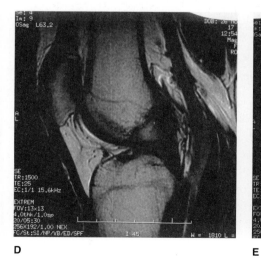

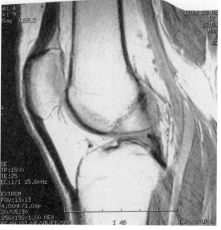

D

E

Figure 12–11. Changes in *window width* and *window level*. Image *A* (center) has a window width of 1810 and window level of 761. In image *B*, the window width is increased to 4174. In image *C*, the window width is decreased to 732, leaving the window level unchanged. The changes in image *gray scale* are evident. Next, images D and E are compared to image A. In image *D*, the window level is increased to 1497. In image *E*, it is decreased to 325. This time the changes in image *brightness* are obvious.

Therefore, windowing and other postprocessing mechanisms permit the radiographer to affect changes in the image and produce "special effects" such as *contrast enhancement, edge enhancement, image stitching* (useful in scoliosis examinations), image inversion, rotation, and reversal.

Image Communication and Interpretation

Using a *picture archiving and communications system* (PACS) and *teleradiology*, digital images can be sent anywhere there is equipment to receive and display them.

Interpretation of digital images can be made from the display monitor ("softcopy display"). In addition, "hardcopies" can be made on a film using a laser printer. A *laser camera* records the displayed image by exposing a film with laser light; it can also record several images on one film. The laser printer is connected for immediate processing of the images.

Summary

- Photostimulable phosphor storage plates (PSPs) are the detectors/receptors used in CR.
- The exposed PSP is placed in the CR reader and scanned with a narrow laser beam.
- Pixel data from the reader is displayed on the monitor as the radiographic image.
- A histogram is a *graphic representation* defining all the grayscale values of a particular image.
- A *processing algorithm* is selected when the radiographer selects the part and projection on the computer.
- A LUT matches the anatomic part being imaged to provide the appropriate gray-scale rendition.
- *Histogram analysis* and the appropriate *LUT* together function to produce predictable image quality in CR.
- The CR image can be *manipulated* by the radiographer (i.e., "windowed") to change contrast and/or brightness.
- When more than one image is made on a PSP, the CR scanner reader uses *exposure field recognition* to analyze each exposure.
- With PACS and *teleradiology*, digital images can be sent anywhere there is equipment to receive and display them.
- "Hardcopies" can be made on (single emulsion) film using a laser printer.

COMPREHENSION CHECK

Congratulations! You have completed the entire chapter. If you are able to answer the following group of very comprehensive questions, you should feel confident that you have really mastered this section. You can refer back to the indicated pages to check your answers and/or review the subject matter.

1. What are the ideal conditions for x-ray film storage (p. 381)?

2. Describe the possible effect of excessive temperature and very low humidity (p. 381).

3. Describe how each of the following can affect the radiographic film (p. 381, 382):

   (A) Chemical fumes

   (B) Radiation

   (C) Storage past the expiration date

   (D) Stacking boxes of film upon each other

   (E) Film bin or darkroom with light leaks

   (F) Safelight too close to work bench

   (G) Too-high-wattage safelight

4. Explain correct care of cassettes and intensifying screens (p. 383).

5. How can suspected flaws in film-to-screen contact be detected (p. 383)?

6. List at least five radiographic artifacts and identify their cause (p. 383)?

7. What information *must* every radiographic image include? Describe two types of film identification systems (p. 384).

8. Define latent and manifest images (p. 385).

9. What is the main function of the developer solution? What are the three important factors in the development process (p. 385)?

10. What are the main functions of the fixer solution (p. 386)?

11. List the order in which a film travels through each of the four sections of the automatic processor (p. 386, 387).

12. Name and describe the location of the structures that function to guide a film in the proper direction through the processor roller systems (p. 387, 388).

13. What are the two functions of the processor replenishment system? What can be the result of inadequate replenishment (p. 387)?

14. Describe the importance of temperature-regulation systems in automatic processing (p. 387, 388).

15. List functions of the processor recirculation system (p. 388).

16. What are the functions of the processor wash-and-dry sections? What can result from an inadequate wash process and inadequate drying (p. 388)?

17. Explain the economic and ecologic importance of silver recovery. Describe the three types of silver recovery methods (p. 388, 389).

18. List at least seven common radiographic problems associated with processing and identify their cause (p. 389).

19. Describe what is meant by the term *filmless radiography* (p. 390).

20. What device functions to transfer the x-ray image from the PSP screen to the display monitor (p. 392)?

21. What does a histogram represent in CR (p. 394)?

22. What is the purpose of a LUT in CR? How does the radiographer modify the LUT (p. 394)?

23. How does the radiographer select a processing algorithm (p. 394)?

24. What is windowing? What does a change in window width and/or window level affect (p. 396)?

25. What can change the appearance of the histogram, and therefore its analysis (p. 395, 396)?

26. In what two ways can a CR reader identify and analyze multiple images on one PSP (p. 395, 396)?

27. What system is used to send digital images anywhere there is equipment available to receive and display them (p. 398)?

28. What device is used to make "hardcopies" of images seen on display monitors (p. 398)?

29. Describe the difference between primary and secondary excitation of barium fluorohalide phosphors. (p. 391)?

30. Identify the cause of PSP fading. (p. 391, 393)?

31. List types of postprocessing functions. (p. 392)?

32. Describe the appearance and cause of aliasing artifact. (p. 392)?

CHAPTER REVIEW QUESTIONS

1. The developer temperature in a 90-second automatic processor is usually approximately:
   (A) 75°F–80°F
   (B) 80°F–85°F
   (C) 85°F–90°F
   (D) 90°F–95°F

2. The exposed PSP screen is subjected to a narrow laser beam:
   (A) On the display monitor
   (B) In the CR reader
   (C) In the cassette
   (D) On the film emulsion

3. The histogram demonstration of pixel value distribution can be changed/affected by the following:
   1. Selection of processing algorithm
   2. Processing delay
   3. Centering
   (A) 1 only
   (B) 1 and 2 only
   (C) 2 and 3 only
   (D) 1, 2, and 3

4. The amount of replenishment solution added to the automatic processor is determined by:
   1. Size of the film
   2. Position of the film on tray feeding into the processor
   3. Length of time required for the film to enter the processor
   (A) 1 only
   (B) 1 and 2 only
   (C) 1 and 3 only
   (D) 1, 2, and 3

5. Types of postprocessing of electronic/digital images include:
   1. Image stitching
   2. Contrast enhancement
   3. Windowing
   (A) 1 only
   (B) 1 and 2 only
   (C) 2 and 3 only
   (D) 1, 2, and 3

6. What is the likely cause of films emerging from the automatic processor in a damp condition?
   (A) Too high air velocity
   (B) Unbalanced processing temperatures
   (C) Insufficient hardening action
   (D) Excessive hardening action

7. The invisible latent image is converted into a visible manifest image in the:
   (A) Developer
   (B) Stop bath
   (C) First half of the fixer process
   (D) Second half of the fixer process

8. Poor storage or handling practices that can result in film fog include:
   1. Outdated film
   2. Exposure to excessive temperatures
   3. Exposure to chemical fumes
   (A) 1 only
   (B) 1 and 2 only
   (C) 2 and 3 only
   (D) 1, 2, and 3

9. Which of the following devices functions to produce hardcopies of digital images?
   (A) Digitizer
   (B) Laser printer
   (C) Histogram
   (D) Display monitor

10. A CR histogram is a graphic representation of:
    (A) Grayscale values of the imaged part
    (B) A characteristic curve of the imaged part
    (C) D_{max}
    (D) D_{min}

Answers and Explanations

1. (D) The advantages of automatic processors are quicker, more efficient operation, and consistent results. Quicker operation is attained with increased solution temperatures. The usual temperature of a 90-second developer is 90°F to 95°F. Excessively high developer temperature can cause chemical fog.

2. (B) CR uses special detector plates inside cassettes to record the radiologic image. No film is used, hence the term *filmless radiography*. The CR cassette is exposed just like a conventional screen–film cassette. Upon exposure, a latent image is produced on the PSP screen, which is located inside the IP. The IP is placed in the CR processor, and the PSP screen is automatically removed. A special *reader* scans the PSP screen with a narrow laser beam to obtain the pixel data, which can then be displayed on a monitor as the radiographic image.

3. (D) Histogram appearance can be affected by a number of things. *Positioning* and *centering accuracy* can have a significant effect on histogram appearance. Other factors affecting histogram appearance include selection of the *correct processing algorithm* (e.g., chest vs. femur), changes in *scatter*, *SID*, *OID*, and *collimation*—in short, anything that affects scatter and/or dose. Another factor affecting histogram appearance is *delay in processing* from the time of exposure. Delay in processing can result in *fading* of the image.

4. (D) When a film first enters the processor from the feed tray, a microswitch signals the replenishment pump to begin sending replenisher solution into the processor. Replenishment continues until the microswitch senses the end (edge) of the film and terminates pump action. So, as long as the film is being fed into the processor, replenishment solution will be added. There is, therefore, more replenisher added with larger size films. There is also more replenisher added when rectangular films are fed into the processor "the long way" because the processor is sensing, for example 17 inches of film rather than 14 inches of film. The film should be put through the processor consistently according to the particular department's preference or routine. A change in film direction can lead to over- or underreplenishment, and hence, a change in film density.

5. (D) The radiographer can manipulate, that is change and enhance, the digital image displayed on the monitor through *postprocessing*. One way to alter image contrast and/or density is through *windowing*. Windowing refers to some change made to *window width* and/or *window level*, that is a change in the LUT. Change in window *width* affects change in the number of gray shades, that is *image contrast*. Change in window *level* affects change in the image brightness, that is *optical density*. Therefore, windowing and other postprocessing mechanisms permit the radiographer to affect changes in the image and produce "special effects," such as *contrast enhancement*, *edge enhancement*, *image stitching* (useful in scoliosis examinations), and image inversion, rotation, and reversal.

6. (C) If the fixer fails to sufficiently reharden the gelatin emulsion, water will remain within the still-swollen emulsion. The dryer mechanism will be unable to completely rid the emulsion of wash water, and the film will emerge from the processor damp and tacky. On the other hand, excessive hardening action may produce brittle radiographs. High air velocity usually encourages more complete drying. Unbalanced processing temperatures can result in blistering of the emulsion.

7. (A) The invisible silver halide image is composed of exposed silver grains. These are "reduced" to a visible black metallic silver image in the developer solution. The fixer solution functions to remove unexposed silver halide grains/crystals from the film.

8. (D) All of those effects listed can result from poor storage practices. The film should be rotated with the oldest being used first to avoid fog from outdated film. By protecting the film from chemical fumes and excessive temperatures, fogging of the sensitive emulsion is prevented.

9. (B) Conventional screen–film images can be scanned and digitized by a special machine called a *film digitizer*. Interpretation of digital images is made from the display monitor; this is referred to as "softcopy display." "Hardcopies" can be made with a *laser printer*. A laser camera records the displayed image by exposing a film with laser light; it can also record several images on one film. The *laser printer* is connected for processing of the images.

10. (A) As in traditional radiography, numerous density values represent various tissue densities, for example, bone, muscle, fat, blood-filled organs, air/gas, metal, contrast media, and pathologic processes. In CR, the CR scanner recognizes these numerous values and constructs a *grayscale histogram* of these values represented in the imaged part. A histogram is a *graphic representation* defining all these values. The radiographer selects a *processing algorithm* by selecting the anatomic part and particular projection on the computer. The CR unit then matches that information with a particular *LUT*—a characteristic curve that best matches the anatomic part being imaged. Hence, *histogram analysis* and use of the appropriate *LUT* together function to produce predictable image quality in CR.

Image Evaluation: Electronic and Screen/Film

13

EVALUATION STANDARDS AND IMAGE CHARACTERISTICS

Overview

It is important to look at x-ray images with a critical eye, evaluating each of the components that contributes to their overall quality. The goal is to have as much information as possible, transferred as accurately as possible from the anatomical part being imaged to the IR.

Recorded Detail and Distortion

The x-ray image should illustrate maximum transference of information without loss of image detail or contrast. As discussed earlier, recorded information can be lost during any step of the transfer. Distortion can be introduced as a result of patient motion, excessive OID, insufficient SID, inappropriate screen/film (SF) combination, or too large a focal spot size. Shape distortion is evidenced as a result of improper alignment of x-ray tube, part, and image receptor.

Spatial resolution in CR is impacted by most of the above and, in addition, the size of the photostimulable phosphors (PSPs), the size of the scanning laser beam, and monitor matrix size. High resolution monitors (2–4 K) are required for high-quality, high-resolution image display. Using a *picture archiving and communications system* (PACS) and *teleradiology*, digital images can be sent anywhere there is the equipment to receive and display them.

Graininess of digital images can be caused by underexposure, incorrect processing incorrect algorithm/LUT selection (from the anatomic menu), inadequate collimation, and grid cutoff.

Digital radiography (DR) does not use IPs or a traditional x-ray receptor; it is a *direct-capture* or *indirect-capture* system of x-ray imaging. DR uses solid-state detector plates as the x-ray image receptor to intercept the x-ray beam.

Causes of CR Graininess

- Underexposure
- Incorrect processing processing algorithm/LUT
- Excess Scattered Radiation
- Inadequate collimation
- Grid misalignment; cutoff

One type of *indirect*-capture flat-panel detector systems uses *cesium iodide* or *gadolinium oxysulfide* as the *scintillator*, that is, a material which captures x-ray photons and emits light. That light is then recorded via a *charge-coupled device* (CCD) or *thin-film transistor* (TFT).

In *direct*-capture flat-panel detector systems, x-ray energy is converted to an electrical signal in a single layer of material such as the semiconductor a-Se (amorphous selenium). Electric voltage is applied to both surfaces of the a-Se, electron–hole pairs are created, and charges are read by *TFT* arrays located on the surfaces. The electrical signal is transferred directly to the analog-to-digital converter (ADC).

Thus, the direct-capture system *eliminates the scintillator step* required in indirect DR. Since selenium has a relatively low Z number (compared to gadolinium [Z #64] or cesium [Z #55]), a-Se detectors are made thicker to *improve detection*, thus compensating for the low x-ray absorption of selenium. There is no diffusion of electrons so *spatial resolution* is not affected in this manner.

DR affords the advantage of *immediate* display of the image; CR is somewhat delayed because the CR must be processed.

It must be emphasized that although the biggest advantage of electronic imaging is its *dynamic range*, patient overexposure can result if the radiographer fails to keep exposure factors within the system's recommended exposure index.

Brightness and Gray Scale

X-ray images must display adequate *brightness* and a *scale of grays* sufficient to make various *tissue densities* visible. Appropriate exposure factors, imaging accessories, and consideration of patient condition, size, and pathology are required.

In *electronic imaging* (CR/DR), the radiographer can alter the digital image displayed on the monitor through *postprocessing*. One way to alter image contrast and/or brightness is through "windowing." *Windowing* refers to some change made to window *width* and/or window *level*. Changes in window *width* affects changes in the contrast/gray scale. Changes in window *level* affects changes in the image *brightness* (analog/SF terminology = *density*).

Windowing and other *postprocessing* mechanisms permit the radiographer to produce "special effects," such as edge enhancement, image stitching (e.g., useful in scoliosis and leg length examinations), and image inversion, rotation, and reversal.

One of the biggest advantages of electronic imaging is the *dynamic range* (in SF imaging referred to as *latitude*) it offers. In SF imaging, there is a "range of correct exposure" limited by the toe and shoulder of the film emulsion's characteristic curve, whereas in electronic imaging, there is a *linear relationship* between the exposure given the PSP and its resulting luminescence as it is scanned by the laser. This affords much greater margin for error; technical exposure inaccuracies can be effectively eliminated (Fig. 13–1).

Overexposure of up to 500% and underexposure of up to 80% are reported as recoverable, thus eliminating most retakes.

CR Resolution Increases As

- PSP phosphor size decreases
- Laser beam size decreases
- Monitor matrix size increases

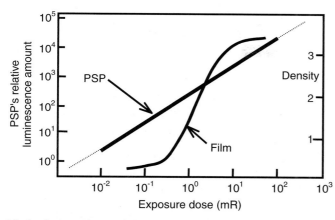

Figure 13–1. Comparison of the characteristic curve of a typical film emulsion with that of a PSP. The *wide dynamic range* (scale of contrast) of the PSP enables the correct detection of slight differences in x-ray absorption characteristics among various tissue densities. (Courtesy of FUJIFILM Medical Systems USA, Inc.)

Screens and Grids: Selection and Use

In *electronic imaging*, CR uses image plates (IPs), whereas DR does not. IPs offer the flexibility of continued use of traditional (SF) x-ray equipment. CR is convenient for mobile radiographic applications, tabletop/nongrid work, and cross-table/horizontal beam work.

As previously mentioned, image *fading* can occur if there is delay in reading the PSP. If an IP and its PSP have been stored, unused, for an extended period of time (i.e., for 48 hours), the PSP should be erased prior to use.

Care and maintenance of CR is discussed in Chapter 15. It is important to protect IPs from unwanted exposure; such exposure can cause artifacts on subsequent images. IPs are subject to double exposure just as SF cassettes (see Fig. 13–14).

Direct *DR* does not use IPs or a traditional x-ray table; it is a *direct-capture* system of x-ray imaging. In DR flat-panel detector systems, x-ray energy is converted to an electrical signal in a single layer of semiconductor material such as a-Se. Electrical signals are transferred directly to the ADC. Thus, DR systems eliminate the scintillator step required in CR and indirect DR.

In SF imaging, the appropriate intensifying screen speed is selected for the particular examination. Slower screens are often employed for examinations of the extremities (e.g., 100 speed), whereas faster screens (e.g., 400 speed) are used for larger body parts. If a grid is required, the appropriate ratio should be selected—a *grid ratio* that is appropriate for the kV (kilovoltage) level employed. X-ray tube centering, angulation, and SID should be suitable for the particular type of grid used.

Image Identification

All essential medicolegal information must be visible on each x-ray image: patient name or identification number, side marker, date, and institution. Much of the demographic information is entered in the console computer. Accurate markers are essential for every image. This

Electronic Imaging

- Brightness changes with changes in window *level*
- Contrast changes with changes in window *width*
- Has wide dynamic range/latitude
- Fading can occur with delayed processing
- IPs are very sensitive to x-ray fog

includes a Left or Right marker, properly placed and not superimposed on essential anatomy. Often special additional markers will be necessary to indicate that the exam was performed upright, decubitus, as a comparison image, and so on.

Exposure index (i.e., exposure dose) values should be identifiable and evaluated for appropriateness on each image.

Anatomic Part, Beam Restriction, and Shielding

The radiograph must include the anatomic *areas of interest* in the desired position and projection. To ensure patient protection, there must be visible evidence of *beam restriction/collimation. Shielding* should be evident when the reproductive organs are in the collimated primary beam, or within 5 cm of it, when the patient has reproductive potential, and when diagnostic objectives permit. Breast and/or thyroid shields should be used when appropriate.

IDENTIFYING AND CORRECTING ERRORS

It is essential that the radiographer be aware of the impact each of the imaging components has on the finished x-ray image. The radiographer must be able to recognize and correct imaging errors.

Each image should be evaluated according to the standards addressed above. If the image is suboptimal in any category, steps must be taken to determine the cause, correct the error, and ensure that the error is not repeated.

It is impossible to address and illustrate here all possible errors in technical factor selection, equipment use and positioning, patient variables, artifacts, and processing—in CR/DR and in SF imaging. Some have been illustrated in earlier portions of this volume and others are illustrated here. Patient-positioning errors are addressed in Part II. Try to identify the illustrated error and then check your answer with that given in the caption.

In CR/DR, we are learning about kinds of artifacts and errors unique to electronic imaging. Some of the more common exposure and processing artifacts are presented here. It is important to remember that PSPs are sensitive to electromagnetic radiations such as ultraviolet and gamma, as well as particulate radiations such as alpha and beta. Exposure of the sensitive PSPs even to normal environmental radiation can result in image *artifacts* appearing as black spots. Therefore, *IPs that have not been used for 48 hours should be subjected to the erasure process before use.*

TECHNICAL FACTOR SELECTION

Most *computed radiography* units use APR—anatomically programmed radiography. The radiographer selects a processing algorithm by selecting the anatomic part and particular projection on the computer workstation/control panel. Workstation menus can come with 100–200 menus, sometimes sorted by tabs, to primary regions of the body. Menus can usually be customized to physician preferences and/or site by site.

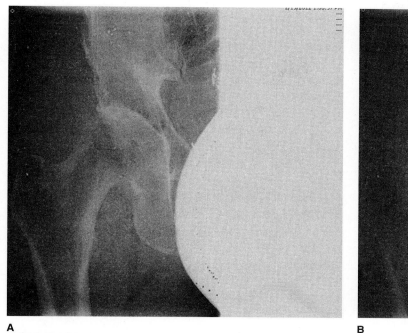

A

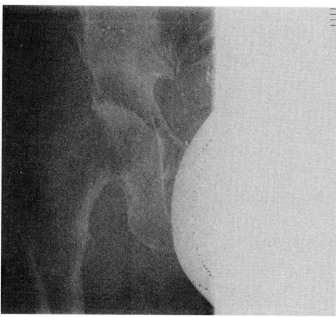

B

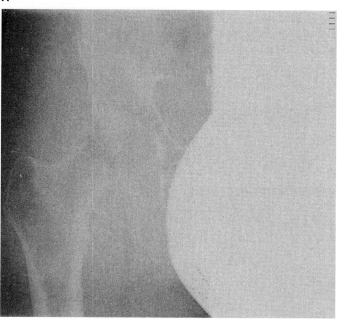

C

Figure 13–2. Image **A** demonstrates correctly selected *AP hip* algorithm and subsequent acceptable image. Image **B** is the same AP hip but with *AP shoulder* selected on the control panel. Image **C** is the same AP hip but with *lateral wrist* algorithm selected. Images **B** and **C** are unacceptable.

If the incorrect anatomical part/menu is selected, histogram analysis will be faulty and the resulting image will be unsatisfactory. Figure 13–2 illustrates this effect. Often, an incorrectly applied part/menu can be switched to the correct part/menu during or after image preview. However, the results can vary, depending on equipment manufacturer. Sometimes the selected new menu will be applied to the original raw data (best results), other manufacturers apply on top of the originally incorrect menu (less optimal results).

SF imaging requires accurate selection of exposure factors, with mAs and kV regulating density and contrast respectively. Figures 13–3, 13–4, 13–5, and 13–6 illustrate the effect of errors in mAs, kV, and SID.

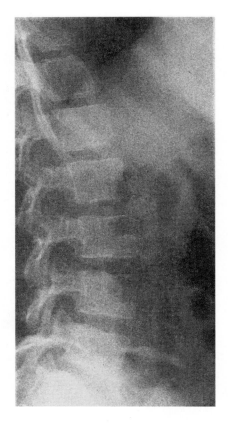

Figure 13–3. Noisy CR image as a result of quantum mottle; usually the result of insufficient mAs. A similar effect occurs in SF imaging with high-speed intensifying screens and insufficient mAs. (Reproduced, with permission, from Shephard CT. *Radiographic Image Production and Manipulation*. New York: McGraw-Hill, 2003.)

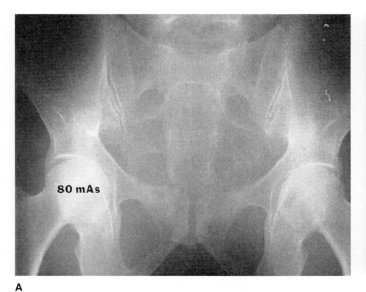

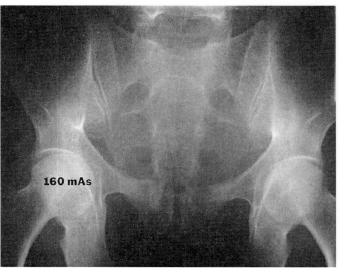

A

B

Figure 13–4. *Excessive optical density*; improper selection of *mAs* (milliampere-seconds). Both images were made at 100-cm SID using 75 kV. **(A)** Image correctly exposed at 80 mAs. **(B)** Image exposed at 160 mAs demonstrates excessive density. (From the American College of Radiology Learning File. Courtesy of the American College of Radiology.)

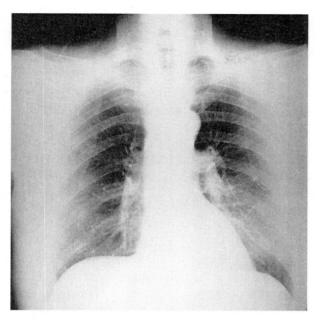

Figure 13–5. *High contrast* as a result of insufficient *kV*. (From the American College of Radiology Learning File. Courtesy of the American College of Radiology.)

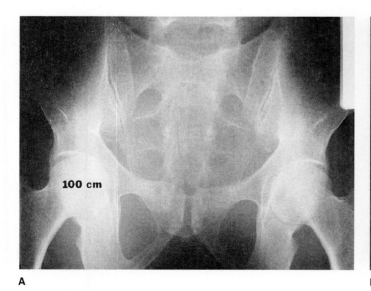

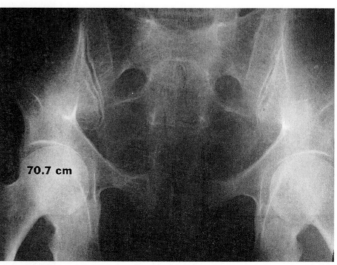

A

B

Figure 13–6. **(A)** X-ray beam intensity at a given point is dependent on the distance from its source. **(B)** Optical *density increases* as a result of *decreased SID*. (From the American College of Radiology Learning File. Courtesy of the American College of Radiology.)

EQUIPMENT USE AND POSITIONING

(A) Digital Imaging

Image plates must be used with the correct side facing up. Figure 13–7 illustrates an image made with the IP inadvertently used upside down. Artifacts from the IP rear panel are imaged superimposed on the anatomic part. Care must be taken to keep exposed IPs separate from unexposed ones. Figure 13–8 is an example of double exposure. Notice that, though double exposed, the image does not look overexposed—as a result of *automatic rescaling*.

Once the PSP reading process is completed in the scanner/reader, any remaining data stored on the PSP is erased by exposing it to high- intensity light (called "erasure"); the PSP is then ready for reuse. If the erasure process is incomplete, remnants of the previous image remain and degrade the new image. Figure 13–9 is an example of incomplete erasure.

Figure 13–10 is another example of a double exposed PSP. The same part was imaged twice using the same PSP. Again, notice that automatic rescaling has corrected the appearance of the image—even though it received *twice* the correct exposure.

When two or more exposures are desired on one IR, the *partition pattern* (or *exposure recognition*) process becomes essential to achieving good images. Unexposed portions of the IP must be well collimated and shielded to protect from exposure to scattered radiation. X-ray fields must not overlap or be too close together without being shielded. Figure 13-11 illustrates the effect of improper partitioning of the IP.

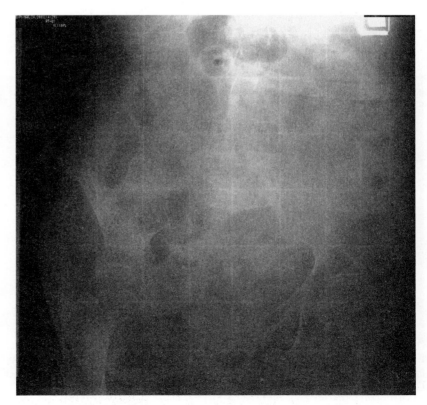

Figure 13–7. IP inadvertently used upside down. Artifacts from IP rear panel are superimposed on anatomic part.

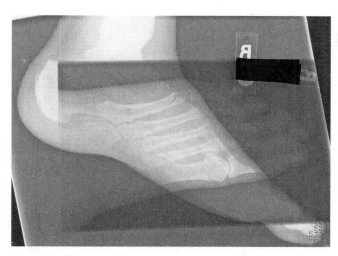

Figure 13–8. Double exposure. Care must be taken to keep exposed IPs separate from unexposed ones. (Courtesy of Stamford Hospital, Department of Radiology.)

Whether digital imaging or SF/analog imaging, motion is the greatest enemy of image detail. Figure 13–12 shows the effect of part motion on recorded detail.

Figure 13–13 illustrates another error that is common to both digital and analog imaging—an upside down focused grid. If a focused grid is placed upside down, the divergent x-ray beam will be absorbed by the grid's lead strips everywhere but the grid's central portion—where lead strips are vertical. An example of another grid error—off focus and lateral decentering—is seen in Figure 13–14.

If two linear grids are superimposed, Moiré effect will occur. In Figure 13–15 the lead strips are aligned in the same direction, yet not exactly superimposed, and this unmistakable moiré effect is seen.

(B) SF Imaging

See Figures 13–12 through 13–15.

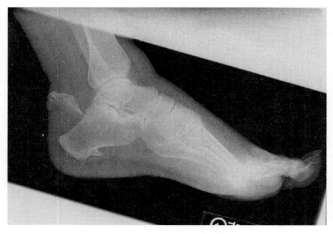

Figure 13–9. Incomplete erasure of PSP. CR reader failed to completely erase the previous image. Faint image of ribs can be seen outside the collimated area, above the foot. (Courtesy of Stamford Hospital, Department of Radiology.)

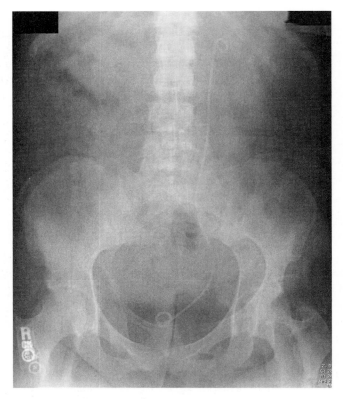

Figure 13–10. Double exposure. Note how CR will "correct" the exposure values; image does not appear overexposed, but second abdomen image is visible. (Courtesy of Stamford Hospital, Department of Radiology.)

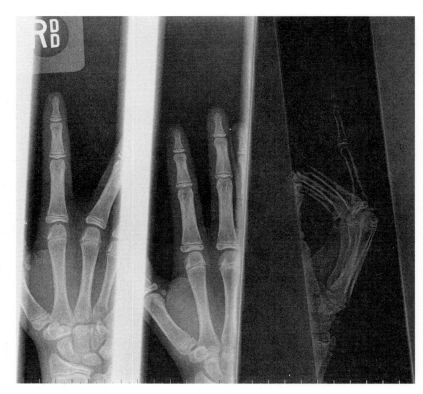

Figure 13–11. The "partition pattern recognition process" in CR will determine if the image is divided, and if so, how it is divided. In the CR image above, one image was not recognized probably because the x-ray field was too close to the adjacent field. (Reproduced, with permission, from Shephard CT. *Radiographic Image Production and Manipulation*. New York: McGraw-Hill, 2003.)

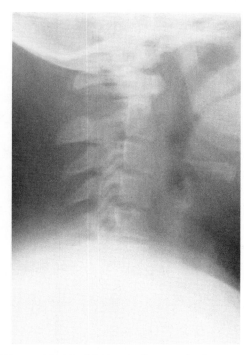

Figure 13–12. Motion is the greatest enemy of image detail. (Courtesy of Stamford Hospital, Department of Radiology.)

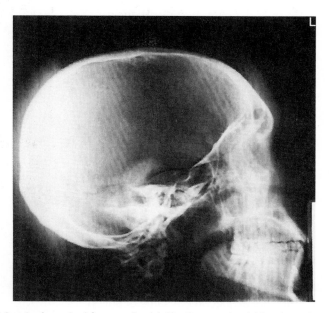

Figure 13–13. *Inverted focused grid.* If a focused grid is placed upside down, the divergent x-ray beam will be absorbed by the grid's lead strips (everywhere but the grid's central portion, where grid lines are vertical). See "Density versus Grids" section of Chapter 12. (Courtesy of Stamford Hospital, Department of Radiology.)

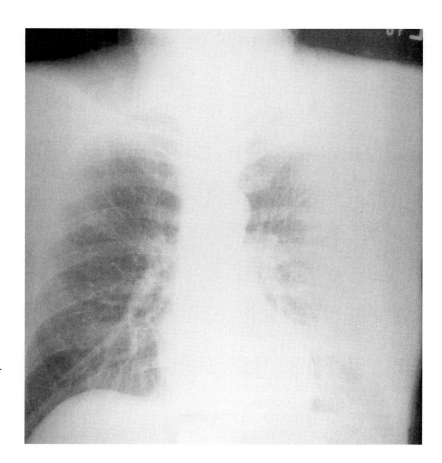

Figure 13–14. *Off-focus and lateral decentering* errors. Notice the asymmetric cutoff from right to left. See "Density versus Grids" section of Chapter 12. (From the American College of Radiology Learning File. Courtesy of the American College of Radiology.)

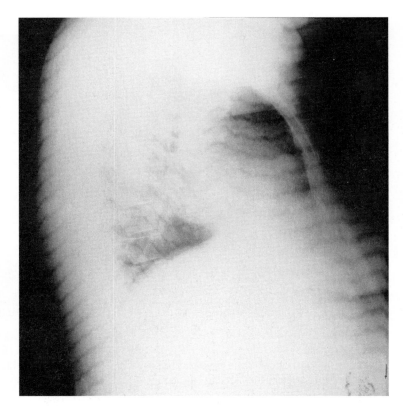

Figure 13–15. *Moiré effect*. This is an example of the effect of *superimposing two linear grids*. When the lead strips are aligned in the same direction, yet not exactly superimposed, this unmistakable moiré effect occurs. (From the American College of Radiology Learning File. Courtesy of the American College of Radiology.)

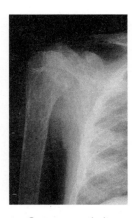

Figure 13–16. *Osteoporotic* bone as a result of thalassemia (Cooley or Mediterranean anemia) requires *reduction of technical factors*. (From the American College of Radiology Learning File. Courtesy of the American College of Radiology.)

PATIENT VARIABLES

Automation or computerization will never completely eliminate patient variables. CR, DR, APR, and AEC, moving tabletops, imaging accessories and mobile equipment can all help us achieve optimal images. But communication, interaction, understanding of individual differences, knowledge, and skill are still essential.

APR, AEC, CR, and DR help us achieve consistent and predictable images by compensating for differences in patient habitus, position, and pathology and by providing computerized preprogrammed equipment.

Figures 13–16 through 13–19 illustrate various abnormal conditions for which our equipment will make compensation. Figures 13–12 and 13–20 illustrate that motion, whether voluntary or involuntary, will affect an x-ray image in a deleterious manner.

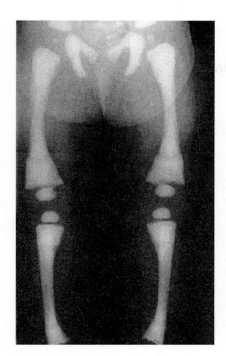

Figure 13–17. *Osteopetrosis* (Albers–Schönberg, or marble-bone, disease) is characterized by *increased bone density*, requiring an appropriate *increase in technical factors*. (From the American College of Radiology Learning File. Courtesy of the American College of Radiology.)

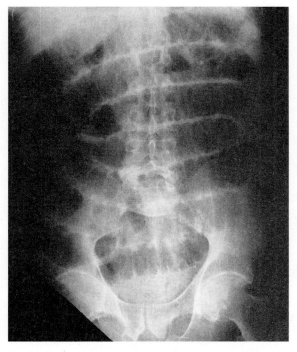

Figure 13–18. Pathology such as *increased amount of air* can require decrease in technical factors. (From the American College of Radiology Learning File. Courtesy of the American College of Radiology.)

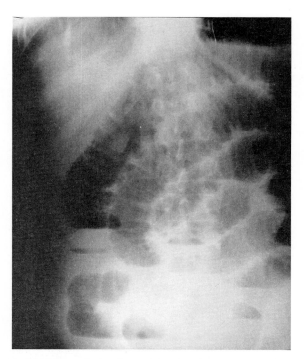

Figure 13–19. A change in *body position* from recumbent to erect will require an increase in technical factors. (From the American College of Radiology Learning File. Courtesy of the American College of Radiology.)

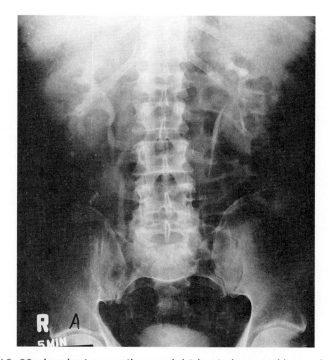

Figure 13–20. *Involuntary motion* on right (ureter) caused by *peristalsis*. Use of the shortest possible exposure time is the best way to avoid loss of detail caused by involuntary motion. (From the American College of Radiology Learning File. Courtesy of the American College of Radiology.)

IDENTIFICATION OF ARTIFACTS

In SF imaging, artifacts have often been classified as exposure, processing, and handling.

Exposure artifacts are even more obvious in CR/DR because of its wide dynamic range. Not only will metallic dentures, hairpins, and prostheses be easily seen, and wrinkled bedding or clothing and braided hair be seen with little difficulty, but even folds of skin and tiny processing artifacts can be readily visualized in CR/DR.

Many artifacts are produced by misuse of imaging equipment, as previously discussed.

Exposure artifacts are seen in Figures 13–21 (tape), 13–22 (gum), 13–23 (hair pin), 13–24 (dentures), and 13–25 (IV pole and necklace).

Handling artifacts such as scratches and dust impact CR images in appearance very similar to SF imaging. Figure 13–30 A illustrates the effect of dust/lint on the PSP, while 13–30 B and 13–31 show the effect of a scratched PSP.

Examples of SF/analog handling artifacts are illustrated in Figures 13–26 (white light leak), 13–27 (crescent marks), and 13–28 (static discharge).

Processing artifacts can be from chemical processing of film or from processing of digital images. The latter will be emphasized here.

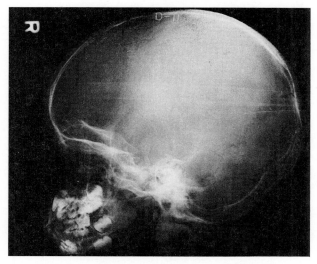

Figure 13–21. *Tape* used for immobilization is often imaged and can impair visualization of details. (From the American College of Radiology Learning File. Courtesy of the American College of Radiology.)

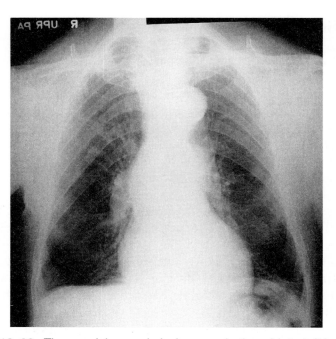

Figure 13–22. The suspicious *coin lesion* seen in the mid- to left lung field was discovered to be a *wad of chewing gum* placed there for safekeeping during this radiographic examination. (From the American College of Radiology Learning File. Courtesy of the American College of Radiology.)

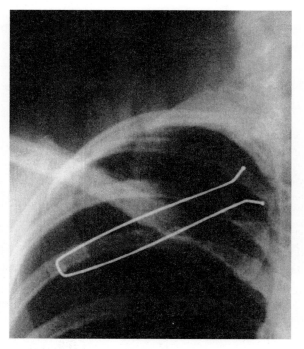

Figure 13–23. Hairpin and braid artifacts. (From the American College of Radiology Learning File. Courtesy of the American College of Radiology.)

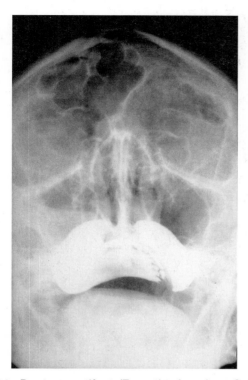

Figure 13–24. *Dentures artifact.* (From the American College of Radiology Learning File. Courtesy of the American College of Radiology.)

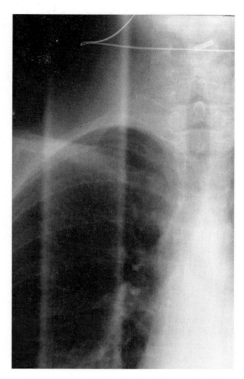

Figure 13–25. Neck chain held in patient's mouth, but (magnified) *I.V. pole* left between the patient and the x-ray tube. (From the American College of Radiology Learning File. Courtesy of the American College of Radiology.)

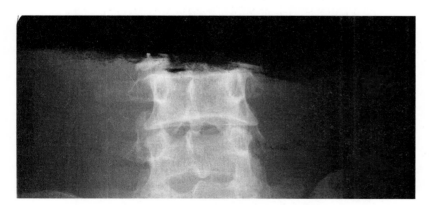

Figure 13–26. *Light leak.* Fogging from *exposure to white light*, such as film bin exposure, resulted in exposed upper edge of film. (From the American College of Radiology Learning File. Courtesy of the American College of Radiology.)

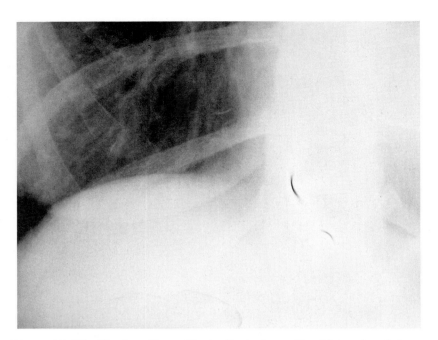

Figure 13–27. *Film handling artifacts*. Typical sensitized (plus density) crescent (kink) mark caused by bending the film acutely. (From the American College of Radiology Learning File. Courtesy of the American College of Radiology.)

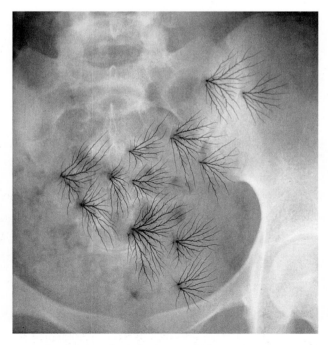

Figure 13–28. *Static electrical discharge*. *Tree* static caused by *low humidity* and *improper handling* of films. (From the American College of Radiology Learning File. Courtesy of the American College of Radiology.)

CR PROCESSOR ARTIFACTS/ERRORS/MALFUNCTIONS

CR processors require adequate care, routine maintenance, knowledgeable troubleshooting, and regular QC evaluation/testing.

After exposure, the IP is placed into the CR scanner/reader and the PSP is automatically removed and scanned by a laser to obtain pixel data. This movement, if not precise, can cause artifact formation. Figure 13–29 illustrates a vertical processing artifact through the shoulder joint; Figure 13–31A illustrates skipped scan lines.

Anhydrous ethanol is recommended for cleaning most PSPs. Unlike isopropyl alcohol, anhydrous ethanol is a water-free liquid. It is a federally controlled HAZMAT and can be acquired from the hospital pharmacy. Cleaning PSPs with any other material can cause breakdown of the protective coat and subsequent artifacts as seen in the Figure 13–32.

If a PSP becomes scratched during processing or at any other time, artifacts such as that seen in Figures 13–30 and 13–33 will occur. If the scratch occurs in an area where imaging is likely to take place (anywhere but the periphery), the PSP should be replaced.

PSPs are exceptionally sensitive to external exposure, like that from scattered radiation. Figure 13–34 illustrates a minus brightness artifact resulting from scattered radiation exposure during processing.

If there is uneven distance between the PSL and light collection device, there will result a shading effect as seen in Figure 13–35.

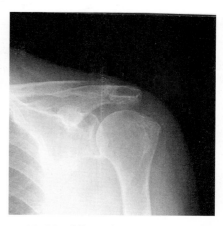

Figure 13–29. CR reader processing artifact seen vertically through the shoulder joint. (Courtesy of Stamford Hospital, Department of Radiology.)

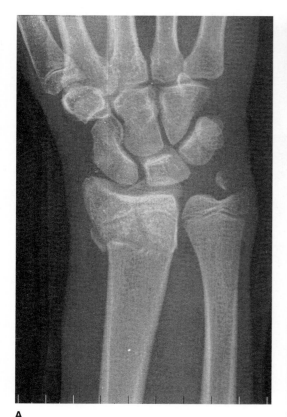

A

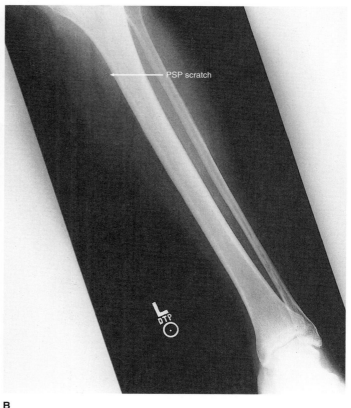

PSP scratch

B

Figure 13–30. Dust/dirt on the PSP creates artifacts similar to those caused by dust on traditional intensifying screens **(A)**. A scratch on the PSP also creates artifact similar to intensifying screen scratch **(B)**. (Reproduced, with permission, from Shephard CT. *Radiographic Image Production and Manipulation*. New York: McGraw-Hill, 2003.)

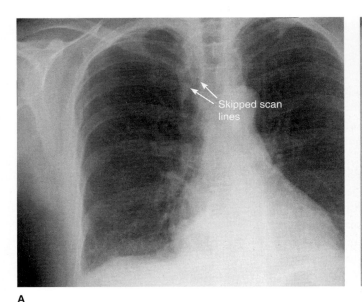

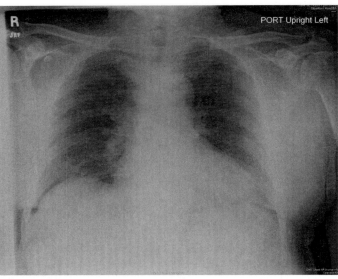

A   B

Figure 13–31. **(A)** Skipped scan line artifact. (Reproduced, with permission, from Shephard CT. *Radiographic Image Production and Manipulation*. New York: McGraw-Hill, 2003.) **(B)** Aliasing artifact. If the direction of the lead strips and the grid frequency matches the scan frequency of the scanner/reader, this artifact can occur. Aliasing (sometimes called Moiré) appears as superimposed images slightly out of alignment, an image "wrapping" effect. This is most common in mobile radiography with stationary grids. (Courtesy of Stamford Hospital, Department of Radiology.)

As rollers grip the PSP travelling through the scanner/reader, the rollers must maintain uniform grip. Should a roller be displaced away from the PSP and increased brightness artifact like that seen in Figure 13–36 can occur.

Dust particles on the PSP can cause a striking artifact during processing. An example is seen in Figure 13–37.

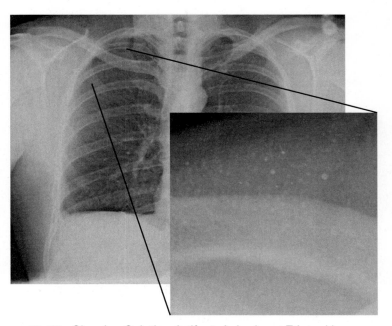

Figure 13–32. Cleaning Solution Artifact. Anhydrous Ethanol is recommended for cleaning many PSPs. Other cleaners can damage the PSP protective coat. (Courtesy of FUJIFILM Medical Systems USA, Inc.)

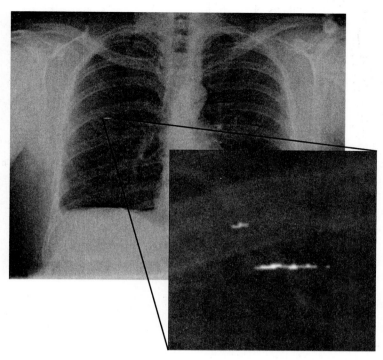

Figure 13–33. Scratch Artifact. The PSP should be replaced if scratch artifact is in region of active imaging. (Courtesy of FUJIFILM Medical Systems USA, Inc.)

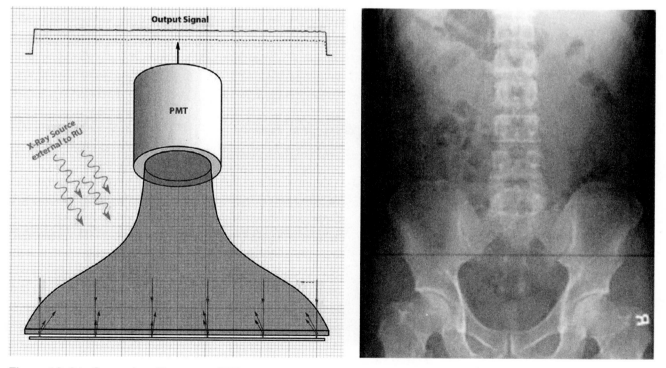

Figure 13–34. Secondary Exposure. PSPs are very sensitive to all external ionizing radiation, such as SR from the x-ray room. Such SR can result in the plus density (minus brightness) artifact seen here. (Courtesy of FUJIFILM Medical Systems USA, Inc.)

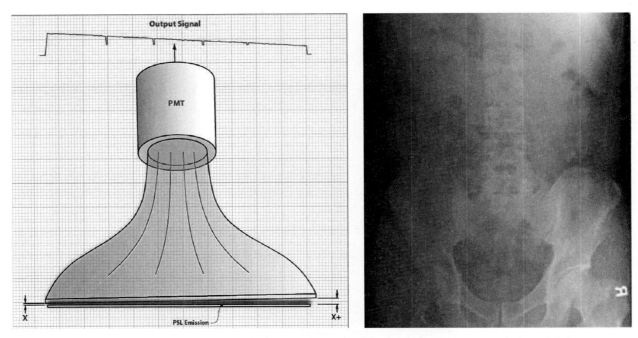

Figure 13–35. Shading. Uneven distance between PSL and light collection can cause obvious brightness variation. (Courtesy of FUJIFILM Medical Systems USA, Inc.)

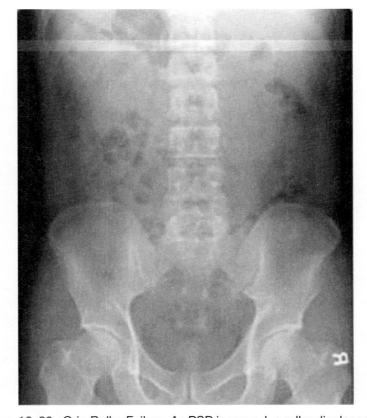

Figure 13–36. Grip Roller Failure. As PSP is moved, a roller displaced away from the PSP will cause a low density (increased brightness) band at the top and/or bottom of the image. (Courtesy of FUJIFILM Medical Systems USA, Inc.)

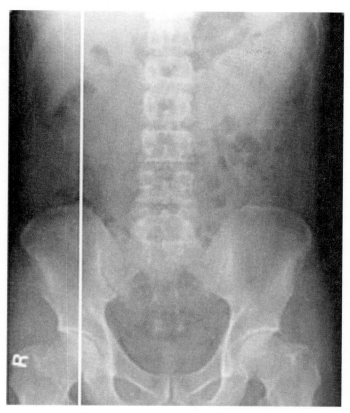

Figure 13–37. Dust Artifact. Dust particle on the light guide of the plate reader will cause a low density (increased brightness) line across the entire image. (Courtesy of FUJIFILM Medical Systems USA, Inc.)

COMPREHENSION CHECK

Congratulations! You have completed this chapter. If you are able to answer the following group of very comprehensive questions, you should feel confident that you have mastered this section.

1. Evaluate radiographs, assessing them for:

    A. Recorded detail and distortion (p. 405)

    B. Image brightness and gray scale/contrast, including structural considerations (p. 406)

    C. Grid selection and use (p. 407)

    D. Image identification requirements (p. 407, 408)

    E. Beam restriction (p. 408)

    F. Patient shielding (p. 408)

    G. Positioning accuracy, including structural considerations (p. 408)

    H. Evidence of artifacts (p. 419)

    I. Processing malfunctions or errors (p. 423)

2. Determine the cause(s) of any problem(s) your evaluation has uncovered and discuss recommendations for corrective action.

PART V

Equipment Operation and Quality Control

CHAPTER 14

Radiographic and Fluoroscopic Equipment | 14

PRINCIPLES OF RADIATION PHYSICS

X-Ray Production

Diagnostic x-rays are produced within the x-ray tube when high-speed *electrons* are rapidly decelerated upon encountering the tungsten atoms of the anode. The *source of electrons* is the heated cathode filament; they are driven across to the anode focal spot when thousands of volts (kV) are applied. When the high-speed electrons are suddenly stopped at the focal spot, their kinetic energy is converted to x-ray photon energy. This happens in two ways:

1. *Bremsstrahlung* ("Brems") or "braking" *radiation*: A high-speed electron, passing near or through a tungsten atom, is attracted and "braked" (i.e., slowed down) by the positively charged nucleus and deflected from its course with a loss of energy. *This energy loss is given up in the form of an x-ray photon* (Fig. 14–1). The electron might not give up all its kinetic energy in one interaction; it can go on to have several more interactions deeper in the anode, each time producing an x-ray photon having less and less energy. This is one reason the x-ray beam is *polyenergetic*, that is, has a *spectrum of energies*. Brems radiation *comprises 70% to 90% of the x-ray beam.*

2. *Characteristic radiation:* In this case, a high-speed electron encounters a tungsten atom within the anode and *ejects* a K shell electron (Fig. 14–2) leaving a vacancy in that shell. An electron from the adjacent L shell moves to the K shell to fill its vacancy, and in doing so *emits a K characteristic ray.* The *energy* of the characteristic ray is equal to the *difference in energy between the K and L shell energy levels.*

X-Ray Beam

Frequency and Wavelength. All *electromagnetic radiations*, including x-rays, can be described as wave-like fluctuations of electric and magnetic fields (Fig. 14–3). The figure illustrates that visible light, microwaves, and radio waves, as well as x-ray and gamma rays, are all part of the *electromagnetic spectrum*. All electromagnetic radiations have the same

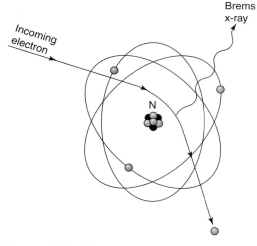

Figure 14–1. Production of Bremsstrahlung (Brems) radiation. A high-speed electron is deflected from its path, and the loss of kinetic energy is emitted in the form of an x-ray photon.

X-Ray Production:

• Brems (70%–90%)
• Characteristic (10%–30%)

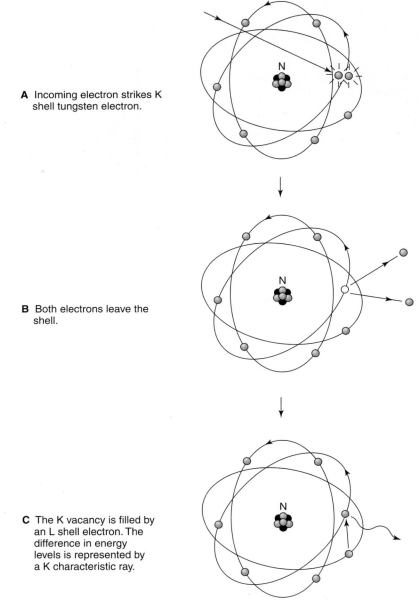

A Incoming electron strikes K shell tungsten electron.

B Both electrons leave the shell.

C The K vacancy is filled by an L shell electron. The difference in energy levels is represented by a K characteristic ray.

Figure 14–2. Production of characteristic radiation. A high-speed electron (**A**) ejects a tungsten K-shell electron, leaving a K-shell vacancy (**B**). An electron from the L shell fills the vacancy and emits a K characteristic ray (**C**).

velocity, 186,000 miles per second (3×10^8 m/s); however, they differ greatly in *wavelength*.

Wavelength refers to the distance between two consecutive wave crests (Fig. 14–4). *Frequency* refers to the number of cycles per second (cps); its unit of measurement is the *hertz* (Hz), which is equal to 1 cps. Frequency and wavelength are closely associated with the relative *energy* of electromagnetic radiations. More energetic radiations have *shorter wavelength* and *higher frequency*. The relationship among frequency, wavelength, and energy is graphically illustrated by the electromagnetic spectrum.

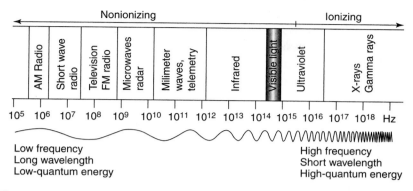

Figure 14–3. The electromagnetic spectrum. Frequency and photon energy are *directly* related; frequency and photon energy are *inversely* related to wavelength.

Beam Characteristics. Some radiations, like x-rays, are energetic enough to rearrange atoms in materials through which they pass, and they can therefore be hazardous to living tissue. These radiations are called *ionizing* radiation because they have the energetic potential to break apart electrically neutral atoms, resulting in the production of negative and/or positive *ions*.

X-rays are infinitesimal bundles of energy called *photons* that deposit some of their energy into matter as they travel through it. This deposition of energy and subsequent *ionization* has the potential to cause chemical and biological damage. Several of the outstanding properties of x-ray photons are listed in the *summary box*.

The possibility of tissue damage as a result of exposure to x-ray photons depends partly on the *quantity* and *quality* of the x-ray beam and the exposure factors that contribute to these factors. The *primary beam* of x-rays refers to the x-ray beam that emerges from the x-ray tube focal spot, before it strikes anything. Many of these photons then encounter

Shorter Wavelength Associated with:

- Higher frequency (cps)
- Higher energy
- Increased ionizing potential

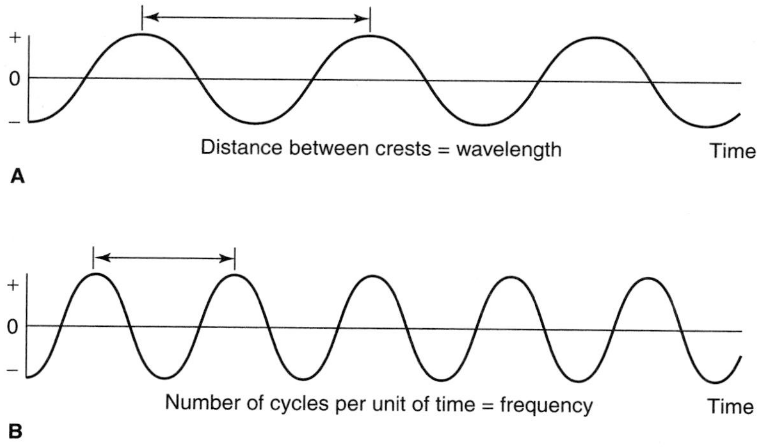

Figure 14–4. Wavelength versus frequency. *Wavelength* is described as the distance between successive crests. The shorter the wavelength, the more crests or cycles per unit of time (e.g., per second). Therefore, the shorter the wavelength the greater the *frequency* (number of cycles/s). Wavelength and frequency are *inversely* related.

Properties of X-Ray Photons

- X-rays are not perceptible by the senses.
- X-rays travel in straight lines.
- X-rays travel at the speed of light.
- X-rays are electrically neutral.
- X-rays have a penetrating effect on all matter.
- X-rays have a physiological effect on living tissue.
- X-rays have an ionizing effect on air.
- X-rays have a photographic effect on film emulsion.
- X-rays produce fluorescence in certain phosphors.
- X-rays cannot be focused.
- X-rays have a spectrum of energies.

X-Ray Photons Can:

- Pass through the part
- Be absorbed by the part
- Scatter within the part

the part to be radiographed. X-ray photons emerging from the part are referred to as the *remnant or exit beam* and help contribute to forming the image. The principal factor affecting beam *quantity* is mAs, whereas the principal factor affecting beam *quality* is kV. Another x-ray beam characteristic is described by the *inverse square law* of radiation. The inverse square law is particularly important in radiation protection considerations and in selection of exposure factors. These factors and many others are thoroughly discussed in Part III *Radiation Protection* and in Part IV *Image Production and Evaluation*.

Photon Interactions with Matter

The gradual decrease in exposure rate as radiation passes through tissues is called *attenuation*. Attenuation is principally attributable to the two major types of interactions that occur between x-ray photons and tissue in the diagnostic x-ray range of energies.

Photoelectric Effect. In the *photoelectric effect*, a relatively *low*-energy (low-kV) x-ray photon uses all its energy (true/total absorption) to eject an *inner shell* electron, leaving an orbital vacancy. An electron from the shell above drops down to fill the vacancy and, in doing so, gives up energy in the form of a *characteristic ray* (Fig. 14–5).

The photoelectric effect is more likely to occur in absorbers having *high atomic number* (e.g., bone and positive contrast media) and contributes significantly to patient dose, as all the photon energy is absorbed by the patient (and, therefore, is responsible for the production of short-scale contrast).

Compton Scatter. In *Compton scatter*, a fairly *high*-energy (high-kV) x-ray photon ejects an *outer shell* electron (Fig. 14–6). Although the x-ray photon is deflected with somewhat reduced energy (modified scatter), it retains most of its original energy and exits the body as an energetic scattered photon.

Because the scattered photon exits the body, it poses little radiation hazard to the patient. Some internal scatter, however, can contribute to patient dose. Compton scatter contributes to *image fog* and poses a *radiation hazard to personnel* (as in fluoroscopic procedures).

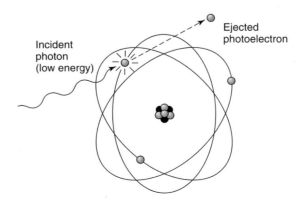

Figure 14–5. In the photoelectric effect, all of the incoming (low-energy) photon's energy is absorbed as it ejects an inner shell electron from orbit.

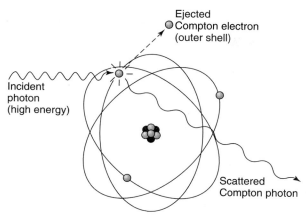

Figure 14–6. In Compton scatter, the incoming (high-energy) photon uses *part* of its energy to eject an outer shell electron; in doing so, the photon changes direction (scatters) but retains much of its original energy.

Coherent (Classical) Scatter. The process of *coherent* scatter is also known as *classical*, *unmodified*, or *Rayleigh* scatter. This interaction between x-rays and matter occurs with very low-energy x-ray photons— energies rarely used in diagnostic radiology. When a very low-energy x-ray photon interacts with an atom of matter, the photon "disappears" as it is absorbed by the atom, leaving the atom in an excited state. As the atom returns to its normal state, it releases an x-ray photon of *identical* wavelength, but travels in a different direction than the incident photon (i.e., a *scattered photon*). It is important to note that this is the only interaction between x-ray photons and matter in which *no ionization occurs*.

Tissue Attenuation. The radiologic image is obtained as a result of the attenuation processes occurring in the body. Tissues that are very dense will allow little or no passage of x-rays—those tissues appear white or light on the image. Other tissues are easy for x-ray photons to penetrate—those tissues appear darker.

Sometimes we use artificial contrast agents to better demonstrate certain parts; depending on the nature of the contrast agent, these parts will look lighter or darker. Some body parts are smaller while others are larger. Various pathologic conditions can alter the nature of the tissues they affect; this can also impact how light or dark the image will be.

All this indicates that the *thickness* or size of body parts, as well as the *atomic number* of the tissue (e.g., bone vs. soft tissue), has a significant influence on photon interactions and, therefore, attenuation of the x-ray beam by various anatomic tissues.

> **X-Ray Photon Interactions with Matter:**
>
> - Coherent/classical scatter
> - Photoelectric effect
> - Compton scatter

Summary

- The radiations of the electromagnetic spectrum all travel at the *same* velocity, 186,000 miles per second, but *differ* in wavelength.
- Wavelength is the distance between two consecutive wave crests.
- The number of cycles and crests per second is frequency; its unit of measure is Hz.

- Wavelength and frequency are inversely related.
- Ionization is caused by high-energy, short-wavelength electromagnetic radiations that break apart electrically neutral atoms.
- Two types of x-radiations are produced at the anode through energy conversion processes: Brems radiation and characteristic radiation; Brems radiation predominates.
- X-rays can interact with tissue cells and cause ionization; interactions between x-rays and tissue cells are the photoelectric effect, Compton scatter, and coherent (classical) scatter.
- Characteristics of photoelectric effect
  - Low-energy x-ray photon gives up all its energy ejecting an inner shell electron
  - Produces a characteristic ray (secondary radiation)
  - Major contributor to patient dose
  - Occurs in absorbers having high atomic number and mass density
  - Produces short-scale contrast
- Characteristics of Compton scatter
  - Predominates in the diagnostic x-ray range
  - High-energy x-ray photon uses a portion of its energy to eject an outer shell electron
  - Responsible for scattered radiation fog to the image
  - Radiation hazard to personnel and to patient as internal scatter
- Characteristics of coherent scatter
  - Very low-energy x-ray photon interacts with the atom, disappears, and sets the atom into an excited state
  - As the atom returns to a normal state, an identical photon is emitted, but in a different direction
  - This is the only interaction that does not cause ionization
- Contributors to exposure dose are beam attenuation and the type of interaction. Exposure dose is, therefore, impacted by radiation quality (kV) and the subject being irradiated (i.e., thickness and nature of part; atomic number of part).

TYPES OF EQUIPMENT

The various kinds of x-ray machines are generally named according to the x-ray energy they produce or the specific purpose(s) for which they are designed, for example, mammographic unit, tomographic equipment, mobile unit, 150 kV (kilovolts) chest unit, 1,200 mA (milliampere) general diagnostic unit, digital fluoroscopy (DF), digital R/F (radiography and fluoroscopy), or computed radiography (CR).

Fixed

Most x-ray equipment is *fixed*, or stationary, that is, it is installed in a particular place and cannot be moved. Most general radiographic and fluoroscopic equipment in the radiology department is fixed.

Mobile

Mobile x-ray equipment is designed to be taken to patients who are unable to travel to the radiology department, for example, the very ill, incapacitated patients, and patients in surgery. Mobile equipment is available for radiographic and/or fluoroscopic x-ray procedures.

Dedicated

X-ray equipment that is designed for a specific purpose or type of examination is referred to as *dedicated equipment*. Examples of dedicated equipments are head units, mammography equipment, chest units, tomographic equipment, bone densitometry, and dental units.

Digital/Electronic

CR, DR, and DF units are examples of equipment whose images can be manipulated and stored for transfer via electronic means and/or printed as hard copies. Detailed discussion of CR/DR is given in Chapters 11 and 12, and later in this chapter.

ELECTRICITY, X-RAY TRANSFORMERS, AND RECTIFIERS

Fundamental to the study of x-ray equipment is a basic understanding of magnetism and electricity. The relationship between magnetism and electricity is central to the operation of many x-ray circuit components; therefore, it is important to review these concepts prior to reviewing x-ray circuit components.

Generators function to change mechanical energy to electrical energy (whereas *motors* convert electrical energy to mechanical energy). Electrical current flowing through a conductor in only one direction and with constant magnitude is called *direct current* (DC). A familiar source of DC is the *battery*.

Electricity is more efficiently transported over long distances at low-current and high-voltage values to avoid excessive power loss (according to the power, or heat, loss formula: $P = I^2R$). Most applications of electricity require the use of *alternating current* (AC), in which the amplitude and polarity of the current vary periodically with time (Fig. 14–7).

AC consists of sinusoidal waves. One *wavelength* consists of two half-cycles: a *positive half-cycle* and a *negative half-cycle*. A *wavelength* is defined as the distance between two consecutive *crests*. A crest is the positive half-cycle peak and a *trough* is the negative half-cycle peak. The maximum height of the wave/impulse is referred to as its *amplitude* and represents electrical potential, or voltage. *AC is therefore characterized by varying amplitude and periodic reversal of polarity.* The number of cycles per unit of time (e.g., second) is called *frequency* (Fig. 14–7), and its

---

Generators:

- Change mechanical energy to electrical energy

Motors:

- Change electrical energy to mechanical energy

Alternating Current

- *Amplitude* and *polarity* vary periodically
- *Wavelength:* Distance between two consecutive crests; one positive and one negative half-cycle
- *Crest:* Positive half-cycle peak
- *Trough:* Negative half-cycle peak
- *Amplitude:* Height of the wave
- *Frequency:* Number of cycles per second
- *Hertz:* Unit of frequency

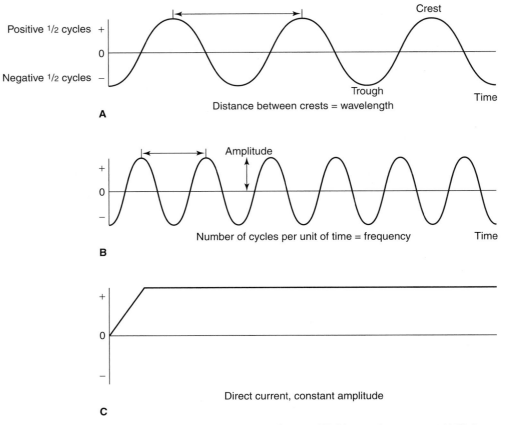

Figure 14–7. Alternating and direct current waveforms. **(A)** Alternating current (AC), low frequency. **(B)** High-frequency AC. Compare the distance between crests and troughs in (B) with those in (A). **(C)** Direct current, like that supplied by a battery, is characterized by constant amplitude (peak potential).

unit of measurement is the *hertz* (Hz). In the United States, AC is generated at 60 Hz or cps, that is, 60 cycles (60 positive half-cycles and 60 negative half-cycles) occur each second. One half second, therefore, would include 30 cycles ($\frac{1}{2} \times 60 = 30$); consequently, 4 cycles represent a $\frac{4}{60}$ or $\frac{1}{15}$ second time interval.

X-rays are produced when high-speed electrons are suddenly decelerated upon encountering the tungsten atoms of the anode. To produce x-rays of diagnostic value, high voltage (thousands of volts, i.e., kV) must be available. To produce high-quality images, a selection of x-ray energy levels (kV) must be available.

The use of AC and electromagnetic principles are fundamental to the operation of the high-voltage transformer and the autotransformer. These are the x-ray circuit devices responsible, respectively, for producing the required high voltage and permitting a selection of kilovoltages.

It has long been known that there is an important relationship between magnetism and electricity. Famous scientists, including Volta, Oersted, Lenz, and Faraday, performed various experiments demonstrating the relationship, making important observations, and formulating principles that explain the operation of electromagnetic devices.

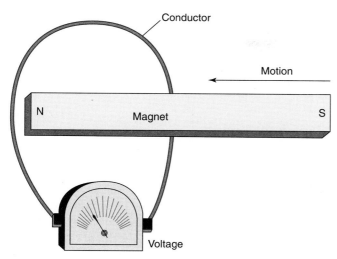

Figure 14–8. Electromagnetic induction. An electric current will be induced in a conductor whenever there is relative motion between a conductor and magnetic field; that is, if a conductor moves through a magnetic field, if a magnetic field moves across a conductor, or if the magnetic field is constantly changing (as in AC).

Faraday's observation that a *magnetic field* will induce an electric current in a conductor if there is motion of either the magnetic field or the conductor (Fig. 14–8) is the fundamental principle of operation of the high-voltage *transformer*. If a coiled conductor is supplied with an AC, a magnetic field expands and collapses around the coil, accompanying the peaks and valleys of the AC waveform. If a second coiled conductor is placed near, but not touching, the first (primary) coil, the moving magnetic field will interact similarly with the second coil and an electric current will be induced in it. Thus, the moving magnetic field from the primary coil can be used to induce a current in another circuit with whom it has no physical connection; this is called *mutual induction*. An AC, producing a continuously moving magnetic field, is necessary for mutual induction to occur.

A conductive wire shaped into a coil is called a *helix*; a helix supplied with a current is a *solenoid*. If an iron core is inserted within the coil, a simple *electromagnet* is formed and the magnetic lines of force are intensified. Thus, a transformer's conductor is frequently coiled around an iron core to increase its efficiency.

Summary

- X-ray equipment may be described as either fixed or mobile.
- X-ray equipment designed for a particular purpose (e.g., mammographic, head, and chest units) is termed *dedicated.*
- A generator converts mechanical energy to electrical energy; a motor converts electrical energy to mechanical energy.
- Electricity is transported over long distances at high-voltage and low-current values to minimize energy loss, according to the heat loss formula: $P = I^2R$.

- AC is characterized by constantly changing polarity and amplitude.
- A coil of wire is a helix; supplied with current it is a solenoid; with an iron core, it is the simplest type of electromagnet.
- X-ray transformers operate on the principle of mutual induction.

High-Voltage Transformers

X-ray transformers are used to increase the incoming voltage to the more useful *kilovoltage* required for x-ray production. Transformers that increase the voltage are called *step-up transformers* or high-voltage transformers. The degree to which transformers increase the voltage is determined by their *turns ratio*, that is, the number of turns in the secondary (high-voltage) coil compared with the number of turns in the primary (low-voltage) coil; the higher the ratio, the greater the voltage increase. As voltage increases, however, current decreases proportionally according to the (*transformer law*) equations that follow:

$$\frac{V_s}{V_p} = \frac{N_s}{N_p} \quad \frac{N_s}{N_p} = \frac{I_p}{I_s}.$$

Note that the relationship between the turns ratio and the *voltage* is a *direct one*, while there is an *inverse* relationship between the turns ratio and the *current*. So, as voltage increases, current decreases proportionally.

For example, if a particular x-ray transformer has a turns ratio of 500:1 and is supplied with 50 A and 220 V, *what is its kV and mA output?*

$$\frac{x}{220} = \frac{500}{1} \qquad \frac{500}{1} = \frac{50}{x}$$
$$x = (500)(220) \qquad 500x = 50$$
$$x = 110,000 = 110\,kv \qquad x = 0.1\,A = 100\,mA.$$

Transformers can also be the *step-down* type, like that found in the x-ray filament circuit.

Although transformers operate at approximately 95% efficiency, energy loss varies according to transformer design. An *open-core* transformer consists of two parallel iron cores with conductive windings; however, a loss or leaking away of magnetic flux occurs at the ends of the iron cores. A *closed-core* transformer (Fig. 14–9) consists of a ring-shaped core of iron that serves to reduce leakage flux energy loss. A *shell*-type transformer has a central partition, effectively dividing it into two halves. The transformer primary and secondary coils are wound around the center bar (but not touching each other) and this arrangement serves to reduce energy loss still further.

Autotransformers

The x-ray circuit transformer is a *fixed*-ratio transformer, that is, the turns relationship is constant. How, then, are we able to have a selection

Types of Energy Loss Inherent in All Transformers

- *Copper losses* are caused by the resistance to current flow that is characteristic of all conductors and are reduced by using larger *diameter* conductive wire.
- *Hysteresis losses* are a result of the continually changing magnetic domains of the core material (as a result of changing polarity of AC) and can be reduced by using core material of greater *permeability* (e.g., silicon).
- *Eddy current* losses are a result of small currents (eddy currents) built up in the core material as a result of the continually changing magnetic fields. Eddy current losses are reduced by *laminating* the core material; any current generated can travel only the small distance between laminations and, therefore, represent a smaller energy loss.

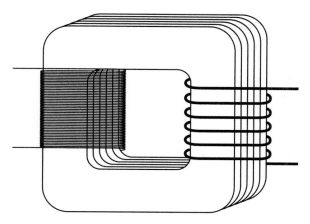

Figure 14–9. The *closed-core* transformer reduces loss of magnetic flux. Note the *laminated* silicon steel that serves to reduce *eddy current* losses.

of kilovoltages from which to choose? It is through the use of an *auto-transformer*, which sends the correct amount of *voltage* to the primary of the high-voltage transformer to be stepped up to the required *kilovoltage* level.

The autotransformer consists of an iron core with a single coil wrapped around it (that serves as its primary and secondary winding) and operates on the principle of *self-induction*. Each coil turn has a contact or tap. A movable contact (corresponding to the kV selector dial on the control panel) makes connection with the appropriate tap on the autotransformer. The voltage sent to the primary coil of the high-voltage transformer depends on the number of coils "tapped." For example, a particular autotransformer has 2,000 windings and is supplied with 220 V. If 500 windings are tapped, *what voltage is sent to the primary of the step-up transformer?* The solution can be determined by using the *autotransformer law* (which is the same as the transformer law):

$$\frac{V_s}{V_p} = \frac{N_s}{N_p}$$

$$\frac{x}{220} = \frac{500}{2,000}$$

$$2,000x = (500)(220)$$

$$2,000x = 110,000$$

$$x = 55\,\text{V sent to the primary coil of step-up transformer.}$$

Transformers:

- Step-up transformers increase voltage (and decrease amperage proportionally)
- Step-down transformers decrease voltage (and increase amperage proportionally)
- Require AC for operation
- Operate on the principle of mutual induction

Autotransformers:

- Select the amount of voltage sent to the transformer (kV selector)
- Operate on the principle of self-induction
- Require AC for operation

Summary

- High-voltage (step-up) transformers function to provide the necessary kilovoltage for x-ray production.
- As the high-voltage transformer steps up voltage to kilovoltage, it proportionally steps down current according to the primary to secondary turns ratio and the transformer law.

- The transformer and autotransformer laws are expressed by the following equations:

$$\frac{V_s}{V_p} = \frac{N_s}{N_p}$$

$$\frac{N_s}{N_p} = \frac{I_p}{I_s}.$$

- Step-down transformers are also called filament transformers; they function on the same principles as step-up transformers, and are placed in the filament circuit.
- Transformers can be designed as open core, closed core, or shell type; transformers are approximately 95% efficient.
- Types of transformer losses include copper losses, eddy current losses, and hysteresis losses.
- The autotransformer, operating on the principle of self-induction, functions to provide a selection of kilovoltages.
- Both the transformer and autotransformer require AC for operation.

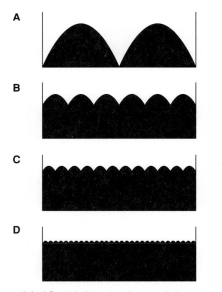

Figure 14–10. (A) Single-phase, full-wave rectified waveform. Note the 100% voltage ripple as each pulse starts at 0 potential, makes its way to 100%, and returns to 0 potential. (B) The three-phase/six-pulse waveform exhibits a 13% voltage drop between peak potentials. (C) Three-phase/12-pulse has only a 4% voltage drop between peak potentials. (D) High-frequency generators are most efficient and produce less than 1% voltage ripple.

Rectification

Some x-ray circuit devices, such as the transformer and autotransformer, operate only on AC. The efficient operation of the x-ray tube, however, requires the use of *unidirectional* current, so current must be *rectified* before it gets to the x-ray tube. The process of full-wave *rectification* changes the nonuseful negative half-cycle to a useful positive half-cycle.

An x-ray circuit rectification system is located between the secondary coil of the high-voltage transformer and the x-ray tube. Rectifiers are solid-state diodes made of *semiconductive materials* such as silicon, selenium, or germanium that conduct electricity *in only one direction*. Thus, a series of rectifiers placed between the transformer and x-ray tube function to change AC to a more useful unidirectional current.

Although rectification remedies the changing polarity problem of single-phase AC, the problem of constantly varying *amplitude* remains. The continually changing voltage from zero to maximum potential and back to zero produces a pulsating beam of x-rays having a wide range of energies. *Three-phase rectification* superimposes three AC waveforms, each separated from the other two by 120 degrees and resulting in a nearly constant potential waveform. Although *single-phase rectification* produces a waveform having 100% "ripple" (i.e., 100% drop in potential between pulses), the three-phase waveform exhibits only a slight drop between pulses (Fig. 14–10).

High-frequency generators first appeared in mobile x-ray units and were then adopted by mammography and CT equipment. Today, more and more radiographic equipment uses high-frequency generators.

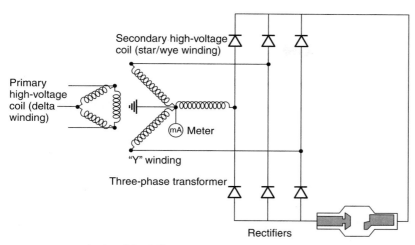

Figure 14–11. A simplified diagram of the secondary (high-voltage) side of a 3φ 6p rectified x-ray circuit. 3φ equipment requires the use of three autotransformers (not shown) and one transformer having three windings arranged in *delta* and *star* (or wye) configuration.

Their compact size makes them popular, and the fact that they produce nearly constant potential voltage helps to improve image quality and decrease patient dose (fewer low-energy photons to contribute to skin dose) (Fig. 14–10).

Three-phase/6-pulse rectification presents a 13% ripple; 3-phase/12-pulse presents only a 4% ripple. The average beam energy therefore increases. For example,

1φ 2p — 100 kV — approximately 70-keV (kilo-electron volt) beam

3φ 6p — 100 kV — approximately 95-keV beam

3φ 12p — 100 kV — approximately 98-keV beam.

Three-phase rectification requires the use of *three autotransformers* (one for each incoming current) and *one transformer* having three windings. A transformer winding can be arranged in either *star* (wye) or *delta* configuration (Fig. 14–11).

Remember that a change in technical factors is required when changing among Sφ to 3φ 6p to 3φ 12p rectified equipment.

Comparison of Technical Factors Required		
Single φ	3φ 6p	3φ 12p
mAs	⅔ × mAs	½ × mAs

Summary

- The x-ray tube operates most efficiently on unidirectional current.
- The rectification system changes AC to unidirectional current and is located between the secondary coil of the high-voltage transformer and the x-ray tube.
- Rectifiers are solid-state diodes made of semiconductive materials such as silicon, selenium, or germanium that permit the flow of electricity in only one direction.
- 3φ rectification uses three ACs out of phase with each other by 120 degrees; 3φ rectified equipment requires three autotransformers and one high-voltage transformer.

- In 3φ rectification, only the peak values of the waveform are used, thus creating a nearly constant potential current.
- 3φ rectification may be 6 pulse (13% ripple) or 12 pulse (4% ripple), depending on the number of rectifiers employed.
- 3φ high-voltage transformer windings are arranged in either star (wye) or delta formation.

THE X-RAY TUBE

X-rays are produced when high-speed electrons emitted from the cathode filament are suddenly decelerated as they encounter tungsten atoms of the x-ray tube anode or target. This can happen in two ways; a review of the two processes follows:

1. *Bremsstrahlung* ("Brems") or "braking" *Radiation*. A high-speed electron, passing through a tungsten atom, is attracted and "braked" by the positively charged nucleus, and deflected from its course with a resulting loss of energy. *This energy loss is given up in the form of an x-ray photon* (Fig. 14–1). Very often, the electron does not give up all its kinetic energy in one such interaction; it goes on to have several more interactions deeper in the target, each time giving up an x-ray photon having less and less energy. This is one reason the x-ray beam is polyenergetic (i.e., having a spectrum of energies). Brems radiation comprises 70% to 90% of the x-ray beam.

2. *Characteristic Radiation*. In this case, a high-speed electron encounters the tungsten atom and ejects a K shell electron, leaving a vacancy in that shell. An electron from an adjacent shell (i.e., the L or M shell) fills the vacancy and in doing so *emits a K characteristic ray* (see Fig. 14–2). The energy of the characteristic ray is equal to the difference in energy level between the K shell and the shell that gave up the electron to fill the K vacancy.

Component Parts

X-ray tubes are used for both radiographic and fluoroscopic purposes. Their basic components are the *anode* (positive electrode) and *cathode* assembly (negative electrode), enclosed within an evacuated (vacuum) *glass envelope* (Fig. 14–12).

The *glass envelope* enclosure creates a *diode* (two electrodes) tube somewhat reminiscent of early radio and television tubes. The x-ray tube glass enclosure, however, is made of glass that is extremely heat resistant to maintain the necessary *vacuum* for the production of x-rays. Should the vacuum begin to deteriorate, air molecules within the tube would collide with, and decelerate, the high-speed electrons traveling to the anode, thus diminishing the production of x-rays. Air within the glass envelope is referred to as a "gassy tube" and will eventually cause oxidation and burnout of the cathode filament.

The cathode assembly consists of one or more *filaments*, their supporting wires, and a *focusing cup*. The filament is a fine (approximately 0.2-mm diameter) 1- to 2-cm coil of tungsten wire that, when heated to

X-Ray Tube:

- Anode (positive electrode)
- Cathode (negative electrode)
- Glass envelope (vacuum)

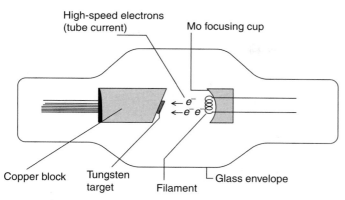

Figure 14–12. A simplified illustration of a *stationary* anode x-ray tube. The tungsten target is embedded in a solid block of copper that serves to conduct heat away from the tungsten and into the oil coolant that surrounds the glass envelope. Most x-ray tubes today use *rotating* anodes as a means of more even heat distribution.

incandescence by approximately 4 A of current, boils off (i.e., liberates) outer shell tungsten electrons. This event is called *thermionic emission*. Most x-ray tubes actually have two or more filaments and are called *double-focus tubes*. The typical x-ray tube has two filaments, one small and one large, to direct electrons to either the small or large anode focal spot. Each filament is closely embraced by a negatively charged molybdenum-focusing cup that serves to direct the electrons toward the anode. The two filaments are arranged in a three-wire/conductor system. A low-voltage conductor carries low voltage to heat the selected (large or small) filament. The third conductor is common to both filaments and carries the high voltage necessary to propel liberated electrons to the anode (Fig. 14–14B).

As the filament boils off electrons, small quantities of tungsten can be vaporized and deposited on the inner surface of the glass envelope. If tungsten is deposited on the port window, it acts as a filter and reduces the intensity of the x-ray beam; it can also affect the tube vacuum and ultimately leads to tube failure.

The filament is heated with the required 3 to 5 A and 10 to 12 V by the *filament circuit*. The filament current is kept at a standby quantity until the rotor is activated; at that time, the *filament booster circuit* brings it up to the level required for exposure. The rotor switch should not be activated for extended periods because the filament current is at maximum potential and tungsten vaporization can increase. Extended activation can also result in bearing damage and decreased tube life.

The anode is a 2- to 5-in. diameter lightweight molybdenum or graphite disk with a beveled edge. The beveled surface has a *focal track* of tungsten and rhenium alloy. The anode rotates at approximately 3,600 rpm (high-speed anode rotation is approximately 10,000 rpm), so that heat generated during x-ray production is evenly distributed over the entire track. *Rotating anodes* can withstand delivery of a greater amount of heat for a longer period of time than *stationary anodes*.

The anode is made to rotate through the use of an *induction motor*. An induction motor has two main parts, a *stator* and a *rotor*. The stator

Anode:

- Graphite/molybdenum disk with beveled edge
- Tungsten/rhenium alloy focal track (0.6–1.2 mm)
- Copper stem (conducts heat away from anode face)

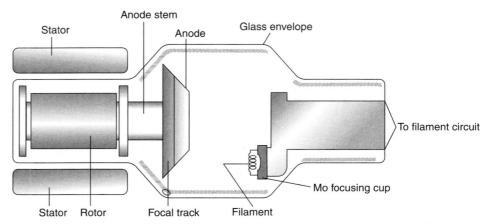

Figure 14–13. The component parts of a rotating anode x-ray tube. Note the position of the stator and rotor. Note the beveled edge of the anode, forming the focal track, and the position of the filament directly across from the rotating focal track.

Induction Motor:

- Rotates anode
- Stator (outside glass envelope)
- Rotor (inside glass envelope)

Characteristics of Tungsten (W) As Target Material

- High atomic number (74) increases x-ray production
- High melting point (3,410°C) to resist pitting and cracking
- Thermal conductivity for heat dissipation

---

is the part located outside the glass envelope and consists of a series of electromagnets occupying positions around the stem of the anode. The stator's electromagnets are supplied with current and the associated magnetic fields function to exert a drag or pull on the rotor within (Fig. 14–13).

Tungsten (W) is usually chosen as target material because of its *high atomic number* ($Z = 74$), *high melting point* (3,410°C), and *thermal conductivity* (equal to that of copper). The high atomic number serves to increase the efficiency of x-ray production; its high melting point makes it resistant to pitting and cracking; its thermal conductivity helps it dissipate the heat produced during x-ray production. Rhenium is added to further resist anode pitting at high temperatures (Fig. 14–14A).

Summary

- X-rays (Brems and characteristic) are produced by the abrupt deceleration of high-speed electrons by tungsten atoms within the focal track.
- The x-ray tube is a diode, that is, it has a negative electrode (cathode) and a positive electrode (anode).
- The x-ray tube's electrodes are enclosed within a vacuum glass envelope; a "gassy" tube produces x-rays less efficiently and results in filament oxidation/burnout.
- The cathode assembly consists of tungsten filament(s) with supporting wires and a (negatively charged) molybdenum-focusing cup.
- Most x-ray tubes have at least two filaments, one for each focal spot.
- Heating of the filament to incandescence (with 3–5 A, 10–12 V) and subsequent "boiling off" of electrons is called thermionic emission.
- The anode is a 2- to 5-in. molybdenum or graphite disk with a peripheral focal track of tungsten and rhenium alloy.

- Tungsten is the target material of choice because of its high atomic number, high melting point, and thermal conductivity; rhenium helps prevent pitting.
- An induction motor, consisting of stator and rotor, rotates the anode 3,600 to 10,000 rpm.

The production of x-rays involves the generation of significant amounts of heat; *only 0.2% of the kinetic energy of the electron stream is converted to x-rays*, and the rest of the energy is converted to *heat*. Because heat can be very damaging to the x-ray tube and its efficient operation, several features are incorporated to expedite its dissipation. The *thermal conductivity* of tungsten is one feature; however, most cooling is a result of heat diffusion to the oil that surrounds the x-ray tube.

If large quantities of heat were continually directed to a single stationary small spot, that spot would be subjected to all the heat generated and would suffer more abuse and subsequent damage. Large quantities of heat delivered to the x-ray tube, especially in a short period of time, can be very damaging to the tube and can shorten its life span. The focal track of the *rotating* anode serves to *spread generated heat over a large area*. The width of the focal track on the anode's beveled edge is approximately 6 mm. Rotating anodes having a diameter of 2 to 5 in. will, therefore, provide significant surface area for the production and dissipation of heat.

The width of the beveled focal track is referred to as the *actual* focal spot size. A distinction is made between the actual focal spot and the *effective*, projected, or apparent focal spot. The actual focal spot size is the width of the finite area on the tungsten target that is actually bombarded by electrons from the filament. The effective, projected, or apparent focal spot is the *foreshortened* size of the focus as it is projected down toward the image receptor, that is, as it would be seen looking up into the x-ray tube (Fig. 14–15). This is called line focusing or the *line focus principle*. The effective focal spot size is also affected by the degree of focal track bevel, or anode angle. Anode angles are usually 5 to 20 degrees.

When using an x-ray tube with a small anode angle, a larger actual anode area (i.e., actual focal spot) can be bombarded (see Fig. 11–11E) and still maintain a small effective focal spot—anode heat load tolerance is not compromised and recorded detail is improved.

The size of the effective focal spot *varies along the length of the image receptor*, being largest in size (and associated with most blur) at the cathode end of the image receptor and smallest at the anode end (see Figs. 11–12 and 11–13).

A difficulty associated with the use of a small anode angle, however, is a pronounced *anode heel effect* (Fig. 11–14). The anode heel effect illustrates (see Figs. 11–43 and 11–44) how a portion of the divergent x-ray beam is absorbed by the anode resulting in diminished image density at the anode end of the image.

Using a small anode angle, a typical radiographic distance of 40 in. source-to-image-receptor distance (SID), and a 14 × 17 in. image receptor, will result in approximately 2 in. of unexposed area at the

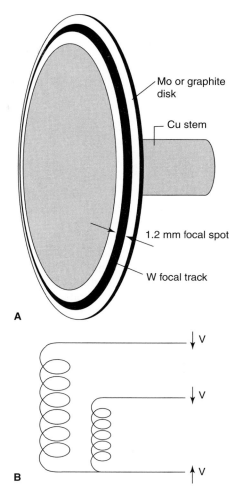

Figure 14–14. (A) A typical rotating anode. The anode disk is usually made of molybdenum and has a beveled edge containing a "band" of tungsten/rhenium alloy that forms the focal track. (B) Two filaments are arranged in a three-supporting wire/conductor system. A *low*-voltage conductor carries low voltage to heat the selected (large or small) filament. The third conductor is common to both filaments and carries the *high* voltage necessary to propel liberated electrons to the anode. The filament is supplied with 3 to 5 A and 10 to 12 V.

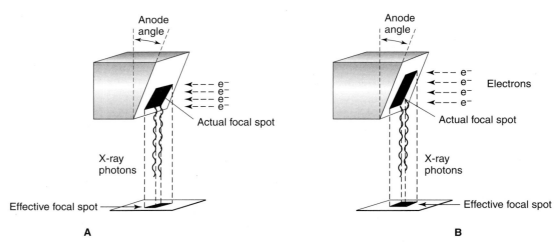

Figure 14–15. Line focus principle. Note how foreshortening of the actual focal spot impacts the effective (projected or apparent) focal spot. **(A)** A square actual focal spot produces a rectangular effective focal spot. **(B)** An elongated actual focal spot produces a square effective focal spot. As the anode *angle* is made smaller, the actual focal spot may be made larger while a small effective focal spot is still maintained.

> **Line Focus Principle:**
>
> The effective focal spot is always smaller than the actual focal spot.

anode end of the image. This can be remedied with an increase in SID, which must be accompanied by an appropriate increase in exposure factors.

When using general x-ray tubes at standard distances, the heel effect is noticeable only when imaging parts of uneven thickness, such as the femur and thoracic spine. In these cases, the heel effect may be used to advantage by placing the thicker body portion under the cathode end of the x-ray beam, thus having the effect of "balancing/evening out" tissue densities.

The *line focus principle* and the *anode heel effect*, and their effects on radiographic quality, are discussed more fully in Part IV. When specifying focal spot size, it is the effective focal spot size that is quoted. We often speak of "double focus" x-ray tubes, meaning that a small (e.g., 0.6 mm) and a large (1.2 mm) focal spot are available to choose from.

These x-ray tubes actually have only *one focal track*, a portion of it is used for the small focus setting. It is more accurate to say that these are *double filament* tubes, for there are two filaments: the smaller one is activated when the small focal spot is selected, and the larger one is activated for the large focal spot.

The amount of heat produced at the target is expressed in terms of *heat units* (HU). Exposure factor selection has a significant effect on the production of heat as expressed in the following equation.

$$HU = mA \times s \times kV \text{ (single phase)}$$

For example,

$$300 \text{ mA} \times 0.4 \text{ second} \times 80 \text{ kV} = 9,600 \text{ HU}$$
$$300 \text{ mA} \times 0.2 \text{ second} \times 92 \text{ kV} = 5,520 \text{ HU}$$

Thus, a greater number of HU are produced with higher mAs and lower kV exposure factors. A *correction factor* is added to the equation when using three-phase equipment.

$$HU = mA \times s \times kV \text{ (single phase)}$$

$$HU = mA \times s \times kV \times 1.4 \text{ (three phase and high frequency)}$$

For example,

$$300 \text{ mA} \times 0.4 \text{ sec} \times 80 \text{ kV} = 9,600 \text{ HU (single phase)}$$

$$300 \text{ mA} \times 0.4 \text{ sec} \times 80 \text{ kV} \times 1.4 = 13,440 \text{ HU (three phase/high frequency)}$$

Operation

Each x-ray tube has its own *tube rating chart* and *anode cooling curve* that illustrate safe tube *heat limits* and the particular *cooling characteristics* of the anode. It is essential that the radiographer know how to use these charts in order to use the x-ray tube properly and safely and to prolong its useful life (Fig. 14–16).

For example, what is the maximum safe kV that may be used with each of the three x-ray tubes using 200 mA and 0.2-second exposure?

Do this for each of the x-ray tubes illustrated: Find the exposure time on the horizontal axis, follow it up until it meets the 200 mA line, and then follow that across to the vertical axis and read the kV.

> A = approximately 147 kV;
> B = greater than 150 kV (off the chart);
> C = approximately 57 kV.

Comparing these answers with the information provided in the legend for Figure 14–16, it can be seen that the *size of the focal spot* and the *type of rectification* significantly impact heat loading characteristics of an x-ray tube.

Next, refer to the anode cooling curve. For example, if the x-ray tube were saturated with 1,300,000 HU, it would take 30 minutes to cool down to 300,000 HU. How long would it take to cool from 700,000 HU to 450,000 HU? (Answer: Approximately 10 minutes.)

Care

Careless treatment or abuse of the x-ray tube, as well as normal wear and tear, will lead to its ultimate demise.

Some Causes of X-Ray Tube Failure

Vaporized tungsten—As a result of thermionic emission, quantities of tungsten can be vaporized and deposited on the inner surface of the glass envelope. When deposited on the port window, tungsten acts as a filter and reduces the intensity of the beam; it can also alter the tube vacuum and finally leads to tube failure.

Pitted anode—Exposures made exceeding the tube rating create enough excessive heat to produce many small melts, or pits, over the surface of the focal track. X-ray photons are absorbed by these surface irregularities and, consequently, x-ray intensity is reduced. Extensive *pitting* also results in *vaporized* tungsten deposited on the inner surface of the tube window that acts as an additional filter and further reduces beam intensity. Arcing can occur between the filament and tungsten deposit, resulting in a cracked glass envelope.

Cracked anode—A single, large, excessive exposure to a cold anode can be severe enough to crack the anode: the large dose of heat creates

---

Safe X-Ray Tube Limits Illustrated in:

- Tube rating charts
- Anode cooling curves

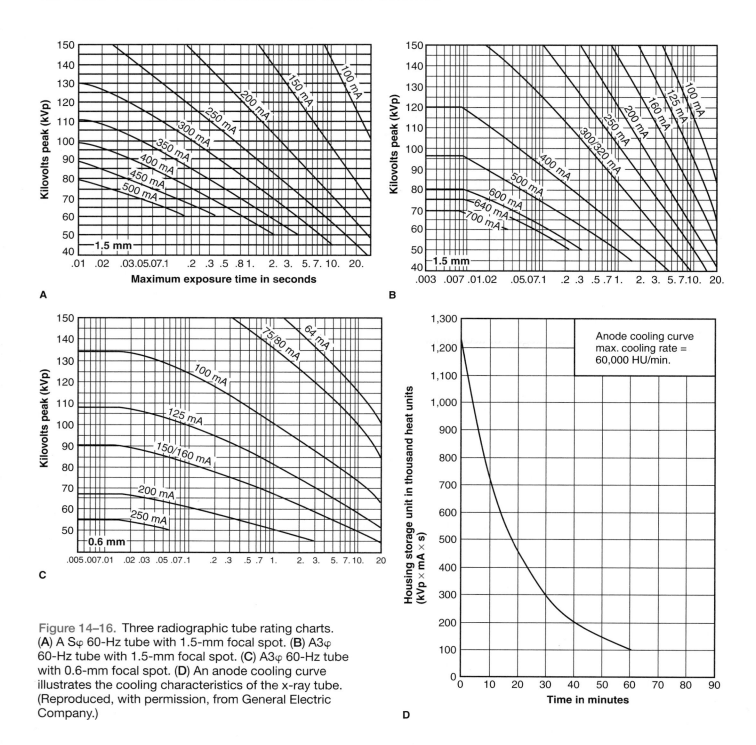

Figure 14–16. Three radiographic tube rating charts. (**A**) A Sφ 60-Hz tube with 1.5-mm focal spot. (**B**) A3φ 60-Hz tube with 1.5-mm focal spot. (**C**) A3φ 60-Hz tube with 0.6-mm focal spot. (**D**) An anode cooling curve illustrates the cooling characteristics of the x-ray tube. (Reproduced, with permission, from General Electric Company.)

sudden expansion of the cold anode. It is therefore advisable to practice tube *warm-up procedures*, as suggested by the manufacturer, prior to starting the day's examinations or after the tube has not been used for several hours. Typical warm-up procedure consists of two exposures made using 100 mA, 2-second exposure, and 70 kV. The long 2-second exposures distribute heat over the entire surface of the anode and promote uniform thermal expansion of the anode.

Gassy tube—If the tube vacuum begins to deteriorate, air molecules collide with and decelerate the high-speed electrons, thus decreasing the efficiency of x-ray production. The condition is referred to as a "gassy tube" and eventually causes oxidation and burnout of the cathode filament.

Summary

- Most of the energy used to produce x-rays is converted to heat; only 0.2% is converted to x-rays.
- Heat is damaging to x-ray tubes; x-ray tubes are surrounded with oil to carry heat away from the anode (also for insulating purposes).
- The width of the focal track is identified as the actual focal spot; its bevel (angle) projects a smaller, effective focal spot to the image receptor according to the line focus principle.
- The degree of anode bevel (angle) influences the degree of heel effect; the smaller the angle, the more pronounced the heel effect.
- HU are used to express the degree of accumulation of anode heat and determined by mA × time × kV; the correction factor for 3φ 6p is 1.35 and for 3φ 12p, it is 1.41.
- Excessive heat loading will cause accelerated tube aging and failure as a result of conditions such as pitted or cracked anode, gassy tube, or vaporized tungsten.
- Tube rating charts and anode cooling curves must be used to determine safe exposures and heat loading.

THE RADIOGRAPHIC CIRCUIT

The x-ray circuit can be divided into three portions:

1. The *low-voltage*, or *primary*, *circuit* contains most of the devices found on the control console.
2. The *filament circuit* varies the current sent to the filament to provide the required mA value.
3. The *high-voltage*, or *secondary*, *circuit* includes the high-voltage transformer, rectification system, and x-ray tube.

Primary Circuit Components

Primary or Low-Voltage Circuit Devices

Main switch and circuit breakers—These are usually located on a wall in or near the x-ray room (Fig. 14–17). Circuit breaker switches must be closed to energize the equipment.

Autotransformer—is a variable transformer that operates on AC and enables the radiographer to select kilovoltage. The function and operation of the autotransformer is discussed earlier in this section.

kV selector—is used by the radiographer to choose the kilovoltage, often as kV major (in increments of 10) and kV minor (in increments of 2). In doing so, the appropriate number of coils (representing V) on the autotransformer is selected by the movable contact.

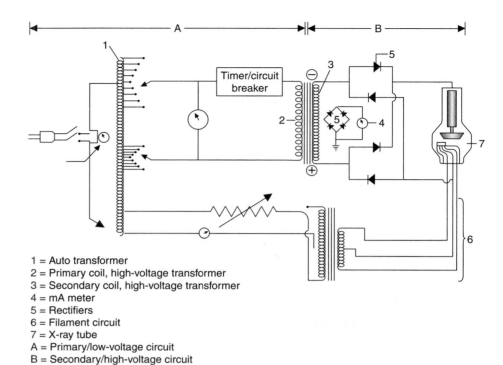

1 = Auto transformer
2 = Primary coil, high-voltage transformer
3 = Secondary coil, high-voltage transformer
4 = mA meter
5 = Rectifiers
6 = Filament circuit
7 = X-ray tube
A = Primary/low-voltage circuit
B = Secondary/high-voltage circuit

Figure 14–17. Simplified x-ray circuit. High-voltage current from the secondary transformer coil is rectified before it reaches the x-ray tube.

Types of X-Ray Timers

- Mechanical
- Synchronous
- Impulse
- Electronic
- mAs
- AEC (phototimer or ionization chamber)

Line voltage compensator—functions to automatically adjust for any fluctuations in incoming voltage supply. A uniformly consistent and accurate voltage supply is required for predictable radiographic results. A small variation in voltage entering the primary transformer coil voltage represents a much larger variation as it leaves the secondary coil. The control consoles of some older x-ray units were equipped with line voltage compensators that were adjustable by the radiographer, but in equipment manufactured today, the process takes place automatically within the machine.

Timer—functions to regulate the length of x-ray exposure. Very simple timers such as the mechanical, synchronous, and impulse timers are rarely used in x-ray equipment manufactured today because they do not permit very fast, accurate exposures. *Mechanical timers* are capable of exposures only as short as $1/4$ second; *synchronous timers* as short as $1/60$ second. *Impulse timers* are more accurate and capable of exposures as short as $1/120$ second.

The *electronic timer* used in x-ray equipment manufactured today is somewhat complex and based on a capacitor–resistor circuit. Electronic timers are very accurate and capable of rapid exposures as short as 1 millisecond (i.e., $1/1,000$ or 0.001 second).

The *milliampere-second timer* (mAs timer) monitors the product of mA and time and terminates the exposure when the desired mAs has been reached. mAs timers are found on some mobile x-ray units. They are also found on some older fixed x-ray units and display the mAs exposure value when exposure time is too short to permit the actual mA to register on the mA meter.

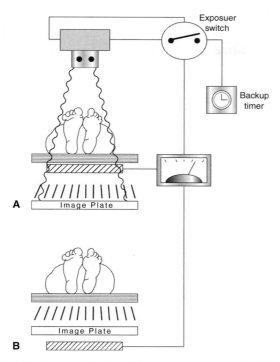

Figure 14–18. Two types of automatic exposure controls. The AEC on the *top* consists of an *ionization chamber* located *under the x-ray tabletop*. The electrometer measures the number of ionizations and terminates the exposure once a predetermined quantity has been reached. The AEC on the *bottom*, the phototimer, consists of a *photomultiplier* tube located *under the image plate*. Note that a backup timer is in place to terminate the exposure, should the AEC fail to do so.

Another type of timer is the automatic exposure device (AED), or *automatic exposure control* (AEC), which functions to produce consistent radiographic results (Fig. 14–18). AECs have sensors that signal to terminate the exposure once a predetermined, known correct, exposure has been reached.

One type of AEC, the *ionization chamber*, is located just beneath the tabletop, above the image plate. The part being imaged is centered to the sensor and exposed. When the predetermined quantity of air ionization has occurred within the chamber, as measured and determined by an electrometer, the exposure is automatically terminated.

Another type of AEC is the *phototimer*, located behind the image plate. The phototimer consists of a special fluorescent screen that, when activated by x-ray, produces light and charges a photomultiplier tube. When the correct charge has been reached, as determined by the electrometer, the exposure is automatically terminated.

A *backup timer* (the manual timer) is used to protect the patient from excessive exposure and x-ray tube from damage should the AEC fail to operate properly. Additional discussion of AECs can be found in Part IV.

X-ray timer malfunction can cause undesirable fluctuation in radiographic density. If the timer terminates the exposure too soon, the image will be underexposed; if the exposure is delayed in terminating, the image will be overexposed. The radiographer should be able to

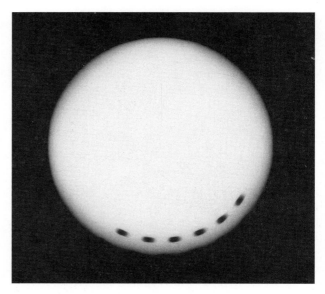

Figure 14–19. The spinning-top test was made using second (50 milliseconds) exposure and correctly produced six dots.

perform a *spinning-top test* to evaluate timer accuracy (Figs. 14–19 and 14–20).

A simple spinning top consists of a circular steel or lead disk with a small hole in its periphery. The disk is mounted on a base that allows the disk to revolve freely. The device is placed on a image plate, the spinning top is set in motion, and an exposure made using the exposure time station to be evaluated.

Recall that with single-phase equipment there are 120 useful x-ray impulses per second using *single-phase full-wave rectified* current. If the x-ray timer is set to use some portion of the impulses, for example, ¼ second, then ¼ of the 120 impulses should be recorded on film if that time station is accurate. Thus, the film should show 30 dots. A minor discrepancy usually indicates a *timer malfunction*; exactly one-half of the correct number of dots indicates a *rectifier problem*. If an exposure of

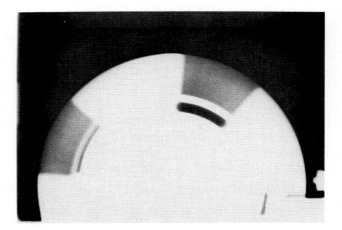

Figure 14–20. Synchronous spinning-top test. An exposure was made using ¹⁄₁₂ second (83 ms). The resulting image correctly demonstrates a 30-degree arc.

$^1/_{10}$ second is made, 12 dots should be recorded, and so on. Simply multiply the number of impulses per second (120 in the case of Sφ full-wave rectified equipment) by the exposure time. In the unlikely event that *half-wave rectified* equipment is being tested, the exposure time is multiplied by 60 (useful impulses/s).

Because most x-ray equipments manufactured today are of three phases, a slightly different approach must be taken when evaluating these timers. Because *three-phase full-wave rectified* equipment produces a *ripple wave*, that is, almost constant potential, the standard spinning-top test does not demonstrate impulses; rather, a *solid arc* is recorded. The use of a *synchronous* (motorized) *spinning top* (or oscilloscope) is required. The exposure is made at the time station to be evaluated, and the resulting image demonstrates a solid arc. If the exposure time made was 1 second, an entire circle (360 degrees) should be demonstrated. For exposure times less than 1 second, the corresponding portion of a circle should be recorded. For example, an exposure made at $^1/_4$ second should record a 90-degree arc (i.e., $^1/_4$ of a 360-degree circle); at an exposure of second, a 36-degree arc should be recorded.

Primary coil of the high-voltage transformer—is the final component of the primary, or low-voltage, circuit. The low voltage entering the primary coil is stepped up to high kilovoltage in the secondary coil by means of mutual induction.

Exposure switch—is a remote control switch that functions to start the x-ray exposure (the timer terminates the exposure).

Filament Circuit Components

The filament circuit is responsible for supplying low-voltage current (3–5 A, 10–12 V) to the filament of the x-ray tube. Because the incoming voltage (110–220 V) is greater than that required, a *step-down transformer* is placed in the filament circuit to make the required voltage adjustment. A *rheostat*, or other type of *variable resistor*, is placed in the filament circuit to adjust amperage and corresponds to the *mA selector* on the control console.

Secondary Circuit Components

Secondary or High-Voltage Circuit Devices

Secondary coil of high-voltage transformer—carries the required high voltage for x-ray production (and proportionally smaller current value).

mA meter—is located at the midpoint of the secondary transformer coil. Because it is grounded, it can be safely placed in the operator's console. The mA meter displays the tube current value.

Rectifiers—a system of diodes located between the secondary coil of the high-voltage transformer and the x-ray tube. Recall from earlier discussion that it functions to change AC to unidirectional pulsating current. Current pulsations decrease with solid-state three-phase rectification (3φ 6p rectification has a 13% ripple; 3φ 12p has a 4% ripple).

X-ray tube—is the final device in the secondary circuit. The filament of its negative electrode, the cathode, is heated by its own circuit to produce *thermionic emission*. As high voltage is applied, the thermionic electron cloud is driven to the anode target. The rapid deceleration of

---

Primary/Low-Voltage Circuit Components:

- Main switch/circuit breaker
- Autotransformer
- kV selector switch
- Line voltage compensator
- Timer
- Primary coil of HV transformer
- Exposure switch

Secondary/High-Voltage Circuit Components:

- Secondary coil of HV transformer
- mA meter (grounded at midpoint of secondary coil)
- Rectifiers
- X-ray tube

electrons, and their interaction with tungsten atoms of the target, results in an energy conversion to heat and x-rays (99.8% heat, 0.2% x-rays).

Circuitry Overview of a Single Exposure

1. X-ray machine is turned on. This activates the filament circuit and heats the x-ray tube filament (10–12 V, 3–5 A).
2. If the machine has been off overnight, warm-up exposures are made to warm the anode throughout (anode cracking can occur when surface heat is applied to a cold anode).
3. Appropriate exposure factors are chosen on the control panel (machines having a line voltage compensator on the control panel should be adjusted to compensate for any incoming voltage fluctuation).
4. The rotor/exposure switch is often a two-stage exposure button that should be depressed completely in one motion; the first click heard after partial depression is the induction motor bringing anode rotation up to speed. At this time, the filament is heated to maximum (thermionic emission) and produces an electron cloud.
5. Upon complete depression of the rotor/exposure switch, the exposure is made. The moment the exposure button is depressed, the voltage selected by the autotransformer is sent to the step-up transformer where it is converted to the high voltage (kV) and low amperage (mA) required. This high-voltage current then passes through the rectification system that changes AC to pulsating DC.
6. The applied high voltage (potential difference) propels the electron cloud to the anode where interactions between the high-speed electrons and tungsten target atoms convert electron kinetic energy to (99.8%) heat energy and (0.2%) x-ray photon energy (see *x-ray production* details in Chapter 8).

Components of Digital Imaging (CR/DR)

Computer Fundamentals. The following is an overview of how we use computers to represent data, and the factors that influence image characteristics.

Computer system. The computer system consists of the *hardware*, which is any physical component of the computer, and the *software*, which is a set of instructions or program to operate the computer.

The hardware consists of input and output devices. These devices allow information to be put into a computer and allow information to be directed outside the computer. The *central processing unit* is the primary control center for the computer consisting of a control unit, arithmetic unit, and memory. The speed is measured in "millions of instructions per second." Most desktop computer speeds are given in MHz. The *memory* is solid state. It is used by the computer during execution of a program. There are two types of memory. The first is *RAM*, or random access memory. This memory is volatile and will lose all information when the computer is turned off unless previously saved. Read-only memory, or *ROM*, is memory that is hardwired into the computer, which means it stays in the computer even when the computer is turned off. ROM usually contains the booting instructions.

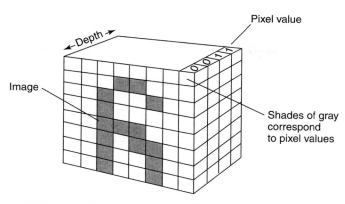

Figure 14–21A. A digital image may be likened to a three-dimensional object made up of many small cubes, each containing a binary digit or bit. The image is seen on one surface of the block, whose depth is the number of bits required to describe each pixel's gray level.

The *software* is a set of instructions the computer uses to function effectively, known as a *program*. Computer programming languages include, but are not limited to

- Fortran: Formula translation. Used mainly in science and engineering applications.
- Basic: A beginner's all-purpose language with symbolic instructions and code.
- Cobol: Common business-oriented language.
- Pascal: High-level mathematics.

Binary numbers. The computer hardware interprets all information as a simple "yes" or "no" decision. Current "on" implies "yes" and current "off" implies "no." This is symbolically represented with digits 1 and 0. A *bit* in computer terminology refers to an individual 1 or 0 and is a single bit of information.

Image storage. Image storage is located in a *pixel* (Fig. 14–21A), which is a two-dimensional "picture element." Pixels are measured in the "XY" direction.

The third dimension in the matrix of pixels is the depth that, together with the pixel, is referred to as the *voxel* (Fig. 14–21B). The voxels are measured in the "Z" direction. The depth of the block is the

Pixel:

- Two dimensional
- *Picture El*ement
- Measured in XY direction

Voxel:

- The third dimension, depth
- *Volume El*ement
- Measured in Z direction

Matrix:

- Number of pixels in XY direction

Field of View (FOV)

- How much of the part/patient is included in the matrix

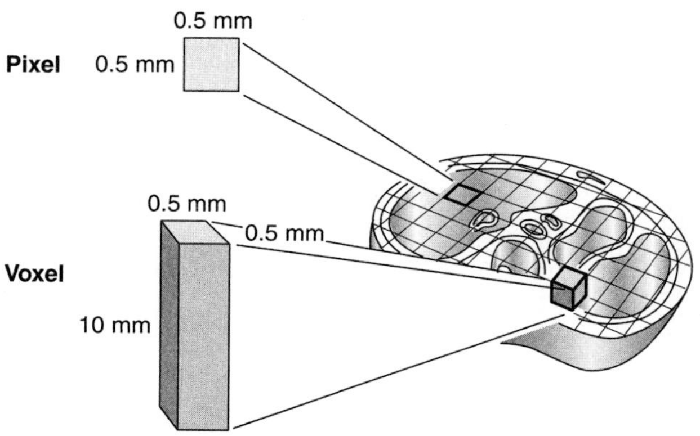

Figure 14–21B. The third dimension in the matrix of pixels is the depth, which together with the pixel is referred to as the voxel (volume element).

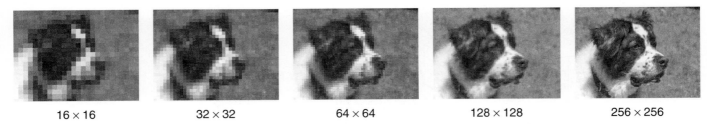

| 16 × 16 | 32 × 32 | 64 × 64 | 128 × 128 | 256 × 256 |

Figure 14–22. The matrix is the number of pixels in the XY direction. The larger the matrix size, the better the image resolution.

Typical Image Matrix Sizes Used in Radiography Are

- Nuclear medicine   128 × 128
- Digital subtraction angiography (DSA) (Fig. 14–23)   1,024 × 1,024
- CT   512 × 512
- Chest radiography   2,048 × 2,048

Digital Image Resolution Improves With:

- Smaller pixel size
- Smaller pixel pitch
- Larger image matrix

number of bits required to describe the gray level that each pixel can take on. This is known as the *bit depth*.

The matrix is the number of pixels in the XY direction. The larger the matrix size, the better the image resolution (Fig. 14–22). The smaller the pixels and *pixel pitch* (i.e., distance between center of one pixel to center of adjacent pixel), the better the resolution.

A digital image is formed by a *matrix* of *pixels* in rows and columns. A matrix having 512 pixels in each row and column is a 512 × 512 matrix. The term FOV is used to describe how much of the patient (e.g., 150-mm diameter) is included in the matrix. The matrix or FOV can be changed without affecting the other, but changes in either will change pixel size. As matrix size is increased, there are more and smaller pixels in the matrix, therefore, improved spatial resolution; *spatial resolution* is measured in line pairs per millimeter (*lp/mm*). Fewer and larger pixels result in a poor resolution "pixelly" image, that is, one in which you can actually see the individual pixel boxes (Fig. 14–22).

One of the most important factors to consider in CR is the ability to transmit images over distances, known as *teleradiography*. The amount of information transferred per unit time is known as the baud rate and is in units of bits per second.

Example: A network is capable of transmitting data at a rate of 9,600 baud. If each pixel has a bit depth of 8 bits, how long will it take to transmit a 512 × 512 image?

Solution:

$$(512 \times 512 \text{ pixels})(8 \text{ bits/pixel})/9,600 \text{ bits/s} = 128 \text{ s.}$$

There are three possible means of image transmission. *Telephone wires* offer low transmission speed while using a modem. *Coaxial cable*

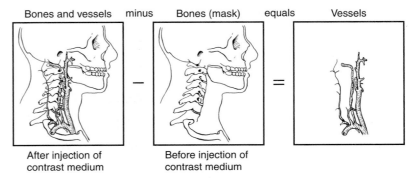

| Bones and vessels | minus | Bones (mask) | equals | Vessels |
| After injection of contrast medium | | Before injection of contrast medium | | |

Figure 14–23. Digital subtraction angiography (DSA). Image details not required for diagnosis can be subtracted from an image. Only vessels containing contrast medium are visualized in the final image.

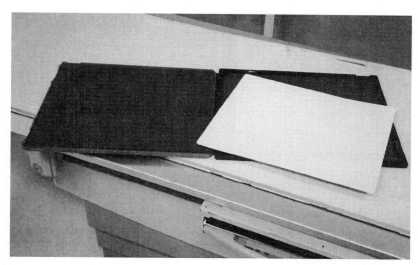

Figure 14–24A. The IP holds a photostimulable storage phosphor (PSP) (the image receptor) between its front and rear panels. (Reproduced, with permission, from Shephard CT. *Radiographic Image Production and Manipulation.* New York: McGraw-Hill, 2003.)

will transmit at approximately 100 MBaud. Finally, there are *fiberoptic cables* that are unaffected by electrical fields and therefore have less error than cables or wires with electrical signals.

Computed Radiography. Computed radiography has been referred to as *filmless radiography*. A *photostimulable storage phosphor* (PSP) within the IP is used as the *image receptor*. The IPs have a *protective* function (for the flexible PSP storage plate within), can be conveniently placed in the Bucky tray or under the anatomic part, and come in a variety of sizes (Fig. 14–24A).

The IPs need not be light tight because the PSP storage plate inside is *not light sensitive*. One corner of the IP's rear panel has a *memory chip* for patient information; the IP also has a thin *lead foil backing* to absorb any backscatter. The computed radiography IP contains a *europium-doped barium fluorohalide* (mixed with a binder) coated screen/storage phosphor plate. When the PSP storage plate receives x-ray photons, the x-ray energy interacts with the $(BaF:Eu^2)$ crystals. As a result of this interaction, a small amount of visible light is emitted, but most of the x-ray energy is stored (hence the term *storage plate*). This *stored energy represents the latent image*.

When the barium fluorohalide absorbs x-ray energy, electrons are released and they divide into two groups. One electron group initiates *immediate luminescence* (primary excitation) during the excited state of Eu^{2+}. The other electron group becomes trapped within the phosphor's halogen ions, forming a "color center." (also called "F center"). These are the phosphors that ultimately form the radiographic image because, when exposed to a *monochromatic* laser light source, these phosphors emit *polychromatic* light (secondary excitation), termed *photostimulated luminescence* (PSL).

The PSP layer can *store* its latent image for several hours; however, after approximately 8 hours, noticeable image *fading* will occur. The europium activator is important for the *storage* characteristic of the

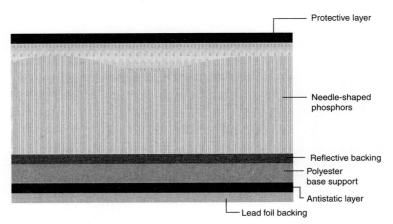

Figure 14–24B. Barium fluorohalide is either granular or "needle shaped." The "needlelike" phosphors have the advantage of *better x-ray absorption and less light diffusion.*

PSPs; it also has a function similar to the sensitization specks within film emulsion—without europium the image will not become visible.

The BaF is usually in the form of *granular* or *turbid* phosphors. Other examples of turbid phosphors are gadolinium oxysulfide and rubidium chloride. *"Needle"*-shaped or *columnar* phosphors (usually cesium iodide) have the advantage of *better x-ray absorption* and *less light diffusion* (Fig. 14–24B).

Just under the barium fluorohalide layer is a *reflective layer* that helps direct emitted light toward the CR reader. Below the reflective layer is the *base*, behind that is an *antistatic layer*, and then the *lead foil* to absorb backscatter. Over the top of the barium fluorohalide is a *protective layer*.

Some PSP storage plates are manufactured specifically for better resolution (e.g., for mammography). Some higher-resolution PSPs "read" the information from *both* sides of the PSP storage plates.

After exposure, the IP is placed into the CR *scanner/reader* (Figs. 14–25A&B), where the PSP screen is automatically removed. The latent image on the PSP is changed to a *visible image* as it is moved at a *constant* speed and scanned by a narrow monochromatic *high-intensity helium–neon laser* or a *solid-state* laser to obtain the pixel data.

The longer wavelength light from the newer *solid-state lasers* has the advantage of being unlikely to interfere with the light being emitted by the PSPs. This appropriate (red, 430–550 nm) wavelength is absorbed by the "color center" and the electrons trapped there, causing PSL to occur during the excited state of Eu^{2+} (secondary excitation). The phosphors are activated by a *mono*chromatic laser light; however, PSL is a *different* color (bluish-purple, blue–green, etc.). These two lights (PSL and laser) must not interfere with each other.

To improve the image SNR, the PSL (carrying the x-ray image) must be a different wavelength/color than, and physically separate from, the laser excitation light. An *optical filter* is used that permits *transmission* of the PSL but *attenuates* the laser light; this filter is mounted in front of a photomultiplier tube (PMT) (Fig. 14–25B).

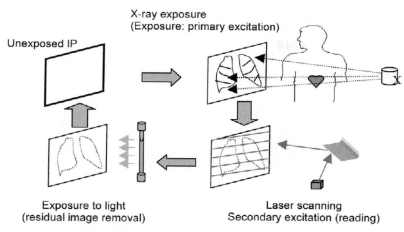

X-ray exposure
(Exposure: primary excitation)

Unexposed IP

Exposure to light
(residual image removal)

Laser scanning
Secondary excitation (reading)

Figure 14–25A. The *recording, reading,* and *erasure cycle* of a CR PSP storage plate. The PSP is exposed to x-ray photons, scanned/read, and then erased for reuse. (Courtesy of FUJIFILM Medical Systems USA, Inc.)

The PMT or photodiode (PD) is used to detect the PSL and convert it to electrical signals (Fig. 14–28). The electrical energy is sent to an *analog-to-digital converter (ADC)* where it becomes the *digital* image that is displayed, after a short delay, on a high-resolution monitor and/or printed out by a laser printer (hard copy). The digitized images can also be manipulated in *postprocessing*, electronically *transmitted*, and stored/ *archived.* Postprocessing manipulation can include *edge enhancement*; a technique that can be used to improve the visibility of structures such as chest tubes by accentuating their edges.

An artifact associated with digital imaging and grids is "aliasing" or the "Moiré effect." If the direction of the lead strips and the grid lines per inch (i.e., grid frequency) matches the scan frequency of the scanner/ reader, this artifact can occur. Aliasing (or Moiré effect) appears as superimposed images slightly out of alignment, an image "wrapping" effect (Fig. 14–26). This most commonly occurs in mobile radiography with stationary grids and can be a problem with DR flat panel detectors.

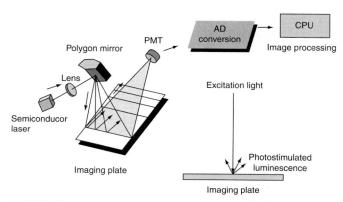

Polygon mirror

PMT

AD conversion

CPU

Image processing

Lens

Semiconducor laser

Excitation light

Photostimulated luminescence

Imaging plate

Imaging plate

Figure 14–25B. The latent image on the PSP screen is changed to a manifest image as it is moved at a constant speed and scanned by a narrow high-intensity helium–neon laser or a solid-state laser to obtain the pixel data. (Courtesy of FUJIFILM Medical Systems USA, Inc.)

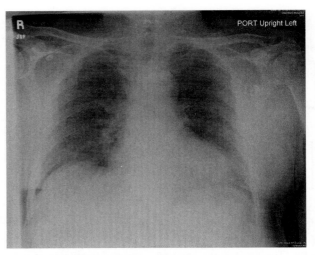

Figure 14–26. Aliasing artifact. If the direction of the lead strips and the grid frequency matches the scan frequency of the scanner/reader, this artifact can occur. Aliasing (sometimes called Moiré) appears as superimposed images slightly out of alignment, an image "wrapping" effect. This is most common in mobile radiography with stationary grids. (Courtesy of Stamford Hospital, Department of Radiology.)

Once the PSP storage plate reading process is completed, any remaining data stored on the PSP are erased by exposing it to high intensity light (called "erasure"); the PSP storage plate is then ready for reuse (see Fig. 14–25A)

Image "*fading*" occurs if there is a delay in reading the PSP. After a time, trapped photoelectrons are released from the "color center" and are therefore unable to participate in PSL. PSL intensity *decreases* in the interval between x-ray exposure and the image-reading process. If the exposed PSL is not delivered to the reader/processor for 8 hours, PSL decreases by approximately 25%. Fading also increases as environmental temperature increases.

This PSL signal represents varying tissue densities and the latent image, which is then transferred to an *analog-to-digital converter* (ADC)—converting the (analog) electrical signal to digital data. This digital data is then transferred to a *digital-to-analog converter* (DAC) to be converted to a perceptible analog image on the display monitor. The monitor image can be electronically transmitted, manipulated, post-processed, and stored efficiently (archived).

After the scanning/reading process has been completed, any remaining information on the PSP is *erased* by exposing the PSP screen to high-intensity laser light; the IP and its PSP storage plate is then ready for reuse.

PSP storage plates are very sensitive (more than film emulsion) not only to x-rays but ultraviolet, gamma, and particulate radiation. Environmental conditions are therefore an important consideration in their storage. Building materials such as concrete, marble, and others constantly emit natural radiation; bedrock in some geographic areas contributes significantly to background radiation. If PSPs are stored for extended periods of time, the possibility of artifacts must be considered. These artifacts typically appear as randomly placed small black spots. *If an IP and its PSP storage plate has been stored, unused, for 48 hours or more), the PSP storage plate should be erased prior to use.*

The mechanical consistency and accuracy of the laser optics and transport systems of the CR scanner/reader is extremely important for image quality—inconsistent scanning motion can result in a wavy, or otherwise distorted, image. This is sometimes referred to as *"laser jitter"* and should be evaluated monthly as part of the CR QA monitoring.

Another advantage of CR is postprocessing, that is, the ability to *manipulate the image after exposure*. Image manipulation postprocessing can be used for *contrast modification, image subtraction* (Fig. 14–23), and *windowing*. Image subtraction is used primarily in angiography to remove superimposed bone structures from contrast-filled vessels.

The digital images' *scale of contrast*, or *contrast resolution*, can be changed electronically through *windowing* of the image. *Windowing* is a process of changing the contrast and density setting on the monitor image. The window *width* controls the *number* of shades of gray in the image, whereas the window *level* corresponds to the *density/brightness* (Fig. 14–27). Narrower windows result in higher (shorter scale) contrast. Pixel values *below* the window range will be displayed as *black*, whereas pixel values *above* the window range will be displayed as *white*. Pixel values between the two limits are spread over the full scale of gray.

Applications for digital imaging include radiography, computed tomography, nuclear medicine, magnetic resonance imaging, sonography, and DSA.

Spatial Resolution. Spatial resolution in digital imaging improves with smaller pixel size, smaller pixel pitch, and larger image matrix. Hence, a 2,000 × 2,000 (2 K) monitor will demonstrate better spatial resolution than a 1,000 × 1,000 (1 K) monitor. Another way to describe monitor resolution that is gaining favor is simply in terms of *megapixels*.

Other factors contributing to image resolution in CR are the *size of the laser beam* and the *size of the* barium fluorohalide *phosphors*. Smaller phosphor size improves resolution in ways similar to that of intensifying screens—anything that causes an increase in light diffusion will result in a decrease in resolution. Smaller phosphors in the PSP screen allow less light diffusion. In addition, the scanning laser light must be of correct intensity and size. A narrow laser beam is required for optimum resolution.

Contrast Resolution. The terms *dynamic range* and *contrast resolution* are commonly used to describe the range of grays a particular digital system is capable of resolving/demonstrating. The *higher* the contrast resolution, the better the ability to see similar adjacent gray shades. As mentioned earlier, the greater the number of bits per pixel, the greater the capability of displaying many shades of gray.

Noise. *Noise* is an electronic term for anything that interferes with visualization of the image we wish to see. We see noise in traditional radiography as a result of fast imaging systems. CR images are even more subject to noise; as in traditional radiography, it appears as *graininess* referred to as *quantum mottle*. Insufficient mAs can cause image noise, and it cannot be removed in postprocessing. Intelligent selection of exposure factors is still required and radiographers must be even more vigilant in minimizing patient exposure. In digital/electronic imaging, high signal and low noise are desired, that is, a high SNR (signal-to-noise ratio).

CR Resolution Is Improved by

- Smaller barium fluorohalide phosphors
- Narrower width laser beam
- Larger monitor matrix

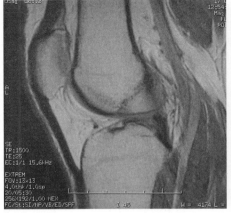

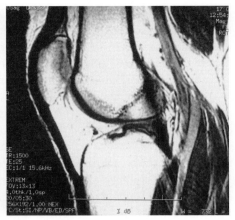

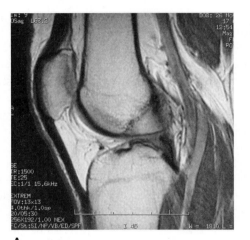

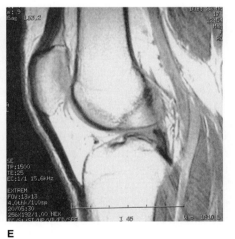

Figure 14–27. Changes in *window width* and *window level.* Image **A** (*center*) has a window width of 590 and window level of 270. In image **B** the window width is increased to 1,340, and in image **C** the window width is decreased to 302, leaving window level unchanged. The changes in image *contrast* are evident. Next, images D and E are compared with A. In image **D** the window level is increased to 441, and in image **E** it is decreased to 45. This time the changes in image *density/brightness* are obvious.

Flat Panel Detectors—Indirect and Direct Digital Radiography. Using flat panel detectors, there are no IPs with PSP detectors within. As its name suggests the digital detector is a flat, plate-like, panel—both x-ray *detection and digitization* take place in the flat panel. Flat panel detectors are a *fixed* part of the x-ray unit—there is no physical transportation of IPs, no wear and tear on PSPs through a scanner/reader. There are two types: *indirect* conversion systems and *direct* conversion systems.

In the *indirect* systems, remnant x-rays transmitted through the imaged part are *converted to light* through a scintillating phosphor such as cesium iodide. The light is collected by CCDs or TFTs where it is then changed to an electrical (analog) signal. The analog electrical signals are then digitized (by the ADC) and processed by the computer, producing an image.

The CCD system is indirect, but it is not an actual flat panel system. The true *indirect flat panel system* is the TFT system. The TFT indirect flat panel system is composed of a *scintillator layer* usually CsI (cesium iodide) or Gd_2O_2S (gadolinium oxysulfide)—also used in fluoroscopic systems and rare earth intensifying screens, respectively. These phosphors absorb x-ray energy and change it into luminescent light energy. Below the scintillator phosphor layer is an a-Si (amorphous silicon) *photodiode layer*. The a-Si is a liquid coated on a thin layer of glass, and it functions to absorb the scintillation light energy and convert it into electrical charges (electrons). Immediately adjacent to the a-Si flat-panel layer is the *TFT array*, which functions to collect and store electrical charges produced by the a-Si flat panel layer.

In Indirect conversion detectors, x-rays are converted to light scintillations and that light is converted to electric signals. However, in *direct* conversion flat-panel detectors, x-rays are *directly* converted to electric signals. The first layer is the *photoconductor*—usually a-Se (amorphous selenium); most commonly used because of its reported excellent x-ray absorption/conversion properties and spatial resolution. The a-Se absorbs x-ray photons and changes them into electric charges. Below the a-Se layer is a *TFT array* that functions to collect and store the electrical charges. Electric charges are transmitted to the ADC for digitization.

Portable detectors are available that can be used in conjunction with a mobile x-ray unit.

Summary

- The x-ray circuit has three major portions: the primary, or low-voltage, side; the filament circuit; and the secondary, or high-voltage, side.

- Primary circuit devices include the main switch and circuit breaker, the autotransformer and kV selector, line voltage compensator, timer, primary coil of the high-voltage transformer, and exposure switch; most of the control console devices are in the primary circuit.

- The timer regulates the length of the x-ray exposure; types of timers include mechanical, impulse, synchronous, mAs timer, electronic timer, and AEC.

- There are two types of AECs: the phototimer, located *behind* the Image Receptor (IR), and the ionization chamber, located *above* the IR.

- A *backup timer* terminates the exposure should the AEC fail, thereby protecting the patient from excessive exposure, and prolonging the life of the x-ray tube.

- Timer accuracy can be tested with a spinning-top test: a simple *spinning top* for single-phase equipment and a *synchronous* spinning top for three-phase equipment.

- Single-phase spinning-top tests show a series of *dots*, each representing an x-ray impulse; three-phase spinning-top tests show a *solid-arc* exposure in a portion of a circle (measured in degrees) representative of a portion of a second.

- A step-down transformer and rheostat (or other variable resistor) are placed in the filament circuit to supply the x-ray tube with low-voltage current.

- Secondary circuit devices include the secondary coil of the high-voltage transformer, mA meter, rectifiers, and x-ray tube; the grounded mA meter displays the tube current value on the control console.

- Rectifiers are located between the transformer's secondary coil and the x-ray tube; they change AC to unidirectional current.

- There are two types of computer memory: RAM and ROM.

- A two-dimensional picture element is a pixel; a three-dimensional picture element is a voxel.

- CR enables image manipulation after exposure ("postprocessing").

- "Windowing" changes image contrast and/or density; window *width* controls the number of grays, whereas window *level* controls density.

- CR uses special detector plates called a photostimulable phosphor (PSP); CR resolution is determined by size of PSP phosphor, laser beam, monitor matrix.

- The terms *dynamic range* and *contrast resolution* are used to describe the range of grays a digital system is capable of resolving.

- Insufficiency of mAs can cause digital image noise (decreased SNR).

- Indirect conversion detector: x-rays are converted to light scintillations and light is converted to electric signals.

- Direct Conversion Detector: x-rays are directly converted to electric signals.

Terminology:

Outdated: "CAT" scan
- Refers to computerized *axial* tomography

Correct: CT scan
- Computed tomography
- Axial images can be reconstructed and viewed in the sagittal and coronal planes

Computed Tomography (CT)

Computed Tomography equipment (Fig. 14–28) and images differ considerably from those produced by conventional *Projection Radiography* or by *CR*. Both conventional radiography and CR are based on the absorption of x-rays as they pass through the different tissues of a patient's body and the exiting x-rays interacting with a detection device (i.e., x-ray film or other IR). This produces two-dimensional images that are made with reference to the *long axis of the body*, with anatomic structures *superimposed* upon one another, and often degraded by *scattered radiation fog*. In CR, analog images are changed to digital images with an *ADC*, though they are generally viewed as analog images for monitor display (Figs. 14–25A&B).

Conventional tomography is referred to as *axial tomography* because the image plane parallels the body's long axis, providing coronal and/or sagittal images. This procedure is infrequently performed today.

Computed tomography images are *cross sectional* (i.e., axial, perpendicular to the body's long axis), individual slices—referred to as *transaxial* (or *transverse*) *images*. The process of CT imaging allows very much improved perception of small tissue density differences; slice thickness is measured in millimeters.

In brief, an x-ray tube and the rows of detectors opposite it rotate around the patient (Fig. 14–29A–C). The CT images (two dimensional or three dimensional) are obtained by detecting and measuring the exit radiation from each slice, determining its attenuation and transmission characteristics, converting to electrical signals, which are then changed to digital data. The digital data is transferred to a computer for reconstruction. The reconstructed images can then be displayed on a monitor, transmitted elsewhere, printed, and archived. The acquisition and reconstruction process in a seventh generation CT unit can normally be accomplished in under 20 seconds.

Sir Godfrey Newbold Hounsfield created the first CT unit, describing the reconstruction of data taken from multiple projection angles. Alan MacLeod Cormack worked with the complex mathematical algorithms required for image reconstruction. Their first commercial CT

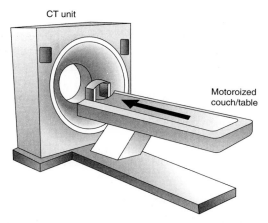

Figure 14–28. A typical computed tomography unit.

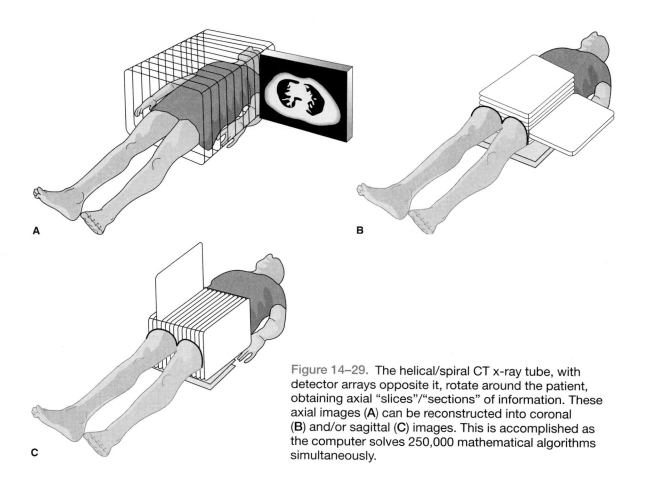

Figure 14–29. The helical/spiral CT x-ray tube, with detector arrays opposite it, rotate around the patient, obtaining axial "slices"/"sections" of information. These axial images (**A**) can be reconstructed into coronal (**B**) and/or sagittal (**C**) images. This is accomplished as the computer solves 250,000 mathematical algorithms simultaneously.

head scanner was available in 1971. In 1979, Hounsfield and Cormack shared the Nobel Prize in Medicine for their historic work with this new imaging science.

To express the beam attenuation characteristics of various tissues, the *Hounsfield Unit* (HU) is used. HUs can also be referred to as *CT numbers* or density values. Godfrey Hounsfield assigned a value of 0 to distilled water, a value of +1,000 to dense osseous tissue, and a value of −1,000 to air. There is a direct relationship between the HU and tissue attenuation coefficient. The greater the attenuation coefficient of the particular tissue, the higher the HU value. One HU represents a 0.1% difference between the particular tissue attenuation characteristics and that of distilled water. HU value accuracy can be affected by equipment calibration, volume averaging, and image artifacts.

Axial images (demonstrating *superior/inferior* structural relationships) are *reconstructed* to *coronal* images (demonstrating *anterior/posterior* relationships) and/or *sagittal* images (demonstrating *medial/lateral* relationships)—see labeled Figure 14–30A–E. The reconstruction is accomplished by resolving 250,000 computerized mathematical algorithms simultaneously!

Component Parts. A CT imaging system has four component parts—a *couch/table* for patient support, a (doughnut-shaped) *gantry*, a *computer*, and *operating consoles* with display.

Couch/Table. The *Couch*, or *Table*, provides positioning support for the patient. Its motorized movement should be smooth and accurate. Inaccurate indexing can result in missed anatomy and/or double-exposed anatomy.

The *Couch*, or *Table*, provides positioning support for the patient. It is located on top of the pedestal containing its motorized mechanism, allowing its horizontal and vertical movement. Its motorized movement should be smooth and accurate; inaccurate *indexing* can result in missed anatomy and/or double-exposed anatomy.

The couch is made of strong but low atomic number materials—so as not to hinder x-ray photon transmission. The material is often a carbon fiber, capable of weight limits up to 450 pounds. Precise table motion is essential, and exceeding the weight limit can affect/damage the table's precise moving mechanism.

In CT, the term "*Pitch*" refers to the relationship between the distance the couch travels during one x-ray tube rotation and the width of the beam/slice (in millimeters). *The Pitch determines the amount of tissue included in the scan.* Pitch values less than 1.0 indicate *oversampling* and can result in excessive exposure. Pitch values above 1.0 indicate *undersampling* and can result in missed data (i.e., anatomy/pathology).

Gantry. The *gantry* component generally includes an x-ray tube, a detector array, a high-voltage generator, a collimator assembly, slip rings, DAS, and laser beams to assist positioning.

The patient/part on the motorized couch is surrounded by the circular gantry opening. Within the circular gantry assembly is the x-ray tube, facing an array of thousands of detectors (up to 60+ rows). In

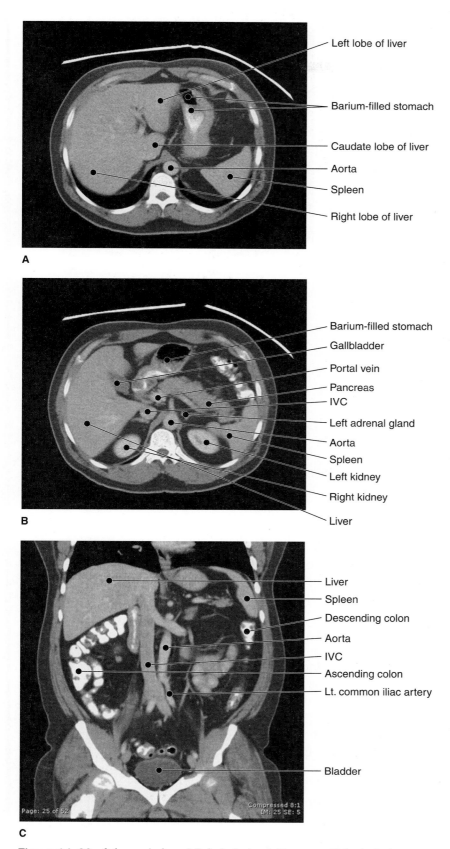

Figure 14–30. A (superior) and **B** (inferior) *axial* images; **C** (anterior) and **D** (posterior) *coronal* images; **E** (medial) and **F** (lateral) *sagittal* images. (*continued*)

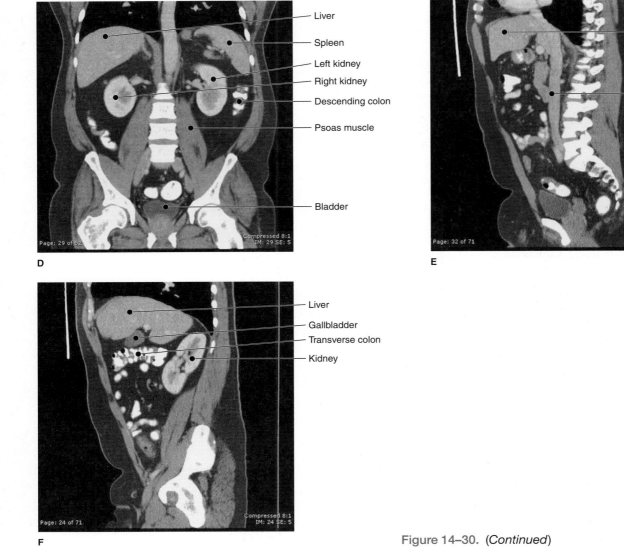

- Liver
- Spleen
- Left kidney
- Right kidney
- Descending colon
- Psoas muscle
- Bladder

D

- Liver
- IVC

E

- Liver
- Gallbladder
- Transverse colon
- Kidney

F

Figure 14–30. (*Continued*)

sixth generation CT, the x-ray tube and detectors move around the patient within the gantry.

Seventh-generation CT can acquire data from multiple sections—up to 320 sections per rotation—the x-ray tube making many *pulsed exposures*, and the detector array receiving the transmitted photons.

In earlier generations of CT, the x-ray tube rotated 360 degrees around the patient lying on a stationary couch, to obtain a "slice" image. The couch would then advance a particular distance (called *indexing*), stop, and then the x-ray tube rotated 360 degrees in the opposite direction for the next "slice" image, and so on.

The several generations of CT scanners have had various combinations of fixed and/or rotating x-ray tubes and detector arrays, and examination times have changed considerably during the evolution of CT.

Gantry Components:

- X-ray tube
- Detector array
- High-voltage generator
- Collimator assembly
- Slip rings
- DAS
- Laser beams for positioning

Generations of CT:

- 1st: *pencil* beam
  - Head scans only
  - Detectors opposite finely collimated beam
  - "Translation" time: time taken for x-ray tube and two detectors to travel from one side of part to other side
  - After one translation, the x-ray tube/detector assembly rotated 1 degree ("indexing")
  - Translation and indexing were repeated until examination completion, followed by computer reconstruction
  - Exam time more than 30 minutes; 1 to 4 sections acquired per rotation
- 2nd: divergent (but flat) *fan* beam (approximately 10°)
  - More data collected with about 30 detectors
  - 30-degree indexing
  - Reduced examination time (one-tenth of first generation time!)
  - 1 to 4 sections acquired per rotation
- 3rd: *rotating tube and detector* array
  - This was recognized as the first multidetector CT
  - Had *thicker* fan beam (i.e., not flat) that now required different reconstruction algorithms
  - *Curved array* of approximately 250 to 900 detectors (covers at least 20 mm in the Z axis)
  - *Greater coverage* and *thinner slices* provide *higher resolution* images
  - Continuous tube operation—*no stop for translation*
  - 360 degrees of data collected
  - *Pause* between each scan for table indexing
  - Reduced scan time; 1 to 4 sections acquired per rotation
- 4th: *stationary detector ring* with rotating tube
  - Clockwise motion, followed by counter clockwise motion for next section
  - Greatly reduced examination time
  - 1 to 4 sections acquired per rotation
- 5th: *Electron beam*; ultra high-speed CT
  - 400 to 800 fixed detectors
  - For cardiac imaging specifically because of its speed
  - Four sections acquired per rotation
- 6th: *helical or spiral CT*
  - Similar to third generation because *x-ray tube and detectors rotate continuously* 360 degrees around the patient (Fig. 14–31)
  - Couch/table is *simultaneously* moving through gantry (no stop for indexing)
  - *Made possible by slip ring technology*

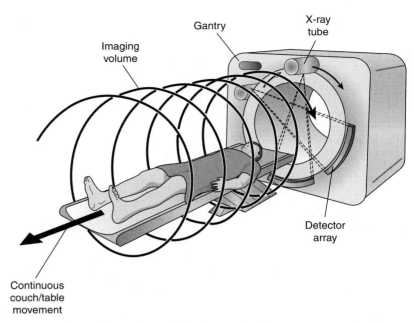

Figure 14–31. Achievement of *slip ring technology* allows *continuous* x-ray tube rotation and *simultaneous* couch movement, permitting acquisition of volume multislice scanning. The method of image acquisition lends itself to the term *helical* (or spiral) CT.

- Complete volume of part (chest/abdomen) can be scanned in 30 s/one breath hold
- Slices of data can be adjusted by table speed—this is referred to as "*pitch*," that is, slices and their data can be right next to each other (referred to as a pitch of 1); a pitch greater than 1 allows fast acquisition but can result in a thicker slice or a gap between slice data (information can be missed, image quality can decrease); a pitch less than 1 indicates overlap of slice data (can result in excessive patient exposure)
- Some helical/spiral CT units have a dual source (i.e., two x-ray tubes) for better resolution and for better balance
- 7th: *multidetector/multisection CT*
  - Images *more than one section (16–320) per rotation*
  - *Multiple rows of detectors* collect the data
  - Thereby decreasing patient dose and total scan time
  - Total scan time (e.g., for chest/abdomen) reduced to approximately 15 seconds

Advantages of Helical Multislice CT:

- Reduced motion blur/artifacts
- Greatly reduced scan time
- Increase in tissue volume imaged
- Lower volume contrast media needed
- High-quality reconstruction

Types of Three-Dimensional MPR:

- MIP (maximum intensity projection)
- SSD (shaded surface display)
- SVD (shaded volume display)

In the 1990s, the implementation of *slip ring technology* allowed *continuous* rotation of the x-ray tube (through elimination of cables) and simultaneous couch movement. Sixth-generation CT scanning is termed *helical* (or spiral) CT—permitting acquisition of volume multislice scanning. Today's helical multislice scanners, employing two or more rows of detectors, can obtain uninterrupted data acquisition of 128 "slices" per tube rotation and can perform *three-dimensional multiplanar reformation* (MPR).

Although the *CT x-ray tube* is similar to direct projection x-ray tubes, the objective is a fan-shaped beam. The CT x-ray tube also has several particular requirements; it must have a very high short-exposure rating and must be capable of tolerating several million HU while still having a small focal spot for optimal spatial resolution. To help tolerate the very high production of HU, the anode must also be capable of high-speed rotation. The x-ray tube produces a pulsed x-ray beam (1–5 ms) using up to approximately 1,000 mA and 140 kV.

The *scintillation detector array* is made of thousands of solid-state photodiodes. If the scintillation crystals are packed tightly together so that there is virtually no distance between them, efficiency of x-ray absorption is increased, and patient dose is decreased. Detection efficiency is extremely high—approximately 90%. These scintillation crystal assemblies (cadmium tungstate or rare earth oxide ceramic crystals) convert the transmitted x-ray energy into light. The light is then converted into electrical energy (by a semiconductor photodiode) and finally converted into an electronic/digital signal by the DAS. From the DAS, binary data are sent to the array processor computer. The computer *reconstructs* the "raw" data into cross-sectional images. Here, additional processing operations and image manipulation can also be carried out, for example, windowing, enhancement, measurements, three-dimensional postprocessing, volume rendering, and multiplanar reconstruction.

The *high-voltage generator* provides high-frequency power to the CT x-ray tube, enabling the high-speed anode rotation and the production of high-energy pulsed x-ray photons. Similar to the high-frequency x-ray tubes used in projection radiography, conventional 60-Hz full-wave rectified power is converted to a higher frequency of 500–25,000 Hz. The CT generator can be located in the CT room, outside the gantry. However, a *high-frequency CT generator* is usually mounted within the gantry's rotating wheel, is solid state and small in size, and produces an almost constant potential waveform.

The *collimator assembly* has two parts: The prepatient, or predetector, collimator at the x-ray tube consists of multiple beam restrictions so that the x-ray beam diverges little. Collimation (and therefore, scan volume) varies according to the procedure being performed. It serves to reduce patient dose and reduce the production of scattered radiation, thereby improving CT contrast resolution. The postpatient collimator, or predetector collimator, confines the exit photons before they reach the detector array, resulting in a nearly parallel beam, and determines slice thickness.

Computer. The CT computer must be capable of performing tens of thousands calculations, simultaneously, per slice—for considerably more than 100 slices per second.

A microprocessor or array processor is used for the all-important function of reconstruction. *Reconstruction* is defined as the time lapse between completion of imaging to the appearance of images.

Operating Consoles. The CT technologist uses one console to operate the CT machine, selecting the correct exam protocols, and entering patient demographics. Another console might be required for technologist postprocessing, archiving, and other administrative tasks. There may be a third display console available for the physician to view and manipulate images.

Summary

- Correct terminology is "CT" (Computed Tomography)
- Axial images can be reconstructed and viewed in the sagittal and coronal planes
- The infrequently performed *conventional tomography* is referred to as *axial tomography* because the image plane parallels the body's long axis, providing coronal and/or sagittal images
- CT images are axial images that can be reconstructed into coronal and/or sagittal images
- In CT, the x-ray tube and detector arrays opposite it, rotate around the patient, obtaining "slices"/"sections" of information
- Exit radiation from each slice is measured; attenuation and transmission characteristics are determined and converted to electrical signals, then changed to digital data and transferred to computer for reconstruction
- In 1979, Hounsfield and Cormack shared the Nobel Prize in Medicine for their historic work with CT imaging
- The HU is used in CT to express the beam attenuation characteristics of various tissues
- A CT imaging system has four component parts—a *couch/table* for patient support, a (doughnut-shaped) *gantry*, a *computer*, and *operating consoles* with display
- The CT gantry is composed of the x-ray tube, detector array, high-voltage generator, collimator assembly, slip rings, DAS, and laser beams for positioning
- The term "*Pitch*" refers to the relationship between the distance the couch travels during one x-ray tube rotation and the width of the beam/slice (in millimeters)
- The seven generations of CT scanners have had various combinations of fixed and/or rotating x-ray tubes and detector arrays, and exam times have changed considerably during the evolution of CT
- *Slip ring technology* allows *continuous* rotation of the x-ray tube (by elimination of cables) and simultaneous couch movement
- *Helical* (or spiral) CT—permits acquisition of volume multislice scans; helical/spiral multislice scanners employ two or more rows of detectors
- Advantages of *Helical Multislice CT* include reduced motion blur/artifacts, decreased scan time, increased tissue volume imaged, lower volume contrast media needed, high-quality reconstruction
- CT x-ray tubes have high-speed anode rotation, produce a pulsed, fan-shaped beam that emerges from a small focal spot for optimal spatial resolution; they have a high short-exposure rating and can tolerate several million HU
- The scintillation detector array is made of thousands of very sensitive/efficient solid-state photodiodes

- The scintillation assemblies convert the transmitted x-ray energy into light, which is next converted into electrical energy by photo-diodes, and finally converted into a digital signal by the DAS

- From the DAS, binary data are sent to the array processor computer, where "raw" data are reconstructed into cross sectional images. This is where additional processing operations and image manipulation can be carried out as well, for example, windowing, enhancement, measurements, three-dimensional postprocessing, volume rendering, and multiplanar reconstruction

- The small size, solid-state high-frequency CT generator is usually mounted within the gantry's rotating wheel, and produces an almost constant potential waveform

- The *collimator assembly* has two parts: *prepatient/predetector* collimator at the x-ray tube has multiple beam restrictions so that the x-ray beam diverges little; it reduces patient dose, reduces the production of scattered radiation (SR), and improves contrast resolution. The *postpatient/predetector* collimator, confines the exit beam before it reaches the detector array, results in a nearly parallel beam, and determines slice thickness

- The CT computer performs tens of thousands of calculations, simultaneously, per slice—for considerably more than one hundred slices per second

- *Reconstruction* is defined as the time lapse between completion of imaging to the appearance of images

- The console is used by the CT technologist to operate the CT machine, select the exam protocols, and enter patient information; another console might be required for postprocessing, archiving, and other administrative tasks

THE FLUOROSCOPIC SYSTEM

Fluoroscopic x-ray examinations are performed to study the dynamics of various parts in *motion*. Fluoroscopy was performed almost exclusively in the very early days of radiology because of the lack of dependable x-ray tubes and image-recording systems (Fig. 14–33). In the late 1940s and early 1950s, image intensification was developed and served to provide much brighter images at lower exposures. *Image intensifiers* (IIs) brighten (intensify) the conventional, or "dark," fluoroscopic image 5,000 to 20,000 times. Today's fluoroscopic procedures are much safer (lower exposure/mA) and brighter; the fluoroscopic image can be photographed still or moving or viewed with a television camera/CCD and projected onto a nearby or remote television monitor.

A fluoroscope has two principal components, an x-ray tube and a fluorescent screen, attached at opposite ends of a *C-shaped arm* (Figs. 14–33 and 14–34). The fluoroscopic *table* accommodates the patient and must be able to move to an upright position (90 degrees) and to a Trendelenburg position (up to approximately 40 degrees). Therefore, a 90/30 fluoroscopic table refers to one that will move upright (90 degrees) and angle Trendelenburg up to 30 degrees.

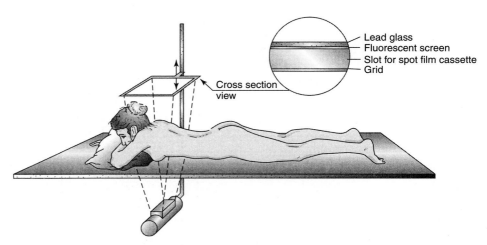

Lead glass
Fluorescent screen
Slot for spot film cassette
Grid

Cross section view

Figure 14–32. Basic early fluoroscope.

Fluoroscopic x-ray tubes are standard rotating anode tubes, usually installed under the x-ray table, but operated at much lower tube currents than radiographic tubes. Over-the-table fluoroscopic x-ray tubes result in higher radiation exposure to personnel than under-the-table x-ray tubes. Instead of the 50 to 1,200 mA used in radiography, traditional image-intensified fluoroscopic tubes are operated at currents that range from 0.5 to 5.0 mA (averaging 1–3 mA). Higher mA is often used in pulsed and/or flat panel fluoroscopy.

Patient dose is much higher in fluoroscopic than radiographic procedures because of the considerably shorter source-to-object distance used in fluoroscopy. Fluoroscopic *entrance exposure* is significantly greater than exit exposure as a result of attenuation processes within the patient. The typical entrance skin exposure rate is 2 R/min; a *"boost"* mode is often available for special situations—employing exposure rates of *up to 20 R/min*. Use of the "boost" mode is permitted for only short periods of time and an *audible signal* is activated during its use.

In digital fluoroscopy (DF), the image-intensifier output screen image is coupled via a charge-coupled device (CCD) for viewing on a display monitor. A CCD converts visible light to an electrical charge that is then sent to the analog-to-digital converter (ADC) for processing. When output screen light strikes the CCD cathode, a proportional number of electrons are released by the cathode and stored as digital values by the CCD. The CCD's rapid discharge time virtually eliminates image lag and is particularly useful in high-speed imaging procedures such as cardiac catheterizations. CCD cameras have replaced analog cameras (such as the vidicon and plumbicon) in new fluoroscopic equipment.

CCDs are more sensitive to the light emitted by the output phosphor (than the analog cameras) and are associated with less "noise." DF eliminates the need for cassette-loaded spot films and/or 100-mm spot films. DF photospot images, which are simply still-frame images, need no chemical processing, require less patient dose, and offer postprocessing capability.

DF also offers "road-mapping" capability. "Road-mapping" is a technique useful in procedures involving guidewire/catheter placement.

Advantages of Flat Panel Fluoroscopy:

- Pulsed x-ray beam
- Decreased patient dose
- Increased sensitivity to x-rays (DQE)
- Increased temporal resolution; decreased motion unsharpness
- Improved contrast resolution

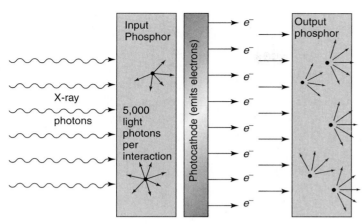

Figure 14–33. Conceptualization of relationship and function of an image intensifier input screen, photocathode, and output screen. For every one x-ray photon interacting with the input screen, 5,000 fluorescent light photons are emitted. Note the close (but not touching) relationship between the input screen and photocathode for maintenance of resolution. The light photons interact with the photocathode and approximately 150 electrons are emitted by the photoemissive metal. The photoelectrons then interact with the output screen, and 2,000 fluorescent light photons are emitted for every electron.

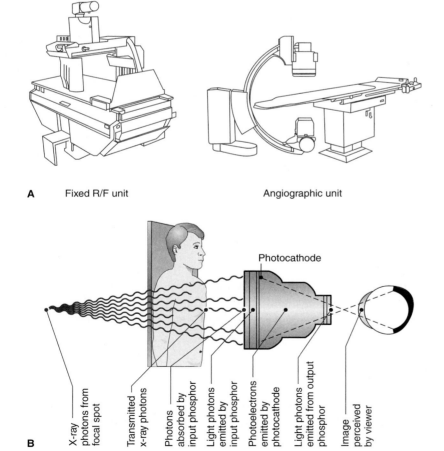

Figure 14–34. (A) *C-arm:* A fluoroscope has two principal components, an x-ray tube and a fluorescent screen, attached at opposite ends of a C-shaped arm. **(B)** Transition of x-ray photons emerging from x-ray tube, through part under study, into image intensifier, to human eye.

During the fluoroscopic examination, the most recent fluoroscopic image can be stored on the monitor ("image hold"), thereby reducing the need for continuous x-ray exposure. This technique can offer significant reductions in patient and personnel radiation exposure.

Since DF images are obtained using a pulsed (rather than continuous) x-ray beam, this significantly decreases patient dose—as long as the pulse rate is below 30 pps. Most DF static images can also be made with a lower mA because of the greater sensitivity of the CCD. Image acquisition rates are usually between 1 and 10 images per second. *Fewer frames per second result in lower patient dose*. Dose reduction advantages can be nullified by taking superfluous digital spot images.

Additionally, instead of the fluoroscopic image being received by an image intensifier, it can be received by a *flat panel detector*. The use of a fluoroscopic flat panel detector can offer the benefit of further reduction in patient dose because of increased sensitivity to x-rays Detective Quantum Efficiency (DQE). There is also increased temporal resolution, helping to reduce motion unsharpness. There is also better contrast resolution, though spatial resolution is the same as, or not as good as, image intensification fluoroscopy.

In this system, *the x-ray tube must be able to turn on and off very quickly*. The term *interrogation time* refers to the time it takes the tube to reach the required exposure factors. The term *extinction time* refers to the time it takes the tube to turn off. The required time is less than 1 millisecond.

For radiation protection purposes, the fluoroscopic tabletop exposure rate must not exceed 10 *R/min* and all fluoroscopic equipment must provide *at least* 12 *in.* (30 cm), and preferably 15 in. (38 cm), between the x-ray source (focal spot) and the x-ray tabletop. Positioning the II *closer* to the patient *decreases the SID* and *decreases patient dose*. Patient dose decreases because as the SID is *decreased* the number of x-ray photons at the input phosphor *increases*; this results in the automatic brightness control *decreasing the mA* to compensate for the increase in x-ray photons.

A *5-minute timer* is used to measure accumulated fluoroscopic examination time and make an audible sound or interrupt exposure after 5 minutes of fluoroscopy. X-ray production is usually activated by a foot switch (*dead man switch*), thus leaving the fluoroscopist's hands free to handle the carriage and position and palpate the patient. The fluoroscopic tube is usually equipped with electrically driven collimating *shutters*. Leaded glass provides shielding from radiation passing through the intensifying screen, and the II is lead lined. A *Bucky slot cover* and *protective curtain* also help reduce exposure to the fluoroscopist.

Older fluoroscopes are often equipped with a *spot film* device to record fluoroscopic images. To expose a spot film, a motor is activated that brings a cassette from a lead-lined compartment within the carriage over into the fluoroscopic field between the intensifying screen and grid (Fig. 14–34A). The fluoroscopic x-ray tube current then automatically increases to a conventional radiographic level of approximately 300 mA or more for the cassette exposure. The lead shutters usually adjust automatically, but may be operated manually.

Some Radiation Safety Features of Fluoroscopic Equipment

- Maximum of 5 mA in traditional II fluoro
- 12 in. minimum between focal spot and tabletop
- 10 R/min maximum tabletop exposure
- 5-minute cumulative timer
- "Dead man" switch
- Automatic collimation
- Bucky slot cover
- Protective curtain

Summary

- Fluoroscopes are used to examine moving parts and are ocassionally equipped with a device to take cassette-loaded spot films.

- A fluoroscope has two major parts: an x-ray tube and a fluorescent screen, attached at opposite ends of a C-shaped arm.

- The fluoroscopic tube is usually located (at least 12 in.) under the x-ray table and usually operated at 1 to 3 mA (upto a maximum of 5 mA); mA automatically increases for fluoroscopic images.

- Fluoroscopic patient dose depends on exposure rate, tissue thickness or density, and length of exposure.

- Fluoroscopic patient dose decreases as the II is moved closer to the patient.

- Fluoroscopic "boost" mode can deliver up to 20 R/min.

- Many guidelines regulate the operation of fluoroscopic equipment because of the unavoidable high patient dose inherent in fluoroscopic procedures (because of the short focus-to-patient distance).

- IIs brighten the conventional, dark fluoroscopic image 5,000 to 20,000 times.

- DF images are obtained using a *pulsed* x-ray beam; this can significantly decrease patient dose.

- DF image acquisition rates are usually between 1 and 10 images per second; fewer frames per second result in lower patient dose.

- In DF the fluoroscopic image can be received by a flat panel detector; in this system, the x-ray tube must be able to turn on and off very quickly.

The Image Intensifier

The fluorescent layer of early conventional (or "dark") fluoroscopic screens was made of *zinc cadmium sulfide* (Patterson B-2 screen). The *input screen* of today's II tube is made of a thin layer of *cesium iodide*, is 5 to 12 in. in diameter, and slightly convex in shape.

Cesium iodide is much more efficient than zinc cadmium sulfide because it absorbs, and converts to fluorescent light, a greater number of the x-ray photons striking it. For each absorbed x-ray photon, approximately 5,000 light photons are emitted (Fig. 14–33). This fluorescent light strikes a *photocathode* made of a photoemissive metal. A number of electrons are subsequently released from the photocathode and focused toward the output side of the image tube. Although this step actually represents a *deamplification*, it has very little effect on the end result. A thin (0.2-mm) layer of glass or other transparent material is placed between the input screen and photocathode to prevent chemical reaction between the two; otherwise, the two must be as close as possible for maximum transfer of accurate information.

The electrons emitted from the photocathode are focused toward the output end of the tube by negatively charged *electrostatic focusing lenses*. They then pass through the neck of the tube where they are accelerated through a potential difference of 25,000 to 35,000 V and strike the small (0.5–1 in.) fluorescent *output screen* that is mounted on a flat glass support (Figs. 14–34 and 14–35).

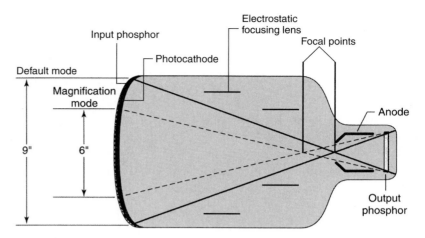

Figure 14–35. As field of view (patient area/normal vs. magnification mode) decreases, magnification of the output screen image increases and contrast and resolution improve. Note that the focal point on the 6-in. field, or mode, is further away from the output phosphor; therefore, the output image appears magnified. Because less minification takes place in this instance, the image is not as bright. Exposure factors are automatically increased to compensate for the loss in brightness.

The entire assembly is enclosed within a 2- to 4-mm thick vacuum glass envelope. The glass is then coated to prevent the entry of light. The glass tube is enclosed within a metal housing that functions to attenuate magnetic fields from outside the tube that would distort the electron paths within.

For there to be undistorted focusing of electrons onto the output screen, each electron must travel the same distance, thus the slight curvature of the input screen.

There are several occasions of information transfer within the II: from x-ray beam to input screen, from input screen to photocathode, from photocathode to electron beam, from electron beam to output screen, and from output screen to the human eye (Fig. 14–34). Thus, an electrical image is transformed to a light image, then back to an electron image, and finally back to a light image.

Electrons from the photocathode are accelerated as they travel toward the output screen. The gain in brightness achieved by the II is the result of this *electron acceleration (flux gain)* and *image minification*. *Flux gain* is defined as the ratio of light photons at the output phosphor to the number at the input phosphor. A typical II has a flux gain of approximately 50.

The image produced on the input screen of the II is reproduced as a minified image on the output screen. Because the output screen is much smaller than the input screen, the amount of fluorescent light emitted from it per unit area is significantly greater than the quantity of light emitted from the input screen. This process is referred to as *minification gain*, and is equal to the ratio of the diameters of the input and output screens squared:

$$\text{Minification gain} = \left(\frac{\text{Input screen diameter}}{\text{Output screen diameter}}\right)^2.$$

For example, the minification gain for an II with an input screen of 11 in. and output screen of 1 in. is 121:

$$\text{Minification gain} = \left(\frac{11''}{1''}\right)^2$$

$$= 121.$$

The total *brightness gain* of an II is the product of flux gain and minification gain:

$$\text{Total brightness gain} = \text{flux gain} \times \text{minification gain.}$$

For example, the total brightness gain for an II with a flux gain of 50 and minification gain of 121 is 6,050:

$$\text{Total brightness gain} = 50(121)$$

$$= 6,050.$$

The brightness, resolution, and contrast of an intensified image are greatest in the center of the image. Because the exposure rate is reduced at the periphery of the input screen, and because there is less-than-exact peripheral electron focusing from the photocathode, brightness, resolution, and contrast are reduced (up to 25%) toward the periphery; this characteristic of IIs is called *vignetting*.

Input screen diameters of 5 to 12 in. are available. Although smaller diameter input screens improve resolution, they do not permit viewing of large patient areas.

A type of image distortion, called *pincushion distortion*, is common to intensified images and is caused by the curvature of the input screen and diminished electron focusing precision at the image periphery.

There will always be some degree of magnification in image intensification (just as in radiography); the degree depends on the distance of the II from the patient.

Dual- and triple-field IIs are available that permit magnified viewing of fluoroscopic images. Magnified images are reduced in brightness unless the mA is automatically increased when the II is switched to the magnification mode (Fig. 14–35). Entrance skin exposure (ESE) can increase dramatically as the FOV decreases (i.e., as magnification increases).

Fluoroscopy units are frequently equipped with a last-view freeze-frame feature. This permits the fluoroscopist a longer view of on-screen anatomy without the need for continuous x-ray exposure.

Summary

- The basic parts of the II are the input screen, photocathode, electrostatic focusing lenses, accelerating anode, and output screen, within a vacuum glass envelope.
- The process of energy conversion within the II is from electrical to light, to electrical, and back to light.
- Cesium iodide is the preferred phosphor for the II's input screen; for each x-ray photon it absorbs, it emits approximately 5,000 light photons.

Comparisons Between Large and Small Fields of View and Modes

Larger field of view
- Focal point closer to output screen
- Less magnification of perceived image
- Brighter image; less exposure required

Smaller field of view
- Focal point farther from output screen
- Magnified image
- Less brightness; more exposure required

- Light photons strike the photocathode, which releases a number of electrons that are directed toward the neck of the II by the negatively charged focusing lenses.
- The input screen and photocathode are slightly curved so that each electron travels the same distance to the output phosphor, to prevent distortion.
- Electrons are accelerated by the anode's 25 to 30 kV potential, thus making the output image brighter (*flux* gain); the electrons strike the output screen and are converted to a much brighter, smaller (minification gain), and inverted fluorescent image.
- *Minification* gain is determined by dividing the input screen diameter by the output screen diameter and squaring the result; *total brightness* gain is equal to the product of flux gain and minification gain.
- Diminished resolution and contrast at the image periphery is called vignetting.
- Magnification results in some loss of brightness; mA is automatically increased to compensate.
- Last-view freeze-frame feature can significantly decrease patient dose.

Viewing Systems

The optical system of the II can transfer the output screen image to a mirror viewing apparatus. Mirror viewing offers good resolution, but its disadvantages include limited viewing by one person at a time and limited fluoroscopist movement. In comparison, *closed-circuit television fluoroscopy* is far more convenient, allows the fluoroscopist freedom of movement, and permits simultaneous viewing by a number of people.

As body areas of different thicknesses and density are scanned with the II, image brightness and contrast require adjustment. The *automatic brightness control* functions to maintain constant brightness and contrast of the output screen image, correcting for fluctuations in x-ray beam attenuation with adjustments in kV and/or mA. There are also brightness and contrast controls on the monitor that the radiographer can regulate. Positioning the II *closer* to the patient *increases the SSD* and *decreases patient dose (ESE)*.

The image on the output screen can be transferred via a television camera to a display *monitor*. The II output screen image is *coupled* via a *television camera* (in analog fluoroscopy) or a CCD (in DF) for viewing on a display monitor. This is an example of closed-circuit TV. The *Vidicon* and *Plumbicon* are currently the most frequently used analog television cameras. They are approximately 6 in. in length and 1 in. in diameter.

Recording and Storage Systems

In addition to being transmitted to nearby or remote monitors, traditional images can be recorded on *videotape* or *cine* film. Television monitors do not offer the very good image resolution obtained from the II, so film recording systems such as spot film cameras and cine cameras can be used to record better resolution images directly from the II (Fig. 14–36).

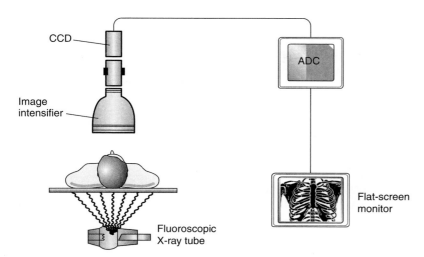

Figure 14–36. Image-intensified fluoroscopic unit with ancillary imaging devices.

Digital images can be stored on magnetic tape and disks, digital videotape, and optical disks and tape.

Cinefluorography. The fluorescent image on the II's output screen can be photographed with a 16- or 35-mm movie camera. Approximately 85% to 95% of the light from the II's output screen is transmitted to the cine camera when it is in use. The rest of the light is used for television monitor viewing. During cinefluorography, x-ray exposure is on only when the film is in proper position for exposure (i.e., no exposure during film movement between frames). Grid-controlled x-ray tubes are used to synchronize x-ray exposure with proper film position. Cine "flickering" is noticeable only with frame rates below 30 frames per second.

Film used in cine cameras must be sensitive to the fluorescent light emitted by the output screen. *Panchromatic* film is sensitive to all wavelengths (i.e., colors) of visible light; *orthochromatic* film is sensitive to all but red light. These are the two film types most often used in cine cameras. Higher quality images are obtained with 35-mm film (rather than 16 mm) because the film size is four times greater than 16-mm frames; however, for that same reason, 35-mm film requires greater patient exposure and is more expensive. Another reason patient dose is significantly greater in cinefluorography than in routine image-intensified fluoroscopy is that the output screen image must be bright enough to expose the cine film (hence, increased mA). Typical doses measured at the II input phosphor are approximately 10 μR/frame.

Spot Films. Spot films in 70-mm, 90-mm, and 105-mm sizes can be made from the image on the output screen of the II. This method of recording static (still) images gained acceptance over the cassette-loaded spot filming procedures (taken from the input screen of the II). The film used for spot-film cameras is less expensive and easier to store, can be exposed in rapid succession, and requires less patient exposure. Typical doses measured at the II input phosphor are approximately 50 to 100 μR/spot film. Image quality is slightly less than that of cassette-loaded spot films, whose typical doses measured at the II input phosphor are approximately 300 to 400 μR/film.

Video Recording. Fluoroscopic procedures can also be recorded on videotape. The most significant advantage of videotape recordings is that it allows immediate playback of dynamic (motion) images (eliminating film processing). Other advantages include the availability of sound and capabilities of playing at slower speeds and viewing single frames. Its biggest disadvantage is loss of some resolution with regular VHS equipment. High-resolution systems (VHS-S) require the use of high-resolution accessories such as high-resolution cameras and monitors, and thus provide a superior image quality. New video disk recorders are similar to videotape machines, sharing all their advantages and having the added advantage of improved image quality (resolution).

Digital Fluoroscopy. In DF, the II output screen image is *coupled* via a CCD for viewing on a display monitor. A CCD converts visible light to an electrical charge, which is then sent to the ADC for processing. When output screen light strikes the CCD cathode, a proportional number of electrons are released by the cathode and *stored as digital values* by the CCD. The CCD's rapid discharge time virtually eliminates image lag and is particularly useful in high-speed imaging procedures such as cardiac catheterizations. CCD cameras have replaced analog cameras (i.e., the Vidicon and Plumbicon) in fluoroscopic equipment. CCDs are very sensitive to the light emitted by the output phosphor and are associated with less "noise;" the CCD SNR is approximately 1,000:1; the TV camera SNR is approximately 200:1.

DF eliminates the need for cassette-loaded spot films and/or 100-mm spot films. DF photospot images, which are simply still-frame images, need no chemical processing, require less patient dose (unless more than necessary are taken), and offer postprocessing capability. DF also offers "road-mapping" capability—a technique useful in procedures involving guidewire/catheter placement. During the fluoroscopic examination, the most recent fluoroscopic image can be stored on the monitor ("image hold"), thereby reducing the need for continuous x-ray exposure. This technique can offer significant reductions in patient and personnel radiation exposure.

DF offers significantly lower patient dose—its x-ray beam is "pulsed," rather than continuous. Most DF static images can also be made with a lower mA because of the greater sensitivity of the CCD (over film emulsion). It is important to take advantage of these patient dose reduction features—they can be nullified by taking excessive digital spot images.

Instead of the fluoroscopic image being received by an II, it can be received by a *flat panel detector*. DF flat panel detector images are obtained using a pulsed x-ray beam, which can significantly decrease patient dose, even though the exposures might be made at traditional high mA—as long as the pulse rate is below 30 pps. Image acquisition rates are usually between 1 and 10 images per second. Fewer frames per second result in lower patient dose.

The use of a fluoroscopic flat panel detector can offer the benefit of further reduction in patient dose because of increased sensitivity to x-rays (DQE). There is also increased temporal resolution, helping to reduce motion unsharpness. There is also better contrast resolution, though spatial resolution is the same as, or not as good as, image intensification fluoroscopic images.

In the flat panel system, *the x-ray tube must be able to turn on and off very quickly.* The term *interrogation time* refers to the time it takes the tube to reach the required exposure factors. The term *extinction time* refers to the time it takes the tube to turn off. The required time is less than 1 millisecond.

Information Storage. The quantity of patient information and diagnostic image data stored by hospitals is ever increasing. It is essential that this information be stored, managed, and utilized efficiently. There are radiology information systems that centrally process and store image data within a hospital, enabling image retrieval from the server by any department over the hospital network, and display image at the requesting department site. This eliminates the cumbersome task of sorting, conveying, and storing films. Hospital information system's networks allow the archiving and distribution of vast amounts of image information from all modalities, managing it all with a single system. Using multiple connections over a network (e.g., Picture Archiving and Communication System [PACS]), image data can also be shared by multiple hospitals.

Advantages of Flat Panel Fluoroscopy:
• Pulsed x-ray beam
• Decrease patient dose
• Increased sensitivity to x-rays (DQE)
• Increased temporal resolution; decreased motion unsharpness
• Improved contrast resolution
• Somewhat less spatial resolution

Advantages of DF Photospots
• No chemical processing needed
• Decreased patient dose
• Postprocessing capability
• "Road-mapping" capability

Summary

- The optical system transfers the output screen image to either mirror viewing or television monitor (via Plumbicon or Vidicon camera).
- Television monitor viewing is more practical and convenient, although it involves some loss of image quality.
- Automatic brightness control automatically adjusts kV or mA; brightness and contrast controls are also available for adjustment on the TV monitor.
- The output screen image is usually coupled to the television camera via a series of complex and precisely adjusted lenses and mirror.
- When used in conjunction with cine and spot-film cameras, the largest portion of the output screen light is diverted to the spot film or cine camera; the remainder goes to the television monitor.
- Cineradiographic film is either 16-mm or 35-mm panchromatic or orthochromatic film; better quality images are obtained with 35 mm, but patient exposure dose is greater.
- Spot-film cameras use 70-mm, 90-mm, or 105-mm film, and are preferable to cassette-loaded spot films because the film is more economical and easier to store and requires less patient exposure.
- Videotape recordings, permitting immediate playback, may be made during the fluoroscopic procedure, although there is some loss of image resolution.
- In DF, the II output screen image is coupled via a CCD for viewing on a display monitor.
- Advantages of DF include no chemical processing, higher SNR, less patient dose, postprocessing capability, and "road-mapping."

COMPREHENSION CHECK

Congratulations! You have completed your review of the entire chapter. If you are able to answer the following group of very comprehensive questions, you should feel confident that you have really mastered this section. You can refer back to the indicated pages to check your answers and/or review the subject matter.

1. Define and give examples of dedicated x-ray equipment (p. 437).

2. Distinguish between an AC and DC waveform (p. 437).

3. Discuss the following characteristics of AC: amplitude, polarity, wavelength, and frequency (p. 437).

4. Define helix, solenoid, electromagnet (p. 439).

5. Describe the function of the transformer, and identify the principle on which it operates (p. 440).

6. Using the transformer law, determine the voltage and current delivered to the x-ray tube (p. 440).

7. Identify four types of x-ray transformer construction (pp. 440).

8. Describe three types of transformer energy losses and methods by which they can be reduced (p. 440).

9. Describe the function of the autotransformer, and identify the principle on which it operates (p. 440, 441).

10. Using the autotransformer law, determine the voltage sent to the transformer primary (p. 441).

11. Identify the type of current required for operation of the transformer and autotransformer (p. 440, 441).

12. Define the function of the generator; motor (p. 437).

13. Describe the rectification process (p. 442, 443).

14. Identify and give examples of the type of material of which solid-state diodes are made (p. 442).

15. Differentiate among single-phase, 3-phase/6-pulse, and 3-phase/12-pulse waveforms (p. 442, 443).

16. Identify the pulse ripple for single-phase, 3-phase/6-pulse, and 3-phase/12-pulse rectification (p. 442, 443).

17. Identify the number of autotransformers and transformers required for three-phase rectification (p. 443).

18. Identify the two types of transformer winding configurations (p. 443).

19. List the three basic component parts of the x-ray tube (p. 444).

20. Discuss the importance of the evacuated glass envelope (p. 444).

21. Identify the component parts of the cathode assembly (p. 444, 445).

22. Describe thermionic emission (p. 444, 445).

23. Describe how a double or dual focus tube differs from a single focus tube (p. 445).

24. Explain why x-ray tube inherent filtration increases as the x-ray tube ages (p. 445).

25. Identify the current and voltage required by the filament circuit (p. 445).

26. Discuss why prolonged periods of rotor activation should be avoided (p. 445).

27. Describe the construction of the anode (p. 445, 446).

28. Discuss the composition and function of the anode focal track (p. 445, 446).

29. Discuss the value of anode rotation (vs. stationary anode) (p. 445).

30. Identify the device responsible for anode rotation and its two major parts (p. 445, 446).

31. Identify two characteristics of tungsten that make it a desirable target material (p. 446).

32. Describe the line focus principle; distinguish between actual and effective focal spot (p. 447).

33. Describe the anode heel effect; relate it to focal track bevel (anode angle) (p. 447, 448).

34. Discuss why heat removal mechanisms are important in x-ray tube construction; give examples of heat reduction features (p. 447).

35. Determine heat units for $S\varphi$, 3φ 6p, and 3φ 12p x-ray equipment (p. 448, 449).

36. Determine safe exposure limits using tube rating charts and anode cooling curves (p. 449).

37. Discuss at least three causes of x-ray tube failure (p. 449, 450).

38. Identify the three portions of the x-ray circuit (p. 451).

39. Identify the components of the primary, or low-voltage, circuit (p. 451, 452).

40. Describe the various types of x-ray timers and identify their accuracy (p. 452, 453).

41. Describe the two types of AECs and identify the location of each (p. 453).

42. Discuss the importance of a backup timer (p. 453).

43. Describe the tests used to evaluate $S\varphi$ and 3φ timers (p. 453-455).

44. Evaluate $S\varphi$ and 3φ timer tests for accuracy (p. 453-455).

45. Identify the function of the rheostat and transformer in the filament circuit (p. 455).

46. Identify and describe the components of the secondary, or high-voltage, circuit (p. 455, 456).

47. What is the primary control center for the computer consisting of a control unit, arithmetic unit, and memory (p. 456)?

48. What are the two types of computer memory (p. 456)?

49. What term is used to describe how much of the patient is included in the matrix (p. 458)?

50. How does matrix size influence resolution (p. 457, 458, 463)?

51. What is the computed radiography PSP (p. 459)?

52. Describe how the image on the PSP is converted to the image seen on the monitor (p. 459, 460).

53. What is the value of postprocessing (p. 461)?

54. Describe how *windowing* (width and level) affects the contrast and density of the diagnostic image (p. 463).

55. What term is commonly used to describe the range of grays a particular digital system is capable of resolving (p. 463)?

56. List three things that determine CR resolution (p. 463).

57. Define *noise;* explain how it might be encountered in CR (p. 463).

58. Describe the two types of indirect capture digital images; identify which is a true flat panel system (p. 465).

59. What portion of the indirect capture system is absent in the direct capture system (p. 465)?

60. What is a scintillator and where is it used in digital imaging; give examples of scintillators used (p. 465)?

61. Describe the direct capture digital imaging process (p. 465).

62. Discuss why the term "CT scan" is correct and the term "CAT scan" outdated (p. 466, 467).

63. Who were the two individuals most instrumental in the development of CT, and how were they recognized (p. 467)?

64. List the four component parts of a CT unit (p. 468).

65. List the seven components of the CT gantry (p. 470).

66. What kind of technology allows continuous rotation of the CT x-ray tube and simultaneous movement of the exam couch (p. 472)?

67. Describe what is meant by the CT term *pitch*, and how it is related to *undersampling* and *oversampling* (p. 468).

68. What is meant by CT *translation* time (p. 471)?

69. What is the shape of the CT x-ray beam (p. 473)?

70. What rotates directly opposite the x-ray tube in the CT gantry (p. 473)?

71. What is the function of the CT prepatient collimator; the postpatient collimator (p. 473)?

72. What is meant by the CT term *reconstruction* (p. 473)?

73. What is meant by the term *indexing*, when applied to the CT couch (p. 470)?

74. Explain the function of fluoroscopy (p. 475).

75. Identify the usual location of the fluoroscopy tube (p. 476).

76. Identify the fluoroscopic mA range of operation; what is "boost mode"? (p. 476).

77. List at least six fluoroscopic equipment features designed to reduce patient and personnel exposure (p. 478).

78. Explain why fluoroscopic exposure dose is greater than radiographic dose (p. 476).

79. Identify, with respect to the image intensifier (II), the: (p. 479-481)?

   A. Composition of the input screen, and its characteristics and advantages

   B. Action of the photocathode

   C. Function of the electrostatic focusing lenses

   D. Function and potential difference of the accelerating anode

   E. Function and size of the output screen

   F. Two components of total brightness gain

80. Determine minification gain (p. 481).

81. Define vignetting (p. 481).

82. Discuss advantages and disadvantages of magnified images (p. 481).

83. Identify ways in which the fluoroscopic image can be recorded (p. 482, 483).

84. Identify by what means the II compensates for varying body thicknesses (p. 482).

85. Define what is meant by coupling (p. 476).

86. Identify the fluoroscopic monitor controls that can be regulated by the radiographer (p. 482).

87. Define/describe the terms *interrogation time* and *extinction time* (p. 485)

88. Identify the sizes of cine film available and compare each with regard to patient dose and image quality (p. 483).

89. Differentiate between panchromatic and orthochromatic film (p. 483).

90. Identify the spot film sizes available and relate each to patient dose and image quality (p. 483).

91. Describe the advantages and disadvantages of videotape image recording (p. 484).

92. What device couples the II and TV monitor in DF (p. 484)?

93. Describe the operation of CCDs (p. 484).

94. Compare the SNR of cameras such as Plumbicon and Vidicon to the SNR of CCDs (p. 484).

95. List four advantages of DF over analog fluoroscopy (p. 484).

96. Explain how/why DF can offer considerably less patient dose (p. 484).

97. What is the advantage of "last image hold"? What is "road-mapping" technique (p. 484)?

98. What are the advantages of flat panel detector fluoroscopy (p. 484-485)?

CHAPTER REVIEW QUESTIONS

1. Advantages of digital radiography (computed radiography) include all of the following, *except* the ability to:

   (A) Compensate for exposure factors

   (B) Make changes in contrast characteristics

   (C) Improve geometric detail

   (D) Store images in binary form

2. A three-phase timer can be tested for accuracy using a synchronous spinning top. The resulting image looks like a:

   (A) Series of dots or dashes, each representative of a radiation pulse

   (B) Solid arc, the angle (in degrees) representative of the exposure time

   (C) Series of gray tones, from white to black

   (D) Multitude of small mesh-like squares of uniform sharpness

3. In the production of Bremsstrahlung radiation, the incident electron:

   (A) Ejects an inner shell tungsten electron

   (B) Ejects an outer shell tungsten electron

   (C) Is deflected with resulting energy loss

   (D) Is deflected with resulting energy increase

4. Which of the following will occur as a result of decreasing the anode target angle?

   1. Anode heel effect will be less pronounced

   2. Effective focal spot size will decrease

   3. Greater photon intensity toward the cathode side of the x-ray tube

   (A) 1 only

   (B) 1 and 2 only

   (C) 2 and 3 only

   (D) 1, 2, and 3

5. Which of the following image matrix sizes will result in the best spatial resolution?

   (A) 128 × 128

   (B) 512 × 512

   (C) 1,089 × 1,089

   (D) 2,048 × 2,048

6. The device used to ensure reproducible images, regardless of tissue density variations, is the:

   (A) Ionization chamber

   (B) Penetrometer

   (C) Grid

   (D) Rare earth screen

7. Changes in window width in digital imaging result in changes in:

   (A) Contrast

   (B) Density/brightness

   (C) Resolution

   (D) Distortion

8. If the primary coil of the high-voltage transformer is supplied by 220 V and has 150 turns, and the secondary coil has 75,000 turns; what is the voltage induced in the secondary coil?

   (A) 75 kV

   (B) 110 kV

   (C) 75 V

   (D) 110 V

9. Which of the following circuit devices operate(s) on the principle of self-induction?

   1. Autotransformer

   2. Choke coil

   3. High-voltage transformer

   (A) 1 only

   (B) 1 and 2 only

   (C) 2 and 3 only

   (D) 1, 2, and 3

10. All of the following are components of the CT gantry, except:

    (A) Collimator assembly

    (B) Slip rings

    (C) High-voltage generator

    (D) Console

Answers and Explanations

1. (C) All other factors can be changed in the computer to manipulate the image. Geometric detail is controlled only by source-to-image-receptor distance (SID), object-to-image-receptor distance (OID), and focal spot size. These factors are fixed during the x-ray exposure.

2. (B) When a spinning top is used to test the efficiency of a single-phase timer, the result is a *series of dots* or dashes, with each dot or dash representing a pulse of radiation. With full-wave rectified current, and a possible $\frac{1}{20}$ dots (pulses) available per second, one should visualize 12 dots at $\frac{1}{10}$ second, 24 dots at $\frac{1}{15}$ second, 6 dots at $\frac{1}{20}$ second, and so on. But because three-phase equipment is almost constant potential, a synchronous spinning top must be used, and the result is a *solid arc* (rather than dots). The number of degrees formed by the arc is measured and equated to a particular exposure time. A multitude of small mesh-like squares describes a screen contact test. An aluminum step-wedge (penetrometer) may be used to demonstrate the effect of kV on contrast (demonstrating a series of gray tones from white to black), with a greater number of grays demonstrated at higher kV levels.

3. (C) Bremsstrahlung (or Brems) radiation is one of the two kinds of x-rays produced at the tungsten target of the x-ray tube. The incident high-speed electron, passing through a tungsten atom, is attracted by the positively charged nucleus; therefore, it is *deflected from its course with a resulting loss of energy.* This energy loss is given up in the form of an x-ray photon.

4. (C) Target angle has a pronounced geometric effect on the effective, or projected, focal spot size. As target angle *decreases* (i.e., gets steeper or smaller), the effective (projected) focal spot becomes smaller. This is advantageous because it will improve radiographic detail without creating a heat-loading crisis at the anode (as would be the case if the actual focal spot size were reduced to produce a similar detail improvement). There are disadvantages, however. With a smaller target angle the anode heel effect increases; photons are more noticeably absorbed by the "heel" of the anode, resulting in a smaller percentage of x-ray photons at the anode end of the x-ray beam and a concentration of x-ray photons at the cathode end of the image.

5. (D) A digital image is formed by a *matrix* of *pixels* in rows and columns. A matrix having 512 pixels in each row and column is a 512 × 512 matrix. As in traditional radiography, *spatial resolution* is measured in line pairs per millimeter (*lp/mm*). As matrix size is increased, there are more and smaller pixels in the matrix, which means improved resolution. Fewer and larger pixels result in a poor resolution "pixelly" image, that is, one that you can actually see the individual pixel boxes (Fig. 14–23).

6. (A) Radiographic reproducibility is an important concept in producing high-quality diagnostic films. Radiographic results should be consistent and predictable, not only in positioning accuracy but with respect to exposure factors as well. Automatic exposure devices (phototimers and ionization chambers) automatically terminate the x-ray exposure once a predetermined quantity of x-ray has penetrated the patient, thus ensuring consistent results.

7. (A) One advantage of computed radiography is the ability to *manipulate* the image after exposure ("postprocessing"). Image manipulation postprocessing can be used for *windowing, contrast and/or density modification*, or *image subtraction*.

Windowing is a process of changing the contrast and density setting on the finished image. The window *width* controls the *number of shades of gray* in the image (contrast), whereas the window *level* corresponds to the image *density*.

8. (B) The high-voltage, or step-up, transformer functions to *increase voltage* to the necessary kilovoltage. It *decreases the amperage* to milliamperage. The amount of increase or decrease *depends on the transformer ratio*, that is, the number of turns in the primary coil to the number of turns in the secondary coil. The transformer law is as follows:

To Determine Secondary V	To Determine Secondary I
$\dfrac{V_s}{V_p} = \dfrac{N_s}{N_p}$	$\dfrac{I_s}{I_p} = \dfrac{V_p}{V_s}$

Substituting known values,

$$\frac{x}{220} = \frac{75{,}000}{150}$$
$$150x = 16{,}500{,}000$$
$$x = 110{,}000 V \ (=110 kV)$$

9. (B) The principle of self-induction is an example of the second law of electromagnetics (Lenz's law), which states that an induced current within a conductive coil will oppose the direction of the current that induced it. It is important to note that self-induction is a characteristic of AC *only*. The fact that AC constantly changes direction accounts for opposing currents set up in the coil. Two x-ray circuit devices operate on the principle of self-induction: The *autotransformer* operates on the principle of self-induction and enables the radiographer to vary the kilovoltage. The *choke coil* also operates on the principle of self-induction; it is a type of variable resistor that may be used to regulate filament current. The high-voltage transformer operates on the principle of mutual induction.

10. (D) The *gantry* component generally includes an x-ray tube, a detector array, a high-voltage generator, a collimator assembly, slip rings, digital acquisition system (DAS), and laser beams to assist positioning.

The patient/part on the motorized couch is surrounded by the circular gantry opening. Within the circular gantry assembly is the x-ray tube, facing an array of thousands of detectors. In sixth generation CT, the x-ray tube and detectors move around the patient within the gantry.

Seventh generation CT can acquire data from multiple sections—up to 320 sections per rotation—the x-ray tube making many *pulsed exposures*, and the detector array receiving the transmitted photons.

In earlier generations of CT, the x-ray tube rotated 360 degrees around the patient lying on a stationary couch, to obtain a "slice" image. The couch then advanced/indexed, stopped, and the x-ray tube rotated 360 degrees in the opposite direction for the next "slice" image, and so on.

The CT technologist uses the *console* to operate the CT machine, select correct exam protocols, and enter patient demographics.

Standards of Performance and Equipment Evaluation | 15

National Council on Radiation Protection and Measurements (NCRP) Report No. 102 serves as a guide to good medical radiation practices by describing the federal regulations on equipment design, performance, and use. Manufacturers of x-ray equipment must follow guidelines that state maximum x-ray output at specific distances, total quantities of filtration, positive beam limitation, and other guidelines. Radiographers must practice safe *principles of operation*; *preventive maintenance* and *quality control* (QC) checks must be performed at specific intervals to ensure continued safe equipment performance.

Radiologic QC involves monitoring and regulating the variables associated with image production and patient care. Every radiologic facility today must establish QC guidelines and conduct QC programs to provide a consistent standard of care. A properly documented, ongoing, and effective QC program is required by hospital accrediting agencies and state departments of health.

The rationale behind QC is that a radiographic imaging system performing in an erratic and undependable manner results in repeat exposures, thus contributing to unnecessary patient dose and uneconomical use of time, equipment, and supplies. *Radiographic QC* is an organized and methodical evaluation of imaging components from the x-ray tube to the automatic film processor, with the purpose of decreasing repeat exposures, thereby decreasing patient radiation exposure and increasing cost-effectiveness. The *frequency of testing* ranges from daily processor checks to quarterly, semiannual, and annual equipment performance testing. Processor QC was discussed in Chapter 12.

The position of QC technologist is an increasingly important one, requiring advanced knowledge and skills. In recognition of this, the ARRT (American Registry of Radiographic Technologists) has implemented an advanced certification examination in QC.

The QC program requires the combined efforts of the radiographer, QC technologist, service engineer, and medical physicist. The radiographer must be alert to any equipment malfunctions or unusual occurrences and report them to the QC technologist without delay. The QC technologist, service engineer, and medical physicist are responsible for equipment testing, correlation of test results, any necessary corrections or modifications, and accurate documentation of their activities.

QC in digital/electronic imaging is relatively new. There are some established parameters for consideration, but there is much more to be experienced and learned. Established maintenance procedures will be discussed.

EQUIPMENT CALIBRATION

Quality Control refers to our equipment and its safe and accurate operation. Various components must be tested at specified intervals and test results must be within specified parameters. Any deviation from those parameters must be corrected. Examples of equipment components that are tested annually are the focal spot size, linearity, reproducibility, filtration, kV, and exposure time.

Kilovoltage

Kilovoltage accuracy is essential to achieve the desired radiographic contrast. *Calibration* of kV was formerly evaluated using a Wisconsin test tool and cassette. The *digital kV test meters* used today are more convenient and simple to use. When various kilovoltages are tested in the normal diagnostic range (40–150 kV), the selected kilovolt and actual kilovolt value should not differ by more than ±4 kV for *general diagnostic* equipment and by 5% of the nominal kV for *mammography* equipment (Fig. 15–1); for example, at 30 kV, a margin of error of 1.5 kV would be within specifications.

> ### Elements of a Typical QC Program
>
> - Timer accuracy testing
> - Milliampere (mA) linearity testing
> - Kilovolts peak (kV) accuracy testing
> - Half-value layer (HVL) testing
> - Exposure reproducibility testing
> - Focal spot size testing
> - X-ray beam/light field/Bucky tray alignment evaluation
> - Intensified screen cleaning and testing
> - Illuminator cleaning and evaluation
> - Automatic processor maintenance and control
> - X-ray evaluation of lead aprons and gloves

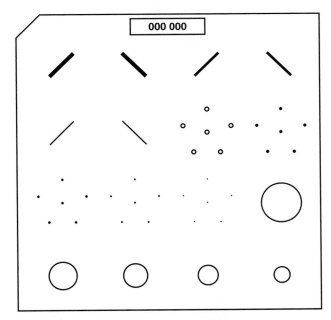

Figure 15–1. A mammographic phantom contains mylar fibers, simulated masses, and specks of simulated calcifications. American College of Radiology accreditation criteria states that a minimum of 10 objects (4 fibers, 3 specks, and 3 masses) must be visualized on test films. (Courtesy of Gammex Inc.)

Milliampere

The accuracy of individual mA stations is related to *patient dose* and is essential for production of expected radiographic *density* levels.

An *aluminum step-wedge* (penetrometer) can be used to evaluate each mA station. A series of exposures is made at a particular kV *using the same mAs* (milliampere-seconds) *value at each mA station*, with exposure time adjusted to maintain a constant mAs. The resulting step-wedge images should be identical. Performance of this test on properly calibrated equipment is a good illustration of the *reciprocity law*. *Linearity* of mA is frequently evaluated using a digital dosimeter (ionization chamber). Exposures are made at a particular mAs with various combinations of mA and time; x-ray output is measured in mR/mAs and should be accurate to within 10%.

Linearity testing is performed after generator modification or calibration, and at least annually.

Timer

Timer accuracy is related to patient dose and the production of expected radiographic density, and should be tested at least on an annual basis. *Spinning-top tests*, for determination of timer accuracy, were described in Chapter 14 (p. 453-455). The use of a digital dosimeter, however, is favored by many as a more simple and accurate measure of timer accuracy. The selected exposure time should be within 5% of the actual exposure time. Similar tests are used to evaluate the accuracy of automatic exposure devices.

Timer accuracy testing is performed after generator modification or calibration, when troubleshooting under- or overexposed images, and at least annually.

Beam Restriction

The collimator assembly (Fig. 15–2) includes a series of lead shutters, a mirror, and a light bulb. The mirror and light bulb function to project the size, location, and center of the irradiated field. The bulb's emitted beam of light is deflected by a mirror placed at an angle of 45 degrees in the path of

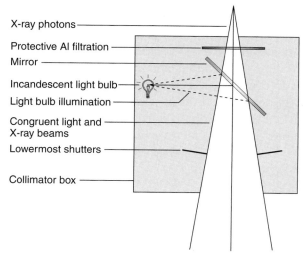

X-ray photons
Protective Al filtration
Mirror
Incandescent light bulb
Light bulb illumination
Congruent light and X-ray beams
Lowermost shutters
Collimator box

Figure 15–2. X-ray and light beams.

the light beam. In order for the projected light beam to be the same size as the x-ray beam, the focal spot and the light bulb *must be exactly the same distance* from the center of the mirror.

Congruence is a term used to describe the relationship between the collimator light field and the actual x-ray field—they must be congruent (i.e., match) to within 2% of the SID. *Centering* indication is required and must be to within 1% of the central ray. PBL must not permit field size to exceed IR size. Collimators should be inspected and verified as accurate *semiannually*, that is, twice a year.

X-ray Tube Overload Protection

Warm-up procedures are performed at the beginning of the day to prevent excessive heat to a cold anode (which could crack the anode). Single exposure overloads are avoided by programmed prevention of an exposure in excess of a particular predetermined amount. The *overload protection circuit testing* is performed after generator modification or calibration, and at least annually.

Reproducibility

This test should be performed annually to evaluate *consistency* of x-ray tube output. A particular group of technical factors is selected and a series of consecutive exposures (at least five) is made. The factors are changed between exposures and then changed back to the original technique. The digital radiation meter should register radiation output that does not vary more than 5%. If a radiographer notices an exposure fluctuation while using a particular group of technical factors, the *reproducibility* test is performed using those factors but, alternately, changing to other technical factors between exposures.

Reproducibility testing is performed when troubleshooting a problem, and at least annually.

Half-Value Layer

HVL testing provides beam quality information that is different from that obtained from kV testing. HVL is defined as the thickness of any absorber that will reduce x-ray beam intensity to one-half its original value. It is determined by measuring the beam intensity without an absorber and then recording the intensity as successive millimeters of aluminum are added to the radiation field. It is influenced by the type of rectification, total filtration, and kV. An x-ray tube HVL should remain almost constant. If HVL decreases, it is an indication of a decrease in the actual kV. If the HVL increases, it indicates the deposition of vaporized tungsten on the inner surface of the glass envelope (as a result of tube aging) or an increase in the actual kV.

Focal Spot Size

Focal spot size accuracy is related to the degree of *geometric blur*, that is, edge gradient or penumbra. Manufacturer tolerance for new focal spots is surprisingly large, 50%; that is, a 0.3-mm focal spot may actually be 0.45 mm (which can significantly impact magnification radiography). Additionally, the focal spot can increase in size as the x-ray tube ages;

hence, the importance of *testing* newly arrived focal spots and periodic testing to monitor focal spots changes.

Focal spot size can be measured with a *pinhole camera, slit camera,* or *star-pattern–type resolution device*. The *pinhole camera* is rather difficult to use accurately and requires the use of excessive tube (heat) loading. With a *slit camera*, two exposures are made: one measures the length of the focal spot and the other measures the width. The *star-pattern–type*, or similar, resolution device can measure focal spot size *as a function of geometric blur* and is readily adaptable in a QC program to monitor focal spot changes over a period of time. It is recommended that focal spot size be checked on installation of a new x-ray tube and annually thereafter.

RADIOGRAPHIC AND FLUOROSCOPIC ACCESSORIES

Cassettes

The exterior of all cassettes should be checked periodically for damage and signs of wear. Loose latches or hinges, damaged frames, or deteriorated felt or sponge should be repaired or replaced.

Intensifying Screens

Intensifying screens should first be visually inspected for abrasions, stains, and other signs of wear. Screens need regular periodic cleaning according to the manufacturer's recommendations. In general, a nonabrasive, lint-free cloth is used with a special antistatic screen cleaner. Care must be taken not to use excessive solution and to allow the screens to dry thoroughly before use.

Adequate screen care includes periodic *screen-to-film contact testing* using the special wire-mesh test device. The cassette to be tested is placed on the x-ray table and the wire-mesh device on top of the cassette, and an exposure is made of approximately 5 mAs and 40 kV. The processed film should be viewed at a distance of at least 6 feet. Any blurry areas are indicative of poor screen-to-film contact and representative of diminished image detail. Cassettes having areas of poor screen-to-film contact must be repaired or replaced, as poor contact will seriously impair *recorded detail*.

Grid cassettes should be evaluated periodically to identify any damage to the fragile lead strips within. The film-loaded grid cassette is slightly exposed, just enough to make the lead strips visible. The processed radiograph is examined for any areas of uneven density or evidence of damaged, misaligned lead strips.

Grids

Frequent rigorous use or mishandling of clip-on/slip-on grids or grid cassettes can result in damage and shifting of the lead strips. These unapparent structural changes result in artifacts that can hide or mimic pathology. Repeat exposures, with resultant patient dose increase, are often necessary. NCRP Report #99, Quality Assurance for Diagnostic Imaging, recommends that grid uniformity be evaluated periodically by imaging a homogeneous phantom with an exposure that will produce an optical density of approximately 1.2.

The report further states that moving grids in x-ray tables should be evaluated before installation and annually thereafter, and that clip-on/slip-on grids and grid cassettes be evaluated every 6 months—or sooner if the grid is damaged or suspected of creating artifacts.

Illumination

One of the most frequently overlooked components of an adequate QC program is radiographic illumination. Radiographic density and contrast can be significantly misrepresented on illuminators providing different degrees of brightness. A radiographic image viewed by the QC technologist in the processor room can look very different on the radiologist's illuminator. A simple light meter, held at the same distance from each illuminator (approximately 3 feet), reveals any differences in illumination.

Illuminator surfaces need to be cleaned periodically to remove buildup of dust and grime. When one bulb in a bank of illuminators requires changing, *all* the bulbs should be changed to guarantee uniform brightness.

Fluoroscopic Exposure Rates

Maximum exposure rate in manual fluoroscopy should not exceed 5 R/min, and 10 R/min in automatic exposure mode—according to the 1986 FDA ruling. Entrance exposure for average size patients undergoing diagnostic fluoro exams commonly receive exposures of up to 25 rad (25cGy). In interventional procedures, entrance doses of 100 rad can be delivered. In consideration of these potentially high doses, it is imperative that the exposure rates are checked regularly. *Generator output testing* is performed whenever the fluoroscopic system is serviced and at least every 6 months.

Lead Aprons and Gloves

Personal fluoroscopic shielding apparel such as lead aprons, gloves, and thyroid shields should be *fluoroscoped annually* to detect any cracks that may have developed in the leaded vinyl.

Proper care is required to help prolong the useful life of lead apparel. If soiled, it can be cleaned with a damp cloth. Lead aprons should not be folded or carelessly dropped to the floor, for that facilitates the development of cracks in the leaded vinyl. Lead aprons and gloves should be hung on appropriate racks when not in use.

DIGITAL IMAGING CONSIDERATIONS

Compared to long-used film/screen imaging, digital/electronic imaging is still relatively new, but a good QC program is essential to consistent, effective operation. There are some established parameters for consideration, but there is much more to be experienced and learned. Established maintenance procedures will be covered here.

A *daily density check* on the printer/processor should be performed according to the manufacturer's recommendations. The air intakes on the *reader* should be cleaned weekly or according to the manufacturer's recommendations.

The *laser* in the computed radiography (CR) reader should be checked monthly for evidence of "jitter." Regular *contrast evaluation* is recommended; this confirms the consistency of the x-ray exposure, CR reader, workstation display, and hardcopy printer. A *sharpness* test is performed to evaluate the x-ray tube performance, CR reader optics, monitor display, and hardcopy printer. The assessment of the exposure index/sensitivity checks the calibration and consistency of the actual x-ray exposures as well as the photomultiplier tube of the CR reader. Other tests include assessment of image *noise*, *artifacts*, *erasure* thoroughness, and *linearity* testing. A special phantom is provided to evaluate all system components/characteristics (Fig. 15–3).

CR image plates (IPs) should be visually checked on a regular basis for any physical damage. Inserting a damaged IP into the reader can result in mechanical failure and system shutdown. The photostimulable phosphor (PSP) storage screen should be removed before cleaning the IP. IPs should be treated in the same way as traditional screen–film cassettes in the presence of blood–body fluids (placed in plastic bag for use). Never place a damp, wet IP into the reader.

The *PSPs* should be cleaned monthly. It is important that *anhydrous ethanol* be used for cleaning most CR PSPs; using any other cleaner can cause breakdown of the PSPs protective coat. A small amount of

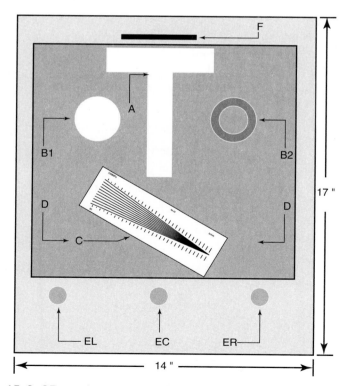

Figure 15–3. CR requires a regular QA program, just as other imaging systems and system components. The figure shows a typical CR test phantom; it is used to evaluate the accuracy of several system components/characteristics. (Courtesy FUJIFILM Medical Systems USA, Inc.)

anhydrous ethanol is placed on a lint-free cloth for cleaning and removal of any dust or other particles. Remnant moisture of any kind must be avoided; it can cause the phosphors to swell. *Dust* on PSPs has the same effect as that of dust on intensifying screens—a clear pinhole artifact. PSPs should be checked for physical damage too. *Scratches* appear as clear areas on the resulting image.

Appropriate care ensures a maximum useful life. The life of the typical PSP is approximately 10,000 exposures

Summary

- The function of QC is to provide consistent high-quality radiographs, thus reducing patient dose and increasing cost-effectiveness.
- QC programs involve evaluation and documentation of all imaging components from the x-ray tube to automatic processor.
- Kilovoltage accuracy can be determined using a Wisconsin test cassette or digital meter, and must be accurate to within 5 kV ($\pm 10\%$).
- Milliamperage accuracy is determined using an aluminum step-wedge or digital dosimeter, and must be accurate to within 10%.
- Timer accuracy is evaluated using a manual spinning top (for $S\varphi$) or synchronous spinning top (for 3φ), and must be accurate to within 5%. Reproducibility refers to tube output consistency and must not vary more than 5%.
- HVL is tested periodically to evaluate x-ray beam quality; HVL should remain almost constant.
- Focal spot size is tested by using a pinhole camera, slit camera, or star-pattern–type resolution device on installation and every year thereafter.
- Cassette exteriors and interiors should be inspected periodically.
- Intensifying screens must be cleaned regularly and screen-to-film contact testing performed periodically.
- Grid cassettes should be tested for damaged lead strips.
- Illuminators must be cleaned and checked for uniformity.
- Lead gloves and aprons must be fluoroscoped annually to detect any cracks; they should be properly hung when not in use.
- CR printer/processors should have a daily density check performed.
- Reader air intakes should be checked weekly.
- IPs and their PSPs should be visually checked and correctly cleaned on a regular basis.
- Dust and scratches on CR PSPs create artifacts similar to those created with screen-to-film cassettes.

COMPREHENSION CHECK

Congratulations! You have completed your review of the entire chapter. If you are able to answer the following group of very comprehensive questions, you should feel confident that you have really mastered this section. You are then ready to go on to "Registry-type" questions that follow. For greatest success, do not go to these multiple-choice questions without first completing the short-answer questions below.

1. Describe the value of a QC program (p. 493).

2. Identify the method used for kV calibration and the required degree of accuracy (p. 494).

3. Describe the method of evaluating mA calibration using an aluminum step-wedge (p. 495).

4. Describe how mA linearity is usually evaluated, and identify the required degree of accuracy (p. 495).

5. Describe how Sφ and 3φ timer accuracy is evaluated, identify the appropriate tool for each, give examples of acceptable results, and identify the degree of accuracy required (p. 495).

6. Explain what is meant by reproducibility, and identify the degree of accuracy required (p. 496).

7. Define HVL and list the three factors that influence it (p. 496).

8. Explain how tube aging can result in increased HVL (p. 496).

9. Identify when the focal spot size should be checked and the three devices that can be used to determine focal spot size (p. 496, 497).

10. Describe the important relationship between the focal spot, mirror, and collimator light bulb (p. 495, 496).

11. Describe the conditions/faults/injuries that cassettes and intensifying screens should be visually checked for (p. 497).

12. Explain the need for, and proper method of, periodic screen cleaning (p. 497).

13. Describe the purpose and method of screen-to-film contact testing (p. 497).

14. Explain when/how to check the condition of a grid (p. 497, 498).

15. Explain the necessity of QA checks on illumination (p. 498).

16. Describe the proper care, storage, and checking of lead apparel (p. 498).

17. How often should density checks be made on CR printer/processors? How often the air intakes be checked (p. 498, 499)?

18. How should CR cassettes be checked and cleaned (p. 499).

19. If a CR IP has particles of dust on it, how will that appear on the digital image (p. 499, 500)?

20. If a CR IP is scratched, how will that appear on the digital image (p. 500)?

CHAPTER REVIEW QUESTIONS

1. Radiographs from a particular three-phase, full-wave rectified x-ray unit were underexposed, using known correct exposures. A synchronous spinning-top test was performed using 100 mA, 1/20 second, and 70 kV, and a 12-degree arc is observed on the test film. Which of the following is *most* likely the problem?

   (A) The 1/20-second time station is inaccurate

   (B) The 100-mA station is inaccurate

   (C) A rectifier is not functioning

   (D) The processor needs servicing

2. Which of the following refers to a regular program of evaluation that ensures proper functioning of x-ray equipment, thereby protecting both patients and radiation workers?

   (A) Sensitometry

   (B) Densitometry

   (C) Quality assurance

   (D) Modulation transfer function

3. Which of the following is used to evaluate focal spot size?

   (A) Spinning top

   (B) Wire mesh

   (C) Slit camera

   (D) Penetrometer

4. Which of the following is usually recommended for cleaning PSPs?

   (A) Denatured alcohol

   (B) Anhydrous ethanol

   (C) Soap and water

   (D) Intensifying screen cleaner

5. Proper care of leaded apparel includes:

   1. Periodic check for cracks

   2. Careful folding following each use

   3. Routine laundering with soap and water

   (A) 1 only

   (B) 1 and 2 only

   (C) 1 and 3 only

   (D) 1, 2, and 3

6. Periodic equipment calibration includes testing of the:

   1. Focal spot

   2. mA

   3. kV

   (A) 1 only

   (B) 1 and 3 only

   (C) 2 and 3 only

   (D) 1, 2, and 3

7. The spinning-top test can be used to evaluate the:

   1. Timer accuracy

   2. Rectifier failure

   3. Effect of kV on contrast

   (A) 1 only

   (B) 2 only

   (C) 1 and 2 only

   (D) 1, 2, and 3

8. Which of the following contribute(s) to inherent filtration?

   1. X-ray tube glass envelope

   2. X-ray tube port window

   3. Aluminum between tube housing and collimator

   (A) 1 only

   (B) 1 and 2 only

   (C) 1 and 3 only

   (D) 1, 2, and 3

9. By which of the following can poor screen-to-film contact be caused?

   1. Damaged cassette frame

   2. Foreign body in cassette

   3. Warped cassette front

   (A) 1 only

   (B) 2 only

   (C) 1 and 3 only

   (D) 1, 2, and 3

10. A quality assurance program includes checks
    on which of the following radiographic
    equipment conditions?
    1. Reproducibility
    2. Linearity
    3. Positive beam limitation
    (A) 1 only
    (B) 1 and 2 only
    (C) 1 and 3 only
    (D) 1, 2, and 3

Answers and Explanations

1. (A) A synchronous spinning-top test is used to test timer accuracy or rectifier function in three-phase equipment. Because three-phase, full-wave rectified current would expose a 360-degree arc per second, a 1/20-second exposure should expose an 18-degree arc. Anything more or less indicates timer inaccuracy. If exactly one-half of the expected arc appears, one should suspect rectifier failure.

2. (C) Sensitometry and densitometry are used in evaluation of the film processor, just one part of a complete QA program. Modulation transfer function is used to express spatial resolution, which is another component of a QA program. A complete QA program includes testing of all components of the imaging system: processors, focal spot, x-ray timers, filters, intensifying screens, beam alignment, and so on.

3. (C) Focal spot size accuracy is directly related to the degree of *geometric blur*; that is, as focal spot size increases, blur increases. Manufacturer tolerance for new focal spots is 50%, and focal spot size can increase in size as the x-ray tube ages; hence, the importance of *testing* new focal spots and periodic testing to monitor any focal spot changes. Focal spot size can be measured with a *pinhole camera*, *slit camera*, or *star-pattern*–type *resolution device*. The pinhole camera and slit camera measure the physical size of the focal spot, whereas the star-pattern–type resolution device measures focal spot size as a function of resolution/geometric blur.

Perfect screen-to-film contact is essential to recorded detail and is evaluated with a *wire-mesh* test. A *spinning-top* test is used to evaluate timer accuracy and rectifier operation. A *penetrometer* (aluminum step-wedge) is used to illustrate the effect of kV on contrast.

4. (B) CR *PSPs* should be cleaned monthly. It is important that *anhydrous ethanol* be used for cleaning most CR PSPs. A small amount of anhydrous ethanol is placed on a lint-free cloth for cleaning and removal of any dust or other particles. Water and remnant moisture must not be used as it can cause phosphor swelling. *Dust* on PSPs has the same effect as that of dust on intensifying screens—a clear pinhole artifact. PSPs should also be checked for physical damage. Scratches appear as clear areas on the

resulting image. CR *IPs* should be visually checked for physical damage; inserting a damaged CR IP into the reader can result in mechanical failure and system shutdown.

5. (A) Protective lead aprons and gloves are made of lead-impregnated vinyl or leather. They should be checked for cracks radiographically from time to time. Otherwise, minimal care is required. Lead aprons and gloves should always be hung on appropriate hangers. Glove supports permit air to circulate within the glove. Apron hangers provide convenient storage without folding. If lead aprons are folded (or just left in a heap), cracks are more likely to form. If lead aprons or gloves become soiled, cleaning with a damp cloth and appropriate solution is all that is required. Excessive moisture should be avoided.

6. (D) Radiographic results should be consistent and predictable not only in positioning accuracy but in exposure factors and image sharpness as well. X-ray equipment should be calibrated periodically as part of an ongoing QA program. The quantity (mAs) and quality (kV) of the primary beam have a big impact on the quality of the finished radiograph. The focal spot should be tested periodically to evaluate its impact on image sharpness.

7. (C) The spinning-top test is used to evaluate *timer accuracy* or *rectifier failure*. With single-phase, full-wave rectified equipment (120 pulses/s), for example, 12 dots should be visualized when using the 1/10-second time station. A few more or less indicate timer inaccuracy. If the test demonstrated 6 dots, one may suspect rectifier failure. With three-phase equipment, a special synchronous spinning top (or oscilloscope) is used and a solid black arc is obtained rather than dots. The length of this arc is measured and compared with the known correct arc.

8. (B) Inherent filtration is that which is "built into" the construction of the x-ray tube. Before exiting the x-ray tube, x-ray photons must pass through the tube's glass envelope and port window; the photons are filtered somewhat as they do so. This inherent filtration is usually the equivalent of 0.5 mm Al. Aluminum filtration *placed* between the x-ray tube housing and the collimator is added to contribute to the total necessary requirement of 2.5-mm Al equivalent. The collimator itself is considered part of the added filtration (1.0-mm Al equivalent) because of the silver surface of the mirror within. It is important to remember that as aluminum filtration is added to the x-ray tube, the HVL increases.

9. **(D)** Perfect contact between the intensifying screens and the film is essential to maintain image sharpness. Any separation between them allows diffusion of fluorescent light and subsequent blurriness and loss of detail. Screen-to-film contact can be diminished if the cassette frame is damaged and misshapen, if the front is warped, or if there is a foreign body between the screens elevating them.

10. **(D)** The accuracy of all three is important to ensure adequate patient protection. *Reproducibility* means that repeated exposures at a given technique must provide consistent intensity. *Linearity* means that a given mAs, using different mA stations with appropriate exposure time adjustments, provides consistent intensity. *Positive beam limitation* is automatic collimation and must be accurate to 2% of the source-to-image-receptor distance. Light-localized collimators must be available and must be accurate to within 2%.

Practice Test | 16

This practice test is intended to simulate the actual certification examination. Set aside special time for this test after your preparations for the actual examination are complete. Try to *simulate the actual examination environment* as much as possible. Choose a quiet place free from distractions and interruptions, gather the necessary materials, and arrange to be uninterrupted for *up to 3 hours*.

Each of the numbered items or incomplete statements in this section is followed by answers or completions of the statement. Select the lettered answer or completion that is *best* in each case.

1. The histogram demonstration of pixel value distribution can be changed/affected by the following:
   1. Selection of processing algorithm
   2. Processing delay
   3. Centering
   (A) 1 only
   (B) 1 and 2 only
   (C) 2 and 3 only
   (D) 1, 2, and 3

2. What is used to account for the relative radiosensitivity of various tissues and organs?
   1. Radiation weighting factors (W_r)
   2. Tissue weighting factors (W_t)
   3. Absorbed dose
   (A) 1 only
   (B) 2 only
   (C) 2 and 3 only
   (D) 1, 2, and 3

3. Which of the following statements regarding Figure 16–1A and 16–1B is true?
   (A) In Figure 16–1A, the CR and plantar surface form a 30-degree angle
   (B) In Figure 16–1A, the CR and plantar surface form a 60-degree angle
   (C) In Figure 16–1B, the CR and plantar surface form a 30-degree angle
   (D) In Figure 16–1B, the CR and plantar surface form a 60-degree angle

4. Photostimulable luminescence (PSL) occurs when the photostimulable phosphor is exposed to:
   (A) Monochromatic laser light
   (B) Barium fluorohalide
   (C) High-energy x-ray photons
   (D) Low-energy x-ray photons

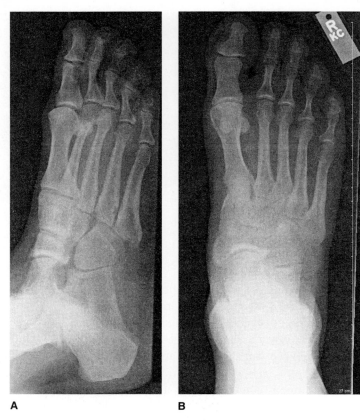

A   **B**

Figure 16–1. **(A)** and **(B)**. Courtesy of Conrad P Ehrlich, MD.

5. What is the relationship between source-to-image-receptor distance (SID), beam intensity, and image density in screen/film imaging?

(A) As SID increases, beam intensity increases and image density increases

(B) As SID increases, beam intensity increases and image density decreases

(C) As SID increases, beam intensity decreases and image density increases

(D) As SID increases, beam intensity decreases and image density decreases

6. When reviewing patients' blood chemistry levels, what is considered the normal creatinine range?

(A) 0.6–1.5 mg/100 mL

(B) 4.5–6.0 mg/100 mL

(C) 8–25 mg/100 mL

(D) Up to 50 mg/100 mL

7. Symptoms of imminent anaphylactic shock include:

1. Dysphasia

2. Itching of palms and soles

3. Constriction of the throat

(A) 1 only

(B) 2 only

(C) 2 and 3 only

(D) 1, 2, and 3

8. Which of the following is (are) well demonstrated in the oblique position/projection of the cervical spine?

1. Intervertebral foramina

2. Apophyseal joints

3. Intervertebral joints

(A) 1 only

(B) 1 and 2 only

(C) 2 and 3 only

(D) 1, 2, and 3

9. Which of the following factors impacts radiation damage to biologic tissue?

   1. Radiation quality
   2. Absorbed dose
   3. Size of irradiated area
   (A) 1 only
   (B) 2 only
   (C) 1 and 2 only
   (D) 1, 2, and 3

10. Which ethical principle below is most closely related to avoidance of deception?
    (A) Autonomy
    (B) Beneficence
    (C) Fidelity
    (D) Veracity

11. *Somatic effects* of radiation refer to effects that are manifested:
    (A) In the descendants of the exposed individual
    (B) During the life of the exposed individual
    (C) In the exposed individual and his or her descendants
    (D) In the reproductive cells of the exposed individual

12. The right colic flexure is formed by the junction of the:
    (A) Transverse and ascending colon
    (B) Descending and transverse colon
    (C) Descending and sigmoid colon
    (D) Cecum and ascending colon

13. Which of the following imaging procedures do *not* require the use of ionizing radiation to produce an image?

    1. Sonography
    2. Computerized tomography
    3. Magnetic resonance imaging
    (A) 1 and 2 only
    (B) 1 and 3 only
    (C) 2 and 3 only
    (D) 1, 2, and 3

14. As a result of the anode heel effect, the intensity of the x-ray beam is greatest along the:
    (A) Path of the central ray
    (B) Anode end of the beam
    (C) Cathode end of the beam
    (D) Transverse axis of the image receptor

15. The position seen in Figure 16–2, used to demonstrate the intercondyloid fossa, requires that the central ray (CR) be directed:
    (A) Vertically to the joint space
    (B) Parallel to the long axis of the tibia
    (C) Perpendicular to the long axis of the tibia
    (D) Perpendicular to the joint space

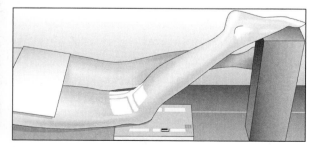

A   B

Figure 16–2. **(A)** and **(B)**.

16. Symptoms of shock include:
    1. Pallor and weakness
    2. Increased pulse rate
    3. Fever
    (A) 1 only
    (B) 1 and 2 only
    (C) 1 and 3 only
    (D) 1, 2, and 3

17. The current term *health care-acquired infection* (HAI) replaces which of the following terms?
    (A) Upper respiratory infection (URI)
    (B) Urinary tract infection (UTI)
    (C) Suppressed infection
    (D) Nosocomial infection

18. The term *effective dose* refers to:
    (A) Whole-body dose
    (B) Localized organ dose
    (C) Genetic effects
    (D) Somatic and genetic effects

19. With the body in the erect position, the diaphragm moves:
    (A) 2–4 inches higher than when recumbent
    (B) 2–4 inches lower than when recumbent
    (C) 2–4 inches superiorly
    (D) Very slightly

20. With all other factors constant, as a digital image's matrix size increases:
    1. Pixel size decreases
    2. Resolution increases
    3. Pixel size increases
    (A) 1 only
    (B) 2 only
    (C) 1 and 2 only
    (D) 2 and 3 only

21. During a gastrointestinal examination, the AP recumbent projection of a stomach of average shape usually demonstrates:
    1. Barium-filled fundus
    2. Double-contrast of distal stomach portions
    3. Barium-filled duodenum and pylorus
    (A) 1 only
    (B) 1 and 2 only
    (C) 1 and 3 only
    (D) 1, 2, and 3

22. The American Hospital Association's Patient Care Partnership includes the essentials of the Bill of Rights and reviews what patients can/should expect during a hospital stay, including:
    1. Protection of patient privacy
    2. Help with billing claims
    3. Help when leaving the hospital
    (A) 1 only
    (B) 1 and 2 only
    (C) 2 and 3 only
    (D) 1, 2, and 3

23. In which of the following positions was the image seen in Figure 16–3 made?
    (A) AP erect
    (B) PA recumbent
    (C) Right lateral decubitus
    (D) Left lateral decubitus

24. Advantages of moving the image intensifier closer to the patient during traditional fluoroscopy include:
    1. Decreased SID
    2. Decreased patient dose
    3. Improved image quality
    (A) 1 only
    (B) 1 and 2 only
    (C) 1 and 3 only
    (D) 1, 2, and 3

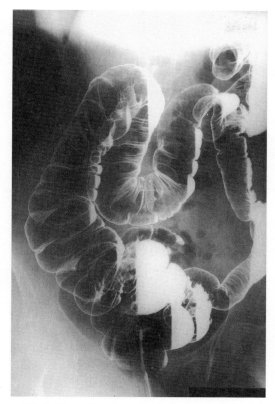

Figure 16–3. From the American College of Radiology Learning File. Courtesy of the American College of Radiology.

25. The exposure factors used for a particular non-grid film/screen x-ray image were 400 mA, 0.02 second, and 90 kV. Another film/screen image using an 8:1 grid is requested. Which of the following groups of factors is *most* appropriate?

    (A) 400 mA, 0.02 second, 110 kV

    (B) 200 mA, 0.08 second, 90 kV

    (C) 300 mA, 0.05 second, 100 kV

    (D) 400 mA, 0.08 second, 90 kV

26. Which of the "curves" seen in Figure 16–4 best illustrates the dynamic range of a CR photostimulable phosphor (PSP)?

    (A) Curve A

    (B) Curve B

    (C) Both represent a CR PSP

    (D) Neither represents a CR PSP

27. Which of the following factor(s) is (are) important in determining thickness of protective barriers?

    1. Distance between x-ray source and barrier

    2. Occupancy factor time

    3. Workload (mA-min/wk)

    (A) 1 only

    (B) 1 and 2 only

    (C) 2 and 3 only

    (D) 1, 2, and 3

28. An autoclave is used for:

    (A) Dry heat sterilization

    (B) Chemical sterilization

    (C) Gas sterilization

    (D) Steam sterilization

29. When examining the fourth and fifth fingers in the lateral position, which side of the forearm should be closest to the image receptor?

    (A) Anterior

    (B) Posterior

    (C) Medial

    (D) Lateral

30. Which image intensifier component emits electrons?

    (A) Input phosphor

    (B) Photocathode

    (C) Focusing lenses

    (D) Output phosphor

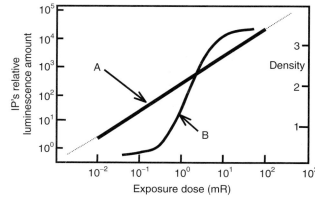

Figure 16–4. Courtesy of FUJIFILM Medical Systems USA, Inc.

31. What artifact, associated with digital imaging, can result if the direction of the grid's lead strips and the grid frequency match the scan frequency of the scanner/reader?

    (A) Phantom image

    (B) Skipped scan lines

    (C) Aliasing

    (D) Grid lines

32. Examples of primary radiation barriers include:

    1. X-ray room walls

    2. Control booth

    3. Lead aprons

    (A) 1 only

    (B) 1 and 2 only

    (C) 2 and 3 only

    (D) 1, 2, and 3

33. Which formula would the radiographer use to determine the total number of heat units produced with a given exposure using three-phase, twelve-pulse equipment?

    (A) mA × time × kV

    (B) mA × time × kV × 3.0

    (C) mA × time × kV × 1.4

    (D) mA × time × kV × 1.6

34. Diseases whose mode of transmission is air include:

    1. Tuberculosis

    2. Mumps

    3. Rubella

    (A) 1 only

    (B) 1 and 2 only

    (C) 1 and 3 only

    (D) 1, 2, and 3

35. Which of the following image matrix sizes will provide the best spatial resolution?

    (A) 256 × 256

    (B) 512 × 512

    (C) 1,024 × 1024

    (D) 2,048 × 2048

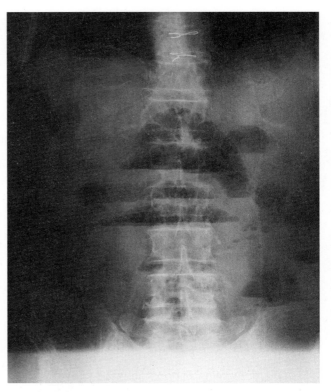

Figure 16–5. Courtesy of Stamford Hospital, Department of Radiology.

36. In which of the following positions was the radiograph seen in Figure 16–5 made?

    (A) AP erect

    (B) PA recumbent

    (C) Right lateral decubitus

    (D) Dorsal decubitus

37. The photoelectric process is an interaction between an x-ray photon and:

    (A) An inner shell electron

    (B) An outer shell electron

    (C) A nucleus

    (D) Another photon

38. What transforms the violet light emitted by the PSP into the image seen on the monitor?

    (A) The photostimulable phosphor

    (B) The scanner/reader

    (C) The analog-to-digital converter (ADC)

    (D) The helium–neon laser

39. When imaging the skull with the orbitomeatal line (OML) perpendicular to the image receptor and the CR directed 25-degrees cephalad:

    1. The occipital bone is well demonstrated
    2. The dorsum sella is seen within the foramen magnum
    3. The petrous pyramids fill the orbits

    (A) 1 only
    (B) 1 and 2 only
    (C) 2 and 3 only
    (D) 1, 2, and 3

40. A profile view of the glenoid fossa can be obtained with the CR directed perpendicular to the glenoid fossa and the patient rotated:

    (A) 20 degree, affected side down
    (B) 20 degree, affected side up
    (C) 45 degree, affected side down
    (D) 45 degree, affected side up

41. Characteristics of nonstochastic effects of radiation include:

    1. They have predictability
    2. They have a threshold
    3. Severity is directly related to dose

    (A) 1 only
    (B) 1 and 2 only
    (C) 2 and 3 only
    (D) 1, 2, and 3

42. Chemical substances that are used to kill pathogenic bacteria are called:

    1. Antiseptics
    2. Germicides
    3. Disinfectants

    (A) 1 only
    (B) 1 and 2 only
    (C) 2 and 3 only
    (D) 1, 2, and 3

43. Potential violations of the ARRT Honor Code include:

    1. Falsification of clinical competency documents
    2. Cheating and/or plagiarism
    3. Violating patient confidentiality

    (A) 1 only
    (B) 1 and 2 only
    (C) 2 and 3 only
    (D) 1, 2, and 3

44. In which of the following locations can the pulse be detected only by the use of a stethoscope?

    (A) Wrist
    (B) Apex of the heart
    (C) Groin
    (D) Neck

45. Mobile fluoroscopic equipment has all of the following features, *except*:

    (A) An image intensifier
    (B) A spot-film device
    (C) A TV monitor
    (D) A TV camera

46. In which position was the radiograph seen in Figure 16–6B made?

    (A) AP erect
    (B) AP recumbent
    (C) PA erect
    (D) PA recumbent

47. What portion of a computed radiography IP records the radiologic image?

    (A) The photostimulable phosphor
    (B) The scanner/reader
    (C) The emulsion
    (D) The helium–neon laser

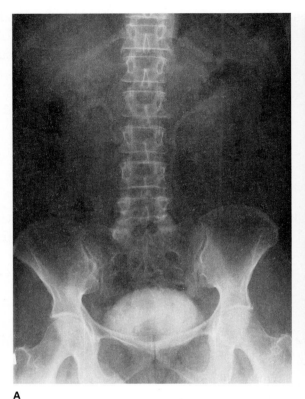
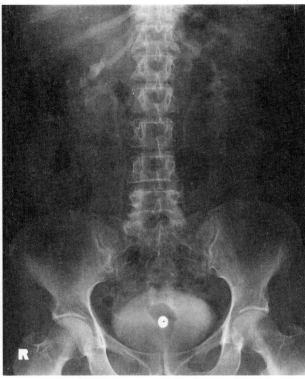

A

B

Figure 16–6. **(A)** and **(B)**. Courtesy of Stamford Hospital, Department of Radiology.

48. The following bones participate in the formation of the knee joint:
    1. Femur
    2. Tibia
    3. Patella
    (A) 1 and 2 only
    (B) 1 and 3 only
    (C) 2 and 3 only
    (D) 1, 2, and 3

49. Which of the following types of adult tissues is (are) relatively insensitive to radiation exposure?
    1. Muscle tissue
    2. Nerve tissue
    3. Epithelial tissue
    (A) 1 only
    (B) 1 and 2 only
    (C) 2 and 3 only
    (D) 1, 2, and 3

50. To better demonstrate ribs below the diaphragm:
    1. Suspend respiration at the end of full exhalation
    2. Suspend respiration at the end of deep inhalation
    3. Perform the examination in the recumbent position
    (A) 1 only
    (B) 2 only
    (C) 1 and 3 only
    (D) 2 and 3 only

51. Any wall that the useful x-ray beam can be directed toward is called a:
    (A) Secondary barrier
    (B) Primary barrier
    (C) Leakage barrier
    (D) Scattered barrier

52. In which of the following positions should you place a patient who is experiencing syncope?

    (A) Dorsal recumbent with head elevated

    (B) Dorsal recumbent with feet elevated

    (C) Lateral recumbent

    (D) Seated with feet supported

53. The phenomenon in which the radiographic information recorded on the photostimulable phosphor/storage phosphor screen (PSP/SPS) upon exposure to x-rays decreases with the elapsed time until it is read by the scanner/reader is termed:

    (A) Excitation

    (B) Photostimulable luminescence

    (C) Scatter

    (D) Fading

54. Arrange the following tissues in order of *decreasing* radiosensitivity:

    1. Liver cells

    2. Intestinal crypt cells

    3. Muscle cells

    (A) 1, 3, 2

    (B) 2, 3, 1

    (C) 2, 1, 3

    (D) 3, 1, 2

55. A particular phosphor's ability to translate absorbed x-ray energy to fluorescent light is termed:

    (A) Density factor

    (B) Intensification factor

    (C) Conversion efficiency

    (D) Detective quantum efficiency

56. Glenohumeral joint dislocation can be evaluated with which of the following?

    1. Inferosuperior axial

    2. Transthoracic lateral

    3. Scapular Y projection

    (A) 1 only

    (B) 1 and 2 only

    (C) 2 and 3 only

    (D) 1, 2, and 3

57. A patient is usually required to drink barium sulfate suspension in order to demonstrate which of the following structure(s)?

    1. Pylorus

    2. Sigmoid

    3. Duodenum

    (A) 1 and 2 only

    (B) 1 and 3 only

    (C) 2 and 3 only

    (D) 3 only

58. Under which of the following conditions is biologic material most sensitive to radiation exposure?

    (A) Anoxic

    (B) Hypoxic

    (C) Oxygenated

    (D) Deoxygenated

59. Which of the following conditions will demonstrate least x-ray penetrability?

    (A) Fibrosarcoma

    (B) Osteomalacia

    (C) Paralytic ileus

    (D) Ascites

60. The image intensifier's input phosphor is generally composed of:

    (A) Cesium iodide

    (B) Zinc cadmium sulfide

    (C) Gadolinium oxysulfide

    (D) Calcium tungstate

61. What does the letter *M* represent in Figure 16–7?

    (A) Scaphoid

    (B) Pisiform

    (C) Trapezium

    (D) Hamate

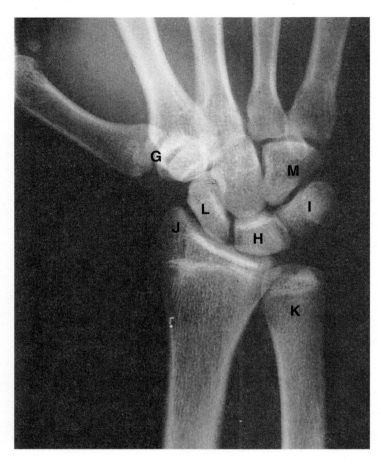

Figure 16–7. Courtesy of Bob Wong, RT.

62. Hysterosalpingography may be performed for the demonstration of:

1. Uterine tubal patency
2. Mass lesions in the uterine cavity
3. Uterine position

(A) 1 and 2 only
(B) 1 and 3 only
(C) 2 and 3 only
(D) 1, 2, and 3

63. Double-contrast examinations of the stomach or large bowel are performed for better visualization of:

(A) Position of the organ
(B) Size and shape of the organ
(C) Diverticula
(D) Gastric or bowel mucosa

64. If the exposure rate at 3 feet from the fluoroscopic table is 40 mR/h, what will be the exposure rate for 30 minutes at a distance of 5 feet from the table?

(A) 7 mR
(B) 12 mR
(C) 14 mR
(D) 24 mR

65. The medical suffix *plasia* refers to:

(A) Embryonic
(B) Condition
(C) Movement
(D) Development

66. The AP axial projection (Towne method) of the skull *best* demonstrates the:

   (A) Occipital bone

   (B) Frontal bone

   (C) Facial bones

   (D) Sphenoid bone

67. Structures found within the mediastinum include all of the following, *except* the:

   (A) Esophagus

   (B) Thymus

   (C) Heart

   (D) Terminal bronchiole

68. A student radiographer who is younger than 18 years must not receive an annual occupational dose greater than:

   (A) 0.1 rem (1 mSv)

   (B) 0.5 rem (5 mSv)

   (C) 5 rem (50 mSv)

   (D) 10 rem (100 mSv)

69. Proper body mechanics includes a wide base of support. The base of support is the portion of the body:

   (A) In contact with the floor or other horizontal surface

   (B) In the midportion of the pelvis or lower abdomen

   (C) Passing through the center of gravity

   (D) None of the above

70. In which of the following projections or positions will subacromial or subcoracoid dislocation be best demonstrated?

   (A) Tangential

   (B) AP axial

   (C) Transthoracic lateral

   (D) PA oblique scapular Y

71. Accurate operation of the automatic exposure control (AEC) device is dependent on:

   1. Thickness and density of the object

   2. Positioning of the object with respect to the ionization chamber

   3. Beam restriction

   (A) 1 only

   (B) 1 and 2 only

   (C) 2 and 3 only

   (D) 1, 2, and 3

72. Major effect(s) of deoxyribonucleic acid (DNA) irradiation includes:

   1. Malignant disease

   2. Chromosome aberration

   3. Cell death

   (A) 1 only

   (B) 1 and 2 only

   (C) 2 and 3 only

   (D) 1, 2, and 3

73. The voltage ripple associated with a three-phase, twelve-pulse rectified generator is approximately:

   (A) 100%

   (B) 32%

   (C) 13%

   (D) 3%

74. When a radiographer is obtaining patient history, both subjective and objective data should be obtained. An example of *subjective* data is:

   (A) The patient appears to have a productive cough

   (B) The patient has a blood pressure of 130/95

   (C) The patient states he or she experiences extreme pain in the upright position

   (D) The patient has a palpable mass in the right upper quadrant of the left breast

75. The exposed PSP is subjected to a narrow laser beam:
    (A) On the display monitor
    (B) In the scanner/reader
    (C) In the cassette
    (D) On the film emulsion

76. What is the best way to reduce magnification distortion?
    (A) Use a small focal spot
    (B) Increase the SID
    (C) Decrease the OID
    (D) Use a slow screen–film combination

77. Which of the following medical abbreviations mean *three times a day*?
    (A) TID
    (B) QID
    (C) QH
    (D) PC

78. The energy of x-ray photons has an inverse relationship to:
    1. Photon wavelength
    2. Applied mA
    3. Applied kV
    (A) 1 only
    (B) 1 and 2 only
    (C) 1 and 3 only
    (D) 1, 2, and 3

79. Cervical spine positions performed to demonstrate the intervertebral foramina closest to the image receptor are:
    (A) Right anterior oblique (RAO) and left anterior oblique (LAO)
    (B) Right posterior oblique (RPO) and left posterior oblique (LPO)
    (C) Anteroposterior (AP)
    (D) Lateral

80. A patient was positioned for a radiographic projection with the x-ray tube, grid, and image receptor properly aligned, but with the body part angled. Which of the following will result?
    (A) Grid cutoff at the periphery of the image
    (B) Grid cutoff along the center of the image
    (C) Increased density at the periphery
    (D) Image distortion

81. It is recommended that PSPs be read soon after exposure, principally, to avoid:
    (A) Aliasing artifacts
    (B) Image fading
    (C) Overdevelopment
    (D) Excessive brightness

82. What does the letter *D* represent in Figure 16–8?
    (A) Fundus
    (B) Pylorus
    (C) Body of stomach
    (D) Bulb of duodenum

83. What does the letter *H* represent in Figure 16–8?
    (A) Jejunum
    (B) Ascending duodenum
    (C) Descending duodenum
    (D) Bulb of duodenum

84. What structure occupies the area represented by the letter *G* in Figure 16–8?
    (A) Gallbladder
    (B) Right lobe of the liver
    (C) Head of the pancreas
    (D) Hepatic flexure of the colon

85. In what position was the radiograph seen in Figure 16–8 made?
    (A) AP
    (B) LPO
    (C) RAO
    (D) Lateral

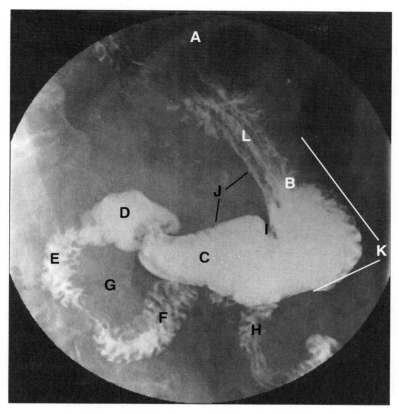

Figure 16–8. Courtesy of Stamford Hospital, Department of Radiology.

86. The purposes of an advanced health care directive, or living will, include all of the following, *except*:

(A) Preserves a person's right to make decisions regarding his or her own health care

(B) Names the individual authorized to make health care decisions for them

(C) Ensures that only the patient's personal physician can make health care decisions for him or her

(D) Includes specifics regarding do not resuscitate (DNR), do not intubate (DNI), and other end-of-life decisions

87. An increase in added filtration will result in:

1. An increase in maximum energy of the x-ray beam

2. A decrease in x-ray intensity

3. An increase in effective energy of the x-ray beam

(A) 1 only

(B) 1 and 2 only

(C) 2 and 3 only

(D) 1, 2, and 3

88. Which of the following will have an effect on radiographic contrast?

1. Beam restriction

2. Grids

3. Focal spot size

(A) 1 only

(B) 1 and 2 only

(C) 2 and 3 only

(D) 1, 2, and 3

89. Which of the following medical equipment is used to determine blood pressure?
    1. Pulse oximeter
    2. Stethoscope
    3. Sphygmomanometer
    (A) 1 and 2 only
    (B) 1 and 3 only
    (C) 2 and 3 only
    (D) 1, 2, and 3

90. Which of the following statements regarding human gonadal cells is (are) accurate?
    1. The female oogonia reproduce only during fetal life
    2. The male spermatogonia reproduce continuously
    3. Both male and female stem cells reproduce only during fetal life
    (A) 1 only
    (B) 2 only
    (C) 1 and 2 only
    (D) 3 only

91. Underexposure of a film/screen x-ray image can be caused by all of the following, *except*:
    (A) Insufficient mA
    (B) Insufficient exposure time
    (C) Insufficient kV
    (D) Insufficient SID

92. Exposure rate increases with an increase in:
    1. mA
    2. kV
    3. SID
    (A) 1 only
    (B) 1 and 2 only
    (C) 2 and 3 only
    (D) 1, 2, and 3

93. Characteristics of anemia include:
    1. Decreased number of circulating red blood cells
    2. Decreased hemoglobin
    3. Hematuria
    (A) 1 only
    (B) 1 and 2 only
    (C) 1 and 3 only
    (D) 1, 2, and 3

94. Grid interspace material can be made of:
    1. Carbon fiber
    2. Aluminum
    3. Plastic fiber
    (A) 1 only
    (B) 1 and 2 only
    (C) 2 and 3 only
    (D) 1, 2, and 3

95. The artifacts seen in Figure 16–9 are representative of:
    (A) Safelight fog
    (B) Inadequate developer replenishment
    (C) Guide shoe marks
    (D) Hair braids

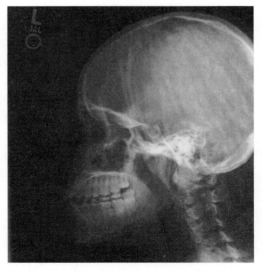

Figure 16–9. Courtesy of Stamford Hospital, Department of Radiology.

96. Which of these radiation exposure situations is likely to be the most harmful?

    (A) A large dose to a specific area all at once

    (B) A small dose to the whole body over a period of time

    (C) A large dose to the whole body all at one time

    (D) A small dose to a specific area over a period of time

97. Which of the following positions would best demonstrate the proximal tibiofibular articulation?

    (A) AP

    (B) 90-degree mediolateral

    (C) 45-degree internal rotation

    (D) 45-degree external rotation

98. Chemical substances that inhibit the growth of pathogenic microorganisms without necessarily killing them are called:

    1. Antiseptics

    2. Germicides

    3. Disinfectants

    (A) 1 only

    (B) 1 and 2 only

    (C) 2 and 3 only

    (D) 1, 2, and 3

99. Which of the following is a vasopressor and may be used for an anaphylactic reaction or cardiac arrest?

    (A) Nitroglycerin

    (B) Epinephrine

    (C) Hydrocortisone

    (D) Digitoxin

100. The absorption of excessive primary radiation by a grid is called:

    (A) Grid selectivity

    (B) Contrast improvement factor

    (C) Grid cutoff

    (D) Latitude

101. Examples of destructive pathologic conditions include:

    1. Emphysema

    2. Pneumoperitoneum

    3. Osteoporosis

    (A) 1 only

    (B) 2 only

    (C) 2 and 3 only

    (D) 1, 2, and 3

102. In which aspect of the orbital wall a "blowout fracture" usually occurs?

    (A) Superior

    (B) Inferior

    (C) Medial

    (D) Lateral

103. Required components of a digital fluoroscopy system include:

    1. Computer

    2. Video monitor

    3. Image manipulation console

    (A) 1 only

    (B) 1 and 2 only

    (C) 2 and 3 only

    (D) 1, 2, and 3

104. What activator is required for barium fluorohalide to retain its luminous properties?

    (A) Cesium

    (B) Iodine

    (C) Europium

    (D) Gadolinium

105. By which of the following dose–response curves are late or long-term effects of radiation exposure generally represented?

    (A) Linear threshold

    (B) Linear nonthreshold

    (C) Nonlinear threshold

    (D) Nonlinear nonthreshold

106. Radiographic *subject unsharpness* is a result of
    1. Object plane is not parallel with CR
    2. Object plane is not parallel with IR
    3. Anatomic details of interest are not in the path of the CR
    (A) 1 only
    (B) 1 and 2 only
    (C) 2 and 3 only
    (D) 1, 2, and 3

107. Typical examples of digital imaging include:
    1. Magnetic resonance imaging (MRI)
    2. Computed tomography (CT)
    3. Pluridirectional tomography
    (A) 1 only
    (B) 1 and 2 only
    (C) 1 and 3 only
    (D) 1, 2, and 3

108. Special beam-shaping optics are used in the CR reader to keep the infrared laser scanning light finely focused in order to:
    1. Collect analog data
    2. Improve signal-to-noise ratio (SNR)
    3. Maintain good spatial resolution
    (A) 1 only
    (B) 1 and 2 only
    (C) 2 and 3 only
    (D) 1, 2, and 3

109. Which of the following is a fast-acting vasodilator used to lower blood pressure and relieve the pain of angina pectoris?
    (A) Digitalis
    (B) Dilantin
    (C) Nitroglycerin
    (D) Cimetidine (Tagamet)

110. Typical characteristics of the android pelvis include:
    1. Pubic angle less than 90 degree
    2. Narrow, vertical
    3. Pelvic inlet large and round
    (A) 1 only
    (B) 1 and 2 only
    (C) 2 and 3 only
    (D) 1, 2, and 3

111. A radiographic image exhibiting few shades of gray between black and white is said to possess:
    (A) No contrast
    (B) High contrast
    (C) Low contrast
    (D) Little contrast

112. A small bottle containing a single dose of medication is termed:
    (A) An ampule
    (B) A vial
    (C) A bolus
    (D) A carafe

113. An increase in kV will have which of the following effects?
    1. More scattered radiation will be produced
    2. The exposure rate will increase
    3. Radiographic contrast will increase
    (A) 1 only
    (B) 1 and 2 only
    (C) 2 and 3 only
    (D) 1, 2, and 3

114. Which of the following is the most proximal structure on the adult ulna?
    (A) Capitulum
    (B) Styloid process
    (C) Coronoid process
    (D) Olecranon process

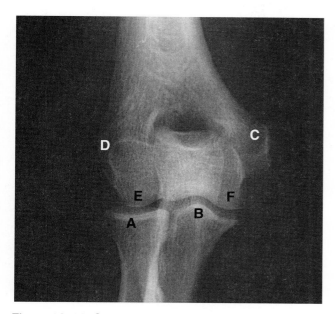

Figure 16–10. Courtesy of Stamford Hospital, Department of Radiology.

115. In Figure 16–10, the letter *E* represents the:
    (A) Trochlea
    (B) Capitulum
    (C) Lateral epicondyle
    (D) Medial epicondyle

116. In Figure 16–10, the letter *D* represents the:
    (A) Trochlea
    (B) Capitulum
    (C) Lateral epicondyle
    (D) Medial epicondyle

117. What is the intensity of scattered radiation perpendicular to and 1 m from the patient, compared to the useful beam at the patient's surface?
    (A) 0.01%
    (B) 0.1%
    (C) 1.0%
    (D) 10.0%

118. Which of the following is demonstrated in a 25-degree LPO position with the central ray entering 1-inch medial to the elevated antero-superior iliac spine (ASIS)?
    (A) Left sacroiliac joint
    (B) Right sacroiliac joint
    (C) Left ilium
    (D) Right ilium

119. A 3-inch object to be radiographed at 36-inches SID lies 4 inches from the image receptor. What will be the image width?
    (A) 2.6 inches
    (B) 3.3 inches
    (C) 26.0 inches
    (D) 33.0 inches

120. The sternoclavicular joints are best demonstrated with the patient PA and:
    (A) In a slight oblique, affected side adjacent to the image receptor
    (B) In a slight oblique, affected side away from the image receptor
    (C) Erect, weight bearing
    (D) Erect, with and without weights

121. Which of the following criteria are required for accurate visualization of the greater tubercle in profile?
    1. Epicondyles parallel to the image receptor
    2. Arm in external rotation
    3. Humerus in AP position
    (A) 1 only
    (B) 1 and 3 only
    (C) 2 and 3 only
    (D) 1, 2, and 3

122. All of the following positions are likely to be employed for both single-and double-contrast examinations of the large bowel, *except*:
    (A) Lateral rectum
    (B) AP axial rectosigmoid
    (C) Right and left lateral decubitus abdomen
    (D) RAO and LAO abdomen

123. In which of the following conditions is protective or "reverse" isolation required?
    1. Tuberculosis
    2. Burns
    3. Leukemia
    (A) 1 only
    (B) 1 and 2 only
    (C) 2 and 3 only
    (D) 1, 2, and 3

124. Which of the following devices functions to produce hard copies of digital images?
    (A) Digitizer
    (B) Laser printer
    (C) Histogram
    (D) CRT

125. In film/screen imaging, with all other factors remaining the same, as grid ratio is increased:
    (A) Recorded detail decreases
    (B) Optical density decreases
    (C) Focal spot distortion decreases
    (D) Scale of contrast becomes longer

126. The *best* way to control voluntary motion is:
    (A) Immobilization of the part
    (B) Careful explanation of the procedure
    (C) Short exposure time
    (D) Physical restraint

127. The manubrial notch, a bony landmark used in radiography of the sternoclavicular joints, is located at the same level as the:
    (A) Vertebra prominens
    (B) First thoracic vertebra
    (C) Third thoracic vertebra
    (D) Ninth thoracic vertebra

128. Which of the following functions to protect the x-ray tube and the patient from overexposure in the event the automatic exposure control fails to terminate an exposure?
    (A) Circuit breaker
    (B) Backup timer
    (C) Rheostat
    (D) Fuse

129. Which of the following would be appropriate cassette front material?
    1. Tungsten
    2. Magnesium
    3. Bakelite
    (A) 1 only
    (B) 1 and 2 only
    (C) 2 and 3 only
    (D) 1, 2, and 3

130. In order to be considered as legitimate legal evidence, each x-ray image must contain certain essential and specific patient information, including:
    1. Date of examination
    2. Side marker
    3. Referring physician
    (A) 1 only
    (B) 1 and 2 only
    (C) 2 and 3 only
    (D) 1, 2, and 3

131. In the lateral projection of the foot, the:
    1. Plantar surface should be perpendicular to the image receptor
    2. Metatarsals should be superimposed
    3. Talofibular joint should be visualized
    (A) 1 only
    (B) 1 and 2 only
    (C) 2 and 3 only
    (D) 1, 2, and 3

132. The x-ray film artifact seen in Figure 16–11 is representative of:
    (A) A processor artifact
    (B) An exposure artifact
    (C) A handling artifact
    (D) Chemical fog

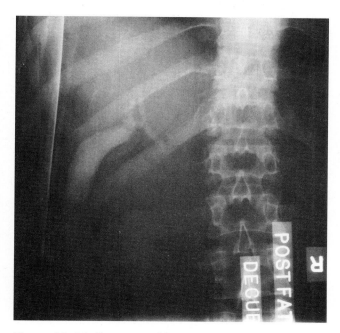

Figure 16–11. Courtesy of Stamford Hospital, Department of Radiology.

133. The factor(s) that can be used to regulate radiographic density in film/screen imaging is (are):

1. Milliamperage
2. Exposure time
3. Kilovoltage

(A) 1 only
(B) 2 only
(C) 1 and 2 only
(D) 1, 2, and 3

134. By which of the following tests is intensifying screen contact evaluated?

(A) Spinning top test
(B) Wire-mesh test
(C) Penetrometer test
(D) Star-pattern test

135. The mechanical device used to correct an ineffectual cardiac rhythm is a:

(A) Defibrillator
(B) Cardiac monitor
(C) Crash cart
(D) Resuscitation bag

136. The term that refers to parts closer to the source or beginning is:

(A) Cephalad
(B) Caudad
(C) Proximal
(D) Medial

137. The blue–green PSL that corresponds to the visible x-ray image occurs:

1. Immediately upon the initial prompt emission of light
2. Some time after the initial prompt emission of light
3. Upon stimulation by finely focused infrared light

(A) 1 only
(B) 1 and 2 only
(C) 2 and 3 only
(D) 1, 2, and 3

138. An abnormal passage between organs is a (an):

(A) Fistula
(B) Polyp
(C) Diverticulum
(D) Abscess

139. The AP projection of the scapula requires that the:

1. Patient's arm be abducted at right angles to the body
2. Patient's elbow be flexed with hand supinated
3. Exposure be made during quiet breathing

(A) 1 and 2 only
(B) 1 and 3 only
(C) 3 only
(D) 1, 2, and 3

140. The type of shock associated with pooling of blood in the peripheral vessels is classified as:

(A) Neurogenic
(B) Cardiogenic
(C) Hypovolemic
(D) Septic

141. What projection of the calcaneus is obtained with the leg extended, plantar surface vertical and perpendicular to the image receptor, and central ray directed 40 degrees caudad?
    (A) Axial plantodorsal projection
    (B) Axial dorsoplantar projection
    (C) Lateral projection
    (D) Weight-bearing lateral

142. The uppermost portion of the iliac crest is approximately at the same level as that of the:
    (A) Costal margin
    (B) Umbilicus
    (C) Xiphoid tip
    (D) Fourth lumbar vertebra

143. Devices that serve to collect PSL and transmit it to an ADC include:
    1. Photomultiplier tube
    2. Photodiode
    3. Charge-coupled device
    (A) 1 only
    (B) 1 and 2 only
    (C) 2 and 3 only
    (D) 1, 2, and 3

144. Which of the following is (are) true when comparing film-screen imaging to that of CR imaging?
    1. CR DQE is better than film-screen DQE
    2. CR has a wider exposure range than film-screen
    3. CR has better spatial resolution than film-screen
    (A) 1 only
    (B) 1 and 2 only
    (C) 2 and 3 only
    (D) 1, 2, and 3

145. The type(s) of radiation produced at the tungsten target is (are):
    1. Photoelectric
    2. Characteristic
    3. Bremsstrahlung
    (A) 1 only
    (B) 1 and 2 only
    (C) 2 and 3 only
    (D) 1, 2, and 3

146. With the patient positioned as for a parietoacanthial projection (Waters method) and the central ray directed through the patient's open mouth, which of the following sinus groups is demonstrated through the open mouth?
    (A) Frontal
    (B) Ethmoid
    (C) Maxillary
    (D) Sphenoid

147. Characteristics of the typical diagnostic x-ray tube and its construction include:
    1. The target material should have a high atomic number and melting point
    2. The useful beam emerges from the port window
    3. The cathode assembly receives both low and high voltages
    (A) 1 only
    (B) 2 only
    (C) 1 and 2 only
    (D) 1, 2, and 3

148. During respiratory motion, the act of:
    1. Expiration raises the diaphragm
    2. Inspiration elevates the ribs
    3. Inspiration depresses the abdominal viscera
    (A) 1 only
    (B) 1 and 2 only
    (C) 2 and 3 only
    (D) 1, 2, and 3

149. The stomach of an asthenic patient is *most* likely to be located:
    (A) High, transverse, and lateral
    (B) Low, transverse, and lateral
    (C) High, vertical, and toward the midline
    (D) Low, vertical, and toward the midline

150. The term *voxel* is associated with all of the following, *except:*
    (A) Bit depth
    (B) Volume element
    (C) Measured in Z direction
    (D) Field of view

151. In which body position would a patient suffering from orthopnea experience the *least* discomfort?
    (A) Fowler
    (B) Trendelenburg
    (C) Recumbent
    (D) Erect

152. The position illustrated in Figure 16–12 can be improved by:
    (A) Bringing the chin up more
    (B) Bringing the chin down more
    (C) Angling the CR caudad
    (D) Opening the mouth more

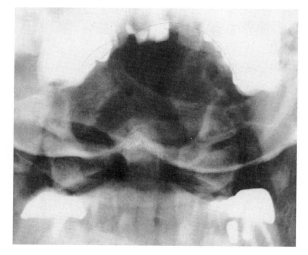

Figure 16–12. Courtesy of Stamford Hospital, Department of Radiology.

153. The medical term referring to *nosebleed* is:
    (A) Vertigo
    (B) Urticaria
    (C) Epistaxis
    (D) Aura

154. Types of positive contrast agents include:
    1. Barium sulfate suspension
    2. Water-based iodinated media
    3. Carbon dioxide
    (A) 1 only
    (B) 2 only
    (C) 1 and 2 only
    (D) 1 and 3 only

155. Which of the following best describes correct hand hygiene?
    (A) The radiographer's hands should be thoroughly washed with soap and warm running water, for at least 15 seconds after each patient
    (B) The radiographer's hands should be thoroughly washed with soap and warm running water, for at least 15 seconds before each patient
    (C) The radiographer's hands should be thoroughly washed with soap and warm running water, for at least 15 seconds before and after each patient
    (D) The radiographer's hands and forearms should always be kept higher than the elbows during cleansing

156. Radiation exposure to the developing fetus can cause:
    1. Mental retardation
    2. Growth retardation
    3. Organ damage
    (A) 1 only
    (B) 1 and 2 only
    (C) 2 and 3 only
    (D) 1, 2, and 3

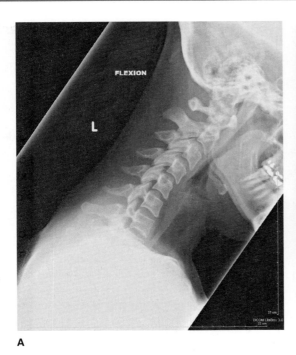
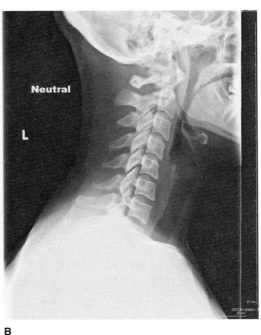

Figure 16–13. (**A**) and (**B**). Courtesy of Conrad P Ehrlich, MD.

157. Characteristics of a 16:1 grid include:

1. Absorbs more primary radiation than an 8:1 grid

2. Has more centering latitude than an 8:1 grid

3. Used with higher kV exposures than an 8:1 grid

(A) 1 only

(B) 1 and 3 only

(C) 2 and 3 only

(D) 1, 2, and 3

158. The automatic exposure device that is located immediately under the x-ray table is the:

(A) Ionization chamber

(B) Scintillation camera

(C) Photomultiplier

(D) Photocathode

159. What device can be used to overcome considerable variation in patient anatomy or tissue density, thus providing more uniform radiographic density?

(A) Compensating filter

(B) Grid

(C) Collimator

(D) Intensifying screen

160. In film/screen imaging, a radiograph demonstrating a long scale of contrast is most likely to be produced by increasing:

(A) Photon energy

(B) Screen speed

(C) mAs

(D) SID

161. Figure 16–13A and 16–13B is most often performed to evaluate the following condition:

(A) Subluxation

(B) Spondyloisthesis

(C) Whiplash injury

(D) Cervical rib

162. Of the following groups of technical factors used in film/screen imagine, which will produce the greatest radiographic density?

(A) 10 mAs, 74 kV, 44-inches SID

(B) 10 mAs, 74 kV, 36-inches SID

(C) 5 mAs, 85 kV, 48-inches SID

(D) 5 mAs, 85 kV, 40-inches SID

163. Which of the following generator types has the advantages of having compact size, producing nearly constant potential voltage, and decreasing patient dose?

(A) Single-phase, full-wave

(B) Three-phase, six-pulse

(C) Three-phase, twelve-pulse

(D) High-frequency

164. *Somatic effects* of radiation refer to effects that are manifested:

(A) In the descendants of the exposed individual

(B) During the life of the exposed individual

(C) In the exposed individual and their descendants

(D) In the reproductive cells of the exposed individual

165. The energy of ionizing electromagnetic radiations is measured in:

(A) mA

(B) mAs

(C) keV

(D) kV

166. The total number of x-ray photons produced at the target is contingent on:

1. Tube current

2. Target material

3. Square of the kilovoltage

(A) 1 only

(B) 1 and 2 only

(C) 2 and 3 only

(D) 1, 2, and 3

167. To produce just a perceptible increase in film/screen radiographic density, the radiographer must increase the:

(A) mAs by 30%

(B) mA-s by 15%

(C) kV by 15%

(D) kV by 30%

168. Which of the following is usually recommended for cleaning CR image storage screens?

(A) Denatured alcohol

(B) Anhydrous ethanol

(C) Soap and water

(D) Intensifying screen cleaner

169. What is the fetal dose limit for pregnant radiographers for the entire gestation period?

(A) 0.1 rem

(B) 0.5 rem

(C) 5.0 rem

(D) 10 rem

170. What type of precaution prevents the spread of infectious agents in aerosol form?

(A) Strict isolation

(B) Protective isolation

(C) Airborne precautions

(D) Contact precautions

171. Which of the following is a condition in which an occluded blood vessel stops blood flow to a portion of the lungs?

(A) Pneumothorax

(B) Atelectasis

(C) Pulmonary embolism

(D) Hypoxia

172. An accurately positioned oblique projection of the first through fourth lumbar vertebrae will demonstrate the classic "scotty dog." What bony structure does the scotty dog's "ear" represent?

(A) Superior articular process

(B) Pedicle

(C) Transverse process

(D) Pars interarticularis

173. Inspiration and expiration projections of the chest may be performed to demonstrate:

    1. Pneumothorax
    2. Foreign body
    3. Atelectasis

    (A) 1 only
    (B) 1 and 2 only
    (C) 1 and 3 only
    (D) 1, 2, and 3

174. What minimum total amount of filtration (inherent plus added) is required in an x-ray equipment operated above 70 kV?

    (A) 2.5 mm Al equivalent
    (B) 3.5 mm Al equivalent
    (C) 2.5 mm Cu equivalent
    (D) 3.5 mm Cu equivalent

175. A CR histogram is a graphic representation of:

    (A) Gray scale values of the imaged part
    (B) A characteristic curve of the imaged part
    (C) D_{max}
    (D) D_{min}

176. Proper care of leaded apparel includes:

    1. Periodic check for cracks
    2. Careful folding following each use
    3. Routine laundering with soap and water

    (A) 1 only
    (B) 1 and 2 only
    (C) 2 and 3 only
    (D) 1, 2, and 3

177. The image seen in Figure 16–14 was made using the following types of x-ray equipment:

    (A) Single-phase
    (B) Three-phase, six-pulse
    (C) Three-phase, twelve-pulse
    (D) High-frequency

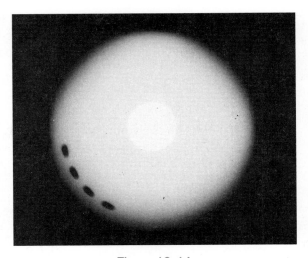

Figure 16–14.

178. If the test image seen in Figure 16–14 is known to represent correctly operating full-wave rectified equipment, then at what exposure time was it made?

    (A) 1/15 second
    (B) 1/30 second
    (C) 1/60 second
    (D) 1/120 second

179. What is meant by the term *controlled area*?

    1. One that is occupied by people trained in radiation safety
    2. One that is occupied by people who wear radiation monitors
    3. One whose occupancy factor is 1

    (A) 1 and 2 only
    (B) 2 only
    (C) 1 and 3 only
    (D) 1, 2, and 3

180. A radiograph made with a parallel grid demonstrates decreased density on its lateral edges. This is most likely caused by:

    (A) Static electrical discharge
    (B) The grid off-centered
    (C) Improper tube angle
    (D) Decreased SID

181. All of the following statements concerning respiratory structures are true, *except*:

    (A) The right lung has two lobes

    (B) The uppermost portion of the lung is the apex

    (C) Each lung is enclosed in pleura

    (D) The trachea bifurcates into mainstem bronchi

182. To demonstrate the pulmonary apices with the patient in the AP erect position, the:

    (A) Central ray is directed 15 to 20 degrees cephalad

    (B) Central ray is directed 15 to 20 degrees caudad

    (C) Exposure is made on full exhalation

    (D) Patient's shoulders are rolled forward

183. The effects of radiation on biologic material are dependent on several factors. If a quantity of radiation is delivered to a body over a long period of time, the effect:

    (A) Will be greater than if it were delivered all at one time

    (B) Will be less than if it were delivered all at one time

    (C) Has no relation to how it is delivered in time

    (D) Is solely dependent on the radiation quality

184. In which quadrant is the sigmoid colon located?

    (A) LLQ

    (B) LUQ

    (C) RLQ

    (D) RUQ

185. In film/screen imaging, a 15% increase in kV accompanied by a 50% decrease in mAs will result in a (an):

    (A) Shorter scale contrast

    (B) Increase in exposure latitude

    (C) Increase in radiographic density

    (D) Decrease in recorded detail

186. The four major arteries supplying the brain include the:

    1. Brachiocephalic artery

    2. Common carotid arteries

    3. Vertebral arteries

    (A) 1 and 2 only

    (B) 1 and 3 only

    (C) 2 and 3 only

    (D) 1, 2, and 3

187. The total brightness gain of an image intensifier is a result of:

    1. Flux gain

    2. Minification gain

    3. Focusing gain

    (A) 1 only

    (B) 2 only

    (C) 1 and 2 only

    (D) 1 and 3 only

188. Radiographers use monitoring devices to record their monthly exposure to radiation. The types of devices suited for this purpose include:

    1. Pocket dosimeter

    2. Thermoluminescent dosimeter (TLD)

    3. Optically stimulated luminescence (OSL)

    (A) 1 only

    (B) 1 and 2 only

    (C) 2 and 3 only

    (D) 1, 2, and 3

189. During gastrointestinal radiography, the position of the stomach often varies depending on:

    1. Respiratory phase

    2. Body habitus

    3. Patient position

    (A) 1 and 2 only

    (B) 1 and 3 only

    (C) 2 and 3 only

    (D) 1, 2, and 3

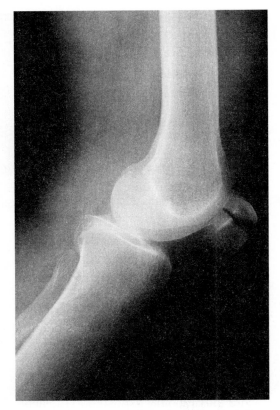

Figure 16–15. Courtesy of Stamford Hospital, Department of Radiology.

190. The radiograph seen in Figure 16–15 illustrates the joint space obscured by the:

(A) Medial femoral condyle

(B) Lateral femoral condyle

(C) Intercondylar eminences

(D) Tibial tuberosity

191. Lateral deviation of the nasal septum may be *best* demonstrated in the:

(A) Lateral projection

(B) PA axial (Caldwell method) projection

(C) Parietoacanthial (Waters method) projection

(D) AP axial (Towne method) projection

192. When a patient is received in the radiology department with a urinary Foley catheter bag, it is important to:

(A) Place the drainage bag above the level of the bladder

(B) Place the drainage bag at the same level as the bladder

(C) Place the drainage bag below the level of the bladder

(D) Clamp the Foley catheter

193. A slit camera is used to measure:

1. Focal spot size

2. Intensifying screen resolution

3. SID resolution

(A) 1 only

(B) 1 and 2 only

(C) 1 and 3 only

(D) 1, 2, and 3

194. The *most* effective method of sterilization is:

(A) Dry heat

(B) Moist heat

(C) Pasteurization

(D) Freezing

195. What should be the radiographer's main objective regarding personal radiation safety?

(A) Not to exceed his or her dose limit

(B) To keep personal exposure as far below the dose limit as possible

(C) To avoid whole-body exposure

(D) To wear protective apparel when "holding" patients for exposures

196. Which of the following conditions would require an increase in exposure factors?

1. Congestive heart failure

2. Pleural effusion

3. Emphysema

(A) 1 only

(B) 1 and 2 only

(C) 1 and 3 only

(D) 1, 2, and 3

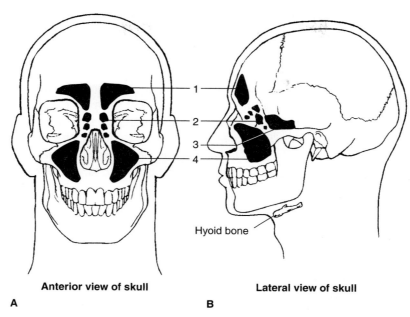

Anterior view of skull

A

Lateral view of skull

B

Hyoid bone

Figure 16–16. **(A)** and **(B)**

197. What structure is indicated by the *number 3* in Figure 16–16?

(A) Maxillary sinuses

(B) Mastoid sinuses

(C) Sphenoid sinuses

(D) Ethmoid sinuses

198. A film/screen exposure was made at 38-inches SID using 300-mA, 30-millisecond exposure, and 80 kV with a 400 film/screen combination and an 8:1 grid. It is desired to repeat the radiograph, and to improve recorded detail, use 42-inches SID and 200 film/screen combination. With all other factors remaining constant, what exposure time will be required to maintain the original radiographic density?

(A) 0.03 second

(B) 0.07 second

(C) 0.14 second

(D) 0.36 second

199. The dose of radiation that will cause a noticeable skin reaction is referred to as the:

(A) Linear energy transfer (LET)

(B) Source skin distance (SSD)

(C) Skin erythema dose (SED)

(D) SID

200. You encounter a person who is apparently unconscious. Although his or her airway is open, there is no rise and fall of his or her chest and you can hear no breath sounds. You should:

(A) Begin mouth-to-mouth rescue breathing, giving two full breaths

(B) Proceed with the Heimlich maneuver

(C) Begin external chest compressions at a rate of 80 to 100 per minute

(D) Begin external chest compressions at a rate of at least 100 per minute

Answers and Explanations

1. (D) Histogram appearance can be affected by a number of things. *Positioning and centering accuracy* can have a significant effect on histogram appearance (see Fig. 12–8). Other factors affecting histogram appearance include selection of the *correct processing algorithm* (e.g., chest vs. femur), changes in *scatter, SID, OID,* and *collimation*—in short, anything that affects scatter and/or dose. Another factor affecting histogram appearance is *delay in processing* from the time of exposure. Delay in processing can result in *fading* of the image (*Shephard, p. 243*).

2. (B) The *tissue weighting factor* (W_t) represents the relative tissue radiosensitivity of irradiated material (e.g., muscle vs. intestinal epithelium vs. bone, etc.). The *radiation weighting factor* (W_r) is a number assigned to different types of ionizing radiations in order to better determine their effect on tissue (e.g., x-ray vs. alpha particles). The W_r of different ionizing radiations is dependent on the LET of that particular radiation. The following formula is used to determine *effective dose* (*E*): Effective dose (*E*) = Radiation weighting factor (W_r) × Tissue weighting factor (W_t) × Absorbed dose (*Bushong, p. 556*).

3. (B) Figure 16–1A is a medial oblique projection of the foot. The foot is rotated medially so that the *plantar surface* and *IR* form a 30-degree angle—the *CR* and *plantar surface* form a 60-degree angle. This position should demonstrate the third through fifth metatarsals completely free of superimposition, when positioned correctly. Articulations around the cuboid and sinus tarsi should be well demonstrated, as well as the tuberosity of the base of the fifth metatarsal. Figure 16–1B is the dorsoplantar projection of the foot. The CR is perpendicular to the plantar surface (*Bontrager & Lampignano, 6th ed., p. 233*).

4. (A) The PSP screen within the IP has a layer of europium-activated barium fluorohalide (BaFX:Eu^{2+}; X = Halogen) mixed with a binder substance. This layer serves as the *image receptor* when exposed to x-rays. Just under the barium fluorohalide layer is first a *reflective layer*, then the *base*, then an *antistatic layer*, and finally a layer of *lead foil* to absorb backscatter. Over the top of the barium fluorohalide is a *protective layer*. When the barium fluorohalide absorbs x-ray energy, *electrons are released and they divide into two groups*. One electron group

initiates *immediate luminescence* during the excited state of Eu^{2+}. The other electron group *becomes trapped* within the phosphor's halogen ions, forming a "color center." These are the phosphors that ultimately form the radiographic image because when exposed to a *monochromatic* (often infrared) laser light source, these phosphors emit *polychromatic* light, termed *photostimulated luminescence* (*Wolbarst, 2nd ed., p. 386*).

5. (D) According to the inverse square law of radiation, the intensity (exposure rate) of radiation from its source is inversely proportional to the distance squared. Therefore, as distance from the source of radiation is increased, exposure rate decreases. Because exposure rate and image density are directly proportional in screen/film imaging, if the exposure rate of a beam directed to an image receptor is decreased, the resulting image density would be decreased proportionally (*Bushong 9th ed., p. 67*).

6. (A) *Creatinine* is a normal alkaline constituent of urine and blood, but increased quantities of creatinine are present in advanced stages of renal disease. Creatinine and *BUN* (blood urea nitrogen) blood chemistry levels should be checked prior to beginning an examination requiring the use of an iodinated contrast agent. Increased levels may forecast increased possibility of contrast media-induced renal effects and poor visualization of the renal collecting systems. Normal creatinine range is 0.6 to 1.5 mg/100 mL (100 mg = 1dL). Normal BUN range is 8 to 25 mg/100 mL (*Bontrager & Lampignano, 7th ed., p. 539*).

7. (C) Adverse reactions to the intravascular administration of iodinated contrast are not uncommon, and although the risk of a life-threatening reaction is relatively rare, the radiographer must be alert to recognize and deal effectively should a serious reaction occur. Minor reaction is characterized by flushed appearance and nausea, occasionally vomiting and a few hives. *Early* symptoms of a possible anaphylactic reaction include *constriction of the throat*, possibly caused by laryngeal edema, *dysphagia* (difficulty swallowing), and *itching of the palms and soles*. The radiographer must maintain the patient's airway, summon the radiologist, and call a "code" (*Adler & Carlton, p. 240*).

8. (A) The cervical *intervertebral foramina* lie 45 degrees to the midsagittal plane (and 15–20 degrees to a transverse plane) and are therefore demonstrated in the *oblique* position. *Intervertebral joints* are well visualized in the *lateral* projection of all the vertebral groups. Cervical articular facets (forming *apophyseal joints*) are 90 degrees to the midsagittal plane and are therefore also well demonstrated in the *lateral* projection (*Bontrager & Lampignano, 7th ed., p. 308*).

9. **(D)** Radiation quality determines the degree of penetration and the amount of energy transferred to the irradiated tissue (LET). Certainly, the larger the absorbed radiation dose, the greater the effect. Biologic effect is increased as the size of the irradiated area is increased. The nature of the effect is influenced by the location of irradiated tissue (bone marrow vs. gonads, etc.) (*Selman, p. 190*).

10. **(D)** *Veracity* is not only telling the truth, but also not practicing deception. *Autonomy* is the ethical principle related to the theory that patients have the right to decide what will or will not be done to them. *Beneficence* is related to the idea of doing good and being kind. *Fidelity* is faithfulness and loyalty (*Adler & Carlton, p. 308*).

11. **(B)** *Somatic effects* of radiation refer to the effects experienced directly by the exposed individual such as erythema, epilation, and cataracts. *Genetic effects* of radiation exposure are caused by irradiation of the reproductive cells of the exposed individual and transmitted from one generation to the next (*Statkiewicz-Sherer & Visconti, pp. 115, 131*).

12. **(A)** The approximately 5-ft-long large intestine (colon) functions in the formation, transport, and evacuation of feces. The colon commences at the terminus of the small intestine; its first portion is the sac-like *cecum* in the RLQ, located inferior to the ileocecal valve. The ascending colon is continuous with the cecum and is located along the right side of the abdominal cavity. It bends medially and anteriorly, forming the right colic (*hepatic*) flexure. The colon traverses the abdomen as the transverse colon and bends posteriorly and inferiorly to form the left colic (*splenic*) flexure. The descending colon continues down the left side of the abdominal cavity, and at about the level of the pelvic brim, in the *left lower quadrant* (LLQ), the colon moves medially to form the S-shaped *sigmoid* colon. The rectum, approximately 5 inches in length, lies between the sigmoid and the anal canal (*Saia, p. 173*).

13. **(B)** Neither ultrasonography nor magnetic resonance imaging requires the use of ionizing radiation to produce an image. Computed axial tomography does require ionizing radiation to produce an image. Ultrasonography requires the use of high-frequency sound waves (ultrasound) to produce images of soft-tissue structures and certain blood vessels within the body. Magnetic resonance imaging relies on the use of a very powerful magnet and specially designed coils that send and receive radiowave signals to produce the image (*Torres et al., p. 7*).

14. **(C)** Because the anode's focal track is beveled (angled, facing the cathode), x-ray photons can freely diverge toward the cathode end of the x-ray tube. However, the "heel" of the focal track prevents x-ray photons from diverging toward the anode end of the tube. This results in varying intensity from anode to cathode, fewer photons at the anode end, and more photons at the cathode end. *The anode heel effect is most noticeable using large image receptor sizes, short SIDs, and steep target angles (Bontrager & Lampignano, 7th ed., p 38).*

15. **(C)** The knee is formed by the proximal tibia, patella, and distal femur, which articulate to form the *femorotibial* and *patellofemoral* joints. The distal posterior femur presents two large *medial* and *lateral condyles* separated by the deep *intercondyloid fossa*. Two small prominences, the medial and lateral epicondyles, are just superior to the condyles. The femoral and tibial condyles articulate to form the femorotibial joint. Figure 16–2 illustrates positioning for the *intercondyloid fossa* (Camp–Coventry method). The patient is posteroanterior (PA) recumbent with knee flexed so that the tibia forms 40-degree angle with the tabletop, with foot rested on support. The CR is directed 40 degrees caudad (perpendicular to the long axis of the tibia) to the knee joint. This results in a *PA axial* (superoinferior) projection of the intercondyloid fossa, tibial plateau, and eminences. It is referred to as the *tunnel view* (*Bontrager & Lampignano, 7th ed., p. 249*).

16. **(B)** A patient going into shock may exhibit *pallor* and *weakness*, a significant *drop in blood pressure*, and an *increase in pulse rate*. The patient may also experience *apprehension* and *restlessness*, and have *cool, clammy skin*. A radiographer recognizing these symptoms should call the patient to the physician's attention immediately. Fever is not associated with shock (*Torres et al., p. 162*).

17. (D) The control and prevention of infection is a hospital-wide effort. Each department has its own infection-control protocol, designed according to the risks unique to their services.

The most susceptible to infection include the sick, infirm, immunocompromised, very young, poorly nourished, weak, or fatigued—all who have a diminished natural resistance to infection. *Health care–acquired infections* (HAIs), formerly referred to as *nosocomial infections*, are infections acquired by *patients* (susceptible hosts) while they are in the hospital, unrelated to the condition for which the patients were hospitalized (*Ehrlich et al. 7th ed., p. 147, 148*).

18. (A) Every radiographic examination involves an *entrance skin exposure* (ESE), which can be determined fairly easily. It also involves a gonadal dose and marrow dose that, if needed, can be calculated by the radiation physicist. If the ESE of a particular examination was calculated to determine the *equivalent whole-body dose*, this is termed *effective dose*. For example, the ESE of a PA chest is approximately 70 mrem, while the effective dose is 10 mrem. The effective (whole-body) dose is much less because much of the body is not included in the primary beam (*Fosbinder & Kelsey, p. 390*).

19. (B) When the body is erect, the diaphragm is more easily moved to a lower position during inspiration. For this reason, chest radiography is performed erect to allow maximum lung expansion. With the body in the supine position, the abdominal viscera exert greater pressure on the diaphragm, and it usually assumes a position 2 to 4 inches higher than that when erect (*Frank, Long, & Smith, 11th ed., Vol. 1, pp. 465-467*).

20. (C) A digital image is formed by a *matrix* of *pixels* (picture elements) in rows and columns. A matrix having 512 pixels in each row and column is a 512×512 matrix. The term *field of view* is used to describe how much of the patient (e.g., 150-mm diameter) is included in the matrix. The matrix and/or field of view can be changed without affecting the other, but changes in either will change pixel size. As in traditional radiography, *spatial resolution* is measured in line pairs per millimeter (*lp/mm*). As matrix size is increased, there are more and smaller pixels in the matrix, and therefore improved resolution. Fewer and larger pixels result in a poor resolution "pixelly" image, that is, one in which you can actually see the individual pixel boxes (*Fosbinder & Kelsey, p. 286*).

21. (B) With the body in the AP recumbent position, barium easily flows into the fundus of the stomach, displacing it somewhat superiorly. The fundus, then, is filled with barium, while the air that had been in the fundus is displaced into the gastric body, pylorus, and duodenum, illustrating them in double-contrast fashion. Air contrast delineation of these structures allows us to see through the stomach to retrogastric areas and structures. Barium-filled duodenum and pylorus is best demonstrated in the RAO position (*Frank, Long, & Smith, 11th ed., Vol. 2, p. 151*).

22. (D) The AHA replaced the patient's Bill of Rights with the *Patient Care Partnership—Understanding Expectations, Rights, and Responsibilities*. Their plain-language brochure includes the essentials of the Bill of Rights and reviews what patients can/should expect during a hospital stay.

The Patient Care Partnership statement addresses *high-quality hospital care*, combining skill, compassion, and respect and the right to know the identity of caregivers. It includes a *clean* and *safe environment*, free from neglect and abuse, and information about anything unexpected that occurred during the hospital stay. The Patient Care Partnership identifies *involvement in your care*: it elaborates on patient discussion/understanding of their condition and treatment choices with their physician, patients' responsibility to provide complete and correct information to the caregiver, understanding who should make decisions for patients if they cannot make those decisions (including "living will" or "advance directive").

The Patient Care Partnership statement identifies *protection of your privacy*, describing the ways in which patient information is safeguarded. It also describes *help when leaving the hospital*—availability of and/or instruction regarding follow-up care. Lastly, the Patient Care Partnership statement addresses *help with your billing claims*, including filing claims with insurance companies and assisting those without health coverage.

These patient rights can be exercised on the patient's behalf by a *designated surrogate* or *proxy* decision-maker. (*Ehrlich et al. 7th ed., p. 64-66*).

23. (D) The pictured radiograph was made in the *left lateral decubitus* position. It is part of a series of radiographs made during an air contrast (double-contrast) barium enema (BE) examination. A *double-contrast examination* of the large bowel is performed to see *through* the bowel to its posterior wall and to visualize any *intraluminal* (e.g., polypoid) *lesions* or *masses*. Various body positions are used to redistribute the barium and air. To demonstrate the medial and lateral walls of the bowel, decubitus positions are performed. The radiograph presents a left lateral decubitus position because the *barium has gravitated* to the left side (the side of the splenic flexure). The *air rises* and delineates the medial side of the descending colon and the lateral side of the ascending colon (*Frank, Long, & Smith, 11th ed., Vol. 2, p. 187*).

24. **(D)** Moving the image intensifier *closer to the patient* during fluoroscopy *reduces* the distance between the x-ray tube (source) and the image intensifier (image receptor); that is, the *SID* is reduced. It follows that the distance between the part being imaged (object) and the image intensifier (image receptor) is also reduced; that is, the *OID* is reduced (Fig. 16–17). The shorter OID produces *less magnification* and *better image quality*. As SID is reduced, the intensity of the x-ray photons at the image intensifier's input phosphor increases, stimulating the automatic brightness control (ABC) to decrease the mA (milliamperage), thereby *decreasing the patient dose* (*Fosbinder & Kelsey, pp. 265-267*).

25. **(D)** The addition of a grid will help clean up the scattered radiation produced by higher kV, but it requires an mAs adjustment in film/screen imaging. According to the grid conversion factors listed

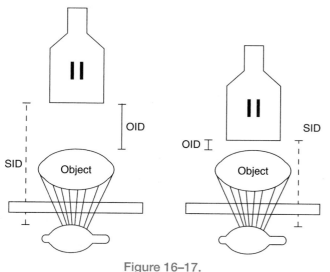

Figure 16–17.

below, the addition of an 8:1 grid requires that the original mAs be multiplied by a factor of 4:

No grid	= 1 × original mAs
5:1 grid	= 2 × original mAs
6:1 grid	= 3 × original mAs
8:1 grid	= 4 × original mAs
12:1 grid	= 5 × original mAs
16:1 grid	= 6 × original mAs

The adjustment therefore requires 32 mAs at 90 kV (*Saia, p. 324*).

26. **(A)** One of the biggest advantages of CR/DR is the *latitude* it offers. In screen–film imaging, there is a "range of correct exposure" limited by the toe and shoulder of the characteristic curve, whereas in CR/DR, the dynamic range is a *linear* relationship between the exposure given the PSP and its resulting luminescence as it is scanned by the laser. This affords much *greater exposure latitude*; technical inaccuracies can be effectively eliminated. In Figure 16–4, *curve A* illustrates the linear relationship between the exposure, given the PSP and its resulting luminescence. *Curve B* illustrates the characteristic curve used in screen–film imaging and its "range of correct exposure" limited by the toe and shoulder of the curve.

Overexposure of up to 500% and underexposure of up to 80% are reported as recoverable, thus eliminating most retakes. *This affords increased efficiency, but this does not mean that images can be exposed arbitrarily* (*Shephard, p. 330*).

27. **(D)** The closer the x-ray source is to the barrier (wall), the greater the thickness necessary. Occupancy factor refers to the degree of occupancy of the department adjacent to the barrier; a stairway would require less shielding than a busy work area. Workload is important in determining barrier thickness and refers to the number of examinations performed in the x-ray room measured in mA-min/wk; the greater the number of examinations per week, the greater the barrier thickness required. Use factor is also important in determining barrier thickness, and refers to the amount of time x-rays are directed to a particular wall; the greater the amount of time, the greater the thickness required (*Sherer et al., p. 204*).

28. **(D)** Sterilization is the complete elimination of all living microorganisms, and can be accomplished by

several methods. *Pressurized steam*, in an *autoclave*, is probably the most familiar means of sterilization; the pressure allows higher temperatures to be achieved. *Gas* or *chemical* sterilization is used for items unable to withstand moisture and/or high temperatures. Other methods of sterilization include *dry heat*, ionizing *radiation*, and microwaves (*non*ionizing radiation) (*Torres et al., pp. 115, 116*).

29. **(C)** When examining the third through fifth fingers in the lateral position, the *medial* side of the forearm (*ulnar side*) should be closest to the image receptor. This *minimizes magnification* by achieving the shortest possible OID. The terms *medial* and *lateral* are identified while viewing the part in the anatomic position (*Bontrager & Lampignano, 7th ed., p. 140*).

30. **(B)** The image intensifier's input phosphor receives the remnant radiation emerging from the patient and converts it into a fluorescent light image. Very close to the input phosphor, separated by a thin, transparent layer, is the photocathode. The photocathode is made of a photoemissive alloy, usually an antimony and cesium compound. The fluorescent light image strikes the photocathode and is converted to an *electron image* that is focused by the electrostatic lenses to the output phosphor (*Fosbinder & Kelsey, p. 260*).

31. **(C)** An artifact associated with digital imaging and grids is *aliasing* or the *Moiré effect*. If the direction of the lead strips and the grid lines per inch (i.e., grid frequency) matches the scan frequency of the scanner/reader, this artifact can occur. Aliasing appears as superimposed images slightly out of alignment, an image "wrapping" effect. This most commonly occurs in mobile radiography with stationary grids, and can be a problem with DR flat-panel detectors. Phantom images are usually associated with incomplete erasure (*Bushong, 9th ed., p. 419, 420*).

32. **(A)** *Primary radiation barriers* protect against direct exposure from the primary (useful) x-ray beam and have much greater attenuation capability than *secondary barriers*, which protect only from leakage and scattered radiation. Examples of primary barriers are the lead *walls* and *doors* of a radiographic room, that is, any surface that could be struck by the useful beam. Primary protective barriers of typical installations generally consist of walls with 1/16-inch (1.5-mm) lead thickness and 7-feet height.

Secondary radiation includes *leakage* and *scattered* radiation. The control booth wall is a secondary barrier; therefore, the primary beam must never be directed toward it. The x-ray tube housing must reduce leakage radiation to less than 100 mR/h at a distance of 1 meter from the housing. Lead aprons, lead gloves, portable x-ray barriers, and the like are also designed to protect the user from exposure to *scattered* radiation, and will not protect from the primary beam (*Sherer et al., pp. 205, 206*).

33. **(C)** The number of *heat units* produced during a given exposure with single-phase equipment is determined by multiplying mA × second × kV. A correction factor is required with three-phase equipment. Unless the equipment manufacturer specifies otherwise, three-phase and high frequency equipment heat units are determined by multiplying mA × second × kV × 1.4. (*Bushong, p. 135*).

34. **(D)** *Indirect contact* involves transmission of microorganisms via *airborne* contamination, *fomites*, and *vectors*. Airborne precaution *requires the patient to wear a mask* to avoid the spread of acid-fast bacilli (in bronchial secretions of tuberculosis patients) or other pathogens during coughing. If the patient is unable or unwilling to wear a mask, the radiographer must wear one. The radiographer should wear gloves, but a gown is required only if flagrant contamination is likely. Patients infected with *airborne precaution* require a *private*, *specially ventilated* (*negative-pressure*) room. A private room is indicated for all patients on *droplet precaution*, that is, diseases transmitted via large droplets expelled from the patient while speaking, sneezing, or coughing. The pathogenic droplets can infect others when they come in contact with mouth or nasal mucosa or conjunctiva. *Rubella* ("German measles"), *mumps*, and *influenza* are among the diseases spread by droplet contact; *a private room is required* for the patient, and health care practitioners must use *gown* and *gloves* (*Adler & Carlton, p. 196*).

35. **(D)** Image storage is located in a *pixel*, which is a two-dimensional "picture element" (see Fig. 14–21) measured in the "XY" direction. The third dimension in the matrix of pixels is the *depth* that together with the pixel is referred to as the *voxel* (see Fig. 14–22), measured in the "Z" direction.

A digital image is formed by a *matrix* of *pixels* in rows and columns. The *matrix* is the number of pixels in the XY direction. *The larger the matrix size, the better the image resolution* (see Fig. 14–23).

A matrix having 512 pixels in each row and column is a 512 × 512 matrix. The term *field of view* is used to describe how much of the patient (e.g., 150-mm diameter) is included in the matrix. The matrix and/or field of view can be changed without one affecting the other, but changes in either will change the pixel size. *As in traditional radiography, spatial resolution is measured in line pairs per millimeter (lp/mm). As matrix size is increased, there are more and smaller pixels in the matrix, and therefore improved resolution.* Fewer and larger pixels result in a poor-resolution "pixelly" image, that is, one in which you can actually see the individual pixel boxes (see Fig. 14–23).

Typical image matrix sizes used in radiography are as follows:

• Nuclear medicine	128 × 128
• Digital subtraction angiography (DSA)	512 × 512
• Computed tomography (CT)	512 × 512
• Chest radiography	2,048 × 2,048

(*Fosbinder & Kelsey, p. 284*).

36. (A) The AP projection provides a general survey of the abdomen, showing the size and shape of the liver, spleen, and kidneys. When performed *erect*, it should demonstrate both hemidiaphragms. The *erect* position is used to demonstrate air/fluid levels (as seen in the radiograph; Fig. 16–4). Air or fluid levels will be clearly demonstrated only if the central ray is directed *parallel* to them. The manner (direction) in which the levels are seen indicates the position in which the image was made (*Frank, Long, & Smith, 11th ed., Vol. 2, p. 102*).

37. (A) In the *photoelectric effect*, a relatively low-energy incident photon uses all of its energy to eject an inner-shell electron, leaving a vacancy. An electron from the next shell will drop to fill the vacancy and *a characteristic ray is given up* in the transition. This type of interaction is more harmful to the patient, as all the photon energy is transferred to the tissue (*Bushong, pp. 176-178*).

38. (C) The exposed CR cassette is placed into the CR scanner reader, where the PSP plate is automatically removed. The latent image appears as the PSP is scanned by a narrow high-intensity *helium–neon laser* to obtain the pixel data. As the plate is scanned in the CR reader, it releases a violet light—a process referred to as *photostimulated luminescence*.

The luminescent light is converted to electrical energy representing the *analog* image. The electrical energy is sent to an ADC where it is digitized and becomes the *digital* image that is eventually displayed (after a short delay) on a high-resolution monitor and/or printed out by a laser printer. The digitized images can also be manipulated in postprocessing, electronically transmitted, and stored/archived (*Shephard, p. 328*).

39. (B) The PA axial projection (Haas method/nuchofrontal projection) of the skull requires that the central ray be angled 25 degrees cephalad to the perpendicular OML. This position is used to demonstrate the *occipital bone* in kyphotic patients and other patients who are unable to assume the AP recumbent position. If positioned accurately, the *dorsum sella* and *posterior clinoid processes* will be demonstrated within the foramen magnum. If the central ray is angled excessively, the *posterior aspect of the arch of C1* will appear in the foramen magnum (*Bontrager & Lampignano, 7th ed., p. 397*).

40. (C) A profile view of the glenoid fossa can be obtained in the AP oblique projection (*LPO or RPO*, Grashey method). In the anatomic position, the bony glenoid fossa is seen to project *posteriorly* and *laterally* approximately 40 degrees. Therefore, if the shoulder is positioned with the body rotated 35 *to 45 degrees toward the affected side*, the glenoid fossa will be placed parallel with the CR (*perpendicular to the image receptor*) and a profile view of the fossa is obtained (*Frank, Long, & Smith, 11th ed., Vol. 1, pp. 192-193*).

41. (D) *Nonstochastic* effects are somatic effects that are predictable, threshold responses; that is, a certain quantity of radiation must be received before the effect occurs, and the greater the dose, the more severe the effect. Examples of nonstochastic effects are erythema, blood changes, cataract formation, and epilation. *Stochastic* effects of radiation are non-threshold and randomly occurring. Examples of stochastic effects include carcinogenesis and genetic effects. The chance of occurrence of stochastic effects is directly related to the radiation dose; that is, as radiation dose increases, there is a greater likelihood of genetic alterations or development of cancer (*Sherer et al., p. 60*).

42. **(C)** Some chemical agents used in health care facilities function to kill pathogenic microorganisms, whereas others function to inhibit the growth/spread of pathogenic microorganisms. Germicides and disinfectants are used to kill pathogenic microorganisms, and antiseptics (like alcohol) are used to stop their growth/spread. *Sterilization* is another associated term, and refers to killing of all microorganisms and their spores (*Frank, Long, & Smith, 11th ed., Vol, 1, p. 16*).

43. **(D)** A question every primary-pathway candidate for certification must answer on their ARRT application, in addition to reading and signing the "Written Consent under FERPA," is, "Have you ever been suspended, dismissed, or expelled from an educational program that you have attended in order to meet ARRT certification requirements?"

The ARRT can obtain specific parts of a graduate's educational records concerning violations to an honor code. If a student has ever been suspended, dismissed, or expelled from an educational program attended in order to meet ARRT certification requirements, he/she should answer "yes" to the question above and include an explanation and documentation of the situation with the completed application for certification. If the applicant is in doubt, he/she should contact the ARRT Ethics Requirements Department at (651) 687–0048, ext. 8580.

Some examples of reportable infractions are listed below:

- Cheating and/or plagiarism
- Falsification of eligibility requirements (e.g., clinical competency information)
- Forgery or alteration of any document related to qualifications or patient care
- Abuse, neglect, or abandonment of patients
- Sexual contact without consent or harassment to any member of the community, including patients
- Conduct that is seriously obscene or offensive
- Practicing in an unsafe manner or outside the scope of professional training
- Violating patient confidentiality (HIPAA)
- Attempted or actual theft of any item not belonging to the student (including patients' property)
- Attending class or clinical setting while under the influence of alcohol, drugs, or other substances

(The American Registry of Radiologic Technologists Standards of Ethics. (Reprinted, with permission, from the ARRT Standards of Ethics. ARRT: 2010.)

44. **(B)** As blood pulsates through the arteries, a throb can be detected. This throb or *pulse* can be readily palpated where the arteries are superficial. (Examples are *wrist*, *groin*, *neck*, and posterior surface of the *knee*.) The apical pulse can be detected with a stethoscope (*Torres, pp. 143-145*).

45. **(B)** The *image intensifier* in mobile fluoroscopic ("C" arm) equipment has the same function as the image intensifier in fixed equipment; that is, it brightens the x-ray image so that it can be viewed in a room having normal lighting. The *TV camera/CCD* transmits the fluoroscopic image from the output phosphor of the image intensifier to the *TV monitor* for viewing. Mobile fluoroscopes/"C" arms have no *spot-film device*, although they frequently have features such as "last image hold" and capacity for digital recording (*Fosbinder & Kelsey, pp. 266-268*).

46. **(B)** Radiograph A was performed *PA* and radiograph B was performed *AP*, as evidenced by the bony pelvis anatomy. The PA projection (image A) shows the ilia more foreshortened, giving the pelvis a "closed" appearance, whereas the AP projection shows the ilia and bladder area more "open." There was an appropriate selection of exposure factors, for the required anatomic structures are well visualized: renal shadows, psoas muscle, lumbar transverse processes, and inferior margin of the liver. There is no evidence of the radiographs having been done erect, as the hemidiaphragms are not included, and the gas patterns appear without leveling (*Bontrager, pp. 109, 110*).

47. **(A)** Inside the CR image plate (IP) is the PSP or SPS. This PSP/SPS with its layer of europium-activated barium fluorohalide serves as the *image receptor* as it is exposed in the traditional manner and receives the latent image. The PSP/SPS can *store* the latent image for several hours; after approximately 8 hours, noticeable image fading will occur. Once the IP is placed into the CR processor (*scanner* or *reader*), the PSP/SPS is automatically removed. The latent image on the PSP is changed to a manifest image as it is scanned by a narrow, high-intensity *helium–neon laser* to obtain the pixel data. As the PSP is scanned in the "reader," it releases a violet light—a process referred to as *photo* (or light)-*stimulated luminescence* (*Shephard, pp. 325-327*).

48. (A) The knee (tibiofemoral joint) is the largest joint of the body, formed by the articulation of the femur and tibia. However, it actually consists of three articulations: (i) the patellofemoral joint, (ii) the lateral tibiofemoral joint (lateral femoral condyle with tibial plateau), and (iii) the medial tibiofemoral joint (medial femoral condyle with tibial plateau). Although the knee is classified as a synovial (diarthrotic) hinge-type joint, the patellofemoral joint is actually a gliding joint, and the medial and lateral tibiofemoral joints are hinge type (*Tortora & Derrickson, p. 282*).

49. (B) Because *muscle* and *nerve* tissues perform specific functions and do not divide, they are relatively *insensitive* to radiation exposure. *Epithelial* cells cover the outer surface of the body and line body cavities as well as tubes and passageways leading to the exterior. They contain very little intercellular substance and are devoid of blood vessels. Because *epithelial* cells constantly regenerate through mitosis, they are very *radiosensitive* (*Sherer et al., p. 108*).

50. (C) Ribs below the diaphragm are best demonstrated with the diaphragm elevated. This is accomplished by placing the patient in a recumbent position and taking the exposure at the end of exhalation. Conversely, the ribs above the diaphragm are best demonstrated with the diaphragm depressed. Placing the patient in the erect position and taking the exposure at the end of deep inspiration accomplishes this (*Frank, Long, & Smith, 11th ed., Vol. 1, p. 492*).

51. (B) Protective barriers are classified as either primary or secondary. Primary barriers protect from the useful, or primary, x-ray beam and consist of a certain thickness of lead. They are located anywhere the primary beam can possibly be directed, for example, the walls of the x-ray room. The walls of the x-ray room usually require 1/16-inch (1.5-mm) thickness of 7-feet-high lead. Secondary barriers protect from secondary (scattered and leakage) radiation. Secondary barriers are control booths, lead aprons and gloves, and the wall of the x-ray room above 7 feet. Secondary barriers require much less lead than do primary barriers (*Bushong, p. 569*).

52. (B) Syncope, or fainting, is a result of a drop in blood pressure caused by insufficient blood (oxygen) to the brain. The patient should be helped into a dorsal recumbent position with feet elevated to facilitate blood flow to the brain (*Adler & Corlton, pp. 247-248*).

53. (D) The phenomenon in which the radiographic information recorded on the PSP/SPS upon exposure to x-rays *decreases* with the elapsed time until it is read by the scanner/reader is termed *fading*. This occurs because the photoelectrons generated by x-ray excitation upon exposure of the photostimulable phosphor are thermally released over time and are therefore unable to contribute to photostimulated luminescence upon scanning/reading. Luminescence decreases by approximately 25% within 8 hours of exposure. The greater the elapsed time and the greater the environmental temperature, the greater will be the degree of fading (*Shephard, p. 325*).

54. (C) According to Bergonié and Tribondeau, the most radiosensitive cells are undifferentiated, rapidly dividing cells, such as lymphocytes, intestinal crypt (of Lieberkühn) cells, and spermatogonia. Liver cells are among the types of cells that are somewhat differentiated and capable of mitosis. These characteristics render them somewhat radiosensitive. Muscle cells, as well as nerve cells and red blood cells, are highly differentiated and do not divide. Therefore, in order of *decreasing* sensitivity (from least to greatest sensitivity), the cells are intestinal crypt cells, liver cells, and muscle cells (*Bushong, p. 495*).

55. (C) Phosphors with a high atomic number have a greater likelihood of interacting with an x-ray photon and therefore possess greater speed. How ably a particular phosphor detects the presence of x-ray photons is referred to as *detective quantum efficiency* (DQE). The phosphor also needs a high *conversion efficiency* (CE); that is, it should emit a liberal measure of fluorescent light for each x-ray photon it absorbs. The greater the conversion efficiency, the greater the speed (*Bushong, p. 209*).

56. (C) Although the *inferosuperior axial* projection can be used to evaluate the glenohumeral joint, the required abduction of the arm would be contraindicated when evaluating a shoulder for possible dislocation. The *transthoracic* lateral projection is used to evaluate the glenohumeral joint and upper humerus when the patient is unable to abduct the arm (as in dislocation). The *scapular Y* projection is an oblique projection of the shoulder and is used in demonstrating anterior or posterior dislocation (*Frank, Long, & Smith, 11th ed., Vol. 1, pp. 181, 184, 189*).

57. (B) *Oral* administration of barium sulfate is used to demonstrate the upper digestive system, esophagus, fundus, body and pylorus of the stomach, and barium progression through the small bowel. The large bowel, including sigmoid colon, is usually demonstrated via *rectal* administration of barium (*Gurley & Callaway, p. 113*).

58. **(C)** Tissue is most sensitive to radiation exposure when in an *oxygenated* condition. Anoxic refers to a general lack of oxygen in tissue; hypoxic refers to tissue with little oxygen. Anoxic and hypoxic tumors are typically avascular (with little or no blood supply) and are therefore more radioresistant (*Sherer et al., pp. 96-97*).

59. **(D)** The ability of x-ray photons to penetrate a body part has a great deal to do with the composition of that part (e.g., bone vs. soft tissue vs. air) and the presence of any pathologic condition. Pathologic conditions can alter the normal nature of the anatomic part. Some conditions such as osteomalacia, fibrosarcoma, and paralytic ileus (obstruction) result in a decrease in body tissue density. When body tissue density decreases, x-rays will penetrate the tissues more readily, that is, more x-ray penetrability. In conditions such as ascites, where body tissue density increases as a result of accumulation of fluid, x-rays will not readily penetrate the body tissues, that is, less x-ray penetrability (*Carlton & Adler, p. 259*).

60. **(A)** The image intensifier's input phosphor receives the remnant beam from the patient and converts it to a fluorescent light image. To maintain resolution, the input phosphor is made of cesium iodide crystals. *Cesium iodide* is much more efficient in this conversion process than the phosphor previously used, zinc cadmium sulfide. Calcium tungstate was the phosphor used in cassette-intensifying screens for many years prior to the development of rare earth phosphors such as gadolinium oxysulfide (*Bushong, p. 360*).

61. **(D)** The wrist is composed of eight carpal bones arranged in two rows (proximal and distal). The proximal row consists of (from lateral to medial) the scaphoid, lunate, triquetrum, and pisiform. The distal row (from lateral to medial) includes the trapezium, trapezoid, capitate, and hamate. The radiograph seen in Figure 16–7 is a *PA projection of the wrist.* The letter *L* represents the *scaphoid*, which is the most *lateral* carpal of the *proximal* row. The letter *M* points out the most *medial* carpal of the *distal* row, the *hamate.* The joints of the wrist include the *inter-*

carpal joints and the *radiocarpal joint* (*Frank, Long, & Smith, Vol. 1, p. 94*).

62. **(D)** Hysterosalpingography may be performed for demonstration of uterine tubal patency, mass lesions in the uterine cavity, and uterine position. Although hysterosalpingography is often performed to check tubal patency, the uterine anatomy, position, and morphology are exhibited. Additionally, polyps, fibroids, or space occupying lesions within the uterus are well demonstrated (*Bontrager & Lampignano, 7th ed., pp. 758-759*).

63. **(D)** Double-contrast studies of the stomach or large intestine involve coating the organ with a thin layer of barium sulfate and then introducing air. This permits seeing through the organ to structures behind it and especially allows visualization of the mucosal lining of the organ. A barium-filled stomach or large bowel demonstrates position, size, and shape of the organ, and any lesion that projects out from its walls, such as diverticula. Polypoid lesions, which project inward from the wall of an organ, may go unnoticed unless a double-contrast examination is performed (*Frank, Long, & Smith, 11th ed., Vol. 2, p. 142*).

64. **(A)** The intensity or exposure rate of radiation at a given distance from a point source is inversely proportional to the square of the distance. This is the inverse square law of radiation and is expressed in the following equation:

$$\frac{t_1}{t_1} = \frac{D_2^2}{D_1^2}$$

Substituting known values:

$$\frac{40 \, mR/h}{x \, mR/h} = \frac{25}{9}$$

$$25x = 360$$

$$x = 14.4 \, mR/h, \text{ therefore } 7.2 \, mR \text{ in 30 minutes}$$

(*Bushong, p. 59*).

65. **(D)** The medical suffix *plasia* refers to development, formation, growth, or proliferation. The suffix denoting embryonic is *blast*. Condition is indicated by the suffix *osis*. The suffix *kinesia* is used to refer to motion or movement (*Taber's, p. 1683*).

66. **(A)** The *AP axial* projection (Towne method) of the skull is used to demonstrate the *occipital* bone. The skull is positioned AP and the CR is directed caudally. This serves to project the anterior structures inferiorly

and away from superimposition on the occipital bone. The frontal bone is best demonstrated in the PA projection, and the facial bones in the parietoacanthial (Waters) position. The sphenoid bone can be seen in the lateral and basal projections (*Frank, Long, & Smith, 11th ed., Vol. 2, p. 316*).

67. **(D)** The mediastinum is the space between the lungs that contains the heart, great vessels, trachea, esophagus, and thymus gland. It is bound anteriorly by the sternum and posteriorly by the vertebral column and extends from the upper thorax to the diaphragm (*Frank, Long, & Smith, 11th ed., Vol. 1, p. 501*).

68. **(A)** Because the established dose-limit formula guideline is used for occupationally exposed persons 18 years of age and older, guidelines had to be established in the event a student entered the clinical component of a radiography educational program prior to age 18 years. The guideline states that the occupational dose limit for students *younger than 18 years* is *0.1 rem* (100 mrem or 1 mSv) in any given year. (*Bushong, p. 559*).

69. **(A)** Proper body mechanics includes a wide base of support. The *base of support* is the part of the body in touch with the floor or other horizontal plane. The *center of gravity* is the midpoint of the pelvis or lower abdomen, depending on body build. The *line of gravity* is the abstract line passing through the center of gravity, vertically. Proper body mechanics can help prevent painful back injuries by making proficient use of the muscles in the arms and legs (*Torres et al., pp. 82-83*).

70. **(D)** The "scapular Y" refers to the characteristic *Y* formed by the body of the scapula, acromion, and coracoid processes. The patient is positioned in a PA oblique position—an RAO or LAO, depending on which is the affected side. The midcoronal plane is adjusted approximately 60 degrees to the image receptor, and the affected arm is left relaxed at the patient's side. The scapular Y position is employed *to demonstrate anterior* (subcoracoid) or *posterior* (subacromial) *humeral dislocation*. The humerus is normally superimposed on the scapula in this position; any deviation from this may indicate dislocation (*Bontrager, p. 185*).

71. **(C)** The AEC automatically terminates the exposure when the proper density has been recorded on the image receptor. The important advantage of the phototimer, then, is that it can accurately duplicate radiographic densities. It is useful in providing accurate comparison in follow-up examinations and in decreasing patient exposure dose by decreasing the number of "retakes" because of improper exposure. The AEC automatically adjusts the exposure required for body parts having different *thicknesses* and *densities*. Remember that proper functioning of the AEC depends on accurate positioning by the radiographer. The correct *ionization chamber*(s) must be selected, and the anatomic part of interest must completely cover the ionization chamber to achieve the desired density. If *collimation* is inadequate, and a field size larger than the part is used, excessive scattered radiation from the body or tabletop can cause the AEC to terminate the exposure prematurely, resulting in an underexposed radiograph (*Shephard, pp. 289-291*).

72. **(D)** *Chromosome aberration, cell death*, and *malignant disease* are major effects of deoxyribonucleic acid (DNA) irradiation, often as a result of abnormal metabolic activity. If the damage happens to the DNA of a germ cell, the radiation response may not occur until one or more generations later (*Bushong, p. 527*).

73. **(D)** Voltage ripple refers to the percentage drop from maximum voltage each pulse of current experiences. In single-phase rectified equipment, the entire pulse (half-cycle) is used; therefore, there is first an increase to maximum (peak) voltage value and a subsequent decrease to zero potential (90-degree past peak potential). The entire waveform is used; if 100 kV were selected, the actual average kilovoltage output would be approximately 70. Three-phase rectification produces almost constant potential with just small ripples (drops) in maximum potential between pulses. Approximately, a 13% voltage ripple (drop from maximum value) characterizes the operation of three-phase, six-pulse generators. Three-phase, twelve-pulse generators have approximately a 4.0% voltage ripple (*Selman, p. 254*).

74. **(C)** Obtaining a complete and accurate history from the patient for the radiologist is an important aspect of a radiographer's job. Both subjective and objective data should be collected. *Objective* data include signs and symptoms that can be observed, such as a cough, a lump, or elevated blood pressure. *Subjective* data relate to what the patient feels and to what extent. A patient may experience pain, but is it mild or

severe? Is it localized or general? Does the pain increase or decrease under different circumstances? A radiographer should explore this with a patient and document additional information on the requisition for the radiologist (*Adler & Carlton, p. 137*).

75. (B) CR uses special phosphor plates inside IPs to record the radiologic image. No film is used, hence the term *filmless* radiography. The IP is exposed just like a conventional screen–film cassette. Upon exposure, a latent image is produced on the PSP, which is located inside the IP. The IP is placed in the CR reader, and the PSP is automatically removed. The PSP is scanned with a narrow laser beam to obtain the pixel data, which can then be displayed on a monitor as the radiographic image (*Shephard, pp. 325-327*).

76. (C) There are two types of distortion: size and shape. *Shape distortion* relates to the alignment of the x-ray tube, the part to be radiographed, and the image receptor. There are two kinds of shape distortion: *elongation* and *foreshortening*. *Size distortion* is *magnification* and is related to the OID and SID. Magnification can be reduced by either increasing the SID or decreasing the OID. However, an increase in SID must be accompanied by an increase in mAs (milliampere-seconds) to maintain density. It is therefore preferable, in the interest of exposure time, to reduce OID whenever possible (*Selman, pp. 348, 356*).

77. (A) Three times a day is indicated by the abbreviation *TID*. The abbreviation *QID* means four times a day. Every hour is represented by *QH*, and *PC* means after meals (*Ehrlich et al., p. 277*).

78. (A) As kV is increased, more *high-energy* photons are produced and the overall energy of the primary beam is increased. *Photon energy is inversely related to wavelength*; that is, as photon energy increases, wavelength decreases. An increase in milliamperage serves to increase the number of photons produced at the target, but is unrelated to their energy (*Selman, p. 177*).

79. (A) The cervical intervertebral foramina lie 45 degrees to the midsagittal plane and 15 to 20 degrees to a transverse plane. When the *posterior oblique* position (LPO and RPO) is used, the cervical intervertebral foramina demonstrated are those *further* from the image receptor. There is therefore some magnification of the foramina. In the *anterior oblique* position (LAO and RAO), the foramina disclosed are those *closer* to the image receptor (*Frank, Long, & Smith, 11th ed., Vol. 1, p. 404*).

80. (D) Proper *alignment* of the x-ray tube, body part, and image receptor is required to avoid image *distortion* in the form of *foreshortening* or *elongation*. *Foreshortening* will usually result when the *part* is out of alignment. *Elongation* is often a result of *angulation of the x-ray tube*. Grid lines or *grid cutoff* will occur when the *grid* itself is off center or is not in alignment with the x-ray tube (*Shephard, p. 232*).

81. (B) Image *fading* will occur if there is delay in reading the PSP. This is because after a time, trapped photoelectrons are released from the "color center" and are therefore unable to participate in PSL. PSL intensity *decreases* in the interval between the x-ray exposure and the image reading process. If the exposed PSL is not delivered to the reader/ processor for 8 hours, PSL decreases by approximately 25%. Fading also increases as environmental temperature increases. It is recommended that the PSP be scanned in the reader at right angles to grid line direction to avoid/reduce aliasing artifacts (*Shephard p. 325*).

82. (D); 83. (A); 84. (C) The *stomach* is the dilated, sac-like portion of the GI tract. When the stomach (or a portion of it) is empty, its mucosal lining forms soft folds called *rugae* (L). Exteriorly, the stomach presents a *greater curvature* (K) on its lateral surface and a *lesser curvature* (J) on its medial surface. The proximal opening of the stomach is the cardiac sphincter; the pyloric sphincter is located at its distal end. The portion of the stomach around the distal esophagus is called the *cardia*; that portion superior to the esophageal juncture is the *fundus* (A). The major portion of the stomach is the *body* (B); the distal portion is the *pylorus* (C). The *incisura angularis* (I) is located on the lesser curvature and marks the beginning of the pylorus (C). The distal opening of the pylorus is the pyloric sphincter. The small intestine is composed of the duodenum, jejunum, and ileum. The duodenum is the shortest portion (approximately 12 inches). It begins just beyond the pyloric sphincter and is divided into four portions: the *duodenal cap* or *bulb* (D), *descending duodenum* (E), transverse duodenum, and *ascending duodenum* (F). These portions form the C-shaped *duodenal loop* that is occupied by the *head of the pancreas* (G). The ascending duodenum terminates at the duodenojejunal flexure that marks the beginning of the 9-foot *jejunum* (H) (*Frank, Long, & Smith, 11th ed., Vol. 2, p. 122*).

85. (C) Because the fundus is the most *posterior* portion of the stomach, it readily fills with barium when the patient is in the *AP* or *LPO* position. With the patient in *PA* or *RAO* position, the barium moves to the more distal portions of the stomach. Figure 16–8 illustrates the RAO position. It is in this position that peristalsis is most active and the stomach's emptying mechanism can be evaluated. To evaluate the stomach adequately, preliminary patient preparation is required. The upper GI tract must be empty; patients should be questioned about their preparation and a preliminary "scout image" taken to check abdominal contents (*Frank, Long, & Smith, 11th ed., Vol. 2, p. 148*).

86. (C) Many people believe that potential legal and ethical issues can be avoided by creating an *advance health care directive* or *living will*. Since all persons have the right to make decisions regarding their own health care, this legal document preserves that right in the event an individual is unable to make those decisions. The directive names the individual authorized to make all health care decisions and can include specifics regarding *DNR, DNI,* and/or other end-of-life decisions (*Ehrlich et al. 7th ed., p. 86*).

87. (C) Added aluminum filtration removes more low energy photons, therefore there is a decrease in the *number* of photons in the x-ray beam—that is, beam *intensity*. Because low energy photons are removed, the overall average energy of the x-ray beam is increased. This process can also be referred to a beam *hardening* because its average energy is increased. The maximum energy of the beam is unchanged as long as the kV remains unchanged (*Bushong, 9th ed, p. 146, 147*).

88. (B) Radiographic contrast is described as the difference between densities, or scale of grays, in the radiographic image. Because the function of *grids* is to collect scattered radiation, they serve to shorten the scale of contrast. *Beam restrictors* function to limit the x-ray field size, thereby reducing the production of scattered radiation, and shorten the scale of contrast. *Focal spot size* is one of the geometric factors affecting the recorded detail and has no effect on the scale of contrast. It is the function of radiographic contrast to make details visible. The sum of subject contrast and film contrast equals radiographic contrast (*Carlton & Adler, pp. 385-389*).

89. (C) A *pulse oximeter* is used to measure a patient's pulse rate and oxygen saturation level. A *stethoscope* and a *sphygmomanometer* are used together to measure blood pressure. The first sound heard is the systolic pressure and the normal range is 110 to 140 mm Hg. When no more sound is heard, the diastolic pressure is recorded. The normal diastolic range is 60 to 90 mm Hg. Elevated blood pressure is called *hypertension. Hypotension*, low blood pressure, is not of concern unless it is caused by injury or disease; in that case, it results in shock (*Adler & Carlton, pp. 161-167*).

90. (C) The development of male and female reproductive stem cells has important radiation protection implications. Male reproductive stem cells reproduce continuously. However, the female reproductive stem cells develop only during fetal life; women are born with all the reproductive cells they will ever have. It is exceedingly important to shield children, whenever possible, as they have their reproductive futures ahead of them (*Bushong, p. 523*).

91. (D) In *film/screen imaging*, insufficient milliamperage and/or exposure time result in lack of radiographic density. Insufficient kV results in underpenetration and excessive contrast. Insufficient SID, however, results in increased exposure rate and radiographic *overexposure* (*Selman, pp. 331-333*).

92. (B) The *quantity* of x-ray photons produced at the target is the function of mAs. The *quality* (wavelength, penetration, and energy) of x-ray photons produced at the target is the function of kV. The kV also has an effect on exposure rate, because an increase in kV increases the number of high-energy x-ray photons produced at the target. Exposure rate *decreases* with an increase in SID (*Selman, pp. 332-333*).

93. (B) Anemia is a blood condition characterized by a decreased number of circulating red blood cells and decreased hemoglobin, and has many causes. Adequate hemoglobin is required to provide oxygen to the body. Anemia is treated according to its cause. Hematuria is the term used to describe blood in the urine and is unrelated to anemia (*Tortora & Derrickson, p. 689*).

94. (C) Grids are composed of alternating strips of lead and radiolucent interspace material. The interspace material is either aluminum or plastic fiber. Aluminum resists moisture, is sturdier, provides a "smoother" appearance with less visible grid lines—but requires a higher mAs and therefore increases patient dose. Plastic fiber interspace material can be affected by

moisture, resulting in warping. Carbon fiber is often used as image plate-front material because of its durability and homogeneity (Bushong, 9th ed, p. 234).

95. (D) Before the radiologic examination begins, patients often need to change their clothing and/or remove radiopaque objects (e.g., jewelry, dentures, and braided hair) from superimposition on structures of interest. *Figure 16–9* illustrates multiple *braids* of hair superimposed on skull structures. While loose hair is radiolucent, hair that is braided becomes more dense and is often imaged radiographically. The ensuing artifacts can interfere with accurate diagnosis (Saia, p. 79).

96. (C) The greatest effect of, and response to, irradiation is brought about by a *large dose of radiation*, *to the whole body*, *delivered all at one time*. Whole-body radiation can depress many body functions. With a fractionated dose, the effects would be less severe because the body would have an opportunity to repair between doses (Bushong, p. 551).

97. (C) In the *AP* projection, the proximal fibula is at least partially superimposed on the lateral tibial condyle. *Medial rotation* of 45 degrees will "open" the proximal tibiofibular articulation. *Lateral rotation* will obscure the articulation even more (Frank, Long, & Smith, 11th ed., Vol. 1, p. 310).

98. (A) Some chemical agents used in health care facilities function to *kill* pathogenic microorganisms, while others function to *inhibit the growth/spread* of pathogenic microorganisms. Germicides and disinfectants are used to kill pathogenic microorganisms and antiseptics (like alcohol) are used to stop their growth/spread. Sterilization is another associated term and refers to killing of all microorganisms and their spores (Torres et al., p. 116).

99. (B) Epinephrine (Adrenalin) is the vasopressor used to treat an anaphylactic reaction or cardiac arrest. *Nitroglycerin* is a vasodilator. *Hydrocortisone* is a steroid that may be used to treat bronchial asthma, allergic reactions, and inflammatory reactions. *Digitoxin* is used to treat cardiac fibrillation (Ehrlich et al. 7th ed., p. 255).

100. (C) Grids are used in radiography to *absorb scattered radiation* before it reaches the image receptor, thus improving radiographic contrast. Contrast obtained with a grid compared to contrast without a grid is termed *contrast improvement factor*. The greater the percentage of scattered radiation

absorbed compared to absorbed nonscattered radiation, the greater the "selectivity" of the grid. If a grid absorbs an abnormally large amount of primary radiation because of improper centering, tube angle, or tube distance, *grid cutoff* occurs (Selman, p. 370).

101. (D) Normal tissue variants and pathologic processes that alter tissue thickness and composition can have a significant effect on image density. The radiographer must be aware of these variants and processes to make an appropriate and accurate selection of technical factors. Normal variants of muscle development result from different lifestyles, occupations, and age, and will affect image density. Other than normal variants that influence image density/brightness, and, consequently the selection of technical factors, are age, gender, and pathology. Various abnormal pathologic conditions, disease processes, and trauma can affect tissue density and, hence, density.

Some pathologic conditions are referred to as *destructive*, such as osteoporosis, osteomalacia, pneumoperitoneum, emphysema, and conditions involving necrosis or atrophy. These conditions can cause an undesirable increase in image density unless they are recognized and appropriate changes made in exposure factors. Other conditions such as ascites, rheumatoid arthritis, and Paget disease are *additive*, and an increase in exposure factors is required to maintain adequate density/brightness.

102. (B) The bony walls of the orbit are thin, fragile, and subject to fracture. A direct blow to the eye results in a pressure that can cause fracture. That fracture is usually to the *orbital floor* (inferior aspect of the bony orbit). Because the fracture results from increased pressure within the eye, it is referred to as a "blowout" fracture (Frank, Long, & Smith, 11th ed., Vol. 2, pp. 295, 298).

103. (D) The advantages of digital fluoroscopy (DF) over conventional fluoroscopy include higher speed acquisition and availability of postprocessing for image/contrast enhancement. Although DF fundamentally appears the same as conventional fluoroscopy, DF has special requirements: a computer, two video monitors, and an operating console that is far more complex than the conventional console. A computer is located between the TV camera (or CCD) and the TV monitor and serves to convert the analog image to a digital image. The operating console has many special function keys for patient data entry, data acquisition, image

display, and image postprocessing manipulation. Two video monitors are required; the second monitor is for display of the subtracted image (*Bushong, p. 408*).

104. (C) When the barium fluorohalide absorbs x-ray energy, electrons are released and they divide into two groups: One electron group initiates *immediate luminescence* during the excited state of Eu^{2+}. The other electron group becomes trapped within the phosphor's halogen ions, forming a "color center." These are the phosphors that ultimately form the radiographic image because when exposed to a *monochromatic* laser light source, these phosphors emit *polychromatic* light, termed *photostimulated luminescence*.

The PSP layer (or SPS) can *store* its latent image for several hours; however, after approximately 8 hours, noticeable image *fading* will occur. The europium activator is important for the *storage* characteristic of the PSPs; it also has functions similar to the sensitization specks within film emulsion. Without europium, the image will not become manifest (*Bushong, 9th ed., p. 413*).

105. (B) Late, long-term, effects of radiation can occur in tissues that have survived a previous irradiation months or years earlier. These late effects, such as carcinogenesis and genetic effects, are "all-or-nothing" effects—either the organism develops cancer or it does not. Most late effects *do not have a threshold dose*; that is, *any* dose, however small, theoretically can induce an effect. Increasing that dose increases the likelihood of the occurrence but does not affect its severity; these effects are termed *stochastic*. *Nonstochastic effects* are those that do not occur below a particular threshold dose and that increase in severity as the dose increases (*Sherer et al., pp. 120-121*).

106. (C) A certain amount of object unsharpness is an inherent part of every radiographic image because of the position and shape of anatomic structures within the body.

For the shape of anatomic structures to be accurately recorded, the structures must be *parallel* to the x-ray tube (*perpendicular* to the CR) and the *image receptor* and *aligned* with the *CR*.

Image details away from the path of the CR will be exposed by more divergent rays, resulting in *rotation distortion*. This is why the CR must be directed to the part of greatest interest.

The shape of anatomic structures lying at an angle within the body or placed away from the CR will be misrepresented on the image receptor. There are two types of shape distortion. If a linear structure is not parallel to the long axis of the part/body and not parallel to the image receptor, that anatomic structure will appear *smaller*—it will be *foreshortened*. On the other hand, *elongation* occurs when the x-ray tube is angled (*Bushong 9th ed., p. 259*).

107. (B) CT and MRI are two common examples of *digital imaging*. Special equipment is also available for digital radiography (DR) or computed radiography (CR): images produced by either a fan-shaped x-ray beam received by linearly arrayed radiation detectors or a traditional fan-shaped x-ray beam received by a light-stimulated phosphor plate. Digital images can also be obtained in digital subtraction angiography (DSA), nuclear medicine, and diagnostic sonography. *Analog* images are conventional images that can be converted to digital images with a device called *digitizer*. Pluridirectional tomography refers to conventional tomographic equipment that is capable of several x-ray tube movements (*Bushong, p. 396*).

108. (C) After exposure, the IP is placed into the CR *reader* where the PSP screen is automatically removed, moved at a constant speed, and scanned by a narrow high-intensity helium–neon (infrared) laser or a solid-state laser to obtain the pixel data. The appropriate wavelength is absorbed by the "color center" and the electrons are trapped there, causing PSL to occur during the excited state of Eu^{2+}.

The phosphors are activated by a monochromatic laser light; however, PSL is a *different* color (bluish-purple, blue–green, etc.). These two lights (PSL and laser) must not interfere with each other. To improve the image SNR, the PSL (carrying the x-ray image) must be of a different wavelength/color than, and physically separate from, the laser excitation light. An *optical filter/beam-shaping optics* is used that permits *transmission* of the PSL, but *attenuates* the laser light; this filter/beam shaper is mounted in front of a PMT.

The PMT or photodiode detects the PSL and converts it to electrical signals that are sent to an ADC where it becomes the digital image displayed on a high-resolution monitor. The digitized images can also be manipulated in postprocessing, electronically transmitted, and stored/archived (*Bushong, 9th ed., p. 420*).

109. (C) Angina pectoris is a spasmodic chest pain frequently caused by oxygen deficiency in the myocardium. The pain often radiates down the left arm and up to the left jaw. Angina pectoris attacks are frequently associated with exertion or emotional stress in individuals with coronary artery disease. Pain may be relieved with a vasodilator such as *nitroglycerin* given sublingually or transdermally. *Digitalis* is used to treat congestive heart failure. *Dilantin* is used in the control of seizure disorders, and *Tagamet* is used to treat duodenal ulcers (*Adler & Carlton, p. 265*).

110. (C) The normal *female (gynecoid) pelvis* differs from the normal *male (android) pelvis* in that it is shallower and its bones are generally more delicate. The pelvic outlet is wider and more circular in the female; the ischial tuberosities and acetabula are further apart; and the angle formed by the pubic arch is also greater in the female. All these bony characteristics facilitate the birth process (see Fig. 6–26).

Following are the male (android) pelvis characteristics:

• Narrower, more vertical

• Deeper from anterior to posterior

• Pubic angle less than 90 degree

• Pelvic inlet narrower and heart-shaped/round

111. (B) Radiographic contrast is described as the difference between densities in the radiographic image. It is the function of radiographic contrast to make details visible. Radiographs exhibiting many shades of gray are said to possess *long-scale*, or *low*, radiographic contrast; that is, there are *many grays*, and there is only *little difference between the various shades of gray*. Conversely, radiographs exhibiting *few shades of gray* are said to possess *short-scale*, or *high*, radiographic contrast. These images have a very *noticeable difference between radiographic densities* (*Shephard, p. 194*).

112. (A) Injectable medications are available in two different kinds of containers. An *ampule* usually holds a single dose of medication. A *vial* is a small bottle that holds several doses of the medication. The term *bolus* is used to describe an amount of fluid to be injected. A *carafe* is a narrow-mouthed container not likely to be used for medical purposes (*Adler & Carlton, p. 279*).

113. (B) An increase in kilovoltage (photon energy) will result in a *greater number* (i.e., exposure rate) of scattered photons (Compton interaction). These scattered photons carry no useful information and contribute to radiation *fog*. This *decreases* radiographic contrast in *film/screen imaging* (*Selman, p. 364*).

114. (D) The distal humerus articulates with the proximal radius and ulna to form the elbow joint. At its proximal end, the ulna presents the *olecranon process*, found at the proximal and posterior end of the *semilunar (trochlear) notch*. The *coronoid process* is seen at the distal and anterior end of the semilunar notch. Specifically, the semilunar notch of the ulna articulates with the trochlea of the distal medial humerus. The *capitulum* is lateral to the trochlea and articulates with the radial head (*Saia, p. 88*).

115. (B); 116. (C) Figure 16–10 shows an AP projection of the elbow joint. The distal humerus articulates with the radius and ulna to form the elbow joint. The lateral aspect of the distal humerus presents a raised, smooth, rounded surface, the *capitulum* (E), that articulates with the superior surface of the *radial head* (A). The *trochlea* (F) is on the medial aspect of the distal humerus and articulates with the semilunar notch of the ulna. Just proximal to the capitulum and trochlea are the *lateral* (D) and *medial* (C) *epicondyles*; the medial is more prominent and palpable. The coronoid fossa is found on the anterior distal humerus and functions to accommodate the *coronoid process* (B) with the elbow in flexion (*Saia, p. 89*).

117. (B) The patient is the most important radiation scatterer during both radiography and fluoroscopy. In general, at 1 m from the patient, *the intensity is reduced by a factor of 1,000*, to approximately 0.1% of the original intensity. Successive scatterings can render the intensity to unimportant levels (*Hendee and Ritenour 4th ed., p. 446*).

118. (B) The sacroiliac joints angle posteriorly and medially 25 degrees to the median sagittal plane (MSP). Therefore, to demonstrate the sacroiliac joints with the patient in the *AP* position, the *affected* side must be elevated 25 degrees. This places the joint space perpendicular to the image receptor and parallel to the central ray. Therefore, the *LPO* position will demonstrate the *right sacroiliac joint* and RPO position will demonstrate the left. When performed with the patient *PA* in position, the *unaffected* side will be elevated 25 degrees (*Bontrager, p. 271*).

119. (B) Magnification is part of every radiographic image. Anatomic parts within the body are at various distances from the image receptor and therefore have various degrees of magnification. The formula used to determine amount of image magnification is:

$$\frac{\text{Image size}}{\text{Object size}} = \frac{\text{SID}}{\text{SOD}}$$

Substituting known values:

$$\frac{X}{3''} = \frac{36'' \, \text{SID}}{32'' \, \text{SOD}} \quad (\text{SOD} = \text{SID} - \text{OID})$$

$$32x = 108$$

$$x = 3.37 \, \text{image width}$$

(*Bushong, p. 321*).

120. (A) Sternoclavicular joints should be performed PA whenever possible to keep OID to a minimum. The *oblique* position (approximately 15 degrees) opens the joint *closest* to the image receptor. The erect position may be used, but is not required. Weight-bearing images are not recommended (*Frank, Long, & Smith, 11th ed., Vol. 1, p. 480*).

121. (D) The greater and lesser tubercles are prominences on the proximal humerus separated by the intertubercular (bicipital) groove. The AP projection of the humerus/shoulder places the *epicondyles parallel to the image receptor* and the shoulder in *external rotation* and demonstrates the *greater tubercle in profile*. The lateral projection of the humerus places the shoulder in extreme internal rotation with the epicondyles perpendicular to the image receptor and demonstrates the lesser tubercle in profile (*Frank, Long, & Smith, 11th ed., Vol. 1, p. 159*).

122. (C) Radiographic examinations of the large bowel generally include the AP or PA axial position to "open" the S-shaped sigmoid colon, the lateral position especially for the rectum, and the LAO and RAO (or LPO and RPO) to "open" the colic flexures. Left and right decubitus positions are usually employed only in double-contrast barium enemas to better demonstrate double contrast of the medial and lateral walls of the ascending and descending colon (*Frank, Long, & Smith, 11th ed., Vol. 2, pp. 170-172*).

123. (C) Protective or "reverse" isolation is used to keep the susceptible patient from becoming infected. Patients who have suffered burns have lost a very important means of protection, their skin, and therefore have increased susceptibility to bacterial invasion. Patients whose immune systems are depressed lose the ability to combat infection, and hence are more susceptible to infection. Active tuberculosis requires airborne precautions (*Gurley & Callaway, p. 153*).

124. (B) Conventional screen–film images can be scanned and digitized by a special machine called a film digitizer. Interpretation of digital images is made from the *CRT* display monitor; this is referred to as "softcopy display." "Hardcopies" can be made with a *laser printer*. A *laser camera* records the displayed image by exposing a film with laser light; it can also record several images on one film. The *laser printer* is connected for processing of the images (*Shephard, p. 360*).

125. (B) Because lead content increases as grid ratio increases, more scattered radiation (*and* nonscattered remnant radiation) is absorbed before reaching the image receptor. There are, therefore, fewer x-ray photons interacting with the image receptor, with a resulting *decrease* in optical/radiographic density as grid ratio increases. *In film/screen imaging*, scale of contrast would *decrease* with an increase in grid ratio (*Carlton & Adler, p. 396*).

126. (B) Patients who are able to cooperate are usually able to control *voluntary* motion if they are provided with an adequate explanation of the procedure. Once patients understand what is needed, most will cooperate to the best of their ability (by suspending respiration and holding still for the exposure). Certain body functions and responses, such as heart action, peristalsis, pain, and muscle spasm, cause *involuntary* motion uncontrollable by the patient. The best way to control involuntary and voluntary motion is by always selecting the shortest possible exposure time. Voluntary motion may also be minimized by careful explanation, immobilization, and (as a last resort and only in certain cases) restraint (*Frank, Long, & Smith, 11th ed., Vol. 1, pp. 18-19*).

127. (C) The *manubrial* or *jugular notch* is the depression on the superior border of the manubrium and is located at the level of the *third thoracic* vertebra. The *vertebra prominens* is at the level of the *seventh* *cervical* vertebra (*Frank, Long, & Smith, 11th ed., Vol. 1, p. 63*).

128. (B) An AEC is calibrated to produce radiographic densities as required by the radiologist for interpretation purposes. Once the part being radiographed has been exposed to produce the required optical density, the AEC automatically terminates the exposure. The manual timer should be used as a *backup timer* should the AEC fail to terminate the exposure, thus protecting the patient from overexposure and the x-ray tube from excessive *heat* load. *Circuit breakers* and *fuses* are circuit devices used to protect circuit elements from overload. In case of current surge, the circuit is broken (opened), thus preventing equipment damage. A *rheostat* is a type of variable resistor (*Shephard, pp. 286-287*).

129. (C) The cassette is used to support the intensifying screens and x-ray film. It should be strong and provide good screen–film contact. The cassette front should be made of a sturdy material with a low atomic number, because attenuation of the remnant beam is undesirable. Bakelite (the forerunner of today's plastics) and magnesium (the lightest structural metal) are the most commonly used materials for cassette fronts. The high atomic number of tungsten makes it inappropriate as a cassette front material (*Selman, p. 274*).

130. (B) X-ray images are often subpoenaed as court evidence in cases of medical litigation. In order to be considered as legitimate legal evidence, each x-ray image must contain certain essential and specific patient information. Essential information that *must* be included on each image is patient identification, the identity of the facility where the x-ray study was performed, the date on which the study was performed, and a right- or left-side marker.

Other useful information that *may* be included, but that is not considered essential, is additional patient demographics such as their date of birth, identity of the referring physician, time of day when the study was performed, and identity/initials of the radiographer performing the examination (*Bontrager & Lampignano, 7th ed., p. 30*).

131. (B) When the foot is positioned for a lateral projection, the plantar surface should be perpendicular to the image receptor so as to superimpose the metatarsals. This may be accomplished with the patient lying on either the affected or unaffected side (usually affected), that is, mediolateral or laterome-

dial. The talofibular articulation is best demonstrated in the medial oblique projection of the ankle (*Frank, Long, & Smith, 11th ed., Vol. 1, p. 266*).

132. (B) Exposure-type artifacts are those that appear on the radiograph as a result of image formation processes. A *foreign body* in the cassette or within the body part will cast its image on the radiographic image. As the exposed film is removed from the cassette, *static electrical discharge* will expose the film in a characteristic manner. These are *exposure-type artifacts*. In *Figure 16–11*, a right lateral decubitus of the gallbladder, a foam pad and sheet have been imaged to produce the exposure artifact. *Processor artifacts* are not placed on the film during image formation, but rather during chemical processing. They can result from mechanical and/or chemical problems. Several kinds of artifacts can be produced by careless *handling* during production of the radiographic image. X-ray film is sensitive and requires proper handling and storage. Tree-like, branching black marks on a radiograph are usually caused by static electrical discharge, especially prevalent during cold, dry weather (*Saia, p. 78*).

133. (D) In film/screen imaging, factors that regulate the number of x-ray photons produced at the target are used to control radiographic density, namely, milliamperage and exposure time (mAs). Radiographic density is directly proportional to mAs; if the mAs is cut in half, the radiographic density will decrease by one-half. Although kV is used primarily to regulate radiographic contrast in film/screen imaging, it may also be used to regulate radiographic density in variable kV techniques, according to the 15% rule (*Selman, p. 332*).

134. (B) Perfect film–screen contact is essential to sharply recorded detail. Screen contact can be evaluated with a *wire-mesh test*. A *spinning-top test* is used to evaluate timer accuracy and rectifier operation. A *penetrometer* (aluminum step-wedge) is used to illustrate the effect of kV on contrast. A *star pattern* is used to measure resolving power of the imaging system (*Selman, pp. 234-235*).

135. (A) The mechanical device used to correct an ineffectual cardiac rhythm is a *defibrillator*. The two paddles attached to the unit are placed on a patient's chest and used to introduce an electric current in an effort to correct the dysrhythmia. A *cardiac monitor* is used to display, and sometimes record, electrocardiogram (ECG) readings and some pressure readings. The *crash cart* is a supply cart with various medications and equipment necessary for treating a patient who is suffering from a myocardial infarction or other serious medical emergencies. It is periodically checked and restocked, usually by nursing staff, although radiographers may be responsible for a daily check of the plastic throwaway locks. These locks are used to ensure that the cart has not been tampered with or supplies inadvertently used in nonemergency situations. A resuscitation bag is used for ventilation, for example, during cardiopulmonary resuscitation (*Tortora & Derrickson, p. 731*).

136. (C) There are many terms (with which the radiographer must be familiar) that are used to describe radiographic positioning techniques. *Cephalad* refers to that which is toward the head, and *caudad* to that which is toward the feet. Structures close to the source or beginning are said to be *proximal*, while those lying close to the midline are said to be *medial* (*Frank, Long, & Smith, 11th ed., Vol. 1, p. 77*).

137. (C) When barium fluorohalide absorbs x-ray energy, *electrons are released, and they divide into two groups*: One electron group initiates *immediate* luminescence during the excited state of Eu^{2+}. The other electron group becomes *trapped* within the phosphor's halogen ions, forming a "color center." These trapped phosphors are the phosphors that ultimately form the radiographic image because when exposed to a *monochromatic* laser light source, these phosphors emit *polychromatic* light, termed *photostimulated luminescence*. The PSP layer *stores* its latent image for several hours; however, after approximately 8 hours, noticeable image *fading* will occur. The europium activator is important for the *storage* characteristic of the PSPs; it also has functions similar to the sensitization specks within film emulsion; without europium, the image will not become manifest (*Bushong, 9th ed., p. 415*).

138. (A) A *fistula* is an abnormal tubelike passageway between organs or an organ and the surface. Fistulas can result from abscesses, injuries, malignancies, inflammation of neighboring tissues, and ionizing radiation exposure. A *polyp* is a tumor with either a pedicle (pedunculated, or having a stalk) or a broad base (sessile), commonly found in vascular organs projecting inward from its mucosal wall. They are usually removed surgically because, although usually benign, they can become malignant. A *diverticulum* is an *outpouching* from the wall of an organ, such as the

colon. An *abscess* is a localized collection of pus as a result of inflammation (*Frank, Long, & Smith, 11th ed., Vol. 2, pp. 66, 129*).

139. (D) With the patient in the AP position, the scapula and upper thorax are normally superimposed. With the arm abducted, elbow flexed, and hand supinated, much of the scapula is drawn away from the ribs. The patient should not be rotated toward the affected side, as this causes superimposition of ribs on the scapula. The exposure is made during quiet breathing to obliterate pulmonary vascular markings (*Frank, Long, & Smith, 11th ed., Vol. 1, p. 212*).

140. (A) The type of shock associated with pooling of blood in the peripheral vessels is classified as *neurogenic shock*. This occurs in cases of trauma to the central nervous system, resulting in decreased arterial resistance and pooling of blood in peripheral vessels. *Cardiogenic shock* is related to cardiac failure, as a result of interference with heart function. It can occur in cases of cardiac tamponade, pulmonary embolus, or myocardial infarction. *Hypovolemic shock* is related to loss of large amounts of blood, from either internal bleeding or hemorrhage associated with trauma. *Septic shock*, as well as *anaphylactic shock*, is generally classified as *vasogenic shock* (*Torres et al., pp. 165-167*).

141. (B) An axial *dorsoplantar* projection is described; the central ray enters the dorsal surface of the foot and exits the plantar surface. The *plantodorsal* projection is done *supine* and requires cephalad angulation. The central ray enters the plantar surface and exits the dorsal surface (*Frank, Long, & Smith, 11th ed., Vol. 1, pp. 277-278*).

142. (D) Surface landmarks, prominences, and depressions are useful to the radiographer in locating anatomic structures not visible externally. The *costal margin* is at about the same level as L3. The *umbilicus* is approximately at the same level as the L3–L4 interspace. The *xiphoid* tip is at about the same level as T10. The fourth lumbar vertebra is approximately at the same level as the *iliac crest* (*Bontrager & Lampignano, 7th ed., p. 111*).

143. (D) In the CR reader, a photomultiplier tube (PMT) or photodiode (PD) is used to detect PSL and convert it to electrical signals. The electrical energy is sent to an ADC where it becomes the *digital* image that is displayed, after a short delay, on a high-resolution monitor.

In indirect-capture DR, a flat-panel detector uses cesium iodide or gadolinium oxysulfide as the scintillator, that is, which captures x-ray photons and emits light. That light is then transferred directly to the ADC via a photodetector coupling agent—a *charge-coupled device* (CCD) or *thin-film transistor* (TFT) (*Bushong, 9th ed., p. 420*).

144. (B) CR systems convert x-ray photons into useful information much more efficiently than film-screen systems, hence a far better DQE. CR also converts that information over a far wider exposure range (about 10^4 times wider) than screen-film. The single negative aspect of CR is its limited spatial resolution (image detail). While film-screen systems resolve about 10–15 lp/mm, CR resolution is about 3–5 lp/mm (*Seeram, p. 10, 11*).

145. (C) X-ray photons are produced in two ways as high-speed electrons interact with target atoms: First, if the high-speed electron is attracted by the nucleus of a tungsten atom and changes its course, the energy given up as the electron is "braked" in the form of an x-ray photon. This is called *bremsstrahlung* ("braking") radiation and is responsible for the majority of x-ray photons produced at the conventional tungsten target. Second, a high-speed electron may eject a tungsten K-shell electron, leaving a vacancy in the shell. An electron from a higher energy level, for example, the L shell, drops down to fill the vacancy, emitting the difference in energy as a K-characteristic ray. *Characteristic radiation* comprises only approximately 15% of the primary beam (*Bushong 9th ed., p. 140-142*).

146. (D) This is a modification of the parietoacanthial projection (Waters method) in which the patient is requested to first open the mouth and then the skull is positioned so that the *OML forms a 37-degree angle* with the image receptor. The central ray is directed through the *sphenoid sinuses* and *exits the open mouth*. The routine parietoacanthial projection (with mouth closed) is used to demonstrate the maxillary sinuses projected above the petrous pyramids. The frontal and ethmoidal sinuses are best visualized in the PA axial position (modified Caldwell method) (*Frank, Long,& Smith, 11th ed., Vol. 1, pp. 343, 400*).

147. (D) Anode target material of *high atomic number* produces higher energy x-rays more efficiently. Because a great deal of heat is produced at the target, the material should have a *high melting point* so as to avoid damage to the target surface. Most of the x-rays generated at the focal spot are directed downward and pass through the x-ray tube's *port window*. The cathode filament receives *low-voltage* current to heat it to the point of thermionic emission. Then *high voltage* is applied to drive the electrons across to the focal track (*Selman, pp. 204-211*).

148. (D) With inspiration, the diaphragm is depressed, that is, moved into a lower position. The ribs and sternum are elevated. As the ribs are elevated, their angle is decreased. Radiographic density can vary considerably in appearance depending on which phase of respiration the exposure is made (*Frank, Long, & Smith, 11th ed., Vol. 1, p. 512*).

149. (D) The four body types (from largest to smallest) are hypersthenic, sthenic, hyposthenic, and asthenic. The abdominal viscera of the *asthenic* person are generally located quite low, vertical, and toward the midline. The opposite is true of the *hypersthenic* person: organs are located high, transverse, and laterally (*Bontrager & Lampignano, 7th ed., p. 458-459*).

150. (D) Digital image storage is located in a *pixel*, which is a *two-dimensional* "*picture element*," measured in the "*XY*" *direction*. The third dimension, "*Z*" direction, in the matrix of pixels is the *depth* that is referred to as the *voxel* (volume *element*). The *depth* of the block is the number of bits required to describe the gray level that each pixel can take on—known as the bit depth.

Bit depth in CT is approximately 2^{12} with a dynamic range of almost 5,000 gray shades, approximately 2^{14} in CR/DR with a dynamic range of more than 16,000 gray shades, and approximately 2^{16} in digital mammography with a dynamic range of more than 65,500 gray shades. The matrix is the number of pixels in the XY direction. As matrix size increases, for a fixed FOV, pixel size is smaller and better spatial resolution results. An electronic/digital image is formed by a matrix of pixels in rows and columns. A matrix having 512 pixels in each row and column is a 512 × 512 matrix (a typical CT image).

The term *FOV* is used to describe how much of the patient is included in the matrix. Either the matrix or the FOV can be changed without one affecting the other, but changes in either will change pixel size. As FOV increases, for a fixed matrix size, the size of each pixel increases and spatial resolution decreases.

Fewer and larger pixels result in a poor-resolution "pixelly" or "mosaicked" image, that is, one in which you can actually see the individual pixel boxes.

151. (D) Orthopnea is a respiratory condition in which the patient has difficulty breathing (*dyspnea*) in any position other than erect. The patient is usually comfortable in the erect, standing, or seated position. The *Trendelenburg position* places the patient's head lower than the rest of the body. The *Fowler position* is a semierect position, and the *recumbent position* is lying down (*Taber's, p. 1535*).

152. (B) The radiograph in *Figure 16–12* shows the odontoid process superimposed on the base of the skull. The maxillary teeth can be seen very superior to the base of the skull. *Bringing the chin down* will move the base of the skull up and permit visualization of the C1 to C2 structures. A diagnostic image of C1 to C2 depends on adjusting the flexion of the neck *so that the maxillary occlusal plane and base of the skull are superimposed*. Accurate adjustment of these structures will usually allow good visualization of the odontoid process and the atlantoaxial articulation. Too much flexion superimposes teeth on the odontoid process; too much extension superimposes the base of the skull on the odontoid process (*Bontrager, p. 292*).

153. (C) The medical word for nosebleed is *epistaxis*. *Vertigo* refers to the feeling of "whirling" or the sensation that the room is spinning. Some possible causes of vertigo include inner ear infection or an acoustic neuroma. *Urticaria* is a vascular reaction resulting in dilated capillaries and edema that cause the patient to break out in hives. An *aura* may be classified as either a feeling or a motor response (such as flashing lights, tasting metal, and smelling coffee) that precedes an episode such as a seizure or a migraine headache (*Adler & Carlton, p. 247*).

154. (C) Contrast media may be described as either positive (radiopaque) or negative (radiolucent). *Positive*, or *radiopaque*, *contrast agents* have a higher atomic number than the surrounding soft tissue, resulting in a greater attenuation or absorption of x-ray photons, thereby producing a higher radiographic contrast. Examples of positive contrast media are iodinated (both water- and oil-based) agents and barium sulfate suspensions. *Negative*, or *radiolucent*, *contrast agents* used are air and various gases. Because the atomic number of air is also

quite different from that of soft tissue, an artificially high subject contrast can be produced. The advantage of carbon dioxide over air is that it is absorbed more rapidly by the body (*Bushong, p. 184*).

155. (C) The most important precaution in the practice of aseptic technique is proper hand hygiene. The radiographer's hands *should be thoroughly washed with soap and warm running water, for at least 15 seconds before and after each patient examination, or by using an alcohol sanitizer*. If the faucet cannot be operated with the knee, it should be opened and closed using paper towels. The hands and forearms should always be kept *lower* than the elbows; care should be taken to wash all surfaces and between fingers. The radiographer's uniform should not touch the sink. Hand lotions should be used to prevent hands from chapping; broken skin permits the entry of microorganisms. Disinfectants, antiseptics, and germicides are substances used to kill pathogenic bacteria; they are frequently used in handwashing substances. Alcohol-based hand sanitizers have been recommended as an alternative to handwashing with soap and water, except when there is visible soiling or after caring for a patient with *Clostridium difficile* (*Ehrlich et al., 7th ed., p. 158-160*).

156. (D) The *developing fetus* is particularly sensitive to radiation exposure. The law of Bergonié and Tribondeau states that *stem cells*, which give rise to a specific type of cell, as in hematopoiesis, are particularly radiosensitive, as are *young cells* and tissues. It also states that *cells with a high rate of proliferation* (mitosis) are more sensitive to radiation. Radiation exposure, especially between the second and sixth week following conception (the period of major organogenesis), can cause *organ damage*, *mental and growth retardation*, *microcephaly*, and *genital deformities* (*Sherer et al., pp. 129, 130*).

157. (B) High-kilovoltage exposures produce large amounts of scattered radiation, and high-ratio grids are often used with high-kilovoltage techniques in an effort to absorb more of this scattered radiation. However, as more scattered radiation is absorbed, *more primary radiation is absorbed* as well. This accounts for the *increase in mAs required* when changing from 8:1 to 16:1 grid. Additionally, precise *centering* and *positioning* become more critical; a small degree of inaccuracy is *more likely to cause grid cutoff* in a high-ratio grid (*Selman, pp. 362-363*).

158. **(A)** AEC devices are used in today's equipment and serve to produce consistent and comparable radiographic results. In one type of AEC, there is an *ionization chamber* just beneath the tabletop above the image receptor. The part to be examined is centered to it (the sensor) and radiographed. When a predetermined quantity of ionization has occurred (equal to the correct density), the exposure terminates automatically. In the other type of AEC, the *phototimer/photomultiplier*, a small fluorescent screen is positioned beneath the image receptor. When remnant radiation emerging from the patient exposes the IR and exits the cassette, the fluorescent screen emits light. Once a predetermined amount of fluorescent light is "seen" by the photocell sensor, the exposure is terminated. A scintillation camera is used in nuclear medicine. A photocathode is an integral part of the image intensification system (*Bushong 9th ed., p. 108, 109, 263, 264*).

159. **(A)** A *compensating filter* is used when the part to be radiographed is of uneven thickness or density (in the chest, mediastinum vs. lungs). The filter (made of aluminum or lead acrylic) is constructed so as to absorb much of the primary radiation that would expose the low-tissue-density area while allowing the primary radiation to pass unaffected to the high-tissue-density area. A *collimator* is used to decrease the production of scattered radiation by limiting the volume of tissue irradiated. The *grid* functions to trap scattered radiation before it reaches the image receptor, thus reducing scattered radiation fog (*Shephard, p. 193*).

160. **(A)** An increase in photon *energy* accompanies an increase in *kilovoltage*. Kilovoltage regulates the penetrability of x-ray photons; it regulates their *wavelength*, the amount of *energy* with which they are associated. The higher the related energy of an x-ray beam, the greater its *penetrability*. (Kilovoltage and photon energy are directly related; kilovoltage and wavelength are inversely related.) *In film/screen imaging*, adjusting kilovoltage is the preferred method of adjusting radiographic contrast: as kilovoltage (photon energy) is increased, the number of grays increases, thereby producing a longer scale of contrast. In general, as *screen speed* increases, so does contrast (resulting in a shorter scale of contrast). An increase in *mAs* is frequently accompanied by an appropriate decrease in kilovoltage, which would also shorten the contrast scale. SID and radiographic contrast are unrelated (*Bushong, p. 167*).

161. **(C)** Fractures and/or dislocations of the cervical spine are usually caused by acute *hyperflexion* or *hyperextension* as a result of indirect trauma. *Whiplash* injury is caused by a sudden, forced movement in one direction and then the opposite direction (as in rear-end automobile impacts). Whiplash symptoms frequently include neck pain and stiffness, headache, and pain and numbness of the upper extremities. Whiplash is often evidenced radiographically by straightening or reversal of the normal lordotic curve and demonstrated in lateral projections performed in flexion and extension.

162. **(B)** If A and B are reduced to 5 mAs for mAs consistency, the kV would increase in both cases to 85 kV, thereby balancing radiographic densities in film/screen imaging. Thus, the greatest density is determined by the shortest SID (greatest exposure rate) (*Shephard, p. 307*).

163. **(D)** Conventional 60-Hz full-wave rectified power is converted to a higher frequency of 500 to 25,000 Hz in the most recent generator design—the *high-frequency generator*. The high-frequency generator is small in size, in addition to producing a nearly constant potential waveform. High-frequency generators first appeared in mobile x-ray units and were then adopted by mammography and CT equipment. Today, more and more radiographic equipment use high-frequency generators. Their compact size makes them popular, and the fact that they produce nearly constant potential voltage helps to improve image quality and decrease patient dose (fewer low-energy photons to contribute to skin dose).

164. **(B)** *Somatic effects* of radiation refer to those effects experienced directly by the exposed individual such as erythema, epilation, and cataracts. *Genetic effects* of radiation exposure are caused by irradiation of the reproductive cells of the exposed individual and transmitted from one generation to the next (*Sherer et al., p. 115*).

165. **(C)** The components of the electromagnetic spectrum are identified in different ways. *Wavelength* is used to identify visible light. *Frequency* is used to identify radiowaves. Units of *energy* are used to identify ionizing electromagnetic radiations. The unit *keV* (kilo-electron volt) is used to identify the x-ray photon energies produced by diagnostic x-ray

equipment. The unit *kV* (kilovolts) describes the voltage required to produce the x-rays within the x-ray tube. The units mA and mAs are quantitative units identifying the number or quantity of x-rays available (*Bushong, p. 63*).

166. (D) The greater the *number of electrons* comprising the electron stream and bombarding the target, the greater the number of x-ray photons produced. Although kV is usually associated with the energy of the x-ray photons, because *a greater number of more energetic electrons* will produce more x-ray photons, an increase in kV will also increase the *number* of photons produced. Specifically, the quantity of radiation produced increases as the *square* of the kV. The material composition of the tube target also plays an important role in the number of x-ray photons produced. The higher the *atomic number*, the denser and more closely packed the atoms comprising the material; therefore, the greater the chance of an interaction between a high-speed electron and target material (*Bushong, pp. 156-158*).

167. (A) In film/screen imaging, if a radiograph lacks sufficient blackening, an increase in mAs is required. The mAs regulates the number of x-ray photons produced at the target. In film/screen imaging, an increase or decrease of at least 30% in mAs is necessary to produce a perceptible effect. Increasing the kV 15% will have about the same effect as doubling the mAs (*Carlton & Adler, p. 370*).

168. (B) CR IP storage screens (PSPs/SPSs) should be cleaned monthly. It is important that *anhydrous ethanol* be used for cleaning most PSPs; use of other materials can cause breakdown of the protective coat. A small amount of anhydrous ethanol is placed on a lint-free cloth for cleaning and removal of any dust or other particles. Water and remnant moisture must not be used as it can cause phosphor swelling. *Dust* on PSPs has the same effect as dust on intensifying screens—a clear pinhole artifact. IPs should also be checked for physical damage. Scratches will appear as clear areas on the resulting image. CR IPs should be visually checked for physical damage; inserting a damaged IP cassette into the scanner–reader can result in mechanical failure and system shutdown (*Fuji Medical Systems CR Users Guide, p. 35*).

169. (B) The pregnant radiographer poses a special radiation-protection consideration, as the safety of the unborn individual must be considered. It must be remembered that the developing fetus is particularly sensitive to radiation exposure. Established guidelines state that the occupational radiation exposure to the *fetus* must not exceed 0.5 rem (500 mrem, or 5 mSv) during the entire gestation period—not to exceed 50 mrem in 1 month (*Bushong, p. 560*).

170. (C) Category-specific isolations have been replaced by *transmission-based precautions*: *airborne, droplet,* and *contact*. Under these guidelines, some conditions or diseases can fall into more than one category. *Airborne precaution* is employed with patients suspected or known to be infected with the *tubercle bacillus* (TB), *chickenpox* (varicella), and *measles* (rubeola). Airborne precaution *requires that the patient wear a mask* to avoid the spread of bronchial secretions or other pathogens during coughing. If the patient is unable or unwilling to wear a mask, the radiographer must wear one. The radiographer should wear gloves, but a gown is required only if flagrant contamination is likely. Patients under airborne precaution require a *private, specially ventilated (negative-pressure) room*.

A private room is also indicated for all patients on *droplet precaution*, that is, diseases transmitted via *large droplets* expelled from the patient while speaking, sneezing, or coughing. The pathogenic droplets can infect others when they come in contact with mouth or nasal mucosa or conjunctiva. *Rubella* ("German measles"), *mumps,* and *influenza* are among the diseases spread by droplet contact; *a private room is required* for the patient, and health care practitioners should use *gown* and *gloves*. Any diseases spread by direct or close *contact*, such as *MRSA* (methicillin-resistant *Staphylococcus aureus*), *conjunctivitis,* and *hepatitis A*, require *contact precaution*. *Contact precaution* procedures require a *private patient room* and the use of *gloves, mask,* and *gown* for anyone coming in direct contact with the infected individual or his or her environment (*Adler & Carlton, p. 215*).

171. (C) Blood pressure in pulmonary circulation is relatively low, and therefore pulmonary vessels can easily become blocked by blood clots, air bubbles, or fatty masses, resulting in a *pulmonary embolism*. If the blockage stays in place, it results in an extra strain on the right ventricle, which is now unable to pump blood. This occurrence can result in congestive heart failure. *Pneumothorax* is air in the pleural cavity. *Atelectasis* is a collapsed lung or part of a lung. *Hypoxia* is a condition of low tissue oxygen (*Torres et al., pp. 167-168*).

172. **(A)** The 45-degree oblique position of the lumbar spine is generally performed for demonstration of the *apophyseal joints*. In a correctly positioned oblique lumbar spine, *scotty dog* images are demonstrated. The scotty's *ear* corresponds to the superior articular process, *nose* to the transverse process, *eye* to the pedicle, *neck* to the pars interarticularis, *body* to the lamina, and *front foot* to the inferior articular process (*Bontrager & Lampignano, 7th ed., pp. 326, 327*).

173. **(D)** Phase of respiration is exceedingly important in thoracic radiography; lung expansion and the position of the diaphragm strongly influence the appearance of the finished radiograph. Inspiration and expiration radiographs of the chest are taken to demonstrate air in the pleural cavity (*pneumothorax*), to demonstrate *atelectasis* (partial or complete collapse of one or more pulmonary lobes) degree of *diaphragm excursion*, or to detect the presence of a *foreign body*. The expiration image will require a somewhat greater exposure (6–8 kV more) to compensate for the diminished quantity of air in the lungs (*Bontrager & Lampignano, p. 80*).

174. **(A)** The x-ray tube's glass envelope and oil coolant are considered inherent ("built-in") filtration. Thin sheets of aluminum are added to make *a total of at least 2.5 mm Al equivalent filtration in equipment operated above 70 kV*. This is done to remove the low-energy photons that serve to contribute only to patient skin dose (*Sherer et al., p. 155*).

175. **(A)** As in traditional radiography, numerous density values represent various tissue densities, for example, bone, muscle, fat, blood-filled organs, air/gas, metal, contrast media, and pathologic processes. In CR, the CR scanner recognizes these numerous values and constructs a *grayscale histogram* of these values represented in the imaged part. A histogram is a *graphic representation* defining all these values. The radiographer selects a *processing algorithm* by selecting the anatomic part and particular projection on the computer. The CR unit then matches that information with a particular *lookup table* (LUT)—a characteristic curve that best matches the anatomic part being imaged. Hence, *histogram analysis* and use of the appropriate LUT together function to produce predictable image quality in CR (*Shephard, p. 243*).

176. **(A)** Protective aprons and gloves are made of lead-impregnated vinyl or leather. They should be checked annually for cracks via radiographic or fluoroscopic means. Otherwise, minimal care is required. Lead aprons and gloves should always be hung on appropriate hangers. Glove supports permit air to circulate within the glove. Apron hangers provide convenient storage without folding. If lead aprons are folded, or left in a careless heap, cracks are more likely to form. If lead aprons or gloves become soiled, cleaning with a damp cloth and appropriate solution is all that is required. Excessive moisture should be avoided (*Bushong, p. 596*).

177. **(A)** The spinning-top test is used to evaluate *timer accuracy* or *rectifier failure*. With *single-phase*, full-wave rectified equipment (120 pulses/s), individual dots are seen that represent x-ray impulses. *Figure 16–14* was made by using single-phase, full-wave rectified equipment. Because three-phase and high-frequency equipment is almost constant potential, a special synchronous spinning top (or an oscilloscope) is used and a solid black arc is obtained rather than dots. The number of degrees formed by the arc is measured and equated to a particular exposure time (*Fosbinder & Kelsey, p. 339*).

178. **(B)** When a spinning top is used to test the timer efficiency of single-phase, full-wave rectified equipment, the result is a *series of dots* or dashes, with each dot representing a pulse of radiation. With full-wave rectified current, and a possible 120 pulses (dots) available per second, one should visualize 12 dots at 1/10 second, 6 dots at 0.05 second, etc.

If 4 dots of a possible 120 are seen, then the exposure time was:

$$\frac{4}{120} = \frac{1}{30}\text{second}$$

The spinning-top test may be used to test timer accuracy in single-phase equipment. A spinning top is a metal disk with a small hole placed in its outer edge, and placed on a pedestal approximately 6 inches high. The exposure is made while the top spins. Because three-phase equipment produces almost constant potential—rather than pulsed radiation—the standard spinning top cannot be used. An oscilloscope or synchronous spinning top must be employed to test timers of three-phase equipment (*Selman, p. 233*).

179. **(D)** A controlled area is one that is occupied by radiation workers trained in radiation safety and who wear radiation monitors. The exposure rate in a *controlled area* must not exceed 100 mR/wk; its occupancy factor is considered to be 1, indicating that the area may always be occupied, and therefore requiring maximum shielding. An *uncontrolled area* is one occupied by the general population; the exposure rate there must not exceed 10 mR/wk. Shielding requirements vary according to several factors, one being *occupancy factor* (*Sherer et al., p. 204*).

180. **(D)** The lead strips in a parallel grid are *parallel to each other* and therefore *not to the x-ray beam*. The more divergent the x-ray beam, the more likely there will be cutoff/decreased density at the lateral edges of the radiograph. This problem becomes more pronounced at short SIDs. If there were a centering or tube angle problem, there would more likely be a noticeable density loss on one side *or* the other (*Shephard, p. 260*).

181. **(A)** The trachea (windpipe) bifurcates into left and right *mainstem bronchi*, each entering its respective lung hilum. The *left* bronchus divides into *two* portions, one for each lobe of the left lung. The *right* bronchus divides into *three* portions, one for each lobe of the right lung (Fig. 6–76). The lungs are conical in shape, consisting of upper pointed portions, termed the *apices* (plural for apex), and the broad lower portions (or *bases*). The lungs are enclosed in a double-walled serous membrane called the *pleura* (*Bontrager & Lampignano, 7th ed., p. 74, 75*).

182. **(A)** When the shoulders are relaxed, the clavicles are usually carried below the pulmonary apices. To examine the portions of the lungs lying behind the clavicles, the central ray is directed cephalad 15 to 20 degrees to project the clavicles above the apices when the patient is examined in the AP position (*Bontrager & Lampignano, p. 96*).

183. **(B)** The effects of a quantity of radiation delivered to a body are dependent on the amount of radiation received, size of the irradiated area, and how the radiation is delivered in time. If the radiation is delivered in portions over a period of time, it is said to be fractionated and has a less harmful effect than if the radiation was delivered all at once. Therefore, cells have an opportunity to repair and some recovery occurs between doses (*Bushong, p. 495*).

184. **(A)** The approximately 5-ft-long large intestine (colon) functions in the formation, transport, and evacuation of feces. The colon commences at the terminus of the small intestine; its first portion is the sac-like *cecum* in the right lower quadrant (RLQ), located inferior to the ileocecal valve. The *ascending colon* is continuous with the cecum and is located along the right side of the abdominal cavity. It bends medially and anteriorly forming the right colic (*hepatic*) flexure. The colon traverses the abdomen as the *transverse colon* and bends posteriorly and inferiorly to form the left colic (*splenic*) flexure. The *descending colon* continues down the left side of the abdominal cavity and at about the level of the pelvic brim, in the *left lower quadrant* (LLQ), the colon moves medially to form the S-shaped *sigmoid* colon. The rectum, approximately 5 inches in length, lies between the sigmoid and the anal canal (*Bontrager & Lampignano, 7th ed., pp. 490, 491*).

185. **(B)** In film/screen imaging, a 15% increase in kV with a 50% decrease in mAs serves to produce a radiograph *similar* to the original, but with some obvious differences. The overall blackness (*radiographic/optical density*) *is cut in half* because of the decrease in mAs. But the loss of blackness is compensated for by the *addition of grays* (therefore, *longer* scale contrast) from the increased kV. In film/screen imaging, the increase in kV also *increases exposure latitude*, a greater margin for error in higher kV ranges. Recorded detail is unaffected by changes in kV (*Shephard, pp. 178, 181*).

186. **(C)** Major branches of the common carotid arteries (internal carotids) function to supply the anterior brain, while the posterior brain is supplied by the vertebral arteries (branches of the subclavian). The brachiocephalic (innominate) artery is unpaired and is one of the three branches of the aortic arch, from which the right common carotid artery is derived. The left common carotid artery comes directly off the aortic arch (*Tortora & Derrickson, p. 767*).

187. **(C)** The brightness gain of image intensifiers is 5,000 to 20,000. This increase is accomplished in two ways: First, as the electron image is focused to the output phosphor, it is accelerated by high voltage. (This is *flux gain*.) Second, the output phosphor is only a fraction of the size of the input phosphor, and this image size decrease represents another brightness gain, termed *minification gain*. *Total*

brightness gain is equal to the product of minification gain and flux gain (Bushong 9th ed., p. 351).

188. (C) The OSL is rapidly becoming the most commonly used personnel monitor today. Film badges and TLDs have been successfully used for years. A pocket dosimeter is used primarily when working with large amounts of radiation and when a daily reading is desired (*Selman, p. 401*).

189. (D) When performing GI radiography, the position of the stomach may vary depending on the respiratory phase, body habitus, and patient position. *Inspiration* causes the lungs to fill with air and the diaphragm to descend, thereby pushing the abdominal contents downward. On *expiration*, the diaphragm will rise, allowing the abdominal organs to ascend. The b*ody habitus* is an important factor in determining the size and shape of the stomach. An asthenic patient may have a long, J-shaped stomach, while the stomach may be transverse in a hypersthenic patient. The body habitus is an important consideration in determining the positioning and placement of the image receptor. The *patient position* can also alter the position of the stomach. If a patient turns from the RAO position into the AP position, the stomach will move into a more horizontal position. Although the cardiac sphincter and pyloric sphincter are relatively fixed, the fundus is quite mobile and will vary in position (*Dowd & Tilson, Vol. 2, p. 778*).

190. (A) The knee is formed by the proximal tibia, patella, and distal femur, which articulate to form the femorotibial and patellofemoral joints. The distal posterior femur presents two large medial and lateral condyles separated by the deep intercondyloid fossa. Two small prominences, the medial and lateral epicondyles, are just superior to the condyles. The femoral and tibial condyles articulate to form the femorotibial joint. In the lateral position, the *medial femoral condyle, being farther from the image receptor, is magnified.* Its magnified image obscures the knee joint space unless correction is made. Angulation of 5 degrees cephalad will *superimpose the magnified medial femoral condyle on the lateral condyle* and permit a *better view of the joint space* (*Bontrager & Lampignano, 7th ed., p 245*).

191. (C) The full length of the nasal septum is best demonstrated in the parietoacanthial projection (Waters method). This is also the single best view for facial bones. The PA axial projection (Caldwell method) superimposes petrous structures over the nasal septum, while the lateral projection superimposes and obscures good visualization of the septum (*Bontrager, p. 395*).

192. (C) When caring for a patient with an indwelling Foley catheter, place the drainage bag and tubing *below the level of the bladder* to maintain the gravity flow of urine. Placement of the tubing or bag above or at level with the bladder will allow backflow of urine into the bladder. This reflux of urine can increase the chance of UTI (*Torres, p. 329*).

193. (A) A quality control program requires the use of a number of devices to test the efficiency of various parts of the imaging system. A *slit camera*, as well as a star-pattern or pinhole camera, is used to test focal spot size. A parallel-line–type resolution test pattern is used to test the resolution capability of intensifying screens (*Selman, p. 326*).

194. (B) The most effective method of sterilization is moist heat, using steam under pressure. This is known as autoclaving. Sterilization by dry heat requires higher temperatures for longer periods of time than moist heat. Pasteurization is moderate heating with rapid cooling and is frequently used in commercial preparation of milk and alcoholic beverages such as wine and beer. It is not a form of sterilization. Freezing can also kill some microbes, but is not a form of sterilization (*Adler & Carlton, p. 208*).

195. (B) Even the smallest exposure to radiation can be harmful. It must, therefore, be every radiographer's objective to keep his or her occupational exposure as far below the dose limit as possible. Radiology personnel should never hold patients during an x-ray examination (*Bushong, p. 8*).

196. (B) *Emphysema* is abnormal distention of alveoli (or tissue spaces) with air. The presence of abnormal amounts of air makes it necessary to decrease from normal exposure factors. *Congestive heart failure* and *pleural effusion* involve abnormal amounts of fluid in the chest and thus require an *increase* in exposure factors (*Carlton & Adler, p. 258*).

197. (C) There are four sets of paranasal sinuses: (i) *frontal*, (ii) *ethmoidal*, (iii) *maxillary*, and (iv) *sphenoidal* (Fig. 16–16). The left and right *frontal* sinuses (*number 1*) are usually asymmetrical and are located behind the glabella and superciliary arches of the frontal bone. The *ethmoidal* sinuses (*number 2*) are composed of 6 to 18 thin-walled air cells occupying the bony labyrinth of the ethmoid bone. The *frontal* and *ethmoidal sinuses* are demonstrated in the PA axial projection (Caldwell position). The *maxillary* sinuses (antra of Highmore; *number 4*) are the largest of the paranasal sinuses and are located in the body of the maxillae. They are particularly prone to infection and collections of stagnant mucus. The maxillary sinuses are well demonstrated in the *parietoacanthial* projection (Waters position). The *sphenoidal* sinuses (*number 3*) are located in the body of the sphenoid bone and are usually asymmetrical. They are well demonstrated in the *SMV* projection. All paranasal sinuses are demonstrated in the *lateral* projection, although the left and right of each group are superimposed. Radiography of the paranasal sinuses must be performed in the erect position so that any *fluid levels* may be demonstrated and to distinguish between fluid and other pathology such as *polyps* (*Bontrager & Lampignano, pp. 408-410*).

198. (B) A review of the film/screen problem reveals that *three changes* are being made: an increase in *SID*, a change from a 400-*speed system* to a 200-speed system, and a change in *exposure time* (to be considered last). Because the original mAs was 9, reducing the speed of the system by half (from 400 to 200) will require a doubling of the mAs to 18, in order to maintain density. Now, we must deal with the distance change. Using the density maintenance formula (and remembering that 18 is now the *old* mAs) we find that the required new mAs at 42 inches is 22:

$$\frac{18\,\text{mAs}}{x} = \frac{1{,}444(38^2)}{1{,}764(42^2)}$$
$$1{,}444x = 31{,}752$$
$$x = 21.98(22)\,\text{mAs}$$

Because we are not changing mA, we must determine the *exposure time* that, used with 300 mA, will yield 22 mAs:

$$300x = 22$$
$$x = 0.07\ \text{second exposure}$$

(*Selman, pp. 332, 335-336*).

199. (C) Erythema is the reddening of skin as a result of exposure to large quantities of ionizing radiation. It was one of the first somatic responses to irradiation demonstrated to the early radiology pioneers. The effects of radiation exposure to the skin follow a *nonlinear, threshold dose–response relationship*. An individual's response to skin irradiation depends on the dose received, period of time over which it was received, size of the area irradiated, and individual's sensitivity. The dose that it takes to bring about a noticeable erythema is referred to as the *skin erythema dose* (*Bushong, p. 521*).

200. (A) The *airway* of the patient is first opened by tilting back the head and lifting the chin. However, if the patient might have suffered a spinal cord injury, the spine should not be moved and the airway should be opened using the jaw-thrust method.

The rescuer next *listens to breathing* sounds and watches for rise and fall of the chest to indicate breathing. If there is no breathing, the rescuer pinches the patient's nose and delivers *two full breaths via mouth-to-mouth rescue* breathing. If rise and fall of the chest is still not present, the Heimlich maneuver is instituted. If ventilation does not take place during the two full breaths, the patient's circulation is checked next (using the carotid artery). If there is no pulse, external chest compressions are begun at a rate of 80 to 100/min for adults and at least 100/min for infants (*Torres, p. 171*).

Index

Note: Page numbers followed by b, f and t indicates box material, figure and table respectively.